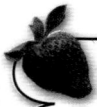

THE CALORIE KING®
Calorie, Fat & Carbohydrate Counter

Extra Diet Guides & Counters

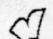

W9-BKA-465

Weight Control Tips

✅ Eat Sensibly

- Avoid fad diets. Eat 3 sensible meals daily with adequate fruit and vegetables.
- Limit portion size. Limit fats and high-fat foods, sugar, soda and alcohol. *(Sample Diet Plan ~ Page 11)*

✅ Exercise Daily

- Get active and exercise every day!
- Include muscle-strengthening exercises. You'll lose more fat and keep it off. You'll also feel and look better, and you can eat a little more! *(Exercise Guide ~ Page 12)*

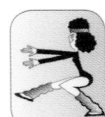

✅ Reshape Eating Behaviors

- Be aware of eating habits and behaviors that lead to overeating.
- Also focus on social and emotional situations that lead you to snack compulsively. *(Extra Notes ~ Page 14)*

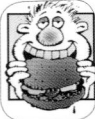

✅ Keep a Food & Exercise Journal

- A journal helps you see exactly what you eat and drink, and how much you exercise. *(Extra Notes ~ Page 15)*
- An excellent motivator and proven weight loss aid. Keeps you honest!

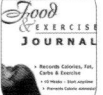

✅ Arrange Moral Support

Gain the support of family and friends. Get extra professional help if required, from your doctor, dietitian, psychologist, exercise trainer, or slimming group. Beware of family saboteurs who discourage you from adopting a healthier lifestyle!

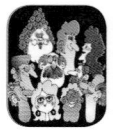

DOCTOR CHECK-UP
Ask your doctor to check your blood pressure, blood sugar and blood cholesterol levels.

HEALTHY WEIGHTS
~ MEN & WOMEN ~
(Over 18 Years)

Based on weights with least risk of disease or death from heart disease, diabetes, stroke and cancer.

Based on Body Mass Index of 20-25

BMI calculated as: $\dfrac{\text{Weight (kg)}}{\text{Height (m)}^2}$

Height (No Shoes) Ft Ins		Healthy Weight Range (Pounds)
4'7"	~	86-108
4'8"	~	88-110
4'9"	~	92-114
4'10"	~	97-121
4'11"	~	99-123
5'0"	~	101-127
5'1"	~	105-132
5'2"	~	110-136
5'3"	~	112-140
5'4"	~	114-145
5'5"	~	119-149
5'6"	~	123-156
5'7"	~	127-158
5'8"	~	129-162
5'9"	~	134-167
5'10"	~	138-173
5'11"	~	143-178
6'0"	~	145-182
6'1"	~	149-187
6'2"	~	156-193
6'3"	~	158-198
6'4"	~	162-202
6'5"	~	170-211
6'6"	~	172-215
6'7"	~	175-220

Body Fat Distribution & Health

Moderate amounts of body fat do not compromise health. However, excess fat above the hips carries a far greater health risk than fat on or below the hips - better to be a 'pear-shape' than an 'apple-shape'.

Abdominal obesity greatly increases the risk of developing diabetes, heart disease, high blood fats, hypertension, stroke, sleep apnea, arthritis and some cancers. So-called **'cellulite'** carries no extra health risk.

Waist Circumference directly reflects the increased health risk of abdominal obesity. Waist size associated with a high health risk:
Men ~ Over 40 inches **Women** ~ Over 35 inches

Body Mass Index (BMI)

BMI is a general (but not specific) indicator of body fatness. Although BMI alone is not diagnostic, the higher the BMI, the greater the health risk of developing diabetes, high blood pressure and heart disease. BMI does not apply to heavily muscled persons. BMI is used in a different way for children.

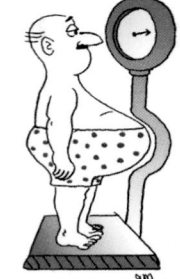

Abdominal obesity greatly increases the risk of ill-health and earlier death.

Check Your BMI: Find your height (no shoes) - look across the row to the weight nearest your own. Then track down to BMI.

Ht	WEIGHT (LBS) ~ ADULTS													
5'1"	100	106	111	116	122	127	132	137	143	148	153	158	185	211
5'2"	104	109	115	120	126	131	136	142	147	153	158	164	191	218
5'3"	107	113	118	124	130	135	141	146	152	158	163	169	197	225
5'4"	110	116	122	128	134	140	145	151	157	163	169	174	204	232
5'5"	114	120	126	132	138	144	150	156	162	168	174	180	210	240
5'6"	118	124	130	136	142	148	155	161	167	173	179	186	216	247
5'7"	121	127	134	140	146	153	159	166	172	178	185	191	223	255
5'8"	125	131	138	144	151	158	164	171	177	184	190	197	230	262
5'9"	128	135	142	149	155	162	169	176	182	189	196	206	236	270
5'10"	132	139	146	153	160	167	174	181	188	195	202	207	243	278
5'11"	136	143	150	157	165	172	179	186	193	200	208	215	250	286
6'0"	140	147	154	162	169	177	184	191	199	206	213	221	258	294
6'1"	144	151	159	166	174	182	190	197	204	212	219	227	265	302
6'2"	148	155	163	171	179	186	194	202	210	218	225	233	272	311
6'3"	152	160	168	176	184	192	200	208	216	224	232	240	279	319
6'4"	156	164	172	180	189	197	205	213	221	230	238	246	287	328

| BMI | 19 | 20 | 21 | 22 | 23 | 24 | 25 | 26 | 27 | 28 | 29 | 30 | 35 | 40 |

BMI Classification:

BMI Below 19
Underweight

BMI 19-24.9
Healthy Weight
(Low Health Risk)

BMI 25-29.9
Overweight
(Moderate Health Risk)

BMI 30-40
Obese (High Health Risk)

BMI Over 40
Morbid Obesity
(Very High Risk)

Interactive BMI Calculator
www.calorieking.com

Calories & Weight Loss

Calories in Food

Calories in food are derived from protein, fat and carbohydrate. Alcohol also provides calories. Vitamins, minerals and water provide no calories.

Calorie Values Per Gram	
Fat/Oil	~ 9 Calories
Carbohydrate	~ 4 Calories
Protein	~ 4 Calories
Alcohol	~ 7 Calories

Note that fats have over double the calories of protein and carbohydrate. The higher the fat content of food, the higher the calories.

Sample Calculation

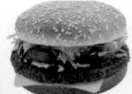

QUARTER POUNDER® WITH CHEESE has 530 calories derived from:

30g Fat (x 9 cals/gram)	= 270
38g Carbohyd.(x 4 cals/gram)	= 152
27g Protein (x 4 cals/gram)	= 108
Total Calories	**= 530**

Calorie Levels for Weight Loss

Start with a calorie-controlled diet that allows a moderate weight loss of $1/2$ - 1 pound per week. Weight loss is usually much greater in the first few weeks due to extra fluid losses.

Note: It is better to increase exercise rather than lessen food calories too drastically.

Suggested Calories for Weight Loss	
Women: Non-active	1000 - 1200
Active	1200 - 1500
Men: Non-active	1200 - 1500
Active	1500 - 1800
Teenagers:	1200 - 1800

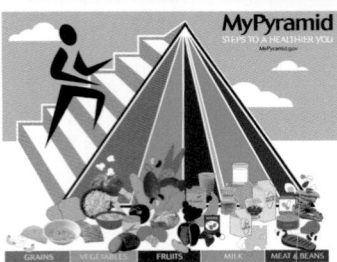

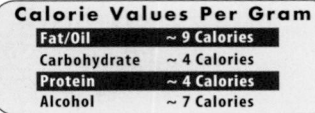

The MyPyramid symbol represents the recommended proportion of foods from each food group and focuses on the importance of making smart food choices in every food group, every day. Daily physical activity is also important. *(More info: www.MyPyramid.gov)*

Examples of Single Serving Sizes

Grains (Eat 6 servings per day):
- 1 slice wholegrain bread (1 oz)
- $1/2$ bun, small bagel or English muffin
- 4 small crackers or 1 tortilla
- 1 oz ready-to-eat wholegrain cereal
- $1/2$ cup cooked cereal, rice or pasta

Vegetable (Eat 3-5 servings per day):
- 1 cup raw leafy vegetables
- $1\frac{1}{2}$ cups raw chopped vegetables
- $1/2$ cup cooked vegetables
- $1/2$ - $3/4$ cup vegetable juice

Fruits (Eat 3-5 servings per day):
- 1 medium apple, orange, banana
- $1/2$ cup canned fruit (in own juice)
- $1/4$ cup dried fruit
- $3/4$ cup fruit juice (unsweetened)
- $1/4$ medium avocado

Milk (2-3 servings per day):
- 1 cup (8 fl.oz) milk/soy (enriched)/yogurt
- $1\frac{1}{2}$ oz cheese or $1/2$ cup cottage cheese

Meat & Beans (Eat 2-3 servings per day):
- 2-3 oz (cooked) lean meat/poultry/fish
- 2 eggs **or** 7 oz tofu **or** $1/4$ cup nuts
- 1 cup (cooked) dried beans **or** chickpeas
- 4 Tbsp peanut butter **or** $1/2$ cup nuts/seeds

Portion Size Counts!

Food portion size is critical to controlling calorie intake for weight control.

Super-sized food servings have become more common when eating out and in the home. This can mean a day's worth of calories being consumed in one meal; or a snack being equivalent to a full meal.

It is easy to underestimate portion size of foods and drinks, and unwittingly consume excess calories – even if the fat content is low or even zero!

To more accurately estimate portion size of different foods, weigh and measure your food with food scales, measuring spoons and cups. Better control of calories will result.

For a visual idea of portion sizes, visit www.CalorieKing.com. See examples (fries and cola) on this page.

Allow for Extra Calories in Packaged Food

The actual weight of packaged foods is usually 5-10% more than the label net weight (the minimum legal weight) - and in some cases up to 50% more. However, manufacturers calculate the calories based on the net weight. For actual calories, weigh the product and calculate the extra calories. **For extra details see www.CalorieKing.com**

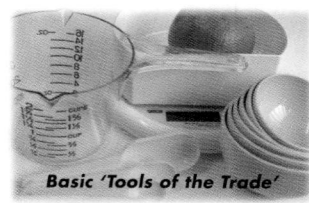

Basic 'Tools of the Trade'

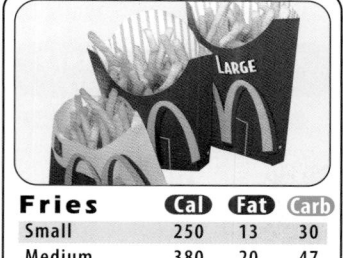

Fries	Cal	Fat	Carb
Small	250	13	30
Medium	380	20	47
Large	570	30	70

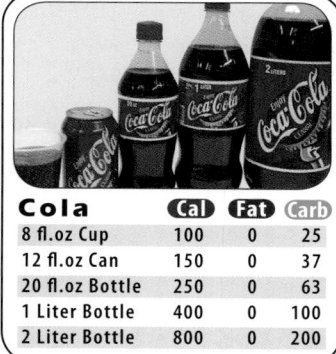

Cola	Cal	Fat	Carb
8 fl.oz Cup	100	0	25
12 fl.oz Can	150	0	37
20 fl.oz Bottle	250	0	63
1 Liter Bottle	400	0	100
2 Liter Bottle	800	0	200

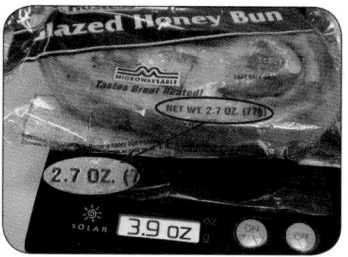

Recommended Fat Intake

Americans consume too much fat with many getting over 40% of total calories from fat – either as fat or oil, or as fat in foods and drinks. A range of 20-30% is healthier.

Fat Intake - Healthy Ranges		
Children	~	30-60g
Teenagers (Active)	~	40-80g
Women	~	30-60g
Men: Active	~	40-80g
Heavy Activity/Athlete	~	80-120g

MAXIMUM DESIRABLE FAT INTAKE (Daily)

Calories	Fat	% Fat Cals
1200 cals	30g fat	23%
1500 cals	40g fat	24%
1800 cals	50g fat	25%
2000 cals	60g fat	27%
2200 cals	70g fat	28%
2500 cals	80g fat	29%
3000 cals	100g fat	30%
4000 cals	135g fat	30%

Percentage Fat Calories Formula:

$$\frac{\text{Grams of Fat Per Serving} \times (900)}{\text{Total Calories Per Serving}}$$

Fat Percent Content

(Grams of fat per 100 grams of food)

Don't be fooled by promotion of foods claiming to have a low percentage of fat. **It's serving size and total grams of fat that count.**

For example, whole milk with 3.5% fat sounds low (3.5g fat/100ml) but an 8 fl.oz cup contains 8g fat; and 2 cups contain 16g fat.

Ice cream with 10% fat seems high, yet a regular scoop (3 fl.oz) has only 5g fat.

(Low-fat ice cream has less than 2g fat/serve.)

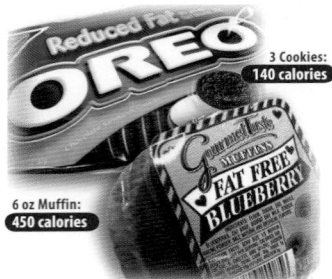

3 Cookies: 140 calories

6 oz Muffin: 450 calories

Reduced fat & fat-free foods are not necessarily low calorie. Portion size is still important.

It is a mistake to think that eating low-fat or fat-free foods allows you to eat double the quantity. You can end up with even more calories than when you eat smaller amounts of regular fat products.

Also fat-free but high in calories are soda drinks, fruit juices, beer, alcoholic spirits, sugar and candy. Bread, rice and pasta also have negligible fat.

Total Calories Count!

Ultimately, **it is food portion size and total calories that count** whether from fat, carbohydrate or protein. Remember, cows get fat on grass!

FOOD LABEL MEANINGS

FDA Nutrition Claim Definitions

(All are on a Per Serving Basis)

Low Calorie: 40 Calories or less

Light or Lite: One third fewer calories or, 50% or less fat than regular product

Fat-Free: Less than half a gram of fat

Low-Fat: 3 grams or less of fat

Reduced Fat: 25% less fat than regular product

Fewer or Less Calories: At least 25% fewer calories than regular product

Hints to Reduce Fat

Meats, Poultry, Fish

- Choose **lean cuts** of meat with little marbling. **Trim all visible fat** from meat and remove the skin from poultry. Removal of fat after cooking, is okay (to prevent dryness). Choose 'extra lean' ground beef.
- **Avoid high-fat meat products** such as salami, bacon, sausage and franks.
- **Broil or bake. Avoid frying in oil.** Allow casseroles to cool and skim off surface fat.
- **Avoid fried fish**, frozen fish in batter and canned fish in oil.

Fats & Oils

- **Use minimal amounts** of all types of fat and oil. All are high in calories.
- **Choose** 'light' and 'reduced fat' spreads but still use sparingly.
- Use minimal amounts of oil when stir-frying. Use no-stick sprays like Pam.

Salad Dressings & Sauces

- **Avoid regular mayonnaise and oil dressings.** Choose 'light', 'reduced fat' or 'fat-free' brands.
- **Choose** low-fat or fat-free sauces (mainly tomato-based). Avoid 'pesto', 'alfredo', 'cheese' and 'creamy' sauces.

Milk, Cheese

- **Choose** low-fat or nonfat milks and yogurts. **Avoid** full-cream milk, cream, Half & Half.
- **Cheese:** Choose fat-free, low-fat and fat-reduced (e.g. cottage, part-skim ricotta). Cheese substitutes can still be high in fat.

Snacks, Cookies, Candy

- **Avoid** high-fat snacks such as potato chips, corn/tortilla chips, cheesy balls, buttered popcorn, chocolate and carob bars.

Desserts/Sweets

- **Avoid high-fat desserts**, such as fruit pies, pastries, cheesecake, cheese board.
- **Choose** fresh fruits, fresh fruit salad, canned fruit in water pack, low-fat ice cream. Use low-fat yogurt in place of cream.

Fast-Foods & Take-Out

Check the Fast-Foods Section of this book for actual fat and calorie counts.

- **Avoid deep-fried chicken**, french fries; onion rings
- **Pizzas:** Avoid sausage/pepperoni. Choose vegetarian topping and modest quantity of cheese. Eat a moderate serving. Eat extra salad and fresh fruit.
- **Hamburgers:** Choose medium size, lower fat burgers. Avoid bacon. Have a side salad (with fat-free dressing).
- **Delis:** Choose sandwiches/bread rolls, pitas with low-fat fillings and plain salad. Limit meat/cheese to small portions.
- **Coffees:** Avoid large sizes of latte and frappuccino. Request nonfat milk and no whipped cream. Avoid cookies.

Extra Information: www.CalorieKing.com

FRYING ADDS FAT!

The greater the surface area of potato exposed to fat or oil, the higher the fat content.

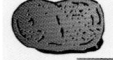

Whole Potato (3 oz)
0g Fat, 65 Cals

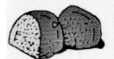

Roast Potato (3 oz)
5g Fat, 155 Cals

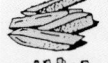

Fries (Large cut, 3 oz)
12g Fat, 220 Cals

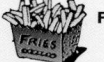

Fries (Small, 3 oz)
15g Fat, 265 Cals

Potato Chips (3 oz)
30g Fat, 450 Cals

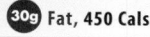

Carbohydrates ~ Friend or Foe?

Naturally Friendly Carbs

- Carbohydrate foods in their more natural forms (not overly processed) are essential to good health. They are the main source of fuel for the body, and also provide important vitamins, minerals, antioxidants and fiber – all of which help protect against heart disease, diabetes, hypertension, constipation-related ailments and many other diseases.

- Carbohydrates even stimulate production of serotonin, the 'feel good' brain chemical that helps control appetite and overeating. Too little serotonin can lead to mood swings and depression.

Carbohydrates are found in different forms in food as:

- Sugars in fruit, sugar cane, milk
- Starches in whole grains, legumes, nuts, seeds and vegetables
- Dietary fiber – (See Fiber Guide ~ Page 276)
  Glycemic Index & Diabetes ~ Page 20

Low carb diets only work if total calories are reduced.

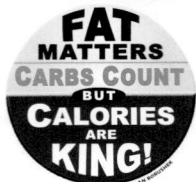

Low Carbohydrate Diets

- Popular low carbohydrate diets are extreme in their recommendations to initially cut carb intake to as little as 20 grams per day – the amount in 1 thick slice of bread, or 1 medium apple, or 1 small potato.

  This greatly increases the risk of nutritional deficiencies and compromises health, particularly if fat intake is excessive through fatty meats, high-fat dairy products, and fried foods.

- While overweight Americans do need to reduce carbohydrate intake, it should be done **sensibly as part of reducing portion size and total calories.**

- Simply eating 'low carb' food products without regard to portion size, calories or fats, will do little to promote weight loss or good health.

- **Low carb diets (and indeed any diet) only work if total calories are reduced.**

- Refined sugars should be one of the first targets in moderating carb intake.

Extra Info ~ www.CalorieKing.com

RECOMMENDED CARBOHYDRATE INTAKE

Calories (Daily)	Carbohydrate (Grams)	Percent Carbohydrate Calories
1200 cals	120g	40%
1500 cals	170g	45%
1800 cals	210g	47%
2000 cals	250g	50%
2500 cals	345g	55%
3000 cals	450g	60%

How Much Do We Need?

- As shown in the chart, well-balanced diets above 2000 calories contain 50-60% of total calories from carbohydrate.

- At lower calorie levels used for weight control (1200-1500 calories), carbohydrates account for as little as 40% of total calories. This is because protein calories have nutritional priority.

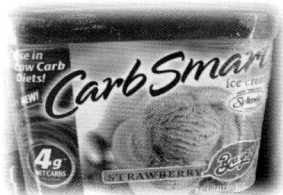

Low carbohydrate products may still be high in calories and fat.

- Many overweight, inactive people consume over 500 calories of refined sugars per day either self-added or as part of food products. This is equivalent to over 30 level teaspoons - a significant amount in weight control terms. Halving this amount would be reasonable and worthwhile.

  Note: Naturally occurring sugars in fruits, vegetables and milk are fine when consumed in normal recommended amounts. These foods are also rich in other nutrients.

  Refined sugar is referred to as having 'empty calories' because it supplies calories but negligible nutrients and no fiber.

- **Most sugar in our diet is 'hidden'** in processed foods such as soft drinks, fruit drinks, candy, cookies, cake, jam, sauces, ice cream, desserts, canned foods, and breakfast cereals.

  Certainly enjoy moderate quantities of these foods, but for serious weight control, look for 'low calorie', 'diet' or 'sugar-free'.

  However, be careful not to substitute sugar-rich foods with high-fat foods which might boost calories even more!

- Be aware that sugar comes in different forms such as sucrose, glucose, fructose, malt, high-fructose corn syrup, molasses, honey and maple syrup. Check the label.

- **Sugar alcohols such as sorbitol,** mannitol and maltitol are carb-based and have $1/2$ - $3/4$ the calories of regular sugar. While not counted as sugar on food labels, they do add to the carb count. Excess amounts can cause bloating, gas and diarrhea.

- **Sugar-free sweeteners** such as *Equal, DiabetiSweet, NutraSweet, Splenda, Sweet'n Low* and *Stevia* make it easy to reduce sugar in drinks and recipes. Use only in moderation.

  Note: Most recipes can be adapted to contain less sugar with little effect on taste or quality.

Extra Info ~ www.CalorieKing.com

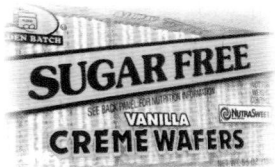

Sugar-free snacks and foods may be higher in fat and calories than the regular product.

Example ~ Creme Wafers (3):
Regular ~ 115 cals, 6g fat
Sugar-Free ~ 160 cals, 10g fat

SUGAR CONTENT OF SOME COMMON FOODS

	Teaspoons of Sugar
Coca Cola or *Pepsi*, 12 fl.oz	10
20 fl.oz size	17
Iced Tea, sweetened, 12 fl.oz	8
Chocolate Milk, 12 fl.oz	6
Honey Smacks Cereal, 1 oz	4
Popcorn, caramel, 1 cup	3.5
Chocolate Bar, 1.5 oz	6
M&M's 1.7 oz pkg	7
Muffin, large, 4 oz	6
Choc Chip Cookie, 1 oz	2
Donut, iced	6
Apple Pie, 1 piece	7
Jell-O, $1/2$ cup	4.5
Jam, 1 Tbsp, 20g	2.5
Syrup, maple, 1 Tbsp	3

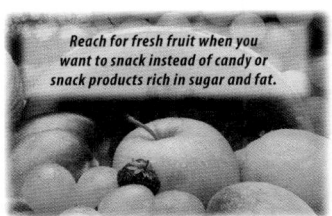

Reach for fresh fruit when you want to snack instead of candy or snack products rich in sugar and fat.

Tips For Overweight Kids & Parents!

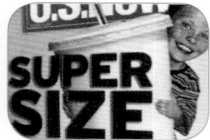

The XL Generation

Some 15% of American kids and adolescents are overweight; and childhood obesity has doubled over the last 20 years. Diabetes, high blood pressure and high cholesterol are major problem areas for overweight children and adolescents, as are depression, low self-esteem, sleep apnea and bone joint problems.

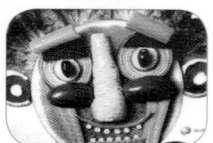

To address this problem, cooperation is required between kids, parents, schools and government. Weight control is a family and community affair.

Some simple tips to get started:

≫ Watch Soda Intake!

Limit soda and sugary drinks to one serving on the weekends. Soda should not be an everyday beverage. Try water instead. When at fast-food restaurants or using a soda fountain, choose small servings with ice or choose diet soda instead. Schools should provide water and restrict access to soda. Parents need to supervise kids at the soda fountain!

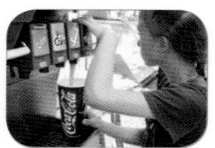

≫ Cut back on Fast-Foods and Eating Out

Many more calories are consumed when you eat out. Healthy meals prepared at home are best for the whole family.

≫ Say "No" to Super-Sizing!

Portion sizes are on the increase, and for just a few cents, meals can be upsized - with loads more calories. Choose sensible portion sizes when dining out and at home. Use smaller plates and choose smaller packages.

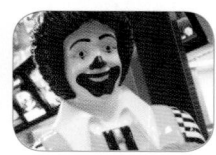

≫ Limit Between-Meal Snacking

Watch out for high-fat and high-calorie snacks – they can have more calories than a meal. Keep your eye on portion sizes and limit foods like chips and candy to parties and special occasions. Choose fresh fruit and vegetables instead.

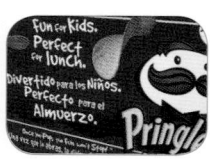

≫ Get Moving ~ Watch Less TV!

Kids need at least 60 minutes of physical activity every day. Limit time spent in sedentary activities (such as playing computer games or watching TV to just one hour per day.) Also limit the accompanying snacks! Include exercise in family activities.

Note: When kids watch TV in a motionless trance, they burn even less calories than if simply sitting, reading or talking.

For extra information and tips see www.CalorieKing.com

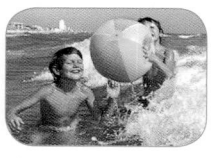

Sample Diet Plan - 1300 Calories

For Overweight Persons. Please Check With Your Doctor.
(Menu contains approximately 30-35 Grams Fat)

 Breakfast (approx. 250 cal)

	1 Small Fruit or ½ oz Dried Fruit
Plus	Cereal: 1½ oz Dry (high fiber)
	or 1 cup cooked Oatmeal
Plus	Milk (from daily allowance)

Daily Milk Allowance (approx. 160 calories)
2 cups Skim Milk or 1½ cups Low-fat (1%) Milk
or equivalent Soy Drink, Yogurt, Cheese, Tofu

Fat Allowance (140 calories; 15g Fat)
4 tsp Fat or 6-8 tsp Diet Margarine or 3 tsp Oil
or 1½ Tbsp Mayonnaise or ½ medium Avocado
or 1½ Tbsp Peanut Butter or 30g Nuts/Seeds

 Breakfast ~ Choice 2

	1 Small Fruit
Plus	1 Egg (no added fat)
	or ¾ oz Cheese
	or 2 oz Cottage Cheese
	or 1 oz Lean Bacon
Plus	1 Toast or ½ Muffin (English)

 Lunch (approx. 440 calories)

	2 slices Bread (2 oz) or 1 medium Roll or Bagel
	or 4 Crispbreads/Crackers or 6" Pita
Plus	2 oz lean Meat, Chicken or Turkey
	or 3½oz Tuna (in water) or 2½ oz Salmon
	or 1 oz Cheese or ½ cup (4 oz) Cottage Cheese
	or ½ cup (4 oz) Ricotta Cheese (low-fat)
	or ½ cup (4 oz) Fruit Yogurt (low-fat)
	or ½ cup (4 oz) Bean Salad
Plus	Large Salad (Oil-free dressing)
Plus	1 small Fruit or ½ oz Dried Fruit

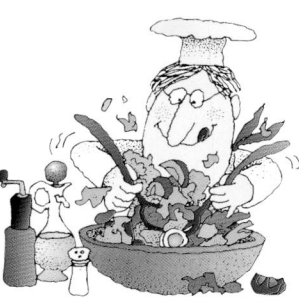

 Dinner (approx. 360 calories)

	Soup (fat-free)
Plus	3 oz lean Meat (cooked weight)
	or 4 oz Chicken Breast (no skin)
	or 3 oz Chicken Thigh/Leg (no skin)
	or 5 oz Fish (grilled, no fat)
	or ¾ cup (6 oz) Beans (Soy, Kidney, Pinto etc)/Lentils
	or Low-fat Entree (e.g. Lean Cuisine) or Recipe Dish
Plus	1 small Potato or ½ cup Rice/Pasta or 1 slice Bread
Plus	2-3 servings Vegetables/Salad
Plus	1 small Fruit + Diet Gelatin Dessert

 Between Meals Water, Coffee, Tea, Diet drinks,

Fruit from main meals; Raw vegetable pieces, Milk from Allowance

Note: Take a multivitamin/mineral supplement daily while dieting.

Exercise & Weight Control

- Persons who exercise regularly lose more weight and keep it off longer than non-exercisers.

- Exercise also improves general health and well-being. Mood, confidence and self-esteem are enhanced by a sense of control and accomplishment.

- **Exercise increases the metabolic rate** of the body even for hours after exercise - a good way to 'wake up' a sluggish metabolism and burn extra fat. Exercise compensates for any decrease in metabolic rate with increasing age and also in some heavy smokers who stop smoking.

- **Strength training** further builds muscle and aids body reshaping. You can also eat a little more food! Note: Each extra pound of muscle burns an extra 50 calories daily ~ even while you sleep! Weight from exercised muscles is okay. It is surplus fat (particularly abdominal fat) that is potentially harmful to health.

- **Avoid injury** by beginning with walking, low impact aerobics, or weight-supported exercise (e.g. swimming, cycling). Avoid competitive sports.

- **How Much?** Start with 10 - 20 minutes/day and progress to 30 - 60 minutes/day.
  Also walk up stairs instead of using elevators. Take a brisk walk at lunch. Use an exercise bike, treadmill or stair machine while watching TV. Walk the dog.

- **How Often?** While aerobic fitness requires only 3 - 4 sessions weekly, **weight control is a daily event which requires daily exercise**.

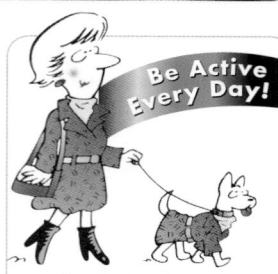

Brisk walking each day is a safe and effective way to keep trim and fit. Try it – you'll like it!

Strength-training with light weights helps to retain or rebuild muscle tissue. It enhances weight control.

FATNESS VS FITNESS

An overweight but fit person can be healthier than a thin, unfit person.

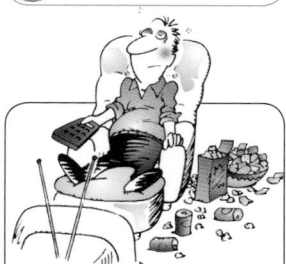

Too little exercise and too much food are the main contributors to middle-age spread.

Daily exercise and sensible eating can minimize middle-age spread. Include some strength-training to retain or build muscle.

TV CAN BE FATTENING!

- Many adults and children spend over 20 hours per week watching TV or at the computer (playing games or 'surfing') – at the same time as eating high calorie snacks and drinks.

- Are you a TV couch potato or computer addict? Limit your TV and computer hours and plan healthy physical activities.

- At home, limit kids to 2 hours daily for TV and computers.

Calories Used in Exercise

LIGHT	MODERATE	HEAVY
130 lbs ~ 3 Cals/Min	130 lbs ~ 5 Cals/Min	130 lbs ~ 8 Cals/Min
170 lbs ~ 4 Cals/Min	170 lbs ~ 6 Cals/Min	170 lbs ~ 10 Cals/Min
220 lbs ~ 5 Cals/Min	220 lbs ~ 7 Cals/Min	220 lbs ~ 12 Cals/Min

LIGHT	MODERATE	HEAVY
Walking, slow	Walking, brisk	Walking (power), Jogging
Cycling, light	Cycling, moderate	Cycling (vigorous), Spinning
Gardening light	Swimming, crawl	Swimming, strenuous
Golf, social	Weight-training, light	Weight-training, heavy
Tennis, doubles	Tennis, moderate	Wrestling/Judo, advanced
Housework, cleaning	Racquetball, beginners	Racquetball, advanced
Calisthenics, Yoga	Aerobics, light	Tae Bo, Kick Boxing
Bowling	Football, Grid Iron	Football, training
Ping-pong, social	Basketball, Baseball	Basketball (Pro)
Ice Skating	Walking Downstairs	Climbing Stairs
Aquarobics, light	Snow Skiing (downhill)	Skipping Rope
Skate Boarding	Shovelling snow	Skiing (cross country)
Line/Square Dancing	Dancing (ballroom)	Aquarobics, advanced
		Dancing (strenuous), Zumba

Note: Only those sports or activities that are sustained over a period of time (e.g running)
qualify for heavy exercise. Stop-start sports such as tennis are considered 'moderate'.

Interactive Calculations ~ www.CalorieKing.com/tools

WALKING PROGRAM

USE DISTANCE, STEPS OR TIME

Weeks	Distance	Steps Pedometer	Time
1-2	1 mile	2000	20 mins
3-5	1.5 miles	3000	18 mins
6-8	2 miles	3500	35 mins
9-10	2.5 miles	4500	45 mins
11+	3.5 miles	6000	60 mins

10,000 STEPS PER DAY

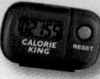

A pedometer can motivate you
to be more active. It clips to
your belt or waist band and
registers each step.

Aim for 8,000 - 10,000 steps per day, instead
of an average of only 3,000 - 4,000 steps.

For Extra Information:
www.CalorieKing.com

Order Details ~ Page 303

Reshaping Eating Behaviors

- Eating is a behavior that is largely controlled by people with whom we live or socialize, places in which we carry out our lives, and our emotions. Become aware of those situations that commonly lead to extra food being eaten.

- We may also be unaware of 'bad' eating habits that can lead to excess calorie intake; e.g. eating quickly, large mouthfuls, eating when tense or bored, finishing a large serving of food when not hungry.

Tips to help uncover and correct those 'bad' eating habits:

- **Don't eat while engaged in other activities;** for example, watching TV, reading. Eat only at the table, not at the fridge or while standing.

- **Don't eat quickly.** Chewing slowly allows time to register a feeling of fullness. Don't use fingers, only utensils. Cut food into smaller pieces. Don't load your fork until the previous mouthful is finished.

- **Don't purchase problem high calorie foods.** Shop from a set list to prevent impulse buying. Avoid shopping with children.

- **Buy snack foods** in the smallest package. The larger the serving size or package, the more you are likely to eat or drink.

- **Plan meals in advance. Stick to a set menu.**

- **Plan a strategy to avoid uncontrolled eating** and drinking at social events, or when your emotions urge you to binge.

  Rehearse repeatedly in your mind exactly what you will do in such situations. Remind yourself several times each day that you are in charge of your actions and that you can be strong-willed. Seek counseling or coaching on various strategies.

- **Promise yourself** that when you feel the urge to snack, you will engage in some activity that will distract you away from food (e.g. go for a walk, brush your teeth, phone a friend.)

  If you eat out of boredom, find some new hobby or interest that gets you out of the house. Even enroll in an adult education class.

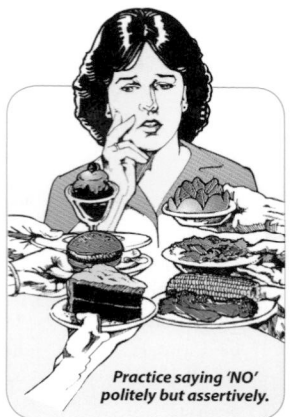

Practice saying 'NO' politely but assertively.

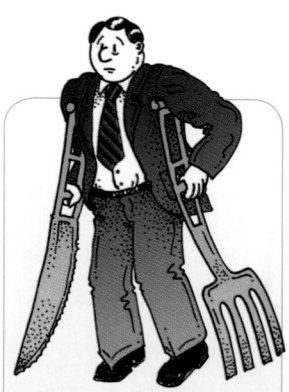

Do you use food as an emotional crutch? If so, professional counseling may be helpful.

The Value of a Food Journal

The food journal is the most powerful proven aid for dieters. Persons who keep a food and exercise journal not only lose more weight they also keep it off. Here are some of the reasons:

- Recording your eating and exercise habits jolts you into realizing just what you do eat and drink each day; and also whether you exercise sufficiently.

- **Helps you identify problem foods** and drinks with excessive calories and fat.

- **Helps identify moods**, situations and events that lead to excessive eating of unwanted calories. You can then plan to overcome or avoid them.

- **Prevents 'calorie amnesia'**, the forgetfulness that leads to rebound weight gain after successful weight loss. Recording puts you back on the right track.

- **Helps you develop greater self-discipline.** You will think twice about overindulging if you have to record it - especially if someone checks your journal regularly. It certainly keeps you honest!

- **Motivates you** to carefully plan your meals and to exercise each day.

- **Serves as a check system** for your doctor, dietitian or counselor to assess your progress and make recommendations.

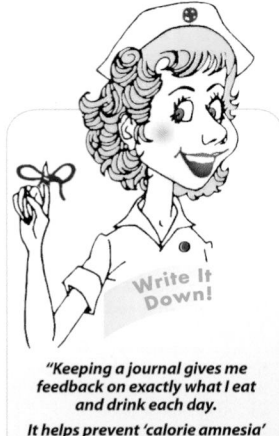

Write It Down!

"Keeping a journal gives me feedback on exactly what I eat and drink each day.

It helps prevent 'calorie amnesia' and reminds me to exercise each day.

It's a must for successful weight control!"

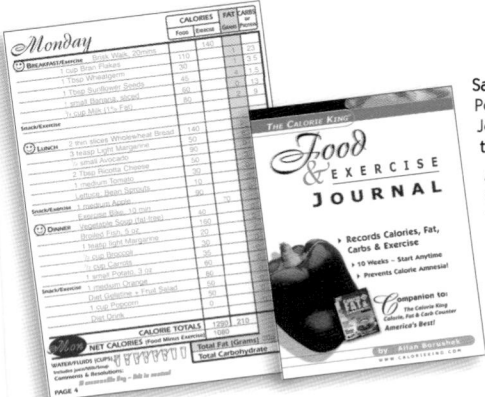

Sample Page from The Pocket Food & Exercise Journal, a 10-week journal to record food and exercise.

At day's end, exercise calories are deducted from food calories.

Includes Weekly Summary Page & Progress Checklist.

EXTRA DETAILS
~ SEE PAGE 302

Diabetes Guide

What is Diabetes?

Diabetes is a disorder in which the body cannot make proper use of carbohydrates (sugar and starches).

- After digestion, sugar and starches are changed into **glucose** – the simplest form of sugar vital for body energy and growth.
- **Insulin** is the hormone which acts like a key that opens the door to body cells and allows glucose to enter.
- **Without sufficient insulin**, unused glucose builds up in the blood and passes into the urine. This produces symptoms of frequent urination, continual thirst and tiredness.
- **Untreated diabetes** increases the risk of damage to nerves and blood vessels. This, in turn, increases the risk of heart disease, stroke, blindness, kidney damage, foot ulcers and gangrene (with amputation), impotence and other complications.

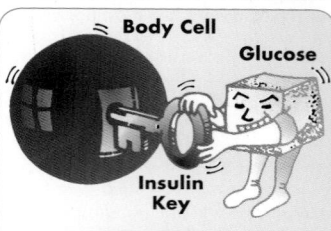

Body Cell

Glucose

Insulin Key

*Insulin acts like a key.
It opens the door to body cells
and allows glucose to enter.*

*People with Type-1 diabetes and some
with Type-2 have too few or no keys and
require insulin injections.*

*Others (most Type-2) have ample keys but
'misshapen' key holes (insulin resistant)
– particularly if obese and inactive.*

TYPE-1 DIABETES

Insulin-Dependent Diabetes

- Occurs in 10% of diabetes cases
- Usually in children and young adults
- Pancreas gland produces little or no insulin. Daily insulin injections are necessary, plus:
- Regular meals with even carbohydrate distribution to match insulin dosage. Regular exercise and weight control are also important.

⚠ WARNING SIGNALS

- Frequent urination
- Continual thirst
- Rapid weight loss
- Unusual hunger
- Extreme weakness/fatigue
- Nausea, vomiting, irritability

TYPE-2 DIABETES

Non-Insulin Dependent

- Occurs in 90% of diabetes cases
- Occurs mainly in adults - particularly in overweight and inactive persons
- Insulin is produced but body cells resist its action and glucose cannot enter cells.
- Usually treated with diet and exercise. Sometimes requires medication (tablets or insulin injections).

⚠ WARNING SIGNALS

- Any Type-1 symptom
- Blurred vision
- Excessive itching
- Skin infections with slow healing
- Tingling/numbness in feet

GESTATIONAL DIABETES • Occurs during pregnancy • Usually disappears on the baby's birth • Over 50% of these mothers develop diabetes within the next 20 years. • Requires weight control, a healthy lifestyle and regular medical checks.

Prediabetes - An Early Warning!

- Prediabetes means you don't have diabetes now but are likely to develop it in the future - if serious preventive action is not taken now! Your risk for heart disease and stroke is also increased by 50%.

- You are prediabetic if your blood sugar level is between 100 and 125 mg/dL (after an overnight fast).

  These levels are higher than normal but not high enough to be diabetes.

- Risk factors for prediabetes include being overweight or obese, a family history of diabetes, high blood lipids, hypertension, and a history of gestational diabetes (during pregnancy).

- Most people with prediabetes can prevent full-blown diabetes (usually Type 2) by adopting a healthier lifestyle. This includes **losing weight if overweight, and exercising for 30 minutes at least 5 days a week.**

- Your doctor and dietitian can plan a preventive lifestyle program for you.

> **NEW BLOOD SUGAR CLASSIFICATION FOR DIABETES**
> (American Diabetes Association, 2003)
>
> **NORMAL:**
> **Below 100 mg/dL**
>
> **PREDIABETES:**
> **100-125 mg/dL**
>
> **DIABETES:**
> **Over 125 mg/dL**

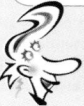

Everyone 45 and over should have a blood glucose test every 3 years.

Importance of Weight Control

- **Type-2 diabetes** occurs 2-3 times more often in overweight persons – particularly if inactive.

- Such persons do not usually lack insulin. Rather, their insulin is less effective. As obesity develops, muscle and other body cells may resist insulin in varying degrees. The resultant build-up of blood glucose may lead to diabetic symptoms.

- **Weight loss alone** often corrects this condition in Type-2 diabetes. If overweight, try a moderate diet of 1200-1500 calories **plus daily exercise.**

  Within several weeks, body cells can lose their resistance and become sensitive once again to the effects of insulin. Insulin and blood glucose levels may normalize, and symptoms may disappear.

  Further, the need for oral antidiabetic drugs might be prevented or much lessened in dosage. **So, give diet and exercise a fair chance** – and maintain them to keep symptoms under control.

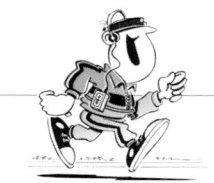

Get Moving! Everyday, do at least 30 minutes of moderate intensity exercise. It's the key to improving insulin sensitivity.

Add strength-training 3-4 times a week to double the benefits.

Diabetes ~ Management

Managing Diabetes

Don't battle diabetes alone. Establish a partnership with your doctor, dietitian, certified diabetes educator and pharmacist. **Extra Support:** • *American Diabetes Association* • *American Diabetes Educators Association* • *National Diabetes Education Program*

Hints to keep blood glucose within safe limits:

- **Control your diet.** Know what and when you will eat. Seek referral to a dietitian for expert advice.
- **Exercise regularly.** It assists weight control and can improve sensitivity of body cells to insulin. Plan exercise into your daily routine.
- **Monitor your blood glucose** at home and work – ideally with a portable blood glucose meter. It will help you become familiar with your blood glucose patterns, and the effects of diet, exercise and medication. Insulin pumps can also help control blood glucose levels around the clock.
- **Don't skip prescribed insulin or oral medication.** If on insulin, know what action to take if hypoglycemia (low blood glucose) occurs. Also educate your family and friends.

Be Heart Smart ~ Know Your ABC's

If you have diabetes, you are at high risk for heart attack and stroke. Heart disease is more likely to strike you – and at an early age – than someone without diabetes.

But you can fight back. Be smart about your heart. **Take control of the ABC's of diabetes** and live a long and healthy live. Talk to your health care provider about your ABC targets.

A is for A1C
The A1C (A-one-C) test – short for hemoglobin A1C – measures your average blood glucose (sugar) over the last 3 months. **Suggested target: below 7**

B is for Blood Pressure
High blood pressure makes your heart work too hard. **Suggested target: below 120/80**

C is for Cholesterol
Bad cholesterol, or LDL, can build up and clog your arteries. **Suggested target: below 100**

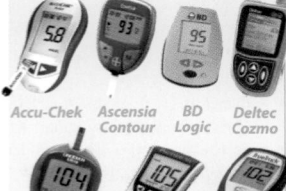

Blood glucose meters and insulin pumps can greatly improve control of diabetes.

BLOOD GLUCOSE METERS

Accu-Chek   Ascensia Contour   BD Logic   Deltec Cozmo

OneTouch Ultra   Medisense Precision Xtra   TrueTrack

INSULIN PUMPS

Medtronic   Animas

Accu-Chek

A1C VALUES	AVERAGE DAILY BLOOD GLUCOSE
6% ▶	**120 mg/dL** Excellent Control
8% ▶	**180 mg/dL** Needs Treatment Change
10% ▶	**240 mg/dL** Poor Control
13% ▶	**330 mg/dL** Seriously Out of Control

Guidelines for choosing a healthy diet apply equally to people with or without diabetes. Eating a wide variety of foods that are mainly low in fat and refined sugars, and high in fiber, is recommended.

However, actual food quantities, as well as when you eat, will also influence control of blood glucose. Your dietitian will individualize a diet plan to suit your food preferences, lifestyle and medical status. Here are a few hints:

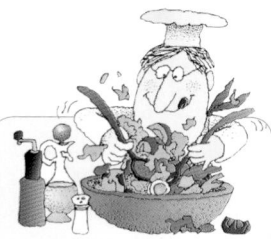

Eat a well-balanced diet, high in fiber-containing foods and low in saturated fat.

- **Maintain a healthy weight.** If overweight, even a modest weight loss plus daily exercise can help to normalize blood glucose in Type-2 diabetes.

- **Don't skip meals.** If you take insulin or an oral hypoglycemic agent, regular meals are important.

- **If on insulin**, eat meals at the same time each day. Eat a similar amount of food at each meal. Even distribution of carbohydrate over the day will make best use of the available insulin and prevent wide variations in blood glucose levels.

  Note: Take your rapid-acting insulin no more than 15 minutes before eating. Regular and combination insulins are best taken with about 30 minutes between insulin injection and breakfast.

- **Choose wholegrain breads, cereals and pasta.** Eat fresh fruits, vegetables and legumes. These foods contain more fiber and slow the release of glucose into your blood after a meal.

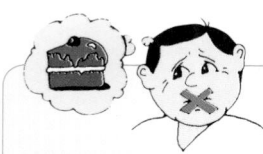

Modest weight loss and daily exercise can greatly improve control of Type-2 diabetes.

- **Limit foods high in saturated fat and cholesterol.** Enjoy fish, soy foods, and other foods rich in omega-3 fats. **Extra Notes** ~ *See Fats & Cholesterol Guide, Page 271*

- **Avoid sugars and foods high in added sugar** particularly if overweight. Small amounts of sugar as part of a meal may occasionally be okay. Check with your dietitian. Use *Equal, Splenda* and *NutraSweet* – sweetened foods and drinks.
  Extra Notes ~ *See Page 9*

- **Foods (and supplements) rich in antioxidant vitamins C, E and beta-carotene**, as well as omega-3 fats, magnesium, zinc and chromium may help prevent long-term complications of diabetes (such as damage to small blood vessels and nerves). Be sure to check with your doctor.

***Excess Alcohol** contributes to obesity, diabetes, and high blood pressure.*

The risk of hypoglycemia (low blood sugar) and drug interactions with alcohol is also increased.

Diabetes ~ Carbs & Glycemic Index

Carbohydrate Type Affects Blood Glucose

The various forms of carbohydrate affect blood glucose levels in different ways. It is difficult to predict the effect of particular foods, sugars or meals, simply by their carbohydrate content.

Thus the same amount of carbohydrate from different foods may affect blood sugar levels very differently. Many factors affect the rate of digestion and absorption – particularly the type of sugar, starch and fiber; the degree of processing and cooking (which increases digestion rate); and the amount of protein and fat (which slows stomach emptying and digestion).

Glycemic Index (GI)

The GI is a method of ranking carbohydrate foods on a scale (0-100) according to how they affect blood glucose levels. (See next column). The higher the GI value, the greater the food's ability to rapidly raise blood glucose levels and the more insulin needed by the body (not desirable).

Eating low GI foods leads to better control of blood glucose and insulin levels (which in turn lowers the risk of damage to blood vessels and nerves). The slower digestion of low GI foods also helps to delay hunger pangs, and benefit weight control.

Of course, choosing low GI foods is not a licence to eat unlimited amounts – **calorie restriction and portion control for weight control is of prime importance.**

Extra Notes: * GI is not meant to be used in isolation without regard to portion size, and other dietary recommendations for healthy eating. Foods are not good or bad on the basis of their GI.

* The GI concept is yet to be adopted by the American Diabetes Assoc. and American Dietetic Assoc. There are other important aspects to consider for wise use of GI, including GL (Glycemic Load).

Extra Information ~ www.calorieking.com

LOWER GLYCEMIC FOODS

Slower Acting Carbohydrates

These foods are more slowly digested and absorbed. They help maintain more even blood glucose levels, as long as excessive amounts are not eaten. Use these foods regularly but still limit portion size for weight control.

Examples:
- Dried beans, peas, lentils
- Nuts and seeds
- Wholegrain breads and pita
- Bran cereals, oats
- Barley, buckwheat, bulgur
- Spaghetti, pasta, Basmati Rice
- Fresh fruit: apples, avocados, bananas (firm), cherries, grapefruit, grapes, olives, oranges, peaches, pears, plums. Fresh juices.
- Vegetables: sweet potatoes, yam
- Milk, yoghurt, soy drinks
- Sugar alcohols (Sorbitol, Maltitol)

HIGHER GLYCEMIC FOODS

Quicker Acting Carbohydrates

These foods more rapidly raise blood glucose levels. Eat only in moderation.

- White bread, rice cakes, bagels, croissants, doughnuts
- Low fiber cereals: Cornflakes, *Rice Krispies, Froot Loops*
- White potatoes, white rice, corn
- Watermelon, ripe bananas, cantaloupe, pineapple
- Soda, sugar-sweetened sports/energy drinks
- Sugar, Sugar Candy
- Ice Cream (low-fat), Frozen Yogurt

EXTRA INFORMATION

- **Book:** The New Glucose Revolution by Jennie Brand-Miller
- www.glycemicindex.com
- www.CalorieKing.com

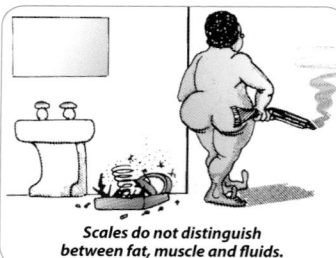

Scales do not distinguish between fat, muscle and fluids.

≫ Body Fluid Changes

Body weight fluctuates from day to day. This is mainly due to changes in body fluids which make up around 70% of total body weight. It can be affected by changes in hormone levels, dietary factors such as salt and carbohydrate, and even exercise.

Weight change over several weeks is more likely to reflect changes in levels of fat and muscle rather than fluid. Unfortunately, the scales do not distinguish between weight changes due to water, fat or muscle. This is why **we shouldn't allow every fluctuation in weight to rule our lives.**

To limit fluid retention, avoid salty foods and go easy on the salt shaker. Eating sufficient fruit and vegetables supplies extra potassium which counteracts sodium and encourages fluid loss. However, **do not limit water intake.** Be sure to drink at least 6-8 glasses of water or other fluids per day.

When dining out, be aware that the extra pound or two that might show on the scales the next morning is not the result of a small dietary indiscretion. It is more likely due to fluid retention resulting from more highly seasoned and salty food.

Monthly hormonal changes in women can also account for a build-up of fluids of several pounds prior to menstruation.

≫ Menopausal Weight Gains

Most women gain an average of 4-5 pounds in the years leading up to menopause – usually in their middle to late 40's. This can occur even when exercise and eating habits have not changed significantly.

With hormonal changes occurring at that time, body fat also tends to be redistributed from thighs, buttocks and hips to the breast and stomach areas (a greater health risk).

Be sure to eat wisely and continue daily physical activity including strength-training to maintain or build muscles – and to boost metabolism and self-esteem.

≫ Underactive Thyroid

Thyroid hormone is made by the thyroid gland in the neck.

When insufficient thyroid hormone is made, metabolism and body processes slow down and weight gain can occur.

Symptoms of hypothyroidism can be subtle and easily overlooked as signs of normal aging. **Early symptoms** may include fatigue, muscle weakness, sluggishness, a swollen tongue that you keep biting, and a puffy face.

As metabolism continues to slow, further **signs can include** chronically cold hands and feet, slow reflexes, constipation, dry skin and coarse hair, brittle nails, heavy menstrual periods, slower pulse, and a husky voice.

Depression-like symptoms may also develop such as forgetfulness, loss of interest, mood swings and irritability.

Weight gains of as much as 10-20 pounds (mainly fluid) can occur, as well as a raised **blood cholesterol level.**

The condition is more common in women, especially following pregnancy, around menopause, or after age 60.

A simple blood test through your doctor can detect hypothyroidism. It is easily treated in most cases with thyroid hormone pills.

Adults 35 and older should have a TSH (thyroid stimulating hormone) test every 5 years. Testing when pregnant is also wise.

Calcium & Osteoporosis Guide

Calcium's Role in the Body

Calcium plays a vital role in nerve and muscle function, clotting of blood, enzyme regulation, insulin secretion and overall bone strength. Bones and teeth store 99% of the body's calcium.

The calcium level in blood is kept at a steady level by the continual exchange of calcium between blood and bone. When insufficient calcium is obtained from food the body draws calcium out of the bones.

This bone loss over a period of years may lead to **osteoporosis** – thinning of the bones (porous bones).

The bones become weak, brittle and easy to fracture, particularly the bones of the wrist, hips and spine. Loss of height and curvature of the spine may also result, as may periodontal disease - the deterioration of the jaw bones that support the teeth.

Common in Women & Men

While osteoporosis also occurs in men, women are particularly vulnerable (1 in 4 by age 60). They have about 30% less bone than men, and a greater bone loss at menopause when oestrogen levels drop. Slender framed women are at greater risk. (A woman in her eighties can have lost up to two thirds of her skeleton.)

Insufficient dietary calcium during pregnancy and breastfeeding will see bone reserves drawn upon, increasing the risk of osteoporosis in later years.

Hip fractures account for 300,000 hospitalizations each year. One in 5 older Americans with hip fracture die within a year – and 1 in 5 end up in a nursing home.

Causes of Osteoporosis

The major factors associated with the bone loss of osteoporosis appear to be:

- hormone changes of menopause
- inadequate dietary intake of calcium and other bone nutrients such as magnesium, vitamin D, zinc and protein
- insufficient exercise (weight bearing - such as walking, cycling ~ 30-60 minutes daily)
- family history of osteoporosis

Other contributing factors may include:

- excessive cola (regular or diet) and alcohol intake
- cigarette smoking
- some drug medications (e.g.steroids, thyroid)

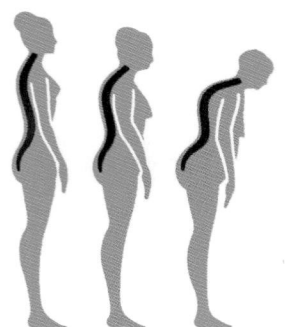

As osteoporosis progresses after menopause, vertebrae may collapse causing the spine to curve and shoulders to hunch.

RECOMMENDED DAILY INTAKE OF CALCIUM

Children:	1-3 yrs	~ 500mg
	4-8 yrs	~ 800mg
	9-12 yrs	~ 1300mg
Teenagers:		
	13-18 yrs	~ 1300mg
Adults:	19-50 yrs	~ 1000mg
	51+ yrs	~ 1200mg
Women:		
Pre-menopausal		~ 1000mg
Menopausal (beginning)		~ 1200mg
Post-menopausal		~ 1500mg
Pregnant & Breastfeeding		
	14-18 yrs	~ 1300mg
	19+ yrs	~ 1000mg

Early Prevention Important

Gradual loss of bone begins in the thirties after maximum bone mass is reached. The stronger the bones at that time, the less trouble is likely to occur later. The earlier that prevention or treatment begins the greater the benefit. **The key to prevention is** to build strong, dense bones early in life. **By age 16,** some 80% of peak bone mass is already reached.

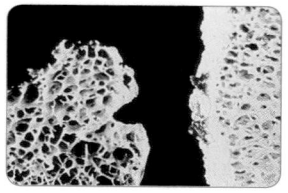

▲ Osteoporotic Fragile Bone   ▲ Healthy Dense Bone

Young women may lessen the risk by:

• eating high-calcium foods as well as adequate fruits, vegetables, wholegrains and nuts
• drinking less soft drink, and more milk
• not engaging in extreme dieting that results in menstrual period cessation (via less estrogen)
• taking regular exercise and not smoking

Good Dietary Sources of Calcium
(Eat 3-4 servings a day of calcium-rich foods)

• Milk, Yogurt, Cheese
• Flavored Milk Drinks & Fruit Smoothies
• Ice Cream (low-fat), Custard (low-fat)
• Soy Drinks (calcium-enriched)
• Orange Juice (calcium-fortified)
• Tofu (with calcium coagulant), Miso, Tempeh
• Canned Salmon or Sardines (with edible bones)
• Breakfast Cereals (calcium-enriched): *Total, Wheaties*
• Broccoli, Dried Beans, Baked Beans
• Almonds, Brazil nuts, Hazelnuts, Seeds

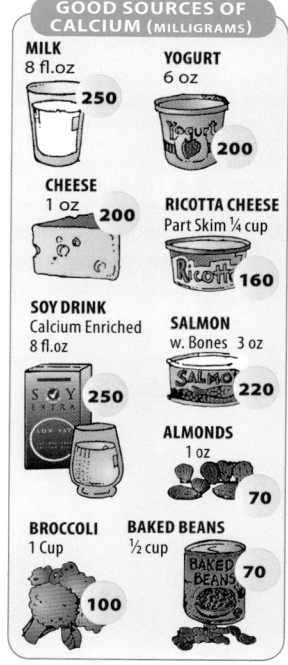

GOOD SOURCES OF CALCIUM (MILLIGRAMS)

MILK
8 fl.oz
250

YOGURT
6 oz
200

CHEESE
1 oz
200

RICOTTA CHEESE
Part Skim ¼ cup
160

SOY DRINK
Calcium Enriched
8 fl.oz
250

SALMON
w. Bones 3 oz
220

ALMONDS
1 oz
70

BROCCOLI
1 Cup
100

BAKED BEANS
½ cup
70

> **Calculating Calcium From Food Labels**
> The calcium content of packaged foods and drinks is shown in the Nutrition Facts label as a percentage of the DRI (dietary reference intake) of 1000 mg calcium.
> To convert this percentage into milligrams of calcium, simply multiply the percent figure by 10 (or add a zero). Examples: 5% = 50 mg calcium; 35% = 350 mg calcium.
> Food Calcium Counter ~ www.CalorieKing.com

Calcium Supplements

Because absorption of dietary calcium decreases with age, prescribed high doses of calcium (1500-2000mg/day) may benefit persons with osteoporosis - as well as vitamin D (preferably in D3 form, not D2), vitamin K, magnesium and zinc. Check with your doctor.

Notes, Abbreviations, Measures

≫ **Calorie and fat values have been rounded off.**
Calories ~ to the nearest 5 or 10 calories.
Fat ~ to nearest half gram. **Note:** Trace amounts of
fat (less than 0.3 grams) have been treated as zero.

≫ **Carbohydrate figures** in this book are for total
carbohydrate, and not **Net Carbs** (which deducts fiber,
polydextrose and sugar alcohols from total carbs).

≫ Because manufacturer's figures on labels are rounded
off, figures in this book may differ slightly from the
label. Serving sizes may also vary.

≫ Food product formulations change occasionally,
and hence the need to regularly update this type of
publication. Many products also come and go. Check
the food label for any changes.

≫ **Seek Professional Advice:** This book is intended
for educational purposes only. It is not a substitute
for professional advice.

≫ **Feedback Welcome:** Please contact the author
directly with your queries, and suggestions for foods
to be included in future editions.
Write to: Allan Borushek (Dietitian)
1001 West 17th Street, Costa Mesa CA 92627.
Email: allan@calorieking.com

≫ **Food Product Updates:** Check the author's website.

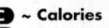

www.CalorieKing.com

C	~ Calories
F	~ Fat (grams)
Cb	~ Carbohydrate (grams)

Abbreviations

tsp	= teaspoon
Tbsp or T	= Tablespoon
oz	= ounce(s)
c	= cup
fl.oz	= fluid ounce(s)
g	= gram(s)
avg	= average
pkg	= package

Volume Measures

(All measures are level)

3 tsp	= 1 Tbsp
2 Tbsp	= 1 fl.oz
½ cup	= 4 fl.oz
1 cup	= 8 fl.oz
2 cups	= 1 Pint
2 Pints	= 1 Quart

Note: 8 oz weight is not the same
as 8 fl oz volume (space occupied).
Dense foods weigh more per set
volume. Examples:
1 cup popcorn weighs ½ oz
1 cup milk weighs 8½ oz
1 cup pudding weighs 10 oz

Metric Conversion

½ oz	= 14 grams
1 oz	= 28.4 grams
2 oz	= 57 grams
3½ oz	= 100 grams
1 fl.oz	= 30 mls
1 cup (8 fl.oz)	= 240 mls
33 fl.oz	= 1 liter (volume)

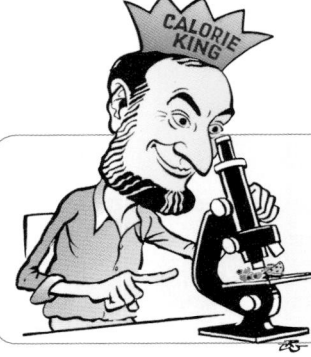

SOURCES OF INFORMATION

• U.S. Dept. of Agriculture
• Food Manufacturers
• Food Industry Boards & Councils
• Independent laboratory analysis
• Scientific publications
• Overseas food composition tables
• Author extrapolations

Milk

Quick Guide   C   F   Cb

Cow Milk ~ *Average All Brands*

Whole (3.5% fat):

	C	F	Cb
2 Tbsp, 1 fl.oz	20	1	1.5
1 Glass, 6 fl.oz	110	6	8.5
1 Cup, 8 fl.oz	150	8	12
1 Pint, 16 fl.oz	300	16	23
1 Quart, 946 ml	600	32	46

Reduced-Fat (2% fat):

2 Tbsp, 1 fl.oz	15	0.5	1.5
1 Glass, 6 fl.oz	90	4	8.5
1 Cup, 8 fl.oz	130	5	13
1 Pint, 16 fl.oz	260	10	26
1 Quart, 946 ml	520	20	52

Light/Low-Fat (1% fat):

2 Tbsp, 1 fl.oz	12	0.3	1.5
1 Glass, 6 fl.oz	75	2	8.5
1 Cup, 8 fl.oz	120	2.5	14
1 Pint, 16 fl.oz	240	5	28
1 Quart, 946 ml	480	10	56

Light/Low-Fat (½ % fat):

2 Tbsp, 1 fl.oz	12	0.1	1.6

Fat Free/Skim:

2 Tbsp, 1 fl.oz	10	0	1.5
1 Cup, 8 fl.oz	90	0.5	13
1 Pint, 16 fl.oz	180	1	26
w. Replace (Oatrim Fiber): 1 cup	85	0	12

Protein-Fortified:

2% fat, 1 cup	140	5	14
1% fat, 1 cup	120	3	14
Skim, 1 cup	100	0.5	14

Acidophilus: *Average All Brands*

Reduced Fat (2%), 1 cup	130	5	13
Low-Fat (1%), 1 cup	100	2	13

Buttermilk: *Average All Brands*

Reduced-Fat (2%), 1 cup	120	5	10
Low-Fat (1%): 1 cup	100	2.5	12

Lactose-Reduced:

Reduced-Fat: *Lactaid,* 1 cup	130	5	12
Dairy Ease 100, 1 cup	130	5	12
Low-Fat: *Lactaid,* 1 cup	110	2.5	13
Fat-Free: *Lactaid/Lucerne,* 1 cup	80	0	13
Lactaid with Soy Protein	110	0	13

Lower Carb Dairy Drinks: *Per 8 fl.oz Cup*

Calorie Countdown (Hood)	130	8	3
2% Reduced-Fat, 1 cup	100	4.5	3
Fat-Free, 1 cup	45	0	3
LeCarb: 2% Low-Fat Dairy, 1 cup	105	4.5	4
Homogenized Dairy	140	9	4

Soy/Non-Dairy Drinks   ~ *See Page 27*

Goat/Sheep Milk, Kefir

Goat's Milk (Meyenberg):   C   F   Cb

	C	F	Cb
Whole, 1 cup, 8 fl.oz	140	7	11
Light/Low-Fat (1%), 8 fl.oz	90	2.5	9
Evaporated, reconst., 8 fl.oz	145	8	11
Kefir: *Steve's Kefir Peach,* 1 cup	220	9	25
Nancy's, fruit flavors, avg, 1 cup	200	8	25
Sheep's Milk: Whole, 1 cup	265	17	13

Canned & Dried Milk

Condensed: Reg. 2 Tbsp, 1 fl.oz	130	3	22
Low-Fat *(Eagle),* 2 Tbsp	120	1.5	23
Fat-Free *(Eagle),* 2 Tbsp	110	0	24
Evaporated: Whole, 2 Tbsp	40	3	3
Whole, ½ cup	170	10	13
Low-Fat *(Carnation),* 2 Tbsp, 1 oz	25	0.5	3
½ cup, 4 fl.oz	115	2.5	14
Fat-Free, 2 Tbsp, 1 oz	25	0	4
Dried: Whole, ¼ cup, 1 oz	150	8	11
Skim/Non-Fat, ⅓ cup	80	0	12
Made-up, 1 cup, 8 fl.oz	80	0	12
Buttermilk sweetcream, 1 oz	110	2	13
Non-Fat, 1 Tbsp	25	0	3
Malted *(Carnation),* dry, 1 Tbsp	30	0.5	6

Whey Drink

Acid: Dry, 1 Tbsp, 3g	10	0	2
Fluid, 1 cup, 8 fl.oz	60	0	13
Sweet: Dry, 1 Tbsp, 8g	25	0	6
Fluid, 1 cup, 8 fl.oz	65	1	13
Nutri Mil: Orig./Low-Fat 8 fl.oz	80	3	11
Chocolate, 8 fl.oz	110	3	19
Fat-Free (Calcium Enriched)	60	0	11

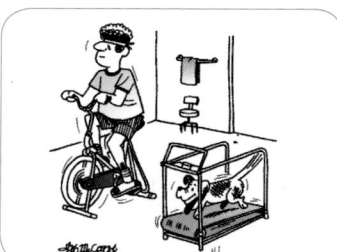

Flavored Milk Drinks

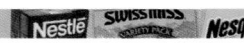

Quick Guide

Chocolate Milk

Average All Brands: Per Cup (8 fl.oz)

	C	F	Cb
Whole Milk (3.3%): 1 cup	200	8	25
1 Pint	400	16	50
Reduced-Fat (2%), 1 cup	175	5	25
Low-Fat (1%), 1 cup	150	2.5	25

Brands ~ Flavored Milk

Ready-To-Drink: Per 8 fl.oz Cup Unless Indicated

	C	F	Cb
Albertson's, low-fat, 1 cup	170	2.5	30
Alta Dena: Chocolate, 1 cup	260	9	36
Low-Fat Chocolate, 1 cup	200	2.5	33
Bravo!: Slim Slammers, 1 cup	110	3	14
Blenders Dble Choc., 11 fl.oz	180	4	19
Milky Way, 1 cup	170	5	22
Dominick's Low-Fat, 1 cup	170	2.5	28
Golden Guernsey, 1 cup	130	2.5	15
Grocers Pride Choc D'Lite, 1 cup	120	3	22
Hershey's			
Chocolate, 1% No Sugar Added, 1 c.	120	2.5	15
Chocolate, Reduced-Fat, 1 cup	200	5	31
Drink Box: Chocolate Drink, 1 box	130	1	29
Chocolate Reduced-Fat, 1 box	200	5	30
Chocolate Shake, 1 box	230	4.5	42
White Reduced-Fat, 1 box	130	5	12
MilkShake: Creamy Choc., 14 fl.oz	465	14	74
Strawb., Cookies'N'Crm, 14 fl.oz	485	12	76
Van. Crm; York Mint, avg., 14 fl.oz	550	12	95
Strawberry, Red-Fat, 14 fl.oz	345	8.5	52
Hood: Low-Fat (1%), Chocolate	170	3	28
Chocolate	230	9	31
Horizon Organic: Smoothies, 6 fl.oz	120	0	25
Chocolate, Low-Fat, 1 cup	170	3	27
Reduced-Fat flavors, avg., 1 cup	180	5	27
Kroger Low-Fat, 8 fl.oz	200	2.5	34
Nesquik: Chocolate, 16 fl.oz bottle	400	10	64
Banana, 16 fl.oz	400	10	60
Choc. Fat Free, 16 fl.oz bottle	320	0	64
Double Choc., 16 fl.oz bottle	400	10	60
Very Vanilla, 16 fl.oz	400	10	60
Oak Farms, 1 cup	210	8	26
Quaker Milk Chillers, 14 fl.oz bottle	250	9	32
Ralph's, 1 cup	240	3	34
Skinny Cow, Chocolate, 1 cup	150	0	26
Starbucks, Strawb. & Creme, 9.5 fl.oz	230	6	38
Viva, Low-Fat (1%), 1 cup	170	2.5	29
Yoo Hoo Choc Drink, 6½ fl.oz	110	1	24

Bottled Coffee

See Coffee Section: *Page 164*

Shakes & Smoothies

Smoothies

Made Up Ready-To-Drink
(8 fl. oz Milk/Soy + Fruit): Per 12 fl.oz

	C	F	Cb
Average all types w. Whole Milk	300	8	50
+ Ice Cream, 1 scoop	400	13	62
with Non-Fat Milk	240	0	50
Freshens; Jamba Juice; TCBY:			
See Fast-Foods Section			

Shakes

	C	F	Cb
Regular: Chocolate, 10 fl.oz	360	11	58
Vanilla/Strawberry, 10 fl.oz	320	9	53
Carb Options, 11.3 fl.oz	185	9	6
Burger King; McDonald's: See Fast-Foods			

Cocoa-Chocolate Mixes

Add extra cals/fat/carbohydrate for milk

Carnation Breakfast Drinks: See Page 158

	C	F	Cb
Ghirardelli			
Choc Mocha, 3 Tbsp	80	1	19
Double Chocolate, 4 Tbsp	140	0.5	34
White Mocha, 2 Tbsp	90	0	23
Hershey's, 1 Tbsp	30	0	7.5
Horlicks, Malt Extract, 1 oz	90	1	18
Land O' Lakes: Per 1¼ oz Pkg			
Choc.Mint/Raspb./Supreme	140	3.5	26
Nestle: French Vanilla, 1 envelope	120	3	22
Milk Chocolate, 2 Tbsp	85	2.5	15
Fat-Free Hot Cocoa, 1 envelope	25	0	1
w. Marshmallows, 1 envelope	35	0	8
Nesquik Powder (Nestle): Per 2 Tbsp			
Choc.; Dble Choc; Strawberry	90	0.5	19
Chocolate, No Added Sugar	40	1	7
Ovaltine Cocoa Mixes, 4 tsp	80	0	20
Swiss Miss: Cocoa Mixes			
Milk Chocolate, 1.2 oz pkg	140	3	27
w. Marshmallows, 1 oz pkg	120	2	24
Choc. Sensation, 1.2 oz pkg	150	3.5	28
Hot Cocoa Sugar Free, 1 pkg	60	0	10
Fat-Free, 0.6 oz	50	0	10
Vending Machine, 1.34 oz pkg	145	2	24

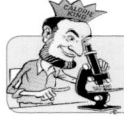

For Full Nutritional Data
~ See Author's Website
www.CalorieKing.com

Soy ~ Ready-To-Drink

Per 1 Cup Serving (8 fl.oz)	C	F	Cb
Eden Blend, 1 cup	125	3.5	19
Edensoy: Original, 1 cup	140	5	14
Vanilla, 1 cup	160	3	25
Light: Original	100	2	14
Vanilla	110	1	22
Extra Original; Unsweetened	140	4	14
Extra, Vanilla	150	3	24
Carob; Chocolate, average	175	4	28
8th Continent: Chocolate, 1 cup	140	3	23
Light Chocolate, 1 cup	90	1.5	13
Original: 1 cup	80	3	8
Fat-Free	60	0	8
Light	50	1.5	2
Vanilla: 1 cup	100	3	11
Fat-Free	70	0	11
Light	60	1	5
Refreshers, all varieties, 1 cup	150	0	30
Hain Soy Supreme: Original	80	3	9
Vanilla, 1 cup	100	3	12
Hansen's Soy Smoothies: See Page 153, 159			
Lifeway: Slim 6 Kefir, 8 fl.oz	110	2	8
SoyTreat, 8 fl.oz	160	4	23
Naked Juice: See Page 155			
Odwalla: Plain, 1 cup	140	4	12
Choc-ahh-lot	150	2.5	27
Vanilla Being	100	3	13
Pacific: Select Plain, Low-Fat	70	2.5	9
Select Vanilla, Low-Fat	80	2.5	9
Organic, Original Unsweetened	90	4.5	4
Ultra (Extra Protein/Calcium): Plain	120	4	12
Vanilla	130	4	14
Pearl			
Orig., Vanilla, Green Tea, avg., 8 fl.oz	110	3.5	12
Chocolate, 8 fl.oz	150	4.5	21
Unsweetened, 8 fl.oz	90	4.5	6
Power Dream: See Page 159			
Silk (White Wave): Plain, regular	100	4	8
Plain, unsweetened	80	4	4
Light: Plain	70	2	8
Vanilla	80	2	10
Chocolate	120	1.5	22
Chai, 1 cup	130	3.5	19
Chocolate; Mocha, average, 1 c.	140	3.5	23
Coffee Soylatte, 1 cup	150	3.5	25
Enhanced, 1 cup	110	5	8
Live! Smoothie, 10 oz	210	4	36
Spice Soylatte, 11 oz bottle	190	5	27
Vanilla	100	3.5	10
Slim-Fast: Soy Shake, avg. 11 fl.oz	230	3	38
Nutritional Drinks: See Page 160			

	C	F	Cb
SoyDream: Orig./Enriched 8 fl.oz	130	4	17
Chocolate Enriched	210	3.5	37
Vanilla; Vanilla Enriched	150	4	22
SoyCoffee, 5.5 fl.oz prepared	5	0	0
Soy Fusion: Berry, 1 cup	120	1.5	24
So Nice: Natural, 1 cup	80	4	3
Original, 1 cup	80	3	7
Chocolate, 1 cup	150	3	24
Vanilla, 1 cup	100	3	11
SunSoy: Chocolate, 1 cup	150	3.5	26
Creamy Original, 1 cup	100	4	8
Vanilla, 1 cup	100	3.5	12
Vitasoy: Smooth Vanilla	110	4	12
Creamy Original	110	4	11
Classic Original	120	4.5	11
Green Tea Soy Drink	120	4	13
Rich Chocolate	160	4	24
Unsweetened Original	80	4	5
Vanilla Delight	120	4	13
Light: Original	60	2	7
Chocolate	110	2	17
Vanilla Soy Drink	70	2	10
WestSoy			
Smoothies: Banana Berry, 1 cup	140	1.5	28
Lite: Plain, 1 cup	90	1.5	15
Vanilla	110	1.5	19
Low-Fat: Plain, 1 cup	90	1.5	14
Vanilla	120	1.5	21
Non-Fat: Plain, 1 cup	70	0	14
Vanilla	80	0	12
Organic: Original, 1 cup	130	3.5	18
Unsweetened	90	4.5	5
Plus: Plain, 1 cup	130	3	17
Vanilla	130	3	19
Smart Plus: Plain, 1 cup	190	5	22
Vanilla	200	5	25
Enriched: Plain, 1 cup	110	3	13
Vanilla	120	3	17
Soy Shakes: Chocolate, 1 cup	170	3.5	30
Vanilla	170	3	28
Soy Slender: Plain	60	3	3
Other varieties, avg., 1 cup	70	3	4
Unsweetened: Almond, 1 cup	90	4.5	4
Chocolate; Vanilla, avg.	100	4.5	6
Vitamite 100: 1 cup, 8 fl.oz	110	5	14
Wild Oats: Original, 1 cup, 8 fl.oz	100	3.5	12
Zen Soy: Plain, 8 fl.oz	90	3.5	9
Chocolate	170	4	25
Cappuccino	150	3.5	22
Vanilla	110	3.5	14

Rice & Cereal Drinks ◆ Yogurt

Soy Powder Mix

	C	F	Cb
1 oz (⅛ cup) mix makes 1 Cup (8 fl.oz)			
Soy Protein Isolate, 1 oz dry	95	1	0
Better Than Milk: Original, 2 T.	100	2.5	16
Chocolate, 3 Tbsp	110	1.5	22
Vanilla, 2½ Tbsp	80	2	17
Joy Soy, Soy Melk, 1 oz	90	2.5	11
Loma Linda Soyagen: Carob, 1 oz	130	6	13
Regular/No Sugar, 1 oz dry	130	6	12
Now Soy, ¼ cup, 22g	95	4.5	6.5
Revival Soy Shakes: *Per Packet*			
Plain; Unsweetened	120	3.5	3
Flavors, average: with Fructose	225	2	33
Unsweetened or Splenda	130	2	4
Soy Quik (Ener-g), 1 oz dry	100	4.5	8

Rice & Cereal Drinks

	C	F	Cb
Amazake, Original, 1 cup, 8 fl.oz	150	0	34
Blue Diamond Natural			
Almond Breeze: Original, 8 fl.oz	60	2.5	8
Chocolate, 8 fl.oz	120	3	22
Vanilla, 8 fl.oz	90	2.5	16
Don Jose: Horchata, 8 fl.oz	140	4	25
Cereal Match, 1 cup	100	3	17
Eden Blend, Rice & Soy, 1 cup	125	3.5	19
Lundberg: Original Rice, 8 oz	120	2.5	22
Vanilla Rice Drink, 8 oz	120	2.5	23
Pacific			
Rice Drinks: Multigrain, 8 fl.oz	160	2	30
Low-Fat Plain/Vanilla, 8 fl.oz	130	2	27
Organic Oat: Original, 8 fl.oz	130	2.5	24
Vanilla	130	2.5	25
Nut Drinks: Hazelnut Orig., 8 fl.oz	110	3.5	18
Almond: Original Low-Fat, 8 fl.oz	80	2.5	14
Almond, Vanilla, 8 oz	100	2.5	15
Rice Dream: Carob, 1 cup, 8 fl.oz	150	2.5	32
Chocolate Enriched, 1 cup	170	3	36
Vanilla/Vanilla Enriched, 1 cup	130	2	28
Original/Original Enriched, 1 cup	120	2	25
Westbrae Rice, Plain/Van., 8 fl.oz	110	2.5	20
WestSoy: Plain Rice, 8 fl.oz	110	2.5	20
Vanilla Rice, 8 fl.oz	110	2.5	20
Wild Oats: Vanilla, 1 cup, 8 fl.oz	120	2	26
Original, 1 cup, 8 fl.oz	100	2	20

Rice/Nut Drink Mixes

	C	F	Cb
Better Than Milk			
Original, 2 Tbsp powder	70	1	16
Vanilla, 2 Tbsp powder	75	2	15

Quick Guide

	C	F	Cb
Yogurt			
Average All Brands: Per 8 oz Cup			
Plain Yogurt: Whole, 8 oz	140	8	10
Low-Fat	145	3.5	16
Fat-Free	125	0	17
Fruit Flavored: Whole, 8 oz	225	8	32
Low-Fat	230	3	43
Fat-Free, regular	215	0.5	43
Fat-Free, no sugar added	80	0	15
Goat's Milk Yogurt ~ Same as Regular Yogurt			

Yogurt ~ Brands

	C	F	Cb
Alex Rod: Fat-Free, all flav., 8 oz	70	0	12
Albertson's			
Swiss, avg. all flavors, 8 oz	240	2	49
Fruit on the Bottom (low-fat):			
Average all flavors, 8 oz	230	2	45
Alta Dena: *Per Cup (8 oz)*			
Low-Fat: Average all flavors	220	2	41
Non-Fat: Fruit Flavors, average	190	0	38
Plain	110	0	16
Vanilla	160	0	30
America's Choice: Swiss Style	210	2.5	41
Non-Fat, all flavors, 8 oz	100	0	15
Berkeley Farms: Non-Fat, avg.	100	0	16
Low-Fat: Boysenberry/Cherry	230	2.5	46
Raspberry	220	2.5	43
Strawberry, Lemon, Vanilla	270	2.5	52
Blue Bunny: Lite85, 6 oz	80	0	14
Low-Carb, avg., all flavors, 6 oz	90	3	5
Swirl'n Sensations, avg., 6 oz	225	5	38
Yo-Pals, avg. all, 6 oz	165	1.5	33
Breyers: Fruit On The Bottom, 8 oz	240	2	46
Light varieties, 8 oz	110	1.5	20
Creme Savers, 8 oz	240	3.5	45
Smooth & Creamy, avg., 8 oz	240	2	48
Brown Cow: *Per 8 oz (Unless Indicated)*			
Cream Top: Plain	170	10	12
Chocolate	270	8	42
Creamy Coffee, Vanilla	210	9	25
Fruit Flavors, average	230	8	33
Whole Fruit & Grains, avg., 6 oz	150	2.5	23
Low-Fat: Plain	130	3	18
Flavors, average	195	2.5	35
Non-Fat: Plain	110	0	16
Fruit Flavors, average	170	0	36
Cabot: Plain, 8 oz	100	0	19
Flavors, 8 oz	130	0	24
Cascade Fresh: Low-Fat, 6 oz	100	0	19
Fat-Free, all flavors, 6 oz ctn	130	0	24
Whole Milk: Plain, 8 oz	170	8	12
Flavored, 8 oz	200	7	24

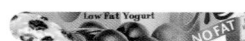
Yogurt ~ Brands (Cont)

C **F** **Cb**

Colombo	C	F	Cb
Light, all flavors, 8 oz	120	0	21
Classic, avg. all types, 8 oz	220	4	42
Fat-Free, Plain, 8 oz	100	0	16
Continental: Vanilla, 8 oz ctn	190	0	38
Fruit on the Bottom, 8 oz	190	0	38
Crowley: Low-Fat Blueberry, 8 oz	240	2.5	48
Dannon: Plain (Natural), 8 oz	170	8	14
Activa, avg. all flavors, 4 oz	110	2	19
Danimals: Super Creamy, 4 oz	110	2	19
XL, 5.75 oz	170	3	29
Drinkable, 3.1 fl.oz	90	1.5	15
Fruit Blends, avg., 6 oz	170	1.5	33
Fruit on the Bottom, avg.,6 oz	150	1.5	28
Frusion Smoothie, 10 fl.oz bottle	260	3.5	50
la Creme: Regular, avg., 4 oz	140	5	19
Mousse, all flavors, 2.6 oz	110	5	14
w. Choc Pieces, 4 oz	170	7	17
Light, 4 oz	140	5	19
Light 'n Fit (0% Fat): Avg., 6 oz	60	0	11
Carb Control + Sugar Control, 4 oz	60	3	3
Creamy, avg. all flavors, 6 oz	100	0	16
Smoothie, 7 fl.oz bottle	70	0	13
w. Fiber, 4 oz	70	0	13
Natural, avg. all flavors, 6 oz	150	2.5	25
Sprinkl'ins, all flavors, 4.1 oz ctn	120	1.5	21
Dominick's: Low-Fat, 8 oz	230	2	40
Fruit on the Bottom, avg, 8 oz	230	2	40
Fat-Free 80 Calories, 8 oz	80	0	13
Plain: Low-Fat, 8 oz	130	2.5	15
Non-Fat, 8 oz	120	0	17
Friendship: Plain, 6 oz	150	3	18
Grocer's Pride: Low-Fat, 4.4 oz	140	1.5	28
Hellios: Kefir Organic, 1 cup	120	5	13
Horizon Organic			
Whole Milk, Plain Vanilla, 8 oz	220	6	32
Low-Fat: Blended, 6 oz cup	160	2	30
Tubes (1)	70	1	12
Fat-Free, all varieties, 6 oz	140	0	27
32 oz Carton, Plain, 8 oz	180	0	33
Yo Yo's, 4 oz	105	1	20

	C	F	Cb
Jerseymaid (Vons)			
Low-Fat: Plain, 8 oz	150	3.5	18
Fruit flavors, average, 8 oz	240	2.5	47
Vanilla	230	2.5	43
Fat-Free: Plain, 8 oz	130	0	18
Light Fat-Free, fruit, 8 oz	120	0	22
YoCups, avg all flavors, 4 oz	130	1	27
Yo On The Go, 2.25 oz tube	80	2	13
Jewel: Low-Fat, average, 8 oz	230	2	45
Kemps: 100 Calories Nonfat, 5 oz	100	0	22
Yo Stix (1), 2.25 oz			
Non-Fat, Light, 6 oz	80	2	13
Knudsen: 70 Calories, 6 oz	70	0	11
Free, average, 8 oz	170	0	33
Kroger: Per 8 oz Ctn			
Lite (Non-Fat) avg. all flavors	100	0	17
Low-Fat: Plain, 8 oz	150	4	17
Blended, average, 8 oz	250	2.5	47
Fruit on the Bottom, 8 oz	220	3	41
La Yogurt			
Original, average, 6 oz	150	1.5	30
Low-Fat, average, 8 oz	130	0	18
Light, average, 6 oz	90	0	15
Rich & Creamy, 6 oz	160	2	30
Enriched, average, 6 oz	160	2	30
Fruit 'N' Cream, avg., 8 oz	200	2	39
Fruit on the Bottom, avg., 8 oz	220	2.5	43
LeCarb: YoCarb Plain, 4 oz	55	2.5	3
YoCarb Flavors, 4 oz	45	1	4
Light n' Lively			
Fruit Flavors, average, 4 oz	110	1	23
Lucerne			
Low-Fat: Plain, 8 oz	150	3.5	18
Fruit flavors, average, 8 oz	240	2.5	45
Vanilla	240	2.5	44
Fat-Free: Plain, 8 oz	110	0	20
Light Fat-Free, fruit, 8 oz			
YoCups, avg all flavors, 4 oz	130	1	27
Yo On The Go, 2.25 oz tube	80	2	13
Meadow Gold: Avg., 6 oz ctn	90	2.5	10
Mountain High			
Original Style, plain, 8 oz	190	8	18
European Delight, all flavors, 4 oz	110	2	19
Low-Fat: Plain, 8 oz	150	2	22
Classic, 6 oz	140	1.5	25
Fat-Free, Plain, 8 oz	120	0	19
Mystic Lake Dairy (Goat Milk Yogurt)			
Plain, 1 cup, 8 oz	120	6	9

Yogurt (Cont)

Brands (Cont)

Nancy's: Per 8 oz Serving

	C	F	Cb
Whole Milk: Honey, plain, 8 fl.oz	170	8	17
w. Fruit Cup, avg, 9.5 oz	230	5	41
Low Fat: Plain/Lemon/Vanilla, avg	150	3	16
Other flavors, average	180	3	27
Non-Fat: Plain, 8 oz	120	0	27
Maple, Vanilla (8 oz ctn)	160	0	27
w. Fruit Cup, avg, 9.5 oz	210	0	40
Vanilla (32 oz ctn), swtn'd, 8 oz	220	0	40
Soy Cultured: (6 oz ctn): Plain	150	3	25
Berry flavors, average	140	3.5	24
Vanilla	120	3	19
Kiwi-Lime; Mango, average	165	3	32
Old Home: 100 Cal., Non-Fat, 6 oz	100	0	20
Old Home Light, average, 6 oz	240	7	39
Publix: Fat-Free, Plain, 8 oz	140	0	23
Swiss Flake (low-fat), 8 oz	240	2.5	41
Redwood Hill Farm (Goat Milk Yogurt)			
Vanilla; Fruit flavors, avg., 8 oz	190	5	31
Plain, 8 oz	130	6	14
Silk (Soy): Plain, 1 cup, 8 oz	140	3	22
Vanilla, 6 oz ctn	140	2.5	25
Other flavors, average, 6 oz	160	2	29
Sky Hill Napa Valley, Plain, 8 oz	130	8	13
Stater Bros: Non-Fat, avg, 8 oz	120	0	20
Stonyfield Farm (Organic)			
All Natural Fat-Free: Plain, 6 oz	80	0	14
Chocolate Underground, 6 oz	170	0	37
Other varieties, 6 oz	130	0	26
All Natural Fat-Free Light, 6 oz	100	0	28
Low-Fat: Caramel	190	1.5	38
Plain	90	1.5	15
Other varieties, average	130	1.5	25
Whole Milk Yogurt: Vanilla Truffle	210	5	37
French Vanilla, 6 oz	190	6	27
Other varieties, avg.	170	6	24
O'Soy: Choc.; Vanilla, avg., 6 oz	160	2	27
Fruit on Bottom, average, 6 oz	170	2	32
Squeezers, all flavors, 57g	60	1	11
Stop & Shop, Blended Lite, 8 oz	120	0	20
Trader Joe's: Low-Fat, 8 oz	220	3	40
Non-Fat: Regular 8 oz	170	0	34
French Village, Vanilla, 8 oz	180	0	34
Organic Vanilla, 8 oz	160	0	27
Organic Low-Fat, average, 6 oz	150	2.5	23
Cultured Soy, all varieties, 6 oz	150	3	28
Fruit on the Bottom, Crm Top, 6 oz	170	6	23

	C	F	Cb
Wallaby (Organic), avg., 6 oz	150	2.5	25
Weight Watchers, all flav., 6 oz ctn	100	0.5	17
Wildwood: Soyogurt Plain, 6 oz	105	5	6
Other varieties, avg., 6 oz	130	3.5	20
Whole Soy & Co: Plain, 6 oz ctn	150	3	27
Other flavors, avg 6 oz ctn	160	3	30
YoCrunch: Low-Fat w. Toppings, 6.5 oz Cup			
Oreo Cookies	200	4	36
Peach/Strawb./Rasp. w. Granola	210	3	40
Average other varieties	220	4	39
Yoplait			
Original, average all flavors, 6 oz	170	1.5	33
99% Fat-Free Original Flavors, 4 oz	110	1	22
Light: Fruit Flavors, 6 oz	100	0	19
Indulgent Flavors, 6 oz	110	0	20
Thick & Creamy: Light, 6 oz	100	0	20
Fridge Pack, 6 oz	190	3.5	32
Thick & Creamy Custard Style, 6 oz	190	3.5	32
Go-Gurt!, Fruit Flavors, 2.2 oz tube	80	2	13
Grande!: Fat-Free Plain, 8 oz cup	130	0	19
99% Fat-Free Flavors, 8 oz cup	250	2.5	48
Trix, Fruit Flavors, 4 oz	120	1.5	20
Whips!: Chocolate Flavors, 4 oz	160	4	26
Fruit Flavors, 4 oz	140	2.5	25
Yoplait Kids, 4 oz	100	2	1

Yogurt Drinks & Probiotics

	C	F	Cb
Actimel (Dannon) Probiotic, 3.3 fl.oz	95	1.5	17
Carbolite, 8 fl.oz	85	2	8
Creme Savers (Breyers), 10 oz	190	3	32
Dannon: Danimals, 3.4 fl.oz bottle	90	1.5	15
Danimals XL, 5.7 fl.oz	170	3	29
DanActive, 3.4 fl.oz	95	1.5	17
Glen Oaks, all flavors, avg, 1 cup	240	3.5	45
Nouriche, Regular, 11 fl.oz	260	0	55
Stonyfield Farm			
Smoothies, avg., 10 oz	250	3	49
Light, all flavors, 10 oz	130	0	41
Weight Watchers, Smoothie, 6.9 oz	80	0	13
WholeSoy, 12 fl.oz bottle	210	3	34
Yo Soy, 8 fl.oz	80	4	4
Yonique: Pina Colada, 6 fl.oz	190	4	30
Peach; Banana; Guava, 6 fl.oz	170	2	30
Yoplait Go Gurt, 5 fl.oz	120	0.5	23
Yoplait: Smoothie, 8 fl.oz	220	2.5	44
Light Smoothie, 8 fl.oz	90	0	16

Quick Guide | C | F | Cb

Ice Cream

Vanilla: *Average All Brands*
Other flavors ~ See Brand Listings.
Regular Ice Cream (10% fat):
(Examples: Borden/Hood)

	C	F	Cb
3 fl.oz scoop	100	5	12
½ cup, 4 fl.oz	130	7	16
1 Pint, 16 fl.oz	520	28	62
½ Gallon (4 Pints)	2100	112	248

Rich (16% fat):

3 fl.oz scoop	130	8	12
½ cup, 4 fl.oz	170	10	17
1 Pint	690	40	64

Super-Rich (20% fat): (Haagen-Dazs/Ben & Jerry's)

3 fl.oz scoop	200	14	16
½ cup, 4 fl.oz	270	18	21
1 Pint	1100	72	84

Reduced-Fat/Light (6% fat):
(Breyer's Light/Hood Light)

3 fl.oz scoop	100	3	14
½ cup, 4 fl.oz	140	4	18
1 Pint	560	16	72

Low-Fat (less than 4% fat):
(Healthy Choice/Weight Watchers/Snackwell's)

3 fl.oz scoop	90	2	17
½ cup, 4 fl.oz	120	2.5	22
1 Pint	480	10	88

Fat-Free: (Baskin-Robbins FF/Borden FF/Breyers FF/Dreyers FF/Hood FF)

3 fl.oz scoop	75	0	17
½ cup, 4 fl.oz	100	0	22
1 Pint	400	0	88

Soft Serve: Regular, ½ cup

	140	5	20
1 cup	280	10	40
Non-Fat, ½ cup	90	0	23
1 cup	180	0	46

Quick Guide

Frozen Yogurt | C | F | Cb

Average All Brands

	C	F	Cb
Hard: Low-Fat, ½ cup	140	3	26
Non-Fat, ½ cup	110	0	29
Soft: Low-Fat, ½ cup	120	2.5	28
Non-Fat, ½ cup	100	0	30

Brands: *See Ice Cream & Ices Section*

Quick Guide | C | F | Cb

Gelato/Ices/Frozen Custard

Gelato: *Per ½ Cup*

	C	F	Cb
Milk base: Vanilla	200	15	18
Choc. Hazelnut	370	29	26
Water base: ½ cup	100	0	25
Frozen Custard: *Per ½ Cup*			
Chocolate	140	6	18
Orange Sherbet	105	2	21
Vanilla	130	6	16
Ice (Milk base): *Average all flavors*			
Hard (4% fat), ½ cup	100	3	15
Soft Serve (3% fat), ½ cup	110	2	19
Shaved Ice: Average, 12 fl. oz	160	0	40
Sherbet: Avg., ½ cup	120	2	28
Sorbet: Fruit (no fat), ½ cup	120	0	30
Fruit Ice Pops	80	0	20

Tofu Frozen Desserts: *See Page 35*

Sundaes | C | F | Cb

Denny's: Sundaes,

	C	F	Cb
Single Scoop, no topping	195	14	14
Double Scoop, no topping	385	27	29
Banana Split	930	43	121
Toppings: Blueberry, 2 oz	105	0	26
Chocolate, 2 oz	340	25	27
Fudge, 2 oz	215	10	30
Strawberry, 2 oz	115	1	26
McDonald's: Sundaes,			
Hot Fudge Sundae, 6.3 oz	350	12	52
Strawberry Sundae	290	7	50
Toppings: Nut/Sundae, ¼ oz	50	3.5	2

Ice Cream Bars & Pops

See Pages 36-38

Ice Cream, Cones & Cups

Average All Brands | C | F | Cb

	C	F	Cb
Wafer Cone/Cup, average	20	0	4
Sugar Cone, average	40	0	9
Waffle Cone:			
Small	60	0	11
Large	100	1	22
Brands:			
Oreo Chocolate Cone	50	1	10
Comet Sugar Cone	50	0	11
Keebler Sugar Cone	45	0	11

Ice Cream & Frozen Yogurt (Cont)

Brands

	C	F	Cb
Atkins: *Per ½ Cup*			
Endulge, average all flavors	155	13	14
Baskin-Robbins: *See Fast-Foods Section*			
Ben & Jerry's: *Per ½ Cup*			
Body & Soul: Cherry Garcia	170	9	22
Chocolate Chip Cookie Dough	190	9	26
Chocolate Fudge Brownie	180	7	25
Half Baked	190	8	29
Singles: *Per Container*			
Cherry Garcia	220	13	22
Chocolate Fudge Brownie	230	11	28
Cookie Dough	240	13	26
Vanilla	200	13	17
Original: Black & Tan Original	230	13	24
Butter Pecan	280	21	20
Cherry Garcia	250	14	26
Chocolate	260	16	25
Chocolate Chip Cookie Dough	270	15	32
Chocolate Fudge Brownie	260	13	32
Chubby Hubby	330	20	31
Chunky Monkey	300	18	30
Coffee	240	15	21
Coffee Heath Bar Crunch	290	18	29
Everything But The...	310	19	30
Fudge Central	300	18	31
Half Baked	280	14	34
Karamel Sutra	280	15	32
Mint Chocolate Cookie	260	16	26
New York Super Fudge Chunk	310	20	29
Oatmeal Cookie Chunk	270	15	31
Peanut Butter Cup	360	26	27
Phish Food	280	13	37
Pistachio Pistachio	260	17	21
Strawberry	230	13	26
Uncanny Cashew	290	19	27
Vanilla	240	16	21
Vanilla Heath Bar Crunch	290	18	29
Vermonty Python	310	19	30
Frozen Yogurt: *Per ½ Cup*			
Phish Food	220	4.5	41
Low-Fat: Black Raspberry	140	1.5	28
Cherry Garcia	170	3	32
Chocolate Fudge Brownie	190	2.5	35
Half Baked	190	3	35
Sorbet: Average all flavors	115	0	30
Bars/Pops: *See Page 36*			

Blue Bunny	C	F	Cb
Fat-Free, No Added Sugar: *Per ½ Cup*			
Brownie Sundae; Burgundy Cherry	90	0	23
Caramel Toffee Crunch	90	0	24
Average other flavors	80	0	19
Reduced-Fat, No Added Sugar: *Per ½ Cup*			
Banana Split; Butter Pecan, avg.	125	5	18
Rocky Road	130	6	18
Turtle Sundae	140	7	20
Other flavors, avg.	120	5	17
Hi Lite: Butter Pecan; Fudge Nut	120	4.5	17
Caramel Pecan	130	4	21
Cookies & Cream; Vanilla, avg.	130	3.5	21
Other varieties, avg.	110	3	18
Carb Freedom: Vanilla Bean	100	7	10
Butter Pecan	110	8	11
Choc. Almond Fudge	120	8	13
Peanut Butter Fudge	150	10	15
Frozen Yogurt, ½ cup	100	0	21
Bars/Pops: *See Page 36*			
Breyers: *Per ½ Cup*			
CarbSmart: Rocky Road	140	10	12
Strawberry; Vanilla	120	9	10
Other varieties, avg.	110	8	12
All Natural: Butter Alm./Pecan, avg.	160	10	14
Caramel Praline Crunch	170	7	22
Chocolate Chip Cookie Dough	160	8	20
Fruit Sherbet, average	130	1.5	26
Lactose Free Vanilla	130	7	14
Rocky Road	160	9	19
Vanilla & Choc. & Strawberry	130	7	16
Vanilla Fudge	150	7	20
Other varieties, avg.	150	8	16
Double Churned Extra Creamy: *Per ½ Cup*			
Chocolate Caramel Brownie	160	7	22
Mint Chocolate	160	9	18
Strawberries & Cream	130	6	16
Other varieties, average	140	7	17
98% Fat Free, all varieties, ½ cup	90	1.5	19
Light: Butter Pecan, ½ cup	120	5	15
Caramel Tracks; Choc. Mocha Silk	130	4.5	19
Mint Chocolate Chip	130	5	18
Rocky Road	170	5	27
Vanilla, Chocolate, Strawberry	100	3.5	16
Other varieties, average	100	3.5	16
No Sugar Added: Butter Pecan	110	6	14
Chocolate Fudge Brownie	90	1.5	20
Peanut Butter; Triple Choc., avg.	115	6	17
Other varieties, avg.	85	4	17
Wild Flavors: Peanut Butter Tracks	180	12	17
Very Chocolate Cherry	150	7	19
Other varieties, avg.	160	8	20

Brands (Cont)

C **F** **Cb**

Brigham's: *Per ½ Cup*

Ice Cream: Big Dig	210	12	24
Chocolate/Chip; Vanilla, avg.	200	12	19
Mocha Almond	210	15	18
Raspberry Lime Rickey Sherbert	130	2	27
Other varieties, avg.	210	13	21

Bruster's

Frozen Yogurt: Chocolate, ½ cup	150	4.5	24
Vanilla, ½ cup	220	6.5	34

No Added Sugar Ice Cream: *Per ½ Cup*

Chocolate; Vanilla, avg.	210	12	24
Choc. Caramel Swirl/Fudge Ripple	120	0	31
Cinnamon; Coffee	100	0	24
Other varieties, average	110	0	30

Carb Promise (Kemps)**:** *Per ½ Cup*

Butter Pecan	150	11	10
Chocolate Peanut Butter Cup	170	12	12
Cow Tracks	150	8	13
Toffee Fudge Chunk	140	9	12
Vanilla	125	8	10
Vanilla Fudge Nut Sundae	170	11	14

Carvel Ice Cream: See Fast-Foods Section

Coldstone Creamery: See Fast-Foods Section

Colombo: *Per ½ Cup*

Frozen, Soft Serve: Non-Fat, avg.	105	0	22
Slender Sensations, average	60	0	15
Low-Fat, Old Worlde; Cookies	120	2	21
Sorbet, all varieties	100	0	25

Costco: (Frozen Yogurt, ½ cup | 100 | 0 | 21 |

CremaLita (Soft Serve)

Calories will vary with density (air in product) and serving size.
Best to weigh product and calculate on 25 cals per 1 oz weight.

Vanilla: Small (4 fl.oz cup):

If 2½ oz weight	60	0	14
If 4 oz weight*	100	0.5	23
If 6 oz weight*	150	1	35
(*) Most common weights			
Medium (8 fl.oz cup), 11 oz wt	275	1.5	63
Chocolate: Small, 6 oz weight	160	1	36

Dairy Queen/Brazier: See Fast-Foods Section

Dippin' Dots

Dots 'n Cream: *Per ½ Cup*

Banana Split; Vanilla	170	10	16
Butter Pecan	180	10	18
Chocolate	165	10	15
Mint Chocolate Chip	200	9	25

Dove: *Per ½ Cup*

C **F** **Cb**

Beyond Vanilla	260	16	25
Caramel Pecan Perfection	310	18	32
Chocolate & Brownie Affair	310	20	30
Irresistibly Raspberry	240	13	30
Toffee Caramel Moment	320	20	32
Other varieties, avg.	300	19	30
Miniatures: All varieties, avg., 5 pcs	300	20	31

Dreyers/Edys: *Per ½ Cup*

Grand: Almond Praline	150	7	20
Chocolate; Vanilla Bean, avg.	150	8	17
Coffee; Neapolitan, avg.	140	8	15
Fudge Tracks; Peanut Butter Cup	185	11	18
Nestle Drumstick Sundae Cone	180	10	19
Real Strawberry	130	6	16
Toasted Almond	150	9	19
Vanilla	150	10	14
Other flavors, avg.	160	9	18
Slow Churned: Neopolitan	100	3	15
Orange & Cream	100	2.5	15
Other varieties, average	100	3.5	15
Fat-Free Frozen Yogurt, average	95	0	20
Sherbet, avg. all flavors	130	1.5	28

Friendly's: *Per ½ Cup Unless Indicated*

Ice Cream: Chocolate Almd Chip	160	10	17
Forbidden Chocolate	160	9	17
Hunka Chunka PB Fudge	240	16	21
Vanilla Choc. Strawberry	140	7	16
Vienna Mocha Chunk	180	9	20
Light: Purely Pistachio	120	5	16
Chocolate PB Swirl	150	7	18
Frozen Yogurt: *Per ½ Cup*			
Fudge Berry Swirl	150	4	24
Mint Chocolate Chip	130	4	21
Sundaes: *Per 3 Scoops*			
Apple Pie	1040	62	118
Royal Banana Split	940	37	136
Jim Dandy	1130	48	159
Reese's Peanut Butter Cup	930	54	90
Friend-Z's: Oreo Cookies, 12 fl.oz	750	23	120
Frostline (Soft Serve): Chocolate	90	1	19
Vanilla, ½ cup	100	1	20

Gelati-da

Gelato: *Per ½ Cup (4 oz)*

Amaretto Chocolate	150	4.5	23
Choc Mint Milano	120	2.5	22
Coffee Fudge Latte	130	2	22
Red Raspberry	130	1.5	25
Vanilla Marsala	120	2	21
White Chocolate	130	3	23

Brands (Cont)

	C	F	Cb
Godiva: *Per ½ Cup*			
Belgian Dark Chocolate	270	17	28
Choc Raspberry Truffle	290	16	32
Classic Milk Chocolate	290	18	28
Milk Chocolate Hazelnut Praline	310	18	35
Vanilla Caramel Pecan	300	16	34
White Choc. Raspberry	260	12	32
Good Humor: *Per ½ Cup*			
Light: Cookies n' Crm	120	6	16
Choc.; Vanilla & Neopolitan, avg.	110	5	14
Strawberry Shortcake	130	4.5	23
Sherbets, all flavors	130	1	28
Haagen-Dazs			
Ice Cream, Sorbet, Frozen Yogurt: *See Fast-Foods Section*			
Bars: *See Page 37*			
Healthy Choice: *Per ½ Cup*			
Cookies 'N Crm; Peanut Butter Cup	120	2	21
Praline & Caramel	120	2	23
Rocky Road	130	2	25
Vanilla	110	2	19
Other flavors, average	120	5	18
Low-Fat, No Sugar Added: Vanilla	100	2	17
Coffee Almond Fudge	110	2	20
Chocolate Fudge Brownie	120	2	21
Mint Chocolate Chip	110	2	18
Hood: *Per ½ Cup*			
Ice Cream: Birthday Party	150	8	19
Butterscotch Blast	160	7	20
Chippedy Chocolaty	150	9	19
Cookie Dough Delight/ 'N Cream	160	8	19
Crunchy Cone N' Peanut Butter	190	11	19
Fudge Twister; Grasshopper, avg.	150	7	21
Heavenly Hash	140	6	21
Maple Walnut	150	9	17
Other varieties, average	140	7	17
Light: Butter Pecan	140	6	18
Caribbean Coffee Royale	110	3	18
Classic Trio; Creamy Vanilla	110	3	18
Raspberry Swirl	120	2.5	22
Other varieties, average	130	4	22
Fat-Free: Double Brownie Sundae	120	0	27
Other varieties, average	100	0	23
Fruit Scoops: Sherbert, all flavors	120	1	27
Fruit Yogurt: Vanilla	110	0	24
Chocolate Almond Praline	140	3	23
Bars: *See Page 37*			

	C	F	Cb
I Can't Believe It's Yogurt: *See Fast-Foods Section*			
Jerseymaid (Vons): *Per ½ Cup*			
After Dinner Mint; Cookies & Crm	170	9	19
Choc Chip; Mint Choc Chip	160	9	17
Heavenly Hash; Nut Chunky Choc.	170	8	22
Mocha Almd Fudge; Rocky Road	160	7	20
Neopolitan; Vanilla	140	7	16
Strawberry	140	6	18
Kilwin's: *Per ½ Cup*			
Almond Toffee Yogurt	135	5	21
Butter Pecan	195	13	17
Chocolate	135	6	16
Chocolate Yogurt	125	3	23
Peach Yogurt	110	3	16
Average other flavors	175	10	20
Topping: Caramel	135	4	26
Fudge	110	5	15
Luigi's Real Italian Ice: *Per Cup (6 fl.oz)*			
All flavors, average	125	0	32
Swirl, all flavors	150	0	38
Rice Dream (Non-Dairy): *Per ½ Cup*			
All varieties, average	160	6.5	25
Tea Dreams, average	145	6.5	25
Soy Delicious: *Per ½ Cup*			
It's Soy Delicious: (Fruit Sweetened)	140	4.5	24
Choc Almond	140	4.5	23
Choc Peanut Butter	135	3.5	24
Pistachio Almond	130	4.5	23
Other flavors, avg.	115	1.5	25
Purely Decadent: PB Zig Zag	230	13	32
Swingin' Anna Bannana	230	13	31
Other flavors, avg.	200	8.5	32
Soy Dream (Non-Dairy): *Per ½ Cup*			
Butter Pecan	160	10	17
Chocolate Fudge Brownie	150	8	20
Mint Chocolate Chip	150	9	19
Average other flavors	140	6	20
Starbucks: *Per ½ Cup*			
Caramel Cappuccino	240	12	30
Classic Coffee	230	12	26
Coffee Almond Fudge; Java Chip	250	13	29
Mud Pie	250	11	33
Low-Fat Latte	170	3	30
Bars: *See Page 38*			

Brands (Cont)

	C	F	Cb

Stonyfield Farm (Organic)
Ice Cream, Super Premium: *Per ½ Cup*

	C	F	Cb
After Dark Chocolate	250	17	21
Brownie Fudge Sundae	250	13	30
Chocolate Raspberry Swirl	230	13	25
Cookies 'n Dream	270	18	27
Creme Caramel	250	14	29
Gotta Have Vanilla; Vanilla Chai, avg.	240	16	21
Javalanche	250	16	22

Sweet Nothings *(Non-Dairy/Fat-Free)*

	C	F	Cb
Average all flavors, ½ cup, 3 oz	120	0	28

TCBY
Soft Serve Frozen Yogurt: *Average all Flavors*

	C	F	Cb
96% Fat-Free: Kids Cup	110	2	18
Junior Cup	200	4	33
Small Cup	290	6	47
Regular Cup	370	8	60
Large Cup	450	10	74
Non-Fat: Junior Cup	160	0	33
Small Cup	220	0	46
Regular Cup	290	0	60
Large Cup	350	0	73
No Sugar Added/Non-Fat: Small	190	0	41
Regular Cup	240	0	53
Large Cup	290	0	65
Low-Carb Lovers: Small	170	10	25
Regular	300	18	45
Large Cup	360	22	56
Kids	70	1	15
Regular	110	2	22

Hand Scooped Frozen Yogurt: *Average all Flavors*

	C	F	Cb
Kids Cup	90	3	14
Junior Cup	140	5	22
Small Cup	180	6	28
Regular Cup	280	10	44
Large Cup	370	13	58

No Added Sugar, Vanilla:

	C	F	Cb
Small Cup	100	1	24
Regular Cup	160	1	38
Large Cup	210	1.5	50

Tasti D-Lite (Soft Serve)

	C	F	Cb

Calories will vary with density (air in product) and serving size.
Best to weigh product and calculate on 25 cals per 1 oz weight.

	C	F	Cb
Vanilla: Small (4 fl.oz cup), 6 oz wt	180	4	35
Medium (8 fl.oz cup), 11 oz wt	330	7	64

Tofutti, Non-Dairy Dessert: *Per ¼ Container (120ml)*

	C	F	Cb
Cheesecake Supreme Pints	200	12	20
Low-Fat Pints: Chocolate Fudge	145	4	25
Coffee Marshmallow Swirl	120	3	24
Vanilla Fudge	140	4	24
No Added Sugar Pints: Chocolate	115	5	12
Strawberry	110	5	12
Premium Pints: Better Pecan	210	13	22
Chocolate Cookie Crunch	190	11	26
Chocolate Supreme	180	11	18
Mint Chocolate Chip	210	13	21
Vanilla	190	11	20
Vanilla Almond Bark	210	13	21
Vanilla Fudge; Wildberry, avg.	190	9	25
Super Soy Supreme Pints: Bella Van.	160	8	20

Turkey Hill: *Per ½ Cup*

	C	F	Cb
Black Cherry	140	7	18
Butter Pecan	170	11	16
Choc Mint	180	11	18
Cookies 'n Crm	160	10	19
Rocky Road	170	8	23
Other flavors, average	150	9	19
Lite: Moose Tracks	130	6	19
Peanut Butter Mania	130	5	19
Vanilla Bean	100	2.5	16
Other flavors, average	115	3	19
All Natural: Average all flavors	145	8	17
CarbIQ: Butter Pecan	140	11	15
Choco Mint Chip	130	9	17
Vanilla Bean	110	8	15
Frozen Yogurt: Graham Canyon	160	7	23
Choc. Chip Cookie Dough	130	3.5	22
Low-Fat: Mint Cookies 'n Cream	110	1.5	22
Vanilla Bean	100	2	19
Fat-Free: Choc. Marshmallow	120	0	25
Other flavors, average	100	0	22
Smoothie, all flavors, average	100	0	22
Sherbet	120	1	26
WholeSoy & Co., ½ cup (70g)	120	1	25

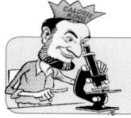

For Full
Nutritional Data
~ See Author's Website
www.CalorieKing.com

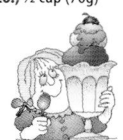

Ice Cream Bars & Pops

Bars & Pops

C F Cb

Per Bar/Serving

	C	F	Cb
Barq's Root Beer & Ice Cream Float, 4 fl.oz cup	120	3	22
Baskin Robbins			
Cappuccino Blast: Low-Fat	220	2	45
Regular, small	300	12	43
Ben & Jerry's			
Peace Pops: Cherry Garcia (1)	270	19	29
Almond Original	340	23	30
Cookie Dough (1)	340	16	46
Vanilla (1)	300	20	26
Novelties: 'Wich Ice Cream, Cookie Sandwich	350	18	45
Big Bear: *See Klondike*			
Big Ed's Super Saucer, 10 fl.oz	590	29	75
Blue Bunny: Ice Pops, avg.	120	0	24
Bomb Pops, avg.	50	0	12
Chocolate Cup, 1.7 oz	100	5	19
Fudge Bar, 2.7 oz	110	1.5	21
Health Smart, 2.2 oz	60	0	15
Sweet Freedom S'wich, avg.	140	1.5	32
Vanilla Nutty Cone, 3 oz	250	11	34
Carb Freedom: Butter Pecan	160	14	11
Almond Bar	160	13	11
White Chocolate Almond Lite	100	7	10
Bon Bons *(Nestlé):* Milk Choc., (8)	330	22	29
Dark Chocolate, 8 pces	310	22	29
Breyers			
Pure Fruit Bars: Banana	110	0	29
Coconut	150	2.5	31
Fruit & Cream	60	0.5	12
Fruit Swirl, all varieties, 1.7 oz	45	0	11
Lime	110	0	27
No Sugar Added Bar	25	0	5
Pineapple	100	0	26
Strawberry	100	0	25
CarbSmart Bar: Fudge Bar	100	7	9
Almond Bar; Vanilla Bar	170	15	9
Vanilla Cone	210	16	14
Vanilla Sandwich	80	4	10
Ice Cream Poppers: Heath (26)	380	27	29
Hershey's (26)	390	29	28
Oreo (26)	420	29	37
Reese's (26)	430	32	32

Per Bar/Serving

	C	F	Cb
Breyers (Cont)			
Double Churned Extra Creamy Bars: *Per Bar*			
No Sugar Added Bar, avg.	145	8	18
Light Bar: Creamy Fudge	90	2.5	14
Other varieties, avg.	170	9	28
Light Sandwich: Creamy Vanilla	130	1.5	28
Creamy Vanilla, Cookie & Cream	140	1.5	30
Bliscotti: Lemon Sandwich	230	12	27
Mint Chip Sandwich	240	13	27
Vanilla Sandwich	260	14	28
Butterfinger Bar, 2.5 oz	210	15	17
Carnation: Sandwich, all types	220	9	32
Sundae Cups, average	205	10	28
Chipwich Jr: Choc. Chip S'wich	220	9	32
Chiquita: Swirls, all flavors	80	3	12
Cool Creations			
Cool Classics: Pops, average	35	0	9
Mini Sandwich	110	4	16
Vanilla Sandwich	170	6	28
Toffee/Chocolate Bar, avg.	155	11	14
Cream Pops, 2 oz	70	0	12
Fudge Pops	100	1	21
Sundae Cones	160	18	36
Creamsicle: Sugar-Free Pops	40	2	10
Orange, 2.8 fl.oz	110	3	20
Crunch: Caramel	210	14	19
Chocolate & Vanilla	230	16	20
Vanilla Flavored	220	15	18
Reduced-Fat	140	8	14
Dove: Caramel Toffee Crunch	270	16	29
Milk Chocolate w. Almonds	340	23	28
Original Dove; Milk Chocolate	260	17	25
Triple Chocolate	340	22	35
Miniatures, 5 pces	300	20	32
Dreyers/Edys			
Dibs: With Chocolaty Coating (26 Pieces)			
Chocolate; Mint; Vanilla	420	32	29
Van. w. Nestle Crunch/Drumstick	310	29	29
Whole Fruit Bars	70	0	17
Whole Fruit Smoothie Bars	100	2	18
Drumstick *(Nestlé):* Chocolate	360	23	33
Original Vanilla	340	21	33
Vanilla Caramel/Fudge	360	22	36
Simply Dipped: Vanilla	320	17	38
Cookies & Cream	360	19	40

Bars & Pops (Cont)	C	F	Cb
Eskimo Pie			
No Sugar Added: Strawb. Bar	110	6	15
Cookies & Cream Cone	140	4.5	29
Cookies & Cream Bar	120	7	17
Vanilla Dark Choc Bar	120	8	14
Vanilla Crisp Rice Bar	110	8	12
Bars: Milk/Dark Choc	160	11	14
Fudge Bar	60	1	11
Peppermint Pattie	240	16	21
Thin Mint Bar	240	17	20
King Size Bar, avg.	220	14	21
Premium Bar	220	13	26
Slender Pie Clamshell, avg.	120	1.5	28
Vanilla Sandwich: Regular	160	4	27
King Size	250	9	38
Fat Boy: Ice Cream Sandwich	220	10	30
Cookies N Cream Sandwich	240	10	34
Nut Sundae on a Stick	310	24	21
FrozFruit: Bar, all flavors	70	0	17
Banana; Strawb. Crm Bar, avg.	124	4	21
Fruit Bars: Mango	80	0	21
Other varieties, avg.	80	0	20
Fruit A Freeze: Coconut	160	9	20
Lime	70	0	17
Banana; Strawberry	120	4	19
Dark Choc-Dipped Strawberry	130	4	22
Fudge Bar (Nestlé)	110	1	23
Fudgesicle: Fudge Bar (1)	100	2	18
Fat-Free (1)	70	0	14
Godiva Belgian Dark Choc Bar	290	19	27
Good Humor: Bubble Play	105	0	26
Candy Center Crunch	310	23	24
Chocolate Eclair	220	11	29
Oreo Bar	250	15	28
Premium Vanilla	260	17	24
Reese's Peanut Butter Cup	310	21	27
Strawb. Shortcake; Tstd Almd, avg.	235	12	30
Cones: Giant King	390	22	44
King	250	13	30
Premium Sundae	260	15	29
Strawberry Shortcake	230	12	30
Sandwiches: Premium Vanilla	160	5	26
Giant Choc Chip Cookie	470	20	71
Giant Neapolitan/Vanilla	250	9	38
Premium Cookie	280	12	41
Swirlwind Cup, 6 oz	160	2.5	31

Per Bar/Serving	C	F	Cb
Haagen-Dazs: Brownie Bar	360	24	30
Chocolate & Dark Chocolate	300	21	24
Coffee & Almond Crunch	310	22	23
Dulce de Leche	300	19	28
Raspberry Sorbet & Vanilla Yogurt	100	0	22
Vanilla & Almonds	320	23	23
Vanilla & Dark Chocolate	300	21	23
Vanilla & Milk Chocolate	290	21	22
Health Smart (Blue Bunny), avg.	60	0	15
Healthy Choice: Fudge Bar	80	1	13
Caramel Swirl Sandwich	140	3	27
Ice Cream Bar w. Fudge Coating	80	1	13
Strawberry & Cream	90	1	18
Swirls, average	90	1.5	17
Vanilla Sandwich	130	3	24
Hood: Chocolate Eclair, 1 bar	150	10	14
Fudge Bar: Chocolate	90	0.5	20
No Added Sugar	50	1.5	12
Nutty Royal	220	12	26
Java Smoothie	100	2.5	7
Vanilla Sandwich	180	6	29
Light Sandwich	160	3	29
Hoodsie Cup Van./Choc.	100	5	12
Orange Cream Bar	90	1.5	19
Hawaiian Punch	50	0	12
Hawaiian Punch Cream Surfer	90	1.5	16
Ice Cream Sandwich (Nestle)	240	10	34
Icee Freeze, 2.25 oz	70	0	17
Klondike: Choco Taco	290	15	36
Dark Chocolate Crunch	250	17	22
Heath Bar	270	19	24
Hershey's Almond Bar	270	19	21
Ice Cream Cup	270	17	26
Krunch Bar	250	17	26
Sara Lee Strawberry Shortcake	290	18	28
Movie Bites	290	21	24
Oreo Bar	260	17	26
Original Bar	250	17	22
Planters Caramel & Peanut Bar	290	19	26
Reese's Peanut Butter Bar	270	18	24
Slim a Bear: Vanilla/Krunch, avg.	170	10	21
Fudge	90	1.5	21
Cookies & Cream	110	1	25
Sandwich: 98% Fat-Free			
Vanilla/Chocolate	130	1.5	29
No Sugar Added Vanilla	110	2.5	22

Ice Cream Bars & Pops (Cont)

Brands (Cont)	C	F	Cb
Klondike (Cont):			
Cones: Klondike Sundae Cone	300	16	35
Vanilla Sundae Cone	280	16	30
Sandwich: Mini Reese's	260	12	38
Choc Chip Cookie	260	12	38
Oreo Cookie	230	9	35
Original Vanilla	190	7	29
King Size Vanilla	300	12	43
Kool-Aid Kool Pops	50	0	13
Krispy Frostick	150	10	13
Juice Flavored Sticks	50	0	13
M&Ms Cookie Ice Cream S'wich	220	11	29
Matterhorn Cone, 10 fl.oz	510	38	19
Milky Way Ice Cream Bar	220	12	25
Minute Maid Fruit Juice Pops	70	0	19
Nestlé: Push Up Pop, average	90	1	19
Crunch Vanilla, 3 oz bar	220	15	18
Drumstick: Cookies n Cream	350	19	40
Strawberry Cheesecake	240	15	25
Vanilla w. Choc Layers	440	24	50
Toll House Sandwich: Choc Chip	520	23	72
Choc Choc Chip	550	29	67
Oreo: Sandwich	230	9	35
Cookies n' Cream Bar	110	1	25
Pathmark Vanilla w. choc. coat.	150	10	14
Pops (water/juice), average	50	0	15
Popsicles: Big Stick Ice Pops	60	0	9
Creamsicle Pop	70	1.5	12
Fudgesicle Fudge Pop	100	2	18
Fat-Free	70	0	14
Firecracker Super Hero	60	1.5	11
Fruit Shots	80	1	9
Minis Ice Cream Pop (3)	40	0	9
Rainbow Floats, 1.75 fl.oz	40	0	10
Sponge Bob Squarepants Pop Up	80	1	16
Scribblers Pops: 2 pces	60	0	15
ACE Juice Pops, 2 pces	50	0	12
Ice Pops: 1 pce	60	0	15
Sugar-Free, 1 pce, 1.9 oz	15	0	4
Reese's Peanut Butter Ice Cream	270	18	24
Rice Dream: Pies, all flavors	330	19	40
Bars: Chocolate	200	12	25
Vanilla	230	14	25
Choc/Vanilla Nutty	320	24	27

Per Bar/Serving	C	F	Cb
Safeway Select Coffee Almd Bar	270	17	26
Skinny Cow			
Fat-Free Chocolate Fudge Bar	100	0	21
Low-Fat Cookies n' Cream Bar	120	1.5	23
Vanilla/Strawberry Sorbet Bar	110	0.5	21
Cones: Chocolate Fudge	150	3	28
Vanilla Caramel	150	2.5	29
Sandwiches: All flavors	140	1.5	30
Snickers: Ice Cream Bar	180	11	18
Cone	280	15	33
Snack Bar (1)	90	6	9
Soy Delicious: Li'l Buddies S'wich	150	3	28
Soy Dream (Non-Dairy):			
Dreamwich Vanilla	130	6	15
Heavenly Pies: Mocha; Vanilla	290	14	40
Lil' Dreamers: Choc; Vanilla	100	4	15
Starbuck's Frappuccino Bars, avg.	125	2	24
Tofutti			
Cuties: Peanut Butter	165	8	20
Other varieties, avg.	130	6	17
Sticks: Treats Bar	30	0	6
Delights	120	7	7
Totally Fudge Pops	95	1.5	19
Too Too's: Vanilla Chocolate Chip	230	11	30
Trader Joe's Fruit Floes,			
Caribbean, 4 oz	80	0	21
Strawberry, 4 oz	110	2	31
Trix: Pops, regular	40	0	10
Sugar Free	15	0	4
Tropicana: Real Fruit Bar	50	0	13
Real Fruit N.A.S. Bar	25	0	6
Twix Bar	170	10	19
Vitari Soft Serve, 4 fl.oz, average	80	0	21
Weight Watchers			
English Toffee Crunch	110	6	13
Fudge Sundae Cups, average	160	1	38
Giant Cookies 'n Cream	140	5	26
Giant Fudge Bar	110	1	25
Wildberry & Orange Bar, avg.	115	0.5	29
Strawb., Passionfr., Lime Sorbet Bar	60	0.5	13
Sandwich: Chocolate Round	140	2	33
Vanilla	120	2	28
Vanilla Round	140	2	32
Yoplait: Froz. Yogurt/Cereal Bars,			
Sandwich	200	4.5	36
Bars	120	1.5	23
Double Fruit Smoothies	45	0	11

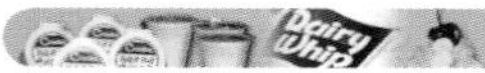

Quick Guide

Cream
Average All Brands

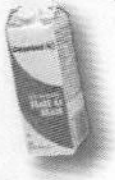

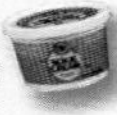

	C	F	Cb
Half & Half Cream:			
1 Tbsp, 0.5 oz	20	2	0.5
2 Tbsp, 1 oz	40	4	1
Light: Coffee/table (20% fat): 1 T.	30	3	0.5
2 Tbsp, 1 oz	60	6	1
Sour Cream:			
Regular: 1 Tbsp, 0.5 oz	25	2.5	0.5
1 cup, 8 oz	490	48	10
Low-Fat/Light: 1 Tbsp, 0.5 oz	20	1.5	1
2 Tbsp, 1 oz	40	3	2
Fat Free: 2 Tbsp, 1 oz	20	0	4.5
Kroger, 2 Tbsp, 1 oz	20	0	3
Naturally Yours; Oak Farm, 2 T.	20	0	3
Knudsen, 2 Tbsp, 1 oz	30	0	5
Sour Cream Substitute:			
Albertson's, 2 Tbsp, 1 oz	60	5	2
Tofutti Sour Supreme, 2 T., 1 oz	85	7	9
Whipping Cream:			
Heavy (37% fat):			
1 Tbsp fluid/2 Tbsp whipped	50	5.5	0.5
¼ cup whipped	100	11	1
½ cup fluid/1 cup whipped	400	44	3.5
Light (30% fat):			
1 Tbsp fluid/2 Tbsp whipped	45	4.5	0.5
½ cup fluid/1 cup whipped	350	37	4

Coconut Cream/Milk

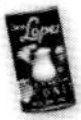

	C	F	Cb
Coconut Cream (Canned),			
Plain/unsweetened: 2 Tbsp, 1 oz	75	6.5	3
½ cup, 4 oz	285	26	12
Sweetened: *Coco Lopez,* 1 oz	120	5	20
½ cup, 4 oz	480	20	80
Coconut Milk (Canned):			
Natural Value: Reg., ¼ c., 2 fl.oz	110	10	2
Lite, ¼ cup, 2 fl.oz	55	5	1
Thai Kitchen: Pure, ¼ c., 2 fl.oz	115	10	4
Lite, ¼ cup, 2 fl.oz	45	4	1
Premium, 2 fl.oz	120	10	4
Coconut Water (Center), 1 cup	45	0.5	9

Whipped Toppings
Average All Brands

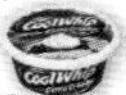

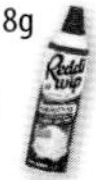

	C	F	Cb
Cream (Pressurized): 2 Tbsp	20	2	1
¼ cup	45	4	2
½ cup	90	8	4
Cream Toppings: *Jewel* Lite, 2 Tbsp	20	1	2
Cool Whip: Extra Creamy, 2 T.	25	1.5	2
Lite, 2 Tbsp, 9g	20	1	2
Free, 2 Tbsp, 9g	15	0	3
Kraft: Dream Whip, 2 Tbsp	15	0	2
Reddi-Wip: Original, 2 T., 8g	15	1	0.5
Chocolate, 2 Tbsp, 8g	15	1	1
Extra Creamy, 2 Tbsp, 8g	15	1.5	0.5
Fat-Free, 2 Tbsp, 8g	5	0	1

Non-Dairy Coffee Creamers

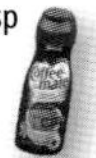

	C	F	Cb
Powder:			
Coffee-Mate/Cremora/N-Rich			
Original, 1 tsp	10	0.5	1
1 heaping tsp	25	2	2
Lite, 1 tsp	10	0	2
Flavors: 1⅓ Tbsp	60	3	9
Fat-Free: Average, 1⅓ Tbsp	50	0	11
Liquid/Refrigerated: *Per Tablespoon*			
Coffee-Mate Non-Dairy Creamer			
Plain: Original/Plain, 1 Tbsp	20	1	2
Fat-Free, 1 Tbsp	10	0	2
Low-Fat, 1 Tbsp	10	0.5	1
Flavors: All flavors, 1 Tbsp	40	2	5
Fat-Free, all flavors, 1 Tbsp	25	0	5
Hood (Non-Dairy), 1 Tbsp	20	1.5	2
International Delight: 1 Tbsp	35	1.5	6
Fat-Free flavors, 1 Tbsp	30	0	7
Mocha Mix: Original, 1 Tbsp	20	1.5	1
Fat-Free, 1 Tbsp	10	0	1
Lite, 1 Tbsp	10	0.5	1
Silk *(White Wave)* Creamer, 1Tbsp	20	1	3
French Vanilla, 1 Tbsp	20	1	3

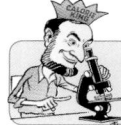

For Full Nutritional Data
~ See Author's Website
www.CalorieKing.com

Fats, Spreads & Oils

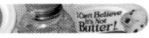

Quick Guide C F Cb

Butter & Margarine
Average All Brands

Regular: 1 tsp (5g) | 35 | 4 | 0
1 Pat (5g)	35	4	0
1 Tbsp, approx. ½ oz	100	11	0
2 Tbsp, 1 oz	205	23	0
1 Stick, ½ cup, 4 oz	815	92	0
1 Pound, 2 cups, 16 oz	3260	368	0

Light (Regular) 40% Fat:

1 tsp (5g)	25	3	0
1 Tbsp, ½ oz	70	8	0
2 Tbsp, 1 oz	140	15	0

Whipped Butter (Regular):

1 tsp (4g)	30	3	0
1 Tbsp (10g)	70	7.5	0
1 Stick, ½ cup, 2 ⅔ oz	545	62	0

Whipped Light Butter 40% Fat:

1 tsp, 5g	25	3	0.5
1 Tbsp, 9g	45	5	1
2 Tbsp, 18g	90	10	2

Unsalted: Same as Regular

Clarified Butter

100% Fat: 1 tsp (5g)	45	5	0
1 Tbsp, 1 oz	180	20	0

Flavored Butter/Spread

Average All Brands

Honey Butter (60% Fat):

1 Tbsp, ½ oz	90	7	4
Downey's, 1 Tbsp, ½ oz	60	1	11

Garlic Butter (80% Fat):

1 Tbsp, ½ oz	100	11	0
Macadamia Butter *(Atkins)*, 1 T.	125	12	2.5

Sweet Cream Butter:

Regular, 1 Tbsp	100	11	0
Stick *(Parkay)*, 70% Fat, 1 Tbsp	90	10	0
Tub *(Land O'Lakes)*, 60% Fat, 1 T.	80	8	0

Other Spreads & Fats

Copha, Dripping, Lard, Suet, Shortening:

1 Tbsp, ½ oz	120	13	0

Chicken, Duck, Goose Fat:

1 Tbsp, ½ oz	115	13	0

Light & Reduced Fat Spreads

Per 1 Tbsp, ½ oz (Unless Stated)	C	F	Cb
Albertson's: Country (48%), 1T.	60	7	0
Butter Blend, 1 Tbsp	80	9	0
Benecol: Spread, 1 Tbsp, 14g	70	8	0
Light, Spread, 1 Tbsp, 14g	50	5	0
Blue Bonnet, Homestyle (48% Veg Oil)	60	7	0
Brummel & Brown, Spread, 1 T.	50	5	0
Canola Harvest, Margarine, 1 T.	100	11	0
Country Crock *(Shedd's):* Regular	60	7	0
Light; Calcium & Vitamins	50	5	0
Spreadable Butter, 1 Tbsp	80	9	0
Country Morning, Soft, 1 Tbsp	100	11	0
Downey's, Honey Butter, 1 Tbsp	60	1	11
Fleischmann's: Soft Spread	70	8	0
Original Stick, 1 Tbsp	100	11	0
Light Spread, 1 Tbsp	50	5	0
'I Can't Believe It's Not Butter': Reg.	80	8	0
Light; Sweet Cream	50	6	0
Imperial: Stick, 1 Tbsp	80	8	0
Tub, 1 Tbsp	60	7	0
Jewel: Country (48%), 1 Tbsp	60	7	0
Butter Blend, 1 Tbsp	80	9	0
Land O'Lakes: Buttery Taste, 1 T.	80	8	0
Honey Butter, 1 Tbsp	90	8	4
Light Butter Whipped, 1 Tbsp	45	5	0
Light Butter, 1 Tbsp	50	6	0
Parkay: Squeeze, 1 Tbsp	70	8	0
Light Stick, 1 Tbsp	50	5	0
Original Stick, 1 Tbsp	90	10	0
Original, 1 Tbsp	60	7	0
Promise: Buttery, 1 Tbsp	45	8	0
Fat-Free, 1 Tbsp	5	0	0
Buttery Light, 1 Tbsp	45	5	0
Smart Balance: 67% Buttery, 1 T.	80	9	0
Light (37%), 1 Tbsp	45	5	0
Smart Beat, Fat-Free, 1 Tbsp	10	0	3
Smart Squeeze, 1 Tbsp	5	0	1
Take Control: Regular, 1 Tbsp	80	8	0
Light Spread, 1 Tbsp	45	5	0

The cheapest slimming exercise is mind over platter. ☺

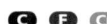

Butter Substitutes

	C	F	Cb
Butter Buds: 1 serving, ½ tsp	5	0	1
Sprinkles, 1 tsp	5	0	0
Earth Balance, Non GMO,1 Tbsp	100	11	0
Molly McButter, ½ tsp	5	0	0
Shedd's Willow Run, Soy, 1 T.	100	1	0
Sunsweet: Baking Butter, 1 Tbsp	35	0	9
Lighter Bake, 1 Tbsp	35	0	9

Spreads Comparison

	C	F	Cb
Mayonnaise: Regular, 1 Tbsp	60	5	3.5
Light, average, 1 Tbsp	50	5	1
Fat-Free, 1 T.	10	0	2
Miracle Whip (Kraft):			
Regular, 1 Tbsp	40	3.5	2
Light, 1 Tbsp	25	1.5	3
Free, 1 Tbsp	15	0	3
Smart Beat Dressing: 1 Tbsp	10	0	2.5

Extra Listings for Mayonnaise & Dressings
~ See Page 89 ~

	C	F	Cb
Avocado, mashed, 1 Tbsp	45	4	2.5
Peanut Butter, 1 Tbsp	100	8	3.5
Nutella, 1 Tbsp	100	5.5	12

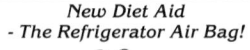

New Diet Aid
- The Refrigerator Air Bag!

POOF!

Animal Fats/Lards

Average All Types
Beef Tallow/Drippings, Lard (Pork), Chicken, Duck, Goose, Turkey.

	C	F	Cb
1 Tbsp (13g)	115	13	0
2¼ Tbsp, 1 oz	255	28	0
1 cup, 7¼ oz	1850	205	0
½ pound, 8 oz	2040	227	0
Ghee/Butter Oil: 1 Tbsp, 13g	110	13	0
2¼ Tbsp, 1 oz	250	28	0

Vegetable Shortening

Average All Types (example, Crisco)

	C	F	Cb
1 Tbsp, 0.44 oz	113	13	0
2¼ Tbsp, 1 oz	250	28	0
1 cup, 7¼ oz	1810	205	0

Vegetable Oils

Includes almond, avocado, canola, corn, coconut, flaxseed, grapeseed, linseed, mustard, olive, palm, peanut, rice-bran, safflower, sesame, sunflower, soybean, wheatgerm. Note: Oil is 100% fat.

	C	F	Cb
1 tsp, 5g	45	5	0
1 Tbsp, ½ oz	120	14	0
2 Tbsp, 1 oz	250	28	0
1 cup, 7¾ oz	1930	205	0

Fish Oils

Average All Types (Includes cod liver, herring, salmon, sardine):

	C	F	Cb
1 Tbsp, ½ oz	125	14	0

Cooking Sprays/Squeezes

Cooking Sprays (Pam, Mazola, I Can't Believe It's Not Butter, Weight Watchers, Wesson):

	C	F	Cb
Per serving	2	0	0
1-3 second spray	6	1	0
I Can't Believe It's Not Butter	0	0	0
Parkay Buttery Spray	0	0	0
Squeeze (Parkay), 1 Tbsp, 0.5 oz	70	8	0

Olestra (Olean)

	C	F	Cb
Olestra (Olean)	0	0	0

Olean is Procter & Gamble's brand name for olestra – a no-calorie cooking oil that gives snacks (like potato chips, tortilla chips and crackers) taste and texture without adding fat or calories.

Cheese

Quick Guide — C F Cb

Firm/Hard Cheeses
(American, Cheddar, Colby, Coon, Swiss)

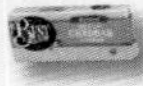

Regular Cheese:

	C	F	Cb
1 oz slice/piece	110	9	0.5
8 oz package	850	72	4
16 oz (1lb) package	1740	144	8
Cubes: 1" cube, ¾ oz	70	5.5	0.5
1¼" cube, 1 oz slice	110	9	0.5
Diced: 1 cup, 4½ oz	525	44	2
Grated: 1 Tbsp, ¼ oz	27	2	0
Shredded:			
¼ cup, 1 oz	105	9	0.5
1 cup, 4 oz	425	35	4
Sliced: 1 thin (3½" sq.), ¾ oz	80	7	0.5
Rectangular (7"x 4"x ⅛"), 1½ oz	165	14	1
Round (3¼" diam. x ⅛"), ¾ oz	85	7	0.5
Semi-circular, 1¼ oz			
(5½" long, 3½" radius, ⅛" thick)	140	11	0.5
Fat-Free: Average all Brands, 1 oz	45	0	4
Low-Fat: Average all Brands, 1 oz	50	2	1
Reduced Fat: Avg. all Brands, 1 oz	80	5	0.5

Cheese — C F Cb

Per 1 oz Unless Indicated

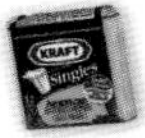

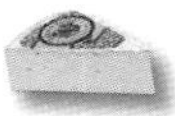

American:

	C	F	Cb
Regular: 1 slice, 1 oz	110	9	0.5
Alpine Lace, 1 oz	90	7	2
Kraft, 0.7 oz slice	60	4.5	0
Shredded, 1 Tbsp, ¼ oz	25	2	0.5
Land O'Lakes, 1 oz	70	5	2
Light: *Kraft* (2% Milk), 0.7 oz slice	50	3	1
Fat-Free: *Kraft,* 0.7 oz slice	30	0	2
HealthyChoice, Singles, 0.7 pce	75	6	0
Babybel (*Laughing Cow*), 21g	70	6	0
Light Original, 21g pce	50	3	0
Bonbel (*Laughing Cow*), 1 pce	70	5	0
Brick (*Land O'Lakes*), 1 oz	110	8	1
Brie, 1 oz	95	8	0
Camembert, 1 oz	85	7	0
Caraway, 1 oz	105	8	1
Castello (*Wegman's*), avg., 1 oz	120	12	0

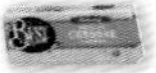

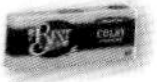

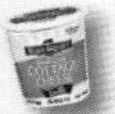

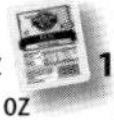

Cheddar: (Also see 'Quick Guide')

	C	F	Cb
Regular: 1 oz	110	9	0.5
Alpine Lace, 1 oz	90	7	0
Reduced-Fat/Low-Fat: 1 oz	50	2	0.5
Cabot Vermont, 50% Light, 1 oz	70	4.5	0.5
Lifetime, 1oz	55	2.5	1
Weight Watchers, 1 oz	80	5	1
Fat-Free, *Weight Watchers,* ¾ oz	30	0	3
Cheese Balls (*Kaukauna*), 1 oz, avg.	100	7	0.5
Cheese Nut, average, 1 oz	100	7	2
Cheese Logs (*Kaukauna*), avg., 1 oz	100	7	0.5
Cheshire, 1 oz	110	9	1.5
Colby: Regular, 1 oz	110	6	0
Reduced-Fat (*Kraft*), 1 oz	80	5	1
Colby-Jack (*Cabot*), 1 oz	110	9	0.5

Cottage Cheese: *Average All Brands*

	C	F	Cb
Creamed (4% milk fat): 2 Tbsp, 1 oz	30	1	1.5
½ cup, 4 oz	120	5	6
w. fruit, ½ cup, 4 oz	130	4	15
Reduced-Fat (2%): 2 T., 1 oz	25	0.5	1
½ cup, 4 oz	100	2	4
Low-Fat (1%): 2 Tbsp, 1 oz	20	.5	1
½ cup, 4 oz	80	1	3
Fat-Free/Non-Fat: 2 Tbsp, 1 oz	25	0	0.5
½ cup, 4 oz	95	0.5	2
Friendship: Low-Fat P'apple, 4 oz	120	1	16
Non-Fat w. Peach, ½ c., 4 oz	110	0	15
Pot Style, ½ cup, 4 oz	90	2.5	3
Hood w. Chive/Onion, 4 oz	90	1	5
Knudsen: Low-Fat w. Fruit, 4.3 oz	120	2	15
Free: Non-Fat, ½ cup, 4.3 oz	80	0	7
2% Milk Fat	100	2.5	6
Cottage Doubles, avg, 5.5 oz ctn	150	2.5	18
On the Go! Free, 4 oz ctn	80	0	7
Low-Fat, 4 oz ctn	90	2.5	6
Light N' Lively: Fat-Free, 4.4 oz	80	0	8
Low-Fat, ½ cup, 4.4 oz	80	1.5	6
Cream Cheese: See Page 45			
Edam, Regular, 1 oz	100	8	0.5
Farmer (*Friendship*), 2 Tbsp, 1 oz	50	2.5	0
Feta: Regular, 1 oz	75	6	1
Crumbled, ½ cup, 2½ oz	190	15	3
Reduced-Fat (*Athenos*), 1 oz	60	4	1
Fontina, 1 oz	110	9	0.5
Gjetost (Goat's Milk, fresh), 1 oz	130	8	12
Wegman's, 1 oz	130	9	11

Goat's Milk Cheese:	C	F	Cb
Chevre, Soft, 1 oz	70	6	0.5
Chavril: 3 Tbsp, 1 oz	60	4.5	0.5
Semi-Soft, 1 oz	100	8.5	1
Hard, 1 oz	130	10	0.5
Gorgonzola, 1 oz	110	9	0.5
Galbani Dolcelatte, 1 oz	95	8	1
Gouda, 1 oz	100	8	0.5
Gruyere, 1 oz	110	8	1
Havarti (Land O'Lakes), 1 oz	120	11	0
Italian Blend (Sargento), 1 oz	90	7	1
Jarlsberg (Wegman's), 1 oz	100	8	1
Jarlsberg Lite shredded, 1 oz	70	4	0
Kefir (Alta Dena), 2 Tbsp, 1 oz	70	6	2
Labneh (Lebanese cream chse), 1.8 oz	70	4	4
Lactose Free Cheese (Lifetime), 1 oz	40	0	1
Limburger, 1 oz	95	8	0
Mascarpone (Wegman's), 1 oz	130	13	1
Mexican (Sargento Recipe Blend),			
Shredded, 1/4 cup, 1 oz	110	9	0.5
Cacique: Cotija, 1 oz	110	9	0
Queso Fresco, 1 oz	80	6	0
Queso Quesadilla, 1 oz	70	5	2
Ranchero, 1 oz	80	6	0
Chi-Chi's: Con Quéso, 2 Tbsp	90	7	4
Hot/Medium/Mild/Acante, 2 T.	10	0	2
Supremo Chihuahua: Quéso Bianco	100	8	0
Quéso Fresco; Rancherito	80	6	0
Monterey, 1 oz	105	8.5	0
Monterey Jack: Regular, 1 oz	110	9	0
Kraft 2% Milk Red. Fat, 1 oz	80	6	1
Alpine Lace, Co-Jack, 1 oz	90	0	7
Weight Watchers, 1 oz	90	6	1
Mozzarella:			
Regular: Kraft, 1 oz	80	6	1
Land O'Lakes/Polly-O, 1 oz, avg.	80	6	1
Shredded, 1/4 cup, 1 oz	90	7	1
Light: Polly-O Lite, 1 oz	60	2.5	1
Kraft 2% Milk Fat, Red. Fat, 1 oz	70	4	1
Sargento Reduced Fat, 1/4 c, 1 oz	80	4.5	0.5
Part Skim: Alpine Lace, 1 oz	70	5	1
Polly-O, 1 oz	70	5	1
Fat-Free: Polly-O, 1 oz	40	0	1
Kraft, shredded, 1/4 cup, 1 oz	45	0	2
Muenster: Regular, 1 oz	105	9	0.5
Low-Fat, 1 oz	80	5	0
Myzithra, 4 Tbsp, 1 oz	80	4	2
Neufchatel: 1 oz	75	6	1
Philadelphia, 1 oz	70	6	1
Flavored: Fruit/Herbs	80	7	1
Chocolate (Hickory Farms), 1 oz	110	8	1

	C	F	Cb
Parmesan: Fresh/Block, 1 oz	110	7	1
Shredded/Grated, 1 Tbsp	20	1.5	0
Grated (Packaged): 1 Tbsp	20	1.5	0
1 oz quantity	115	9	0
1/2 cup, 1 3/4 oz	200	15	0
w. Romano (Frigo), grated, 1 oz	130	9	1
Kraft Reduced-Fat, 1 Tbsp	20	1	2

Note: Packaged grated and shredded Parmesan have more calories (per unit weight) than block Parmesan Parmesan due to lower moisture content.

Pizza Cheese, shredded:	C	F	Cb
Regular (Kraft) 1/4 cup, 1 oz	90	7	1
Port de Salut, 1 oz	100	8	0
Port Wine (Kaukauna), 1 oz	90	6	4
Pot (Sargento), 1 oz	25	0	1
Provolone: Regular, 1 oz	100	8	0.5
Reduced-Fat (Alpine Lace), 1 oz	80	5	1
Pub (Rondele), 1 oz, avg.	95	7	1
Quark: 40% fat, 1 oz	47	3	1
20% fat, 1 oz	32	1.5	0
Skim/Non-Fat, 1 oz	22	0	1.5
Queso: Anejo/Asadero/Blanco	105	9	0
Chichuahua/De Papa	110	9	2
Ricotta Cheese:			
Whole Milk, 2 Tbsp, 1 oz	50	3.5	1
1/2 cup, 4 1/2 oz	215	16	3.5
Part Skim, 2 Tbsp, 1 oz	40	2	1.5
1/2 cup, 4 1/2 oz	170	10	6.5
Light/Low-Fat, 2 Tbsp, 1 oz	25	1	1.5
1/2 cup, 4 1/2 oz	125	5	6
Fat-Free, 1/2 cup, 4 1/2 oz	100	0	10
Baked Ricotta, 2 oz portion	130	9	3
Romano: Block/Loaf, 1 oz	110	8	1
Grated (Pkg), 1 oz	120	9	1
1 Tbsp, 5g	20	1.5	0
Roquefort, 1 oz	105	9	0.5
Sheep's Milk, 1 oz	45	3	1
Smoked: Cabot, Smoky, 1 oz	110	9	0
Kaukauna, Smoky Cheddar, 1 oz	90	6	4
Stilton (Wegman's), 1 oz	110	10	0
String (Frigo/Kraft/Sargento), 1 oz	80	6	0.5
Light String-Ums (Kraft), 1 oz	80	4.5	1
String Lite (Frigo)	60	3	0
Light (Sargento), 1 stick	50	2.5	0.5
Swiss: Regular, 1 oz	110	8	1.5
Reduced-Fat: Alpine Lace, 1 oz	90	6	1
Kraft, 2% Milk, 3/4 oz slice	50	2.5	2
Taco Cheese (Kraft) shredded, 1/4 cup	120	10	1
Tilsit, 1 oz	95	7	0.5
Tybo, 1 oz	100	7	0.5
Vermont (Cabot), 1 oz	110	9	0
Wensleydale, 1 oz	110	9	0
Whey Cheese, 1 oz	125	8	9

Cheese (Cont)

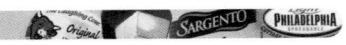

Cheese Products

	C	F	Cb
Cheese Food:			
Average all flavors: ¾ oz slice	70	5	2
1 oz slice	95	7	2.5
Alouette: Sundr. Tomato, 2 T., 0.8oz	80	7	1
Light Garlic, 2 Tbsp, 0.8 oz	50	4	2
Peppercorn Cajun, 2 T., 0.8 oz	80	8	1
Savory Vegetable, 2 T., 0.8 oz	70	5	1
Cabot, Jalapeno, 1 oz	70	4.5	0
Cracker Barrel, Cheddar, 1.1 oz	100	8	0
Handi-Snacks: *(Kraft)*			
Breadsticks 'n Cheez, 1 oz pkg	110	4.5	14
Pretzels 'n Cheez, 1 oz pkg	90	3.5	12
Crackers 'n Cheez, 1 oz pkg	100	5	10
Mozzarella Stringchse Stick, each	80	6	0.5
Healthy Choice, Amer. Singles, 1 sl.	30	0	2
Heluva Good Cheese:			
American, 1 slice	45	5	2
Cheddar w. H/radish, 2 Tbsp, 1oz	90	7	3
Kraft: American shredded, 1Tbsp.	25	2	0.5
Singles, 1 slice, ¾ oz	60	4.5	1
Free Singles, 1 slice, 0.7 oz	30	0	2
Pimento Spread, 2 Tbsp, 1.1 oz	80	6	3
Light String-Ums, 1 stick, 1 oz	80	4	1
Lifetime Cholesterol Reducing,			
Slices, 1 Slice, 19g	30	1	2
Block, 1 oz	55	2.5	1
Lifeway Farmers Kefir, 1 oz	25	1.5	4
Precious String Chse Stuffsters, 1 oz	70	4.5	1
Rondele: Soft Spread., 2 T., 1 oz	100	9	1
Light, 2 Tbsp, 1 oz	60	5	2
SmartBalance Crmy Cheddar, 1 sl.	40	2	2
Spreadery: Vermont, 2 Tbsp, 1 oz	100	9	2
Velveeta: Regular, ⅜" slice, 1 oz	80	6	3
Light, ⅜" slice, 1 oz	60	3	4
Shredded, ¼ cup, 1.3 oz	130	9	3
WisPride: Port Wine,			
Ball/Cup, 2 Tbsp, 1.1 oz	100	7	8
Light, 2 Tbsp, 1.1 oz	80	3	5

Cheese Whiz (Sauce)

	C	F	Cb
Original, 2 Tbsp, 33g	90	7	2
Light, 2 Tbsp, 33g	80	3	6
Salsa Con Queso, 2 Tbsp, 33g	90	7	4

Cheese Substitutes

	C	F	Cb
Per 1 oz Unless Indicated			
Galaxy:			
Veggie Yellow American, 1 sl., ½ oz	35	2	1
Veggy Mozz. Singles, 1 sl., ½ oz	40	2	1
Lifetime Rice Cheese, 1 oz	60	3	5
Mori Nu Tofu: Mozzarella, 1 oz	70	4	2
Fat-Free Mozz./Ched./Jack, 1 oz	40	0	2
Sargento Chef Style,			
Cheddar, shredded, ¼ cup, 1 oz	110	9	1
Mozzarella, shrd, ¼ cup	80	6	0.5
Smart Beat, Fat-Free, 0.6 oz sl.	25	0	3
Soya Kaas: Regular, 1 oz	70	5	1
Fat-Free, all varieties, 1 oz	40	2	1
Soyco: Almond/Oat/Rice Slices,			
1 slice, 0.7 oz	40	2	1
Veggy Singles, 1 slice, 0.7 oz	40	2	1
Grated Parmesan, 2 tsp, 5g	15	0.5	0
Soy Sation: Shredded Cheese, 1 oz	70	4	2
Tofu Rella, avg. all varieties, 1 oz	60	4	0
Tofutti Better Than Cream Cheese	80	8	1
Trader Joe's:			
Soy Cheese: Cheddar Flavor, 1 sl.	45	2	3
Mozzarella Flavor, 1 oz	70	4	3
Sliced Yogurt Cheese, 1 oz	100	8	0
Yves, Good Slice, ¾ oz slice, avg.	35	2	1

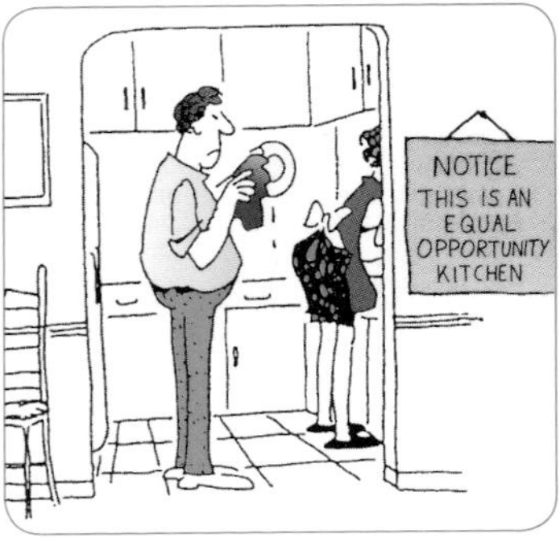

NOTICE
THIS IS AN
EQUAL
OPPORTUNITY
KITCHEN

Snack & Cheese Dips, Spreads

Cream Cheese

	C	F	Cb
Regular/Soft: 2 Tbsp, 1 oz	100	10	1
3 oz pkg	300	30	2.5
w. Chives/Herbs/Pimento, 1 oz	75	2.5	10
w. Fruit/Strawb./P'apple, 1 oz	90	8	4
Lox, 1 oz	90	8	1
Philadelphia *(Kraft): Per 2 Tbsp*			
Original, 1 oz	100	10	1
⅓ Less Fat, 1 oz	70	6	1
Light: Plain, 1 oz	60	4.5	2
Flavors, avg., 0.7 oz	70	4	6
Fat-Free Varieties, 1 oz	30	0	2
Flavored: Blueberry/Raspberry, 1 oz	90	7	5
Honey Nut; Strawberry, 1 oz	90	8	4
Garden Vegetable, 1 oz	90	8	2
Snacks: Bars, avg, all types (1)	180	11	20
Snack Bites (1) 1 oz	130	7	15
Bagel & Crm Chse To Go, 3.2 oz	240	8	36
Swirls, avg., 2 Tbsp, 1 oz	90	8	4
Whipped: Regular, 2 Tbsp, 0.7 oz	60	6	1
Mixed Berry, 2 Tbsp, 0.7 oz	70	6	3
Weight Watchers, 2 Tbsp, 1 oz	40	2.5	1

Dips/Spreads

Per 2 Tbsp (1 oz), Unless Indicated

Average All Brands

	C	F	Cb
Avocado/Guacamole, 2 Tbsp, 1 oz	45	4	2
Baba Ghannoush *(Eggplant/Sesame)*	70	6	2
Cheese Fondue, ½ cup, 4 oz	210	14	4
French Onion Dip, 2 Tbsp	60	6	3
Hummus: 2 Tbsp, 1 oz	50	3	5
½ cup, 4.5 oz	220	4.5	23
Tzatziki *(Cucumber/Yogurt)* 2 T.	40	3	1
Clearman's: Original Spread, 1 oz	150	15	2
Frito Lay: Chili Cheese; Jalapeno	50	3	5
French Onion	60	5	4
Bean/Jalapeno Bean	40	1	6
Guiltless Gourmet: Nacho Dip	25	0	5
Other varieties	30	0	5
Heluva Good Cheese: Chse 'N Salsa	80	3	3
Clam/French Onion	50	5	2
Bacon/Homestyle/Ranch	60	5	2
Light Fr. Onion/Jalapeno Cheddar	40	2	3
De La Casa, 5 Layer Party Dip, 2 T.	40	2.5	4
Kaukauna Nacho Cheese	90	7	4
Knudsen Nacho Cheese	60	4	3
Sour Cream Bacon & Onion	60	5	2
Sour Cream French Onion	50	4	2

Dips/Spreads (Cont)

Per 2 Tbsp (1 oz)

	C	F	Cb
Kroger, The Big Dipper; all flavors	60	5	2
Kraft: Average all flavors, 2 Tbsp	60	5	4
Philly flavors: Bacon & Cheddar	60	5	3
Average other flavors	60	4.5	3
Fat-Free: Strawberry	25	0	2
Garden Veges	30	0	2
Lay's Dip Mix, prepared, 2 Tbsp	60	6	3
Louise's, Sour Crm & On./White Chse	25	0	0
Marie's Dips, average all varieties	90	9	2
Nalley's, all flavors, average	120	12	3
Naturally Fresh: Chocolate Dip	100	0	23
Cream Cheese Dip, 2 Tbsp	80	4.5	10
Fruit Dip, 2 Tbsp	120	11	6
Old Dutch French Onion, 2 Tbsp	50	3	4
Old El Paso: Black Bean, 2 Tbsp	25	0	5
Cheese 'n Salsa: Mild; Medium	40	3	4
Low-Fat, medium	30	1.5	4
Chunky Salsa varieties, avg.	15	0	3
Olys Bagel Spread: Berry	100	8	3
Garden Veg; Garlic & Herb	90	9	1
Prices: Pimiento Cheese Spread	80	7	3
Light Pimiento, 1 oz	55	3	3
Rite, Cream Cheese & Lox Spread	90	8	1
Ruffles, French Onion; Ranch	70	6	4
Snyder's Mustard Pretzel	70	1	15
Stop & Shop: Veggie Dip, 2 Tbsp	110	10	3
Sour Crm French Onion, 2 T.	60	5	2
TGI Fridays, Spinach,Chse,Artichoke	45	3.5	2
T. Marzetti: Choc Fruit, 2 Tbsp	110	2	23
Guacamole	130	13	2
Veggie: Ranch	120	12	2
Light Ranch	60	6	2
Fat-Free Ranch	30	0	6
Toby's: Tofu Pate, 2 Tbsp	80	7	2
Other Spreads, average, 2 Tbsp	40	2.5	2
Tostitos Dip: Con Quéso Salsa	40	2.5	5
Reduced-Fat Zesty Cheese, 2 T.	40	2	4
Wise: French Onion, 2 Tbsp	60	5	3
Nacho Cheese	50	4.5	3
Salsa: *See Page 85*			

Egg & Egg Dishes

Chicken Eggs

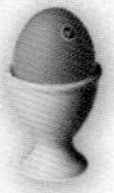

Fresh Eggs

Raw (weight with shell):	C	F	Cb
Small, 40g	65	4	0
Medium, 44g	70	4	0
Large, 50g	75	4.5	0
Extra Large, 56g	80	5	0
Jumbo, 63g	90	5.5	0
Egg Yolk, 1 extra large	63	5	0
Egg White, 1 extra large	16	0	0

Dried Egg Powder

	C	F	Cb
Whole Egg: ¼ cup, 1 oz	170	12	0
1 Tbsp	30	2	0
Egg White, ¼ cup, 1 oz	105	0	0
Egg Yolk, ¼ cup, 1 oz	195	18	0

Egg Substitutes

¼ Cup (Equivalent to 1 Egg) ~ Zero Cholesterol.

	C	F	Cb
Better 'n Eggs (Papetti), ¼ cup, 2 oz	30	0	1
EggBeaters (Fleischmann's) Frozen/Liquid Regular/Flavors, ¼ cup, 2.2 oz	30	0	1
Egg Watchers (Tofutti), ¼ c., 2 oz	30	0	1
Ener-G, Egg Replacer, 1½ tsp, 4 g	15	0	4
Egg Substitute (Jewel), ¼ cup	30	0	1
Nature Egg, Simply Egg White, ¼ c., 2 oz	25	0	0
Scramblers (Morning Star), ¼ cup	35	0	0
Second Nature, Fat-Free, ¼ c., 2 fl.oz	35	0	1

Other Eggs

	C	F	Cb
Duck, 1 large, 2½ oz	130	9.5	0
Goose, 1 large, 5 oz	280	19	0
Quail, 3 eggs, 1 oz	42	3	0
Turkey, 1 large, 3 oz	135	9.5	0
Turtle, 1 egg, 1¾ oz	75	5	0

Omega-3 Fat Enriched

	C	F	Cb
Eggland's Best, 1 large	70	4	0
Eggs Plus (Pilgrim's Pride), 1 large	70	4.5	1

Note: Cholesterol content same as regular eggs, but Omega-3 fats inhibit blood cholesterol increase. (Extra Notes ~ See Page 271)

Cooked Eggs

	C	F	Cb
Boiled Egg: Same as raw egg			
Fried Egg:			
With fat: 1 large egg	105	9	0.5
2 small eggs	175	13	1
No fat/nonstick pan, 1 large	75	5	0.5
Deviled Egg, 2 halves	145	13	0.5
Eggs Benedict (2) on toast or English muffin	860	56	25
Eggs Florentine (2) on toast or English muffin	890	59	25
Pickled Egg, 1 large	80	5.5	0
Poached Egg, 1 large	65	4	0
Quiche (Home-Made):			
Egg & Bacon, 1 slice, 5.3 oz	580	43	27
Ham & Cheese, 1 slice, 5.3 oz	475	33	29
Scotch Egg, 1 egg	300	21	16
Scrambled Eggs: 1 large egg:			
w. 1 Tbsp milk + 1 tsp fat	120	9	1
w. 1 Tbsp skim milk/no fat	85	5.5	1
2 large eggs:			
w. 2 Tbsp milk + 2 tsp fat	260	20	2
w. 2 Tbsp skim milk/no fat	180	11	2

Omelets

	C	F	Cb
1 Egg: Plain (w. 1 tsp fat)	125	10	0.5
with ½ oz cheese	175	15	0.5
w. ½ oz cheese + ½ oz ham	200	16	0.5
2 Eggs: Plain (w. 2 tsp fat)	250	20	1
with 1 oz cheese	360	29	2
w. 1 oz cheese+1 oz ham	410	32	2
3 Eggs: Plain (w. 1 Tbsp fat)	360	29	1.5
w. 2 oz cheese	580	47	2.5
w. 2 oz cheese+2 oz ham	680	53	2.5
Extras: Tomato/Onion/Veges	20	0	4.5
Egg Substitute (EggBeaters):			
2 eggs (½ cup) + 1 tsp fat	100	4	2
3 eggs (¾ cup) + 2 tsp fat	160	8	3
Extras: 1 oz cheese	110	9	1
1 oz ham	50	3	1
Tom./Onion/Veges	20	0	4.5

Egg Nog ~ Per ½ Cup (4 fl.oz)

	C	F	Cb
Average all Brands, ½ cup	170	9.5	17
Regular: Borden	160	9	17
Hood (Golden)	180	9	22
Light/Low-Fat: Horizon; Hood	140	4	22
Fat-Free: Hood	55	0	9

Breakfast Sides

	C	F	Cb
Toast: Plain, 1 thick slice	85	1	13
with 2 tsp butter/marg.	155	9	13
with 3 tsp/1 Tbsp fat	190	13	13
English Muffin: Plain, 2 oz	130	1	26
with 3 tsp fat	230	12	26
Bacon, 2 strips	70	5	0
Ham, Lean, 2 oz	100	3	0
Hash Browns: ½ cup	125	6.5	14
1 cup serving	250	13	28
Sausages, 2 links (1 oz ea.)	180	16	1.5

Frozen Egg Breakfasts

Aunt Jemima Great Starts: *Per Package*

	C	F	Cb
French Toast & Sausage Bkfst	440	27	35
Griddle Cake w. Ham, Egg, Cheese	240	8	33
Pancakes & Sausage Breakfast	470	25	50
Sausage, Egg & Chse Biscuit	340	21	26
Sausage, Egg & Cheese Croissant	350	23	22
Scrambled Eggs & Saus. Bkfst	370	27	18
Jimmy Dean			
Bacon, Egg, Cheese Muffin (1)	230	9	27
Croissant: Egg & Cheese (1)	310	20	23
Egg, Sausage, Cheese (1)	450	33	24
Egg, Sausage, Cheese Biscuit (1)	430	30	28
Omelet: 3 Cheese (1)	290	23	5
Ham & Cheese (1)	280	17	5
Pillsbury: Toaster Scrambles,			
Cheese, Egg & Bacon	180	12	15
Cheese, Egg & Sausage	180	11	15
Red Baron			
Scrambles: Ham (1), 5 oz	330	15	33
Bacon (1), 5 oz	400	22	35
Minis, 4 pieces, 5½ oz	390	17	45
Swanson Great Starts			
Hungryman Hearty Breakfast	1170	61	125
Weight Watchers: Omelet	220	5	30

Frozen Pancake/Waffles: *See Page 122*

Frozen Egg Rolls

Chun King/La Choy: *Average All Brands*

	C	F	Cb
Chicken Egg Rolls: Mini, 6 rolls	210	9	25
Restaurant Style, 1 roll, 3 oz	210	9	25
Pork & Shrimp Egg Rolls:			
Mini, 6 rolls, 3 oz	210	9	27
Shrimp Egg Rolls: Mini, 6 rolls	190	6	28
Restaurant Style, 1 roll, 3 oz	180	7	25
Lotus: Pork, 3 oz	180	7	18
Vegetable, 3 oz	70	1.5	13
Kahiki: Pork, 3 oz	140	3.5	20
Chicken, 3 oz	160	6	19
Vegetarian, 3 oz	130	3.5	21

Fast Food/Restaurants

	C	F	Cb
Au Bon Pain: Egg on a Bagel	400	4	63
w. Bacon & Cheese	560	18	63
Bob Evans: Eggs Benedict	440	21	35
Three Cheese Omelette	770	67	4
Bojangles: Egg Biscuit	400	30	26
Bacon, Egg & Cheese Biscuit	550	42	27
Bruegger's Bagels: Breakfast Sandwiches,			
Egg & Cheese	420	18	71
Egg & Cheese & Sausage	640	38	72
Burger King: Egg & Cheese Biscuit	430	25	36
Egg & Cheese Croissan'wich	300	17	26
Saus., Egg & Chse Croissan'wich	470	32	26
Carl's Jr.: Scrambled Eggs & Sausage	900	56	72
Chick-Fil-A			
Chicken, Egg & Cheese Bagel	500	20	49
Denny's: Two Eggs & More B'Fast	680	55	20
Country Scramble, no syrup/marg.	1040	62	79
All American Slam, no toast	970	76	21
Eat 'N Park: Cheese Omelette	390	30	2.5
Hardee's: Bacon Platter	980	56	90
Steak N Egg Burrito	470	22	38
IHOP: T-Bone Steak & Eggs	1325	86	63
Country Fried Steak/Eggs	1535	105	73
McDonald's: Egg McMuffin	300	12	30
Bacon, Egg & Cheese Biscuit	500	29	42
Scrambled Eggs (2)	170	11	1
Whataburger			
Breakfast Platter w. Bacon (2 sl.)	740	45	53

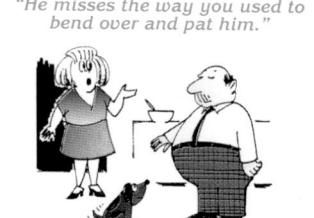

"He misses the way you used to bend over and pat him."

Meat & Beef

Note: Cooking reduces weight of meat by 20-45% due to water and fat losses. Average weight loss is 30%. Actual loss depends on cooking method and cooking time. Examples:

4 oz raw wt. = approx. 3 oz cooked wt.
4 oz cooked wt. = approx. 5½ oz raw wt.

What 3 oz Cooked Meat Looks Like

- Half the size of this book (4¼" x 3" x ⅜" thick)
- Rectangular piece (4" x 2½" x ½" thick)
- Deck of cards (3½" x 2½" x ⅝" thick)

Quick Guide

Steak
Sirloin (Choice Grade)
External fat trimmed to ¼"
Broiled, Edible Portion (no bone)

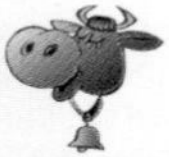

Small Serving, 3 oz (cooked)	C	F	Cb
(3 oz cooked, from 4-4½ oz raw)			
Lean + fat (¼"), 3 oz	**225**	13	0
Lean + marbling, 3 oz	**195**	10	0
Lean only, 3 oz	**160**	6	0
(No external fat or marbling)			
Medium/Regular Serving, 5 oz (cooked wt)			
(from approx. 7 oz raw)			
Lean + fat (¼"), 5 oz	**350**	21	0
Lean + marbling, 5 oz	**325**	17	0
Lean only, 5 oz	**265**	10	0
Large Serving, 8 oz (cooked wt)			
(from 11-12 oz raw)			
Lean + fat, 8 oz	**600**	36	0
Lean + marbling, 8 oz	**520**	27	0
Lean only, 8 oz	**425**	15	0
Extra Large Serving, 12 oz (cooked wt)			
(from approx. 16-17 oz raw)			
Lean + fat (¼"), 12 oz	**900**	52	0
Lean + marbling, 12 oz	**740**	40	0
Lean only, 12 oz	**640**	23	0
Pan Fried			
Sirloin (choice), medium serving:			
Lean + fat (¼"), 5 oz	**460**	32	0
Lean only, 5 oz	**340**	16	0

Other Steaks

	C	F	Cb
Filet Mignon (Tenderloin):			
1 Medium steak, 6 oz raw wt.			
Broiled, with ¼" fat trim			
Lean + fat (¼"), 4 oz	**380**	28	0
Lean only, 3½ oz	**230**	12	0
New York/Club Steak:			
Top Loin/Short Loin			
1 steak, regular (9¼ oz raw, ¼" fat)			
Broiled: Lean + fat (¼"), 6¼ oz	**580**	43	0
Lean + marbling, 5½ oz	**400**	25	0
Lean only, 5¼ oz	**360**	20	0
Porterhouse Steak:			
1 Medium, (6 oz raw wt. no bone), broiled			
Lean + fat (¼"), 4¼ oz	**410**	33	0
Lean only, 3½ oz	**210**	11	0
1 Large (12 oz raw wt. no bone), broiled			
Lean + fat (¼") 8½ oz cooked	**820**	66	0
Lean only, 7 oz cooked	**420**	22	0
With Bone: *See T-Bone Steak*			
T-Bone Steak (Broiled/Grilled): wts. include bone			
Medium, 8 oz raw wt. (with bone)			
Lean + fat (¼")	**410**	32	0
Lean only, 4 oz raw	**230**	12	0
Large, (12 oz raw wt.) ¼" fat	**620**	48	0
Supersize, (20 oz raw wt.) ¼" fat	**1025**	88	0

Also See Fast-Foods & Restaurants Section ~
LoneStar Steakhouse, Outback Steakhouse, WesterN SizzliN

Beef - Average All Cuts

Average All Retail Cuts
Edible weight (no bone)

Raw	C	F	Cb
(1 lb raw yields approx. 11-12 oz cooked)			
Lean + fat (¼" trim), 1 oz	**70**	6	0
½ Pound, 8 oz	**560**	44	0
Lean only, 1 oz	**40**	2	0
½ Pound, 8 oz	**320**	17	0
Fat only, 1 oz	**190**	20	0
Cooked (No Added Fat)			
Lean + fat (¼"), 1 oz	**86**	6	0
Small serving, 3 oz	**260**	18	0
Lean + marbling, (no ext. fat), 1 oz	**78**	5	0
Small serving, 3 oz	**235**	15	0
Lean only, 1 oz	**60**	3	0
Small serving, 3 oz	**180**	9	0
Fat only, 1 oz	**255**	28	0

Beef - Individual Cuts

	C	F	Cb
Average All Grades			
Edible Weight (no bone)			
Brisket, whole, braised:			
Lean + fat ¼", 3 oz	330	27	0
Lean + marbling, 3 oz	280	21	0
Lean only, 3 oz	250	17	0
Chuck, blade, braised:			
Lean + fat (¼"), 3 oz	295	22	0
Lean + marbling, 3 oz	290	21	0
Lean only, 3 oz	245	21	0
Flank: Raw, 4 oz	175	8	0
Braised, 3 oz	225	14	0
Broiled, 3 oz	155	6	0
Ribs, whole (ribs 6-12): Roasted			
(1 lb raw yields 10¼ oz roasted)			
Lean + fat (¼")			
(3.6 oz w. bone, 3 oz no bone)	305	25	0
Lean only 3 oz (no bone)	280	22	0
Round, bottom, braised:			
Lean + fat (¼"), 3 oz	190	7.5	0
Lean only, 3 oz	185	6.5	0
Round, eye/tip, roasted:			
Lean + fat (¼"), 3 oz	205	11	0
Lean, 3 oz	145	4	0
Round, top: Per 3 oz (cooked wt)			
Braised, Lean + fat	210	10	0
Lean only	175	5	0
Broiled, Lean + fat	180	8	0
Lean only	155	5	0
Pan-fried, Lean + fat	235	13	0
Lean only	190	7	0

Ground Beef

	C	F	Cb
Ground Beef, Raw: Per 4 oz			
73% lean (27% fat)	380	34	0
80% lean (20% fat)	290	22	0
85% lean (15% fat)	240	17	0
90% lean (10% fat)	200	11	0
93% lean (7% fat)	170	8	0
96% lean (4% fat)	150	4.5	0
Baked/Broiled: Reg., 3 oz	230	16	0
Lean (80%), 3 oz	230	15	0
Extra lean (90%), 3 oz	185	10	0
Pan-fried: Regular, 3 oz	230	15	0
Lean, 3 oz	230	15	0
Extra lean, 3 oz	195	10	0
Ground Beef Patties: Average (23% Fat)			
Frozen, raw, 4 oz	320	26	0
Broiled, 3 oz	240	17	0

Quick Guide

Roast Beef	C	F	Cb
Round (Eye/Tip, average) Average All Cuts			
Small Serving, 3 oz			
(2 thin slices/1 thick slice)			
Lean + fat (¼"), 3 oz	200	11	0
Lean only, 3 oz	150	5	0
Medium Serving, 5 oz (3-4 thin slices)			
Lean + fat, 5 oz	330	19	0
Lean only, 5 oz	245	9	0
Large Serving, 8 oz (3 thick slices)			
Lean + fat, 8 oz	525	30	0
Lean only, 8 oz	390	14	0

Roast Dinner Extras

	C	F	Cb
Gravy: Thin, 2 Tbsp	20	0.5	3.5
Thick, 2 Tbsp	50	2	0.5
1 Ladle/4 Tbsp	100	4	1
Veges: Beans, green, ½ cup	20	0	4
Cauliflower w. cheese sce, 4 oz	135	9	15
Corn, kernels, ¼ cup	35	0	9
Carrots, ¼ cup	20	0	3
Peas, ¼ cup	35	0	6
Pumpkin baked: w. fat, 4 oz	90	7	5
No added fat, 2 pces, 4 oz	25	0	5
Potato: Roasted w. fat, 1 small	155	8	30
Baked in Jacket, 1 large	280	0	63
with 1 Tbsp whipped butter	350	8	63
with Sour Cream, 2 Tbsp	270	5	64
Sweet Potato/Yam, 1 medium	105	1	24
Beef Kabobs: Beef & Veggies, 2 oz	160	10	4
If very lean meat	100	4	4

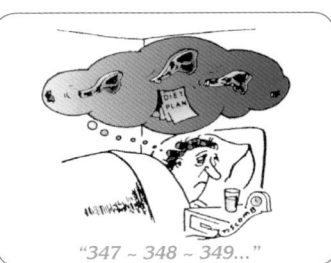

"347 ~ 348 ~ 349..."

Meat • Lamb, Veal, Pork

Lamb | C | F | Cb |

Choice Grade

Leg (Whole), roasted:
	C	F	Cb
Lean + fat, 3 oz	250	18	0
Lean only, 3 oz	155	6	0

Leg (Sirloin Half), roasted:
Lean + fat, 3 oz	250	18	0
Lean only, 3 oz	175	8	0

Leg (Shank Half), roasted:
Lean + fat, 3 oz	190	11	0
Lean only, 3 oz	155	6	0

Loin Chop, broiled:
1 chop (raw wt., 4¼ oz):
Lean + fat (2¼ oz edible)	180	12	0
Lean only (1.6 oz edible)	85	3.5	0

Rib Chop, broiled/roasted:
1 chop (raw wt., 3½ oz)
Lean + fat (2½ oz edible)	255	21	0
Lean only (1¾ oz edible)	105	6	0

Shoulder (Arm/Blade):
Braised: Lean + fat, 3 oz	290	21	0
Lean only, 3 oz	240	12	0
Broiled: Lean + fat, 3 oz	240	16	0
Lean only, 3 oz	170	8	0
Roasted: Similar to Broiled			

Cubed Lamb (Leg/Shoulder):
For stew or kabob
Raw, lean only, 8 oz	305	12	0
Braised, lean only, 3 oz	190	8	0
Broiled, lean only, 3 oz	160	6	0

New Zealand Lamb (Imported):
Similar calories and fat to domestic.

Veal | C | F | Cb |

Edible Weights

Leg (Top Round):
	C	F	Cb
Braised: Lean + fat, 3 oz	180	6	0
Lean only, 3 oz	170	5	0
Pan-fried, breaded:			
Lean + fat, 3 oz	195	8	9
Lean only, 3 oz	175	6	9
Pan-fried, not breaded:			
Lean + fat, 3 oz	180	7	0
Lean only, 3 oz	155	4	0
Roasted: Lean + fat, 3 oz	135	4	0
Lean only, 3 oz	130	3	0

Veal (Cont) | C | F | Cb |

Loin Chop: 1 chop, 7 oz raw wt.
	C	F	Cb
Braised: Lean + fat, 3 oz	240	14	0
Lean only, 3 oz	190	8	0
Roasted: Lean + fat, 3 oz	185	10	0
Lean only, 3 oz	150	6	0

Rib, roasted: Lean + fat, 3 oz
Lean + fat, 3 oz	195	12	0
Lean only, 3 oz	150	7	0

Shoulder, Arm/Blade, roasted:
Lean + fat, 3 oz	155	7	0
Lean only, 3 oz	145	6	0

Sirloin, roasted:
Lean + fat, 3 oz	170	9	0
Lean only, 3 oz	145	6	0

Cubed for Stew, braised:
Leg/Shoulder, lean only, 3 oz	160	4	0

(1 lb raw yields approx. 9¼ oz cooked)

Pork

Figures based on NLMB data (1990)

Fresh Pork (Cooked Wt., no bone)
(4 oz raw wt. = approx. 3 oz cooked wt.)

Blade Steak, broiled:
	C	F	Cb
Lean + fat, 3 oz	220	15	0
Lean only, 3 oz	190	11	0

Country Style Ribs, broiled:
Lean + fat, 3 oz	280	22	0
Lean only, 3 oz	210	13	0

Spareribs, braised: lean & fat, 6 oz
(from 1 lb raw wt)	675	51	0

Leg (Ham), roasted:
Lean + fat, 3 oz	230	15	0
Lean only, 3 oz	180	8	0
(Ham, cured ~ See Cold Meats)			

Loin Chops, broiled: Average
(From 1 chop: 5 oz raw wt. w. bone
or 4 oz raw wt., no bone
Lean + fat, 3 oz	200	11	0
Lean only, 3 oz	165	7	0

Rib Chops, broiled:
Lean + fat, 3 oz	220	14	0
Lean only, 3 oz	185	9	0

Rib Roast, roasted:
Lean + fat, 3 oz	215	13	0
Lean only, 3 oz	180	9	0

Loin Roast, roasted:
Lean + fat, 3 oz	190	10	0
Lean only, 3 oz	160	7	0

Pork (Cont) | C | F | Cb |

Pork (Cont)	C	F	Cb
Sirloin Chop, broiled:			
Lean + fat, 3 oz	175	8	0
Lean only, 3 oz	165	6	0
Sirloin Roast, roasted:			
Lean + fat, 3 oz	175	8	0
Lean only, 3 oz	170	7	0
Tenderloin, roasted:			
Lean + fat, 3 oz	147	5	0
Lean only, 3 oz	140	4	0
Ground Pork			
Raw: Average, ¼ lb, 4 oz	300	24	0
Broiled, 3 oz	250	18	0
Pan-fried, drained, 3 oz	260	19	0

Bacon

Bacon	C	F	Cb
Raw: 1 med. slice (20 lb), ¾ oz	95	9	0
1 thick slice (12 lb), 1⅓ oz	175	17	0
(1 lb raw yields approx. 5 oz cooked)			
Broiled/Pan-Fried: 1 med. sl., 8 g	40	3	0
3 medium slices, 24g	125	10	0
2 thin slices, ½ oz	75	6	0
1 thick slice, 12g	65	5	0
Canadian-style: Cooked, 1 slice	35	1.5	0.5
As purchased, 1 slice, 1 oz	35	1.5	0.5
Bacon Bits, 1 Tbsp, ¼ oz	35	2.5	0
Breakfast Strips, Broil., 1 sl., 12 g	50	4	0

Ham

Ham	C	F	Cb
Boneless Ham, cooked:			
Regular, (approx. 11% fat):			
Unheated (as purch.), 1 oz	50	2.5	0
Roasted, 3 oz	150	8	0
Extra Lean (5% fat):			
Unheated, 1 oz	45	2.5	0
Roasted, 3 oz	125	5	0
Whole Ham, cooked:			
Lean + fat (as purchased)			
Unheated, 1 oz	70	5	0
Roasted, 3 oz	210	15	0
Lean only, unheated, 1 oz	40	2	0
Roasted, 3 oz	135	5	0
Canned Ham, Similar to boneless ham			
Chopped, canned, 3 oz	200	16	0
Ham Patties, ckd, 1 pty, 2¼ oz	215	20	1
Ham Steak, extra lean, 2 oz	70	2.5	0
Luncheon Slices: See Deli Meats, Page 53			

Game & Other Meats

Game & Other Meats	C	F	Cb
Bison Steak,			
lean, 6 oz (raw)	205	4	0
Boar (wild), roasted, 3 oz	140	4	0
Buffalo Steak: New West Foods, 4 oz	70	3	0
Trader Joes, 1 patty	430	30	1
Caribou, roasted, 3 oz	140	4	0
Deer/Venison, roasted 3 oz	135	3	0
Goat (Capretto): Raw, 3 oz	95	2	0
Roasted, 3 oz	120	2.5	0
Ostrich: Blackwing Ostrich Meats,			
Sport Jerky, ½ oz pce	25	0	0
Sausage Patties (2) 2 oz	60	0.5	0
New West Foods:			
Ground Ostrich, 4 oz	165	7	0
Ostrich Steak, 4 oz steak	130	2.5	0
Rabbit: Roasted, 3 oz	165	7	0
Stewed, 1 cup, diced, 5 oz	290	12	0

Variety & Organ Meats

Variety & Organ Meats	C	F	Cb
Brains: Braised, 3 oz	130	9	0
Pan-fried, 3 oz	200	14	0
Chitterlings, pork, simmered, 3 oz	200	17	0
Ears, pork, simmered, 1 ear	185	12	0
Feet, pork: Simmered, 3 oz	200	14	0
Cured, pickled, 3 oz	170	14	0
Hormel, 2 oz	80	6	0
Head Cheese (Pork Snouts/Ears/Vinegar/Spices):			
1 oz slice	50	4	0
Heart: Average, braised, 3 oz	125	5	0
Jowl, pork, raw, 4 oz	750	80	0
Kidneys, simmered, 3 oz	135	4	0
Liver (beef): Raw, 4 oz	150	4	4
Braised, 3 oz	145	4	4
Pan-fried, 3 oz	160	4.5	4
Pancreas, pork, braised, 3 oz	185	8	0
Pork Cracklins, 0.5 oz	80	6	0
Pork Hocks, 1 piece, 6 oz	340	23	0
Scrapple, pork, 2 oz	120	8	8
Spleen, pork, braised, 3 oz	130	3	0
Stomach, pork, raw, 4 oz	185	12	0
Sweetbreads: Beef, ckd., 3 oz	125	9	0
Lamb, cooked, 3 oz	125	9	0
Tail, pork, simmered, 3 oz	340	31	0
Tongue: braised, 3 oz: Veal	170	9	0
Beef/Lamb/Pork, average, 3 oz	235	17	0
Tripe, beef, raw, 4 oz	95	4	0
Lean + fat, 3 oz	80	3.5	1.5

Sausages, Franks

Quick Guide

Franks & Weiners
Average All Brands

	C	F	Cb
Regular/Smoked: *Per Frank*			
Regular, 1.5oz (10/16oz pkg)	140	13	1
Jumbo, 2 oz (8/16 oz pkg)	170	16	0
Bun Length, 2 oz	180	17	2
Extra Long, 2.75 oz	240	21	2
Small/Cocktail (50/lb) each	30	3	0.5
Beef Franks: *Per Frank*			
Regular, 1.6 oz (10/16 oz pkg)	140	13	2
Jumbo, 2 oz (8/16 oz pkg)	170	15	2
Bun Length, 2 oz	180	16	2
¼ lb Dog, 4 oz	300	24	4

Brands

	C	F	Cb
Ball Park			
Reg./Smoked, Fat-Free (1), 1.76 oz	40	0	4
Beef: Fat-Free, 1.76 oz link	45	0	5
Reduced-Fa, 2 oz link	100	7	3
Turkey Franks, 1.76 oz link	45	0	5
Beef Kosher			
Beef: 2 oz link	180	14	4
2.6 oz link (6/16 oz)	230	19	6
Foster Farms			
Chicken Franks, 2 oz (8/16 oz)	140	12	1
Healthy Choice			
Turkey Franks, 1.76 oz link	70	2.5	6
Hebrew National			
Beef: 1.72 oz link	150	14	1
14 lb link, 4 oz	340	32	1
97% Fat-Free, 1.72 oz link	50	1.5	2
Jennie-O			
Turkey Franks: 1 oz link	70	5	1
2 oz link	120	10	2
Oscar Mayer			
Reg./Smoked, Fat-Free, 1.76 oz link	40	0	3
Beef, Reduced-Fat, 2 oz link	110	8	2
Cheese Frank, 1.6 oz link	140	13	1
Turkey Frank: 1.6 oz link	100	8	2
2 oz link	120	10	3
Shelton's			
Chicken Franks, 1.2 oz link	70	6	0
Turkey Franks, 1.2 oz link	60	4.5	1
Zacky Farms			
Chicken Frank, 2 oz link	160	12	1

Vegetarian Sausages

See Frozen/Canned & Packaged Meals

Quick Guide

Fresh Sausages
Pork/Beef: *Average All Types*

	C	F	Cb
Small: Raw, 4" link, 1 oz	85	7.5	0
Broiled/Pan-fried	80	7	0
Medium: Raw, 2 oz	170	15	0
Broiled/Pan-fried	165	14	0
Large: Raw, 3 oz	255	22	0
Broiled/Pan-fried	245	21	0
Italian: Raw, 3.2 oz	315	28	0.5
Cooked, 2.4 oz	230	18	3
Chorizo: Beef Chorizo, 2.5 oz pce	250	23	5
Pork Chorizo, 2 oz piece	250	23	5

Note: Fat is lost in broiling/pan frying. (Cooked wt. = approx. 60-70% raw wt.)

Smoked Sausage

	C	F	Cb
Average All Brands: 2 oz link	170	15	0
3 oz link	255	22	0
Ball Park, Bun Size, 2 oz	180	17	2
Butterball (w. Turkey), 2 oz	100	6	4
Eckrich, 2 oz	180	16	2
Healthy Choice, Beef/Polska, 2 oz	80	2.5	6

Breakfast Sausages/Patties

	C	F	Cb
Armour Brown 'n Serve			
Pork/Turkey, 3 links, 2.1 oz	210	19	2
Lite Original, 3 links	120	8	3
Beef Sausage, 3 links, 2 oz	230	22	1
Butterball: Turkey Brkfast Pats (2)	120	7	2
Turkey Breakfast Links (3)	120	8	2
Healthy Choice, Patties/Links (3), 2 oz	70	3	3
Jennie-O, Italian Turkey Saus. (2)	160	10	0
Jimmy Dean: Pork Saus. Patties (2)	260	24	0
Pork Sausage Links: Original (3)	290	28	0
Country Maple (3)	230	20	3
Breakfast Sandwiches: *See Page 47*			
Jones/Golden Brown:			
Pork Sausage Patties: Original (1)	75	7	0.5
All Natural (1)	95	9	0
Sandwich Patties (1)	170	16	1
Pork Sausage Links: 2 links	180	18	2
Light, 2 links	110	8	1
Swanson 'Great Starts': *See Page 47*			

Vegetarian Patties:
Boca: *See Page 61*
Garden Burger: *See Page 62*

BAR-B-Q CHICKEN & RI...

Bagel, Corn & Hot Dogs

Hot Dogs, Ready-To-Go

	C	F	Cb
(Includes Ketchup/Relish; no Mayo)			
Regular (1.5 oz frank, 1.5 oz bun)	260	15	22
Bun Length (2 oz frank, 1.5 oz bun)	290	18	21
Jumbo Dog (2 oz frank, 2 oz bun)	360	20	36
¼ lb Beef Dog (¼ lb dog, 2 oz bun)	480	15	36
Mile Long Dog (2.6 oz dog, 1.5 oz bun)	360	24	23

Weinerschnitzel: *See Fast-Foods*

Corn Dogs

Beef/Pork Frank: Average, 2.6 oz	170	10	16
Foster Farms Chicken Franks:			
1 dog, 2.6 oz (75g)	180	10	15
Chili Cheese, 1 dog, 2.6 oz (75g)	200	9	24
Mini Corn Dogs (4), 2.68 oz	210	12	18
Oscar Mayer Turkey & Pork, 3.2 oz	260	15	25
State Fair w. Ball Park Franks,			
Corn Dogs, 1 dog, 2.7 oz (76g)	210	12	23
Mini Corn Dogs (4)	230	13	22

Bagel Dogs

Best's Kosher: 1 dog, 1 oz	320	11	43
Mini, 1 piece, 0.8 oz	60	2	8
Vienna Beef: 1 piece, 1 oz	85	3.5	7

Hot Dog Toppings/Extras:

American Chse, 1 slice, 1 oz	110	9	1
Catsup, 1 Tbsp	16	0	4
Chili (w. Beans), ¼ cup	70	3.5	9
Mustard, 1 Tbsp	20	0	1
Pickle Relish, 1 Tbsp	20	0	5
Sauerkraut, ½ cup	20	0	5

WILL-POWER TONIC
~ RECIPE ~

• 1 Cup of Desire
• 1 Quart of Determination
• 1 Tbsp of Common Sense
• 1 Tbsp of Stick-to-itiveness
• 1 Tbsp of Foresight
• 1 Cup of Energy

Deli & Luncheon Meats

Beef Jerky:	C	F	Cb
Bridgeford Beef Jerky, 1 oz	100	0.5	5
Beef Stick (5.5 oz stick), 1 oz	150	13	2
Beef Steak, 1 oz	70	0.5	2
Beef & Cheese (Giant Size),			
½ pkg, 1.5 oz	170	14	1
Pepperoni Sticks (2), 1 oz	160	13	2
Pepperoni (1" diam.), 1 oz	130	12	0
Teriyaki, 1 oz pkg	80	0.5	4
Original; Hot 'n Spicy	70	1	5
Berliner (pork/beef), 1 oz	65	5	1
Beerwurst (Beef):			
Small (2.75"diam), ¹⁄₁₆" slice	20	2	0
Large (4"diam), ⅛" slice	75	7	0.5
Beerwurst (Pork):			
Small (2.75"diam), ¹⁄₁₆" slice	15	1	0
Large (4"diam), ⅛" Slice	55	4	0.5
Bologna: 1 Slice	65	6	1
Fat-Free, 1 slice, 1 oz	20	0	2
Beef Bologna: 1 slice, 1 oz	90	8	1
Light, 1 slice, 1 oz	60	4	2
Light (Oscar Mayer), 1 sl., 1 oz	60	4	2
Red. Fat (Hebrew Nat.), 2 sl.,1 oz	40	2.5	0.5
Fat Free (Osc. M.), 2 sl., 1.6 oz	40	0	1
Healthy Choice, 1 oz	35	1	3
Weight Watchers, 2 sl., ¾ oz	35	2	0
Beef (Tyson), 1 slice	80	7	1
Ring (Boar's Head), 2 oz	145	13	0
Turkey, average, 1 oz	60	5	0.5
Blood Sausage, 1 oz	100	9	0.5
Bratwurst: Average, 1 oz	80	7	1
Boar's Head, cook., 1 wurst, 4 oz	300	25	0
Bob Evan's, Beer, 2.6 oz link	270	21	1
Braunschweiger (Pork/Liver/Sausage),			
Oscar Mayer, 1 oz slice	110	10	1
Chicken, Average All Brands			
1 thick or 2 thin slices, 2 oz	30	1	1
Chicken Roll, 1 slice, 2 oz	90	4	1.5
Corned Beef: Average, full fat, 1 oz	60	5	0.5
Healthy Choice, Hillshire Farm, 1oz	30	1	0
Hebrew National, 4 slices, 2 oz	90	4.5	0
Loaf, jellied, 1 oz	45	2	0
Hash, canned, average, 1 oz	50	3	3
Dutch Brand Loaf, average, 1 oz	70	5	1.5

Continued Next Page

Deli & Luncheon Meats

Ham, Luncheon:	C	F	Cb
Baked/Boiled, sliced, 1 oz	30	1	0.5
Chopped: *Eckrich (97% FF), 1 oz*	25	1	1
Armour: Canned, 1 oz	35	1.5	0.5
97% Fat Free, 1 oz	25	1	1.5
Healthy Choice, 2 sl., 2 oz	60	1.5	1
Hormel (Black Label), 1 oz	70	6	0
Oscar Mayer, 1 oz slice	60	2	0.5
Honey/Brown Sugar: Avg., 1 oz	30	1	1
Healthy Choice Deli Traditions:			
2 slices, 2 oz	60	1.5	2
Prosciutto, average, 1 oz	70	5	0
Ham & Cheese Loaf, avg., 1 oz	70	5	1
Head Cheese *(Osc. Mayer),* 1 oz sl.	50	4	0
Honey Loaf *(Osc. Mayer),* 1 oz sl.	35	1	2
Italian Sausage, 2.6 oz	250	20	3
Kielbasa *(Polish Sausage),* 1 oz	65	5	1
Scott Petersen, 3.4 oz link	320	27	4
Beef, 2 oz link	190	17	1
Boar's Head, 1 oz	60	5	0
Kippered Beefsteak:			
Hickory Farms, 3 slices, 0.75 oz	50	1	1
Knockwurst, 1 oz	90	8	0.5
Linguica *(Gaspar's),* 2 oz	180	8	1
Liverwurst, 1 oz	65	5	2
Liver Pate, fresh, average, 1 oz	90	8	1
Luncheon Loaf *(Foods Co),* 1 oz	65	5	2
Mortadella, 1 oz	105	9	0
Olive Loaf: Average, 1 oz	70	5	3
Oscar Mayer, 1 oz slice	75	6	2
Pastrami (Beef): Average, 1 oz	45	3	0.5
Healthy Deli, 1 oz	34	1	0.5
Hillshire (DeliSelect), 6 sl., 2 oz	60	1	0
Boar's Head, 2 oz	70	4	0
Peppered Beef, 1 oz slice	40	2	0
Pepperoni, 5 slices, 1 oz	140	13	0
Pickle Loaf, average, 1 oz	70	5	5
Pickle & Pimento Loaf			
Oscar Mayer, 1 oz	75	6	3
Polish Sausage: *See Kielbasa*			
Proscuitto/Prosciutti: Avg., 1 oz	70	5	1
Hormel, 1 oz	90	7	1
Roast Beef: Lean, 1 oz	40	2	0
Healthy Choice, all types, 2 oz	60	1.5	4
Salami: Beef, average, 1 oz	80	7	1
Beer Salami, average, 1 oz	50	4	0.5
Cotto: *Oscar Mayer,* 1 slice, 1 oz	70	6	1
Dry: Hard, avg., 4 slices, 1 oz	110	10	3
Oscar Mayer, 2 slices, 1.6 oz	100	8	1

Salami (Cont):	C	F	Cb
Genoa: Average, 1 oz	120	9	1
Stick *(Best's Kosher),* 2, 1.75 oz	180	15	2
Italian *(Bridgeford),* 1 oz	120	11	0
Turkey, average, 1 oz	55	4	1
Spam *(Hormel):*			
Regular: ¼" slice, 1 oz	90	8	1
½" slice, 2 oz	180	16	2
Lite: ¼" slice, 1 oz	55	4	0
½" slice, 2 oz	110	8	1
Turkey: ¼" slice, 1 oz	40	2	1
½" slice, 2 oz	80	4	2
Singles: Classic, 3 oz pkg	210	16	2
Turkey, 3 oz pkg	110	4	3
Summer Sausage:			
Bridgeford, 1 oz	100	9	1
Oscar Mayer, 1 slice, 0.8 oz	70	7	0.5
Treet *(Armour),* canned, 1 oz	100	9	1.5
Turkey: Average, 1 oz slice	30	1	0.5
¾ oz slice	22	0.5	0.5
Turkey Breast:			
Butterball Fat Free, 3 sl., 2 oz	60	0	4
Deli Thin Smoked, 2 sl., 1 oz	50	0.5	2
Hillshire Deli Select, 6 sl., 2 oz	50	0.5	2
Louis Rich Carvery Board,			
2 slices, 1.8 oz (52g)	50	0	2
Free, 2 slices, 2 oz	50	0	2
Healthy Choice: Deli Thin: Per 4 Slices, 52g (1.8 oz)			
Oven-Roasted	60	1.5	2
Smoked/Rotisserie Seasoned	60	1.5	3
Honey Roasted & Smoked	60	1.5	4
Hearty Deli Sliced:			
Oven Rstd Turkey Brst. 1 sl., 1 oz	30	1	1
Turkey Ham, 1 slice, 1 oz	35	1.5	0.5
Turkey Pastrami, 1 oz	35	1.5	1
Turkey Roll, 1 oz	40	2	0.5
Turkey Loaf, 1 oz	30	1	0.5
Vegetarian Deli *(Worthington, Yves): See Page 76*			

Meat Spreads

	C	F	Cb
Average All Brands: Per ¼ Cup (2 oz)			
Chicken	90	10	2
Ham, deviled	140	11	0
Liverwurst	190	16	2
Roast Beef	130	10	2
Sandwich Spread	140	10	9
Turkey	110	7	2

Paté

	C	**F**	**Cb**
Canned: *Average All Brands*			
Chicken Liver, 2 Tbsp, 1 oz	60	4	2
Paté de Foie Gras, goose liver, 1 oz	130	12	2
Fresh (Refrigerated):			
Average all types, 1 oz	110	10	1
Boar's Head Liverwurst Pate, 2 oz	145	12	0
Marcel Henri			
Pate de Champagne	210	18	2
Chicken Liver w. Port Wine, 2 oz	210	18	2
Duck Truffle w. Port Wine, 2 oz	240	24	2
Old Wisconsin Pate			
All types, 1 oz	105	9	1.5
Vegetable Pate; Spin/Mushr., 2 oz	105	7	10
Trois Petit Cochons			
Mediterranean, 2 oz	130	11	3
Smoked Salmon, 2 oz	115	9	2
Wegmans			
Alexian Wild, 2 oz	270	27	1
Cognac; Black Peppercorn, 2 oz	160	17	4

Lunch Packs

	C	**F**	**Cb**
Lunchables *(Oscar Mayer): Per Package*			
Cracker Stackers Ham & Cheddar	420	23	37
Nachos Cheese & Salsa, 4.4 oz	380	21	39
Pizza varieties, avg., 4.5 oz	300	13	28
Taco Bell Beef Tacos, 5.35 oz	310	11	34
Fun Fuel: Ham Bagels, 5.6 oz	410	10	64
Chicken/Ham Wraps, 5.5 oz	435	13	64
Peanut Butter Soft White Bread	600	19	85
Turkey Bagels, 5.6 oz	420	10	64
Pizza Dunks Soft Breadsticks	500	13	84
Beef Taco, 5.7 oz	495	15	69
Waffles & Sausage, 4.8 oz	460	16	66
Fun Snacks: Chips Ahoy!, 3.1 oz	200	9	30
Fudge Brownie, 4.3 oz	260	9	42
Oreo Cookies 'N Frosting, 3.7 oz	230	9	37
S'Mores, 3.4 oz	200	6	35
Star Cookies 'N Frosting, 3.6 oz	230	10	34
Mega Pack: Combo Ham & Ched.	765	32	101
Combo Turkey & Cheddar, 5.4 oz	750	31	101
Pizza: Pepperoni, 6.85 oz	760	28	105
Extra Cheesy, 6.8 oz	700	25	104
Pizza Stix, 7.15 oz	680	16	118
Ultimate Nachos Cheese & Salsa	780	32	113
Lunch Bucket *(Armour)*			
Beans 'n Weiners, 7.5 oz	290	10	37
Chili w. Beans, 7.5 oz	235	9	25
Hearty Beef Stew, 7.5 oz	155	8	15
Rings 'n Franks, 7.5 oz	225	9	30
Lunchmakers *(Armour)*			
Loco Nachos	370	13	59
Cheese Pizza	310	13	36
Smuckers			
Snackers, 3.3 oz package	410	20	47
Uncrustables Sandwiches:			
Grilled Cheese Sandwich, 1.76 oz	150	6	17
Peanut Butter Sandwich, 1.72 oz	200	11	18
Peanut Butter & Honey, 1.76 oz	210	9	26
Peanut Butter & Grape Jelly: 1.76 oz	210	9	25
Large, 80g	320	16	33
Peanut Butter & Strawb. Jam: 1.76 oz	210	9	25
Large, 80g	320	16	33
South Beach Diet *(Kraft)*			
Wraps: *Per Package*			
Deli Ham & Turkey, 1 pkg	220	10	24
Grilled Chicken Caesar, 1 pkg	230	10	24
Southwestern Style Chicken	240	10	26
Turkey & Bacon Club, 1 pkg	250	12	25

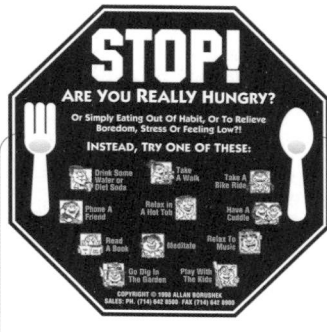

Chicken

Quick Guide

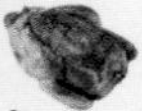

	C	F	Cb
Chicken			
From 3lb ready-to-cook chicken			
Breast/Wing Quarter			
Roasted: With skin	300	15	0
Without skin	185	5	0
Fried, batter dipped	530	30	17
Leg Quarter: Thigh & Drumstick			
Roasted: With skin	270	16	0
Without skin	185	5	0
Fried, batter dipped	435	25	15
KFC: See Fast-Foods Section			

Average - All Meats

	C	F	Cb
Average of Light Meat: Per 4 oz (no bone)			
Roasted: with skin	250	12	0
without skin	190	5	0
Stewed: with skin	225	12	0
without skin	180	4.5	0
Fried: Batter-dipped, 4 oz	310	17	12
Flour coated, 4 oz	275	14	2
Average of Dark Meat: Per 4 oz (no bone)			
Roasted: with skin	285	18	0
without skin	230	12	0
Stewed: with skin	260	16	0
without skin	215	10	0
Fried: Batter-dipped, 4 oz	330	21	12
Flour coated, 4 oz	320	20	5

Chicken Parts

	C	F	Cb
Broilers or Fryers: Edible Weights (no bone)			
Breast: Per ½ Breast			
Raw: With skin, 5 oz	240	13	0
Without skin, 4¼ oz	130	1.5	0
Roasted: With skin, 3½ oz	195	8	0
Without skin, 3 oz	140	3	0
Stewed: With skin, 4 oz	210	8	0
Without skin, 3¼ oz	145	3	0
Fried: Batter-dipped, 5 oz	365	19	12
Flour coated, w. skin, 3½ oz	220	9	7
Drumstick: Per Drumstick			
Roasted: With skin, 2 oz	115	6	0
Without skin, 1½ oz	75	2.5	0
Fried: Batter-dipped, 2½ oz	195	11	7
Flour coated, 1¾ oz	120	7	1
Stewed: With skin, 2 oz	115	6	0
Without skin, 1½ oz	80	3	0

	C	F	Cb
Thigh Portion: Edible Wt. (no bone)			
Raw: With skin, 3.3 oz			
(4¼ oz with bone)	200	14	0
Without skin, 2.4 oz	80	3	0
Roasted: With skin, 2¼ oz	155	10	0
Without skin, 2 oz	110	6	0
Stewed: With skin, 2½ oz	160	10	0
Without skin, 2 oz	105	5	0
Fried: Batter-dipped, 3 oz	240	14	8
Flour coated, 2¼ oz	165	9	2
Wing: Per Wing			
Raw Weight 3.2 oz (with bone)			
Raw: With skin	110	8	0
Without skin	35	1	0
Roasted: With skin	100	7	0
Without skin	45	2	0
Fried: Batter-dipped	160	11	5
Flour coated	105	7	1
Stewed: With skin, 4 oz	100	7	0
Buffalo Wings: See Fast-Foods Section			
Neck: Simmered, with skin	95	7	0
Without skin	30	2	0
Skin Only: Skin from ½ Chicken			
Raw skin, 2¾ oz	275	26	0
Roasted skin, 2 oz	255	23	0
Stewed skin, 2½ oz	260	24	0
Fried, Flour coated, 2 oz	280	24	5
Fried, Batter-dipped, 6¾ oz	750	55	45
Roasters			
Average of Light & Dark Meat:			
Roasted: With skin, 4 oz	250	15	0
Without skin, 4 oz	190	8	0
Light Meat: Without skin, roasted	175	5	0
Dark Meat: Without skin, roasted	200	10	0
Stewing Chicken			
Average of Light & Dark Meat: Per 4 oz Stewed			
With skin	320	21	0
Without skin	265	14	0
Light Meat: Without skin	240	9	0
Dark Meat: Without skin	290	17	0
Capon Chicken			
Roasted: With skin, 4 oz	260	13	0
½ Chicken, with skin	1460	74	0
Chicken Offal & Stuffing			
Giblets: Simmered, 1 cup	230	7	0.5
Fried, flour-coated, 1 cup	400	20	6
Gizzard, simmered, 1 cup	225	4	0
Heart, simmered, 1 cup	270	12	0.2
Liver: Raw, 4 oz	135	5.5	1
Simmered, 1 cup	215	8.5	1
Liver Pate Fresh, 1 Tbsp, ½ oz	30	2	1
Stuffing: Average, ½ cup	180	9	22

Chicken Products   **C** **F** **Cb**

Shop Stop

	C	F	Cb
Blazing Chicken Wings, 3 oz	200	12	1
Breaded Tenderloins (3), 4 oz	240	12	15
Boneless Skinless Breasts (1), 8 oz	210	5	3

Stove Top

	C	F	Cb
Chicken Stuffing Mix: 1 oz	110	1	20
½ cup prepared	170	9	20
Tyson: Breaded Nuggets (5)	280	18	16
Breast Nuggets (5)	280	16	21
Southern Fried Nuggets (6)	270	21	11
Breast Patties: Regular, 2.6 oz	180	11	10
Southern Fried (1), 2.6 oz	240	18	12
Wings: Flavored, average (3)	220	15	1
BBQ Style (3), 3½ oz	250	15	13
Stir Fry Kit: Chicken, 2¾ c. froz.	430	4.5	73

Duck, Goose, Quail

	C	F	Cb
Duck: Roasted, with skin, 3 oz	285	24	0
Without skin, 3 oz	170	10	0
½ whole duck, with skin	1290	108	0
Goose: Roast, with skin, 3 oz	260	19	0
Without skin, 3 oz	200	11	0
Pheasant: ½ bird, raw	725	37	0
Quail: 1 whole, raw	210	13	0

Turkey

Fryer-Roasters: *Per 3 oz Serving*

	C	F	Cb
Roasted: Light Meat, with skin	140	4	0
without skin	120	1	0
Dark Meat: with skin	155	6	0
without skin	140	4	0

½ of Whole Turkey: (Approx. 3¼ lbs raw wt. w/out neck and giblets; 1.8 lbs cooked wt.)

	C	F	Cb
Roasted: With skin	1400	46	0
Without skin	1030	18	0

Ground Turkey, Raw: (4 oz raw wt. = 3 oz ckd wt.)

	C	F	Cb
Regular (85% lean), 4 oz	170	12	0
Lean (90% lean), 4 oz	160	8	0
Foster Farms (94% lean), 4 oz	150	7	0
Jennie-O (93% lean), 4 oz	160	8	0
Breast, no skin, 4 oz	115	1	0
Patties: Small, 3 oz	110	6.5	0
Medium, 4 oz	160	9	0
Large, 5.3 oz	175	10	0

Turkey Parts   **C** **F** **Cb**

Roasted, Edible Weights (no bone)

Breast (½): (from 17¼ oz raw wt. w/bone)

	C	F	Cb
With skin, 12 oz (no bone)	525	11	0
Without skin, 10¾ oz	415	2	0

Back (½):

	C	F	Cb
With skin, 4½ oz	305	18	0
Without skin, 3½ oz	165	6	0

Leg (Thigh & Drumstick): (from 1 lb raw wt. w/bone)

	C	F	Cb
With skin, 8½ oz (no bone)	345	16	0
Without skin, 7¾ oz	235	5	0

Wing: (from 7¼ oz raw wt. w/bone)

	C	F	Cb
With skin, 3 oz (no bone)	185	9	0
Without skin, 2 oz	100	2	0

Neck: Simmered, 1 neck,

	C	F	Cb
(9 oz w. bone)	275	11	0
Giblets, simm., 1 cup, 5 oz	240	7	3

Young Hens (Roasted)

	C	F	Cb
Light Meat: With skin, 3 oz	175	8	0
Without skin, 3 oz	135	3	0
Dark Meat: With skin, 3 oz	200	11	0
Without skin, 3 oz	165	7	0
Young Toms — Similar to Young Hens			

Turkey Products

	C	F	Cb
Banquet: See Frozen Meals, Page 61			
Circle L: Boneless Bacon, 3 oz	120	9	1
Hormel: Turkey Ham & Chunks (canned), ckd:			
Breast & White Turkey, 2 oz	60	1	2
Turkey Ham/Pastrami, 2 oz	70	3	1
Turkey Salami, 2 oz	100	8	0
Jennie-O: Turkey Bacon, 2 slice	35	3	0
Turkey in BBQ Sauce, 5 oz	200	2	17
Louis Rich: 98% Fat Free Breast of Turkey			
Rotiss'd/Smoked/Rstd, 2 oz, 3 sl.	60	0	0
Franks: Medium, 1½ oz	100	8	2
Large, 2 oz	125	10	3.5
Smoked Sausage/Kielbasa, 1 oz	45	2.5	1
Turkey Bacon, 1 oz	70	5	0
Turkey Nuggets/Sticks, ckd, ea.	75	5	4.5
Luncheon Slices: See Deli Meats, Page 54			
Swanson: Frozen Meals, Page 67			
Turkey Store (Jennie-O)			
Gobble Stix (1)	25	0	1

Fish ~ Fresh & Canned

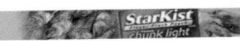

Quick Guide

Fresh Fish

C F Cb

Low Oil (Less than 2.5% fat)
White/pale colored flesh. Examples:
Cod, Flounder, Haddock, Halibut, Mahi Mahi
Perch, Pike, Pollock, Snapper, Sole, Whiting.

Per 4 oz Edible Portion

	C	F	Cb
Raw, 4 oz (no bones)	90	1	0
Steamed, Broiled, Baked	130	1	0
Fried: Lightly Floured	210	8	3.5
Breaded	260	12	8
In Batter	320	16	27

Medium Oil (2.5-5% fat)

C F Cb

Pale colored flesh. Examples:
Bluefin Tuna, Catfish, Kingfish, Orange Roughy,
Salmon (Pink), Swordfish, Rainbow Trout, Yellowtail.

	C	F	Cb
Raw, 4 oz (no bones)	140	4	0
Baked, Broiled, 4 oz	175	6	0
Fried, 4 oz	230	11	8

High Oil (Over 5% fat)

C F Cb

Darker colored flesh. Examples:
Albacore Tuna, Bluefish, Herring, Mackerel,
Salmon (Atl./Chinook/Sockeye), Sardines, Trout,
Whitefish.

	C	F	Cb
Raw, 4 oz (no bones)	230	16	0
Baked, Broiled, 4 oz	275	17	0
Fried, 4 oz	340	23	12

Cooking Yields (Fin Fish):

4 oz Raw wt. = 3 ½ oz Cooked wt.
4 oz Cooked wt. = 5 oz Raw wt.

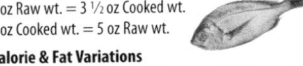

Calorie & Fat Variations

The amount of fat/oil in fish varies with the species,
season and locality. Within the same fish, fat/oil content
is generally higher towards the head.

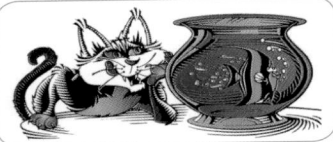

Fish & Shellfish

C F Cb

Edible Weights: (no bones/shell)

	C	F	Cb
Abalone, Raw, 3 oz	90	0.5	5
Ahi Tuna, grilled, 6 oz fillet (no fat)	220	2	0
Anchovy: Paste, 1 Tbsp, ¼ oz	15	1	0.5
Cnd. in oil, drnd., 5 only, ¾ oz	40	2	0
Pickled, 1 oz	50	3	0
Barracuda (Pacific), raw, 4 oz	130	3	0
Bass: Sea, raw, 4.6 oz fillet	125	2.5	0
Striped: Raw, 1 fillet, 5½ oz	150	3.5	0
Baked, 3 oz	105	3	0
Blue Fish: Raw, 1 fillet, 5¼ oz	185	6.5	0
Baked, 3 oz	130	5	0
Butterfish, raw, 3 oz	125	7	0
Cajun & Creole Dishes: *See Page 176*			
Calamari, breaded/fried, 1 serve	360	21	10
Carp, raw, 3 oz	110	5	0
Catfish: Raw, 4 oz	115	6.5	0
Fried, breaded, 1 fillet, 3 oz	200	12	7
Baked, 3 oz	130	7	0
Caviar, black/red, 1 Tbsp, 16g	40	3	0.5
Clams: Raw, 3 oz (4 lge/9 small)	65	1	2
Fried, breaded, 6.6 oz (20 small)	380	21	20
Canned, drained, ½ cup, 2½ oz	105	1.5	3.5
Minced, ¼ cup, 2 oz	25	0	1
Clam Juice: (*Snow's*) 1 Tbsp	0	0	0
Cod, Atlantic/Pacific: Raw, 4 oz	95	1	0
Baked/Broiled, 1 fillet, 6¼ oz	190	2	0
Canned, 3 oz	90	1	0
Minced, ¼ cup, 2 oz	25	0	0
Smoked/Dry Heat, 3 oz	95	1	0
Crab: Alaska King, 1 leg, 6 oz	145	2	0
1 leg, cooked, 4¾ oz	130	2	0
Blue: Raw, 1 crab			
(⅓ lb whole crab, ¾ oz flesh)	20	0.2	0
Steamed, 3 oz	85	1	0
Canned, drained, ½ cup, 2½ oz	65	1	0
Dungeness, 1 crab, 5¾ oz edible			
(from 1½ lb whole crab)	180	2	2
Imitation Crab Legs/Stix, 3oz	85	1	8.5
Crab Cakes (Low-fat), (1), 2 oz	95	4.5	0.5
Regular (1), 3 oz	130	6.5	0.5
Crab Legs, restaurant (*Red Lobster*)	260	4.5	0
Crayfish, raw, 4 oz (edible)	100	1	0
Croaker, raw, 3 oz	90	3	0
Cuttlefish, raw, 3 oz	70	1	1
Dolphinfish, raw, 1 fillet, 7 oz	175	1.5	0
Eel: Raw, 3 oz	155	10	0
Smoked/Dry Heat, 3 oz	200	13	0
Fish & Chips: *Arthur Treacher*	1540	101	132
Denny's, no condiments	960	54	83
Fish S'wich w. Tartar Sce, 5½ oz	430	23	41
Fish Sticks (1), frozen, breaded, 1 oz	70	3.5	6

Fish & Shellfish (Cont)

Edible Weights: (no bones/shell)	C	F	Cb
Fish Oil, 1 Tbsp, ½ oz	125	14	0
Flounder/Sole: Raw, 4 oz	105	1.5	0
Baked, 1 fillet, 4½ oz	150	2	0
Frozen Fish & Entrees: See Page 60			
Gefilte Fish: See Kosher/Deli Foods, Page 179			
Grouper, raw, 4 oz	105	1	0
Haddock, raw, 4 oz	100	1	0
Broiled, 1 fillet, 5¼ oz	170	1.5	0
Smoked, 3 oz	100	1	0
Baked, 3 oz	90	1	0
Halibut: Raw, 4 oz	125	3	0
Baked, ½ fillet, 2¾ oz	225	5	0
Herring: Atlantic, raw, 4 oz	180	10	0
Pickled, 2 pieces, 1 oz	80	5	3
In Sour Cream, 1 oz	55	3	5
Party Snacks, ¼ cup, dr., 2 oz	120	5	0
Rollmops, 1½ oz	110	8	6
Canned: Plain, drained, 3 oz	130	8	0
in Tomato Sauce, 3.5 oz	140	8	2
Smoked, kippered, 4 oz	245	14	0
Jellyfish: Raw, 4 oz	30	0	0
Dried, Salted, 1 cup, 2 oz	20	1	0
King Fish, raw, 4 oz	120	2.5	0
Ling, raw, 4 oz	100	0.5	0
Lobster, Northern: Raw, 4 oz	105	1	0.5
1 Lobster, 6¼ oz			
(from 1½ lb whole lobster)	160	1.5	1
Cooked, 1 cup, 5 oz	140	1	2
Lobster Newberg, ¾ cup	360	20	9
Lobster Thermidor, 1 serving	370	22	15
Lobster Salads, ½ cup	220	13	5
Lobster Tail, restaurant (Red Lobster)	260	3	0
Lomi Salmon, ¼ cup, 4 oz	20	1	3
Lox, Regular/Nova, 2 oz	65	2.5	0
Mackerel: Atlantic, raw, 4 oz	230	16	0
Broiled, 3 oz fillet	230	16	0
Jack, canned, ½ c., 3⅓ oz	150	6	0
King, raw, 4 oz	120	2	0
Pacific/Jack: Raw, 4 oz	180	9	0
Broiled, 3 oz	170	9	0
Spanish, raw, 4 oz	160	7	0
Mahi-Mahi, raw, 4 oz	125	1	0
Milkfish, raw, 4 oz	170	7.5	0
Monkfish: Raw, 4 oz	85	1.5	0
Baked, 3 oz	80	2	0
Mullet, striped, raw, 4 oz	135	4.5	0
Mussels: Raw, 4 oz (edible wt.)	100	2.5	4
1 cup, 5¼ oz (edible wt.)	130	3.5	5
Cooked, moist heat, 3 oz	150	4	6

	C	F	Cb
Ocean Perch: Raw, 4 oz	105	1	0
Baked, 3 oz	100	1	0
Octopus, common, raw, 4 oz	95	1	2.5
Orange Roughy, raw, 4 oz	85	1	0
Oysters: Common, raw, 3 oz	70	2	4
Eastern raw: 6 medium, 3 oz	50	1.5	4.5
1 cup, 8¾ oz	150	4	14
Fried/breaded, 6 med., 3 oz	170	11	10
Pacific, raw, 1 med., 1¾ oz	40	1	2
Oysters Rockerfeller, 3 oysters	220	13	12
Perch, average, raw, 4 oz	105	1	0
Pike: Northern, raw, 4 oz	100	1	0
Walleye, raw, 4 oz	105	1.5	0
Pollock, raw, 4 oz	105	1	0
Pout (Ocean), raw, 4 oz	90	1	0
Pompano, Florida, raw, 4 oz	190	10	0
Porgy/Scup, raw, 4 oz	150	4	0
Quahogs ~ See Clams			
Red-Snapper, raw, 4 oz	115	1.5	0
Rockfish, Pacific, raw, 4 oz	110	2	0
Roe, raw, 2 Tbsp, 1 oz	40	2	0.5
Sablefish: Raw, 4 oz	220	17	0
Smoked, 3 oz	220	17	0
Salmon:			
Raw: Chinook, 4 oz	205	12	0
Atlantic; Coho/Silver, 4 oz	210	12	0
Chum; Pink, 4 oz	135	4	0
Red/Sockeye, 4 oz	190	10	0
Baked: Atlantic/Coho, 3 oz	150	7	0
Smoked Salmon: Chinook, 3 oz	100	4	0
Pacific Supreme, 2 oz	100	4	0
Wild Oats, Pastrami Style, 2 oz	130	9	0
Canned Salmon: Average All Brands			
Pink: 1 oz	40	2	0
¼ cup, 63g (2.2 oz)	90	5	0
3¾ oz can, whole	155	8.5	0
7½ oz can, whole	300	17	0
Skinless/boneless, ¼ c., 2 oz	70	2	0
Red Sockeye: 1 oz	50	3	0
¼ cup, 63g (2.2 oz)	110	7	0
3¾ oz can, whole	190	12	0
Atlantic, ½ cup, 3½ oz	230	14	0
Chinook/King, ½ cup	210	14	0
Chum, ½ cup, 3½ oz	140	5	0
Coho/Silver, ½ cup	155	5	0
Atlantic Steaks: Small, 8 oz	320	14	0
Medium, 12 oz	480	21	0
Large, 16 oz	640	28	0
Salmon Cake, take-out, 3 oz	240	15	6

Fish ~ Fresh & Canned (Cont)

Fish (Cont)

	C	F	Cb
Sardines (Canned): *Average All Brands*			
In Oil, undrained, 1 oz	85	7	0
Drained of oil, 1 oz	60	3	0
3¾ oz can, drained, (3¼ oz)	190	11	0
1 lrg/2 med. ³/₅" small, 0.8 oz	50	3	0
In Tom./ Mustard Sce, 1 oz	45	3	0
3¾ oz can (3 sardines)	210	12	1
Sashimi: *See Japanese Foods, Page 178*			
Scallop: Raw, 6 lge/15 small, 3 oz	80	0.5	2
Breaded/fried, 6 pces, 3½ oz	200	10	10
Sea Bass, raw, 4 oz	110	2	0
Seafood Salad, ½ cup	190	16	7
Shark: Raw, 4 oz	150	5	0
Batter-dipped, fried, 4 oz	260	16	4
Baked, 4 oz	185	7	0
Shark Fin, dried, 1 oz	30	0	0
Shrimp: Raw, in shell, ½ lb	140	2	1.5
Raw, shelled, 3 oz (12 lge)	90	1.5	0.5
Breaded/fried, 3 oz (11 lge)	210	11	10
Canned, 1 oz (10 shrimp)	65	1	0
Tiger, cooked, 1 shrimp, ½ oz	15	0.5	0
Battered, fried, 1 shrimp	60	4	3
Shrimp Cocktail, restaurant-style	140	2	1
Smelt, Rainbow, raw, 4 oz	110	3	0
Snapper: Raw, 3 oz	85	1	0
Cooked, 1 fillet, 6 oz	215	3	0
Sole, Raw, 4 oz	105	1.5	0
Squid: Raw, 4 oz	105	1.5	3.5
Fried, 3 oz	150	6	7
Surimi (Imitation Crab), 4 oz	115	1.5	11
Sweet & Sour Fish, ½ dish, 10 oz	580	29	53
Swordfish raw:			
Small Steak, 4 oz	135	4.5	0
Medium Steak, 6 oz	205	7	0
Tilapia, Rain Forest Fillets, 4 oz	110	2	0
Trout, Rainbow: Raw, 4 oz	135	4	0
Broiled, 3 oz	125	5	0
Smoked, 3 oz	110	6	0
Tuna: *Average All Brands*			
Raw: Albacore, 4 oz	190	8	0
Bluefin, 4 oz	165	5.5	0
Skipjack, Yellowfin, 4 oz	125	1	0
Broiled, 3 oz	115	1	0
Canned:			
In Water, drained:			
Chunk/Solid: 2 oz can	75	1.5	0
3 oz can	110	2.5	0
6 oz can	220	5	0
In Oil, drained:			
Chunk Light: 2 oz	110	5	0
6 oz can, drained	340	14	0

Tuna (Cont)

	C	F	Cb
Solid White, 2 oz	105	4.5	0
6.3 oz can, drained	330	14	0
Tuna Salad: Deli Style, ½ c., 4oz	300	24	15
Lower fat, 4 oz	210	10	11
Whitefish: Raw, 4 oz	150	6.5	0
Baked, 3 oz	145	6.5	1
Smoked, 3 oz	90	1	0
Whiting: Raw, 4 oz	100	1.5	0
Baked, 3 oz	85	1	0
Yellowtail: Raw, 4 oz	165	6	0
Grilled, 3 oz (from 4 oz raw)	160	6	0

Other Canned/Packaged Fish

	C	F	Cb
Bumble Bee: *Incl. Mayo & Crackers*			
Tuna Salad Kit: Original	280	20	18
Fat-Free Kit	150	1.5	24
w. Mayonnaise Kit	420	22	24
Seafood Salad w. Crab Kit	180	5.5	27
Sensations: Spring Thai Chili Kit	250	12	20
Other varieties, average	200	8.5	13
Lunch on the Run, Tuna Salad Kit	320	14	19
Chicken of the Sea			
Albacore Tuna, 3 oz pouch	100	1.5	0
Light Tuna, 3 oz pouch	90	1	0
Shrimp, 2.5 oz pouch	55	0.5	1
Smoked Pacific Salmon, 3 oz pouch	120	3.5	1
Starkist			
Pouch: *Per 3 oz Pouch (Drained)*			
Tuna Chunk Light, in water, 2 oz	90	1	0
Albacore Tuna, in water, 2 oz	105	1.5	0
Lunch-To-Go Kit: Chunk Light Tuna			
w. Mayo/Crackers, 4.5 oz	210	9	27
Tuna Creations, all varieties, 2 oz	60	0	0

Frozen Fish Products

Gorton's: *See Page 63*
Kroger: *See Page 64*
SeaPak: *See Page 66*
Van De Kamp's: *See Page 68*
Fast-Foods & Restaurant Chains: *See Page 183*
Captain D's Seafood: *See Fast-Food Section*
Long John Silvers: *See Fast-Food Section*
Shoney's: *See Fast-Food Section*

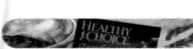

Amy's (Vegetarian)

	C	F	Cb
Per Serving			
Bowls: Brown Rice & Vegs, 10 oz	260	9	36
Santa Fe Enchilada, 10 oz	350	11	47
(Other Varieties ~ www.CalorieKing.com)			
Asian Meals: Thai Stir Fry, 9.5 oz	310	11	45
Asian Noodle Stir Fry, 10 oz	290	7	50
Entrees: Chse Enchilada, 4.5 oz	240	14	8
Cheese Lasagna, 10.3 oz	380	14	44
Macaroni & Cheese, 9 oz	410	16	47
Macaroni & Soy Cheeze, 9 oz	370	15	42
Whole Meals: Chse Enchilada, 9 oz	350	15	38
Black Bean Enchilada, 10 oz	330	8	53
Veggie Loaf, 10 oz	280	7	40
Pot Pies: Country Vege, 7½ oz	370	16	47
Mex. Tamale; Shepherd's Pie, avg.	160	4	27
Vegetable (Non Dairy), 7½ oz	360	13	50
Burgers: Californian, 2½ oz	140	5	19
Other varieties, avg., 2½ oz	120	2.5	14
Burritos: Bean & Rice, 6 oz	280	6	38
Bean & Cheese, 6 oz	280	8	43
Breakfast Burrito, 6 oz	230	6	38
Snacks: Nacho, 5-6 pieces	210	8	26
Cheese Pizza, 5-6 pieces	190	7	22

Extra Product Listings ~ www.CalorieKing.com

Banquet

Pot Pies: Beef, 7 oz	450	27	36
Chicken/Turkey, average, 7 oz	380	21	36
Chicken: Breast Patties (1)	260	19	13
Chicken Brst Tenders/ Nuggets (5)	220	13	14
Crispy Chicken, Skinless, 4.2 oz	330	19	16
Popcorn Chicken, 11 pieces	180	9	18
Wings: Hot & Spicy, 3 oz	260	17	8
Honey Barbecue, 3 oz	270	17	12
Crock Pot Classics: *Per Cup*			
Beef Stew	210	5	23
Chicken & Dumplings	310	14	27
Chicken & Red Potatoes	240	11	21
Creamy Chicken & Pasta	430	20	39
Herb Chicken & Rice, 1 cup	310	3.5	51
Homestyle Pork	200	4	24
Stroganoff Beef & Noodles	350	12	38
Hearty One Dinners: Turkey, 16 oz	520	22	48
Boneless Pork Rib, 16 oz	650	34	55
Chicken Fried Beef Steak, 16 oz	730	40	65
Fried Chicken, 16 oz	820	40	70
Salisbury, 16 oz	600	30	50

Banquet (Cont)

	C	F	Cb
Meals: BBQ Chicken	280	8	35
Boneless Pork Rib, 10 oz	370	18	37
Cheese Enchilada Meal, 11 oz	410	12	64
Chicken Fingers, 7.1 oz	550	26	60
Chicken Fried Beef Steak, 10 oz	380	18	41
Corn Dog Meal, 7.5 oz	490	18	68
Fettuccine Alfredo	420	18	50
Fried Chicken, 9 oz	450	20	35
Fried Rice w. Chicken & Egg Roll	320	7	46
Homestyle Noodles & Chicken	450	20	46
Lasagna w. Meat Sauce, 11 oz	340	9	50
Mac & Cheese, 6.5 oz	400	11	59
Macaroni & Beef, 11 oz	320	6	50
Meatloaf Meal, 9.5 oz	280	14	25
Mexican Style Enchilada Combo	400	15	60
Our Original Fried Chicken	470	27	35
Pepperoni Pizza, 6.75	400	13	61
Salisbury Steak Meal, 9.5 oz	300	15	27
Spaghetti & Meatballs, 10.5 oz	400	17	40
Swedish Meatballs, 10.25 oz	400	19	33
Sweet & Sour Chicken, 10 oz	430	16	60
Turkey Mostly White Meat	230	6	30

Bertolli

Per ½ Package			
Chicken alla Vodka & Farfalle	500	24	40
Chicken Florentine & Farfalle	560	31	40
Chicken Parmesan & Penne	530	25	52
Grilled Chicken Alfredo	710	42	54
Meatballs Pomodoro & Penne	600	31	54
Roasted Chicken & Linguini	420	17	41
Shrimp Asparagus & Penne	480	21	50
Shrimp Scampi & Linguini	500	25	53
Spicy Shrimp Fra Diavolo & Penne	410	19	41
Spinach & Ricotta Cheese Ravioli	500	28	46

Birds Eye – Voila!

Per Cup, Cooked (2 Cups Frozen)			
Chicken Voila!: Garlic Chicken	240	8	21
Other varieties, average	220	7	28
Steak Voila! Beef Sirloin/Potato	190	7	22
Reduced Carb Voila: *Per 1 cup Cooked*			
Chicken & Sausage Tuscano	170	8	10
Chicken Teriaki & Vegetables	160	4	15
Down Home Chicken and Vegetables	180	5	17
Roasted Garlic Chicken & Vege.	120	2.5	13
Teriaki Chicken & Vegetables	150	2.5	15

Frozen Entrees & Meals (Cont)

Boca (Vegetarian)

	C	F	Cb
Burger: Cheeseburger, 1 patty	100	5	5
All American Flame Grilled (1)	90	5	5
Vegan, Original, 1 patty	70	0.5	6
Organic Burgers: Vegan, Orig. (1)	100	2.5	9
Roasted Garlic/Onion, 1 patty	70	1.5	6
Chik'n: Nuggets (4), 3 oz	180	7	17
Hot & Spicy Buffalo Wings (4)	160	7	14
Patties (1), 2.5 oz	160	6	15
Sausages: Bratwurst (1), 2.5 oz	140	7	6
Italian, 2.5 oz	130	6	6
Organic Pizza, ⅓ Pizza	260	8	36

Boston Market

	C	F	Cb
Meals: *Per Serving*			
Beef Sirloin & Noodles	470	12	59
Chicken Pot Pie, 1 cup (½ box)	560	36	43
Meatloaf	670	39	50
Salisbury Steak	720	28	61
Swedish Meatballs	860	49	70

Budget Gourmet (Michelina's)

	C	F	Cb
Classics: *Per Container (8 oz)*			
Escalloped Noodles & White Turkey	300	10	44
Fettuccini Alfredo w. 4 Cheeses	300	9	43
Pizza Snacks, 5 oz	410	21	41
Spicy Szechwan Vege w. Chicken	310	6	51
Stir Fry Rice & Vegetables	450	20	60
Other varieties, average	290	12	37
Premium: Beef Stroganoff, 8 oz	290	7	38
Beef Pepper Steak w. Rice, 8 oz	260	4.5	43
Cheese Manicotti	300	13	31
Chicken and Pasta, 8.5 oz	380	15	43
Lasagne w. Meat Sauce	320	8	47
Stuffed Pepper Casserole	260	10	32
Swedish Meatballs, 10 oz	470	22	50
Lean Gourmet: Shrimp Scampi	220	2.5	44
Salisbury Steak w. Pot. & Gravy	210	7	26
Santa Fe Style Rice & Beans	350	9	59
Shrimp w. Pasta & Veges, 8 oz	260	6	37
Swedish Meatballs, 9 oz	310	9	41

Cedarlane (Vegetarian)

	C	F	Cb
Burrito, Beans, Rice, Chse (1), 6 oz	260	1	48
Eggplant Parmesan, ½ pkg, 5 oz	480	8	16
Dr Sears Zone: Chse Omelet, 1 ctn	350	13	37
Spinach & Cheese Pizza (1)	370	14	40
Vegetable Lasagne, 1 pkg	310	12	33
Enchilada: Garden Vege (1), 4.8 oz	140	3	20
Three-Layer Pie, 5.5 oz	215	7	27
Lasagne: Cheese, ½ ctn, 5 oz	190	6	22
Garden Vege, ½ ctn, 5 oz	180	3	26

Claim Jumper

	C	F	Cb
Meals: Baby Back Pork Ribs (3)	210	14	8
Beef Pot Pie	580	41	39
Beef Pot Roast	500	20	48
Buffalo Wings (2)	160	9	5
Chicken Fried Beef Steak	660	36	68
Chicken Pot Pie, ½ pie, 8 oz	550	37	39
Chicken Tenderloins, 2 pieces	160	6	12
Country Fried Chicken, 19 oz	610	26	72
Lasagna w. Meat Sauce, 8 oz	280	13	26
Meatloaf Dinner	570	36	38
Rst Turkey Brst w. Gravy & Dressing	520	24	53
Salisbury Steak	630	36	43
Spicy Chicken Tenderloins, 3 oz	210	8	20
Turkey Pot Pie, ½ pie, 8 oz	540	39	37
Sauce: Hot Sauce, ½ Tbsp	0	0	0
Original Barbecue, 4 Tbsp	70	0.5	17

Contessa

	C	F	Cb
Meals: *Per Serving*			
Beef Goulash, 8 oz	210	5	32
Burgandy Beef Stew, 8 oz	210	11	22
Chicken Cacciatori, 8 oz	230	7	24
Chicken Chow Mein, 8 oz	320	2.5	55
Chicken Tandoori, 1⅓ cups, 8 oz	200	3.5	27
Kung Pao Shrimp, 8 oz	200	3.5	30
Shrimp Mediteranean, 1¾ cups	180	3	27
Shrimp Primavera, 1½ cups	350	21	30
Shrimp Stir Fry, 1¾ cups	120	2.5	16
Sweet n Sour Shrimp, 1½ cups	180	0	40

Croissant Pockets

	C	F	Cb
Egg, Sausage & Cheese	360	20	37
Five Cheese Pizza (1)	390	20	40
Ham & Cheddar	340	16	39
Pepperoni Pizza	390	20	42
Philly Steak & Cheese	360	19	36
Other varieties, average	320	15	35

El Monterey

	C	F	Cb
Shredded Beef Tamales (1)	310	19	27
Soft Taco: Beef & Cheese (1)	440	22	42
Spicy Beef & Cheese (1)	420	22	40
Spicy Chicken & Cheese (1)	340	11	44
Quesadilla: Gr. Chkn & 3 Chse (1)	260	14	20
Char Broiled Chicken & Chse (1)	230	10	20
Taquitos: Fiesta Appetizers Pack	370	23	29

Essensia (Albertson's)

	C	**F**	**Cb**
Entrees: Corn Souffle, 1 cup	300	19	17
Eggplant Parmesan, 1 cup	310	18	26
Herbed Chicken, 1/3 pkg	180	4.5	17
Jambalaya, 1 cup	220	5	26
Mac & Cheese, 1 cup	300	10	36
2 Meat Lasagna, 1 cup	360	20	31
Pork & Vege Spring Roll (1)	210	10	23
Roast Garlic Mash Potatoes, 5 oz	190	9	26
6 Cheese Cannelloni, 1 cup	180	7	16
7 Cheese Lasagna, 5 oz	310	13	33
Striped Ravioli, 1 cup	360	20	31
Vegetable Lasagna, 1 cup	230	6	32

GardenBurger (Vegetarian)

	C	**F**	**Cb**
Meals: Chicken n Grill, 1 patty	100	2.5	5
Herb Crusted Chicken Cutlet (1)	150	9	10
Mamma Mia Meatballs (6)	110	4.5	7
Riblets, 1 riblet + sauce	230	4.5	27
Burgers: *Per 2½ oz Patty*			
Original Burger; Black Bean, avg	90	3	13
Flame Grilled, Homestyle Classic, avg.	120	4	7
Garden Vegan	100	1	12
Other varieties, average	100	3	1
Wraps: Margherita Pizza	240	8	34
Black Bean Chipotle (1)	240	8	32

Gorton's

	C	**F**	**Cb**
Fish Fillets: Beer Batter (1)	115	7	9
Crispy Battered (1)	130	8.5	8.5
Crunchy Golden (1)	120	6	12
Grilled, average all flavors (1)	100	3	1
Grilled Salmon, average (1)	100	3.5	1
Fish Sticks, Breaded (6), 3.7 oz	250	14	20
Grilled Fillet Meal: Alfredo	160	3	14
Lemon & Herb Butter	240	3.5	34
Popcorn Shrimp (11), 4 oz	280	17	22
Shrimp Bowl: Alfredo, 1 bowl	250	5	49
Fried Rice, 1 bowl	350	2.5	68
Garlic Butter, 1 bowl	260	6	38
Primavera, 1 bowl	270	6	41
Teriyaki, 1 bowl	320	6	57
Tenders: Extra Crunchy, 3½ pieces	260	12	29
Original, 3½ pieces, 4 oz	270	15	25

Green Giant

	C	**F**	**Cb**
Create A Meal: *Prepared with Meat & Oil*			
(Prepared Wt. ~ Approx 10 oz)			
Oven Rstd: Garlic Herb, 1¾ cup	350	9	35
Parmesan Herb Chicken, 1¾ c.	340	11	29
Stir Fry: Lo Mein, 1 cup	270	7	28
Szechuan; Teriyaki, avg., 1 cup	190	9	10

Green Giant (Cont)

	C	**F**	**Cb**
Complete Skillet: *Per 1¼ Cup (Prep.)*			
Beef Stew	180	3.5	27
Chkn Alfredo/& Cheesy Pasta, avg.	270	6	40
Chicken Lo Mein	190	2	31
Chicken Noodle, 1¼ cups	320	6	45
Chicken Teriyaki, 1½ cups	240	1	36
Garlic Chicken & Pasta, 1 cup	230	6	33
Steak Teriyaki, 1½ cup	300	3.5	53
Pasta Accents: *Per Cup (Cooked)*			
Alfredo Pasta	210	4	34
Primavera Pasta	250	11	33
Roasted Garlic Pasta	240	10	31

Healthy Choice

	C	**F**	**Cb**
Entrees/Familiar Favorites: *Per Meal*			
Cheesy Rice & Chicken	230	4	33
Chicken Enchilada	360	7	59
Lasagna Bake	270	7	36
Macaroni & Cheese	270	6	40
Roast Turkey Breast	230	6	25
Dinners: Beef Pot Roast	320	9	39
Beef Tips Portabello	280	8	28
Chicken Enchilada	310	7	46
Chicken Parmigiana	320	9	40
Chicken Teriyaki w. Rice	270	6	37
Lemon Pepper Fish	280	5	49
Roasted Chicken Breast	280	8	32
Salisbury Steak	360	9	45
Sweet & Sour Chicken	340	7	54
Flavor Adventures: Beef Merlot	240	8	26
Chicken Tuscany	330	9	42
Grilled Chicken Baja	270	5	33
Oriental Style Beef	300	9	27

Home Bistro

	C	**F**	**Cb**
Meals: *Per Package*			
Blackened Chkn in Champagne Sce	560	32	8
Chicken Stir Fry	310	7	15
French Toast Breakfast	720	59	28
Grilled Chkn Brst in Caper Parmesan	480	31	7
Poached Salmon Fillet in Sauce	580	44	10
Roasted Turkey Breast w. Stuffing	440	20	19
Sea Scallops in Chili Hollandaise Sce	590	31	51
Shrimp Scampi	710	44	49
Low Carb: Beef Stir Fry	400	17	15
Filet Mignon w. Bearnaise Sce	870	73	14
Grilled Chicken Satay	640	40	20
Roasted Crab Cakes w. Sauce	540	43	10
Roasted Rack of Lamb w. Sauce	700	41	16
Szechuan Beef	390	21	8
Western Omelette w. Sausage	660	57	9

Frozen Entrees & Meals (Cont)

Hot Pockets

	C	F	Cb
Breakfast Pastries: Ham, Egg & Chse	150	7	17
Sausage, Egg & Cheese	170	9	18
Fruit Pastries: Apple/Strawb., avg.	240	9	39
Cream Cheese & Strawb. w. Icing	240	10	34
Pizza Mini's, avg., 5 pces, 3 oz	240	12	29
Sandwiches: Pepperoni Pizza	360	17	44
Barbecue Sce w. Beef; Italian	340	12	50
Chicken Melt with Bacon, 4½ oz	350	17	39
Four Cheese Pizza (no meat), 4½ oz	390	20	44
Steak Fajita, 4½ oz	260	7	39
Other varieties, average, 4½ oz	310	13	36
Subs: Ham & Cheese, 5.6 oz	360	10	49
Meatballs & Mozzarella, 5.6 oz	360	14	44
Other varieties, average, 5.6 oz	390	16	44
Pot Pie Express: Turkey, 1 pce	340	18	35
Other varieties, average, 1 pce	350	17	40

Impromptu Gourmet (Schwan's)

	C	F	Cb
Entrees: Choice Beef Filet Mignon	620	50	0
Choice Bison Rib Eye Steak, 10 oz	410	16	0
French Cut Rack of Pork, 4 oz	150	5	1
Fully Cooked Cajun Turkey, 3 oz	140	8	2
Gourmet Chkn Wellington, 8 oz	420	19	13
New York Strip, 10 oz	660	48	0
Orange Ginger Mahi Mahi, 7 oz	240	6	9
Prime Rib Roast, 12 oz	840	67	2
Spiral Sliced Ham, 3 oz	150	7	7
Stuffed Chkn Breast Saltimbocca	330	14	3
T-Bone Steak, 16 oz	250	18	0

José Olé

	C	F	Cb
Breakfast Burrito			
Egg, Sausage & Cheese, 4 oz	270	11	34
Egg, Ham & Cheese, 4 oz	260	9	34
Taquitos, average, 3 pieces	180	8	22
Mexi-Minis: Beef & Chse Tacos (4)	200	11	19
Chimichangas, 3 pces	240	12	25
Taquitos, 4 pces	180	8	21
Quesadillas, 3 pces	220	8	28
Burrito: Beef & Cheese (1)	300	10	39
Chicken Monterey (1)	270	6	40
Chimichanga: Beef, 1 pce	350	15	39
Chicken , 1 pce	330	12	44

Kid Cuisine

	C	F	Cb
Meals: Cheese Pizza Painter	400	8	68
Chicken Nuggets	440	17	53
Dip & Dunk Cheese Pizza Strips	470	13	65
Fiesta Beef Taco Dippers	390	18	44
Macaroni & Cheese	400	11	61
Pepperoni Pizza	390	7	69
Popstar Popcorn Chicken	420	13	61

Kroger

	C	F	Cb
Stir Fry: Beef Stir Fry, 1¾ cup	180	4	26
Calamari Rings (15)	200	11	19
Chicken Stir Fry, 1½ cup	200	2	30
Chicken Alfredo, 1¾ cup	270	9	30
Coconut Shrimps (5) w. Sauce	360	22	30
Grilled Fillet varieties, avg., 1 pce	100	3	1
Popcorn Shrimp (19)	200	11	16
Shrimp Fried Rice, 1½ cups	190	0.5	36
Shrimp Linguini, 1¾ cups	340	8	51
Swedish Style Meatballs (6)	250	18	7

Lean Cuisine

	C	F	Cb
Cafe Classics Entrees: *Per Meal*			
Beef Portabello	210	5	25
Bow Tie Pasta & Chicken	240	4.5	33
Garlic Beef & Broccoli	170	6	13
Sweet & Sour Chicken	300	3	51
Thai Style Chicken	220	4	30
Cafe Classics Bowls: *Per Bowl*			
Chicken Teriyaki	250	2	44
Grilled Chicken Caesar	230	6	24
Three Cheese Stuffed Rigatoni	240	6	35
Comfort Classics Entrees: *Per Meal*			
Baked Chicken	240	4.5	34
Cheese Lasagna w. Chicken	290	8	35
Honey Roasted Pork	180	6	14
Meatloaf & Whipped Potato	250	7	27
Roasted Turkey Breast	260	2.5	46
Salisbury Steak	270	8	27
Dinnertime Selects: *Per Meal*			
Beef Steak Tips Dijon	320	8	44
Grilled Chicken & Penne Pasta	330	4.5	52
Salisbury Steak	310	8	34
One Dish Favorites: Rstd Chicken	240	6	30
Angel Hair Pasta	260	4	48
Chicken Enchilada	270	4.5	47
Lasagna w. Meat Sauce	320	7	44
Macaroni & Cheese	290	7	41
Santa Fe Rice & Beans	290	6	49
Stuffed Cabbage	200	6	25
Swedish Meatballs	280	7	32
Teriyaki Stir-Fry	300	4.5	49

Frozen Entrees & Meals (Cont)

Lean Cuisine (Cont)

	C	F	Cb
Skillets: Chkn Alfredo	190	4.5	25
Chicken Primavera	180	2.5	28
Garlic Chicken	240	4	40
Herb Chicken & Roasted Potatoes	160	3.5	22
Spa Cuisine: Chicken Pecan	260	6	32
Pork w. Cherry Sauce	260	4	41
Salmon w. Basil	230	6	25

Lean Pockets

Per Piece

	C	F	Cb
BBQ Sauce w. Beef	290	7	48
Ham/Philly Steak & Cheese, 1 pce	280	7	41
Meatballs & Mozzarella	290	7	45
Steak Fajita	260	7	40
Three Cheese & Chicken Quesadilla	280	7	42
Turkey/Broccoli/Cheese	270	7	41
Other varieties, avg.	280	7	43
Lean Pockets Subs, average	310	7	44
Lean Pockets Ultra, 4 oz	200	6	19

Lightlife (Vegetarian)

	C	F	Cb
Smart Menu: Breakfast Patties (1)	45	1.5	3
Burgers (1)	100	1	9
Chick'n Nuggets (4)	220	11	16
Chick'n Patties (1)	160	7	14
Meatless Meatballs (5)	160	7	6
Gimme Lean! Meals, avg., 2 oz	50	0	4
Grab'n Go: Smart Pretzel Dog (1) 5 oz	350	8	50
Smart Tortilla Wrap Burrito:			
Breakfast Scramble (1) 6 oz	320	1	41
Chick'n Ranchero (1) 6 oz	300	6	48
Mexican Beef Style (1) 6 oz	340	7	54
Hot Dogs, Tofu Pups, 1 link, 1.5 oz	60	2.5	2
On The Go: Smart BBQ, ¼ cup, 2 oz	70	0	13
Smart Chili, 1 cup, 8.3 oz	210	0	34
Smart Garlic Teriyaki Chick'n	290	4	50
Smart Orange Sesame Chick'n	270	5	46
Smart Veggie Bolognese	220	1	37
Smart Tex Mex, ¼ cup, 2 oz	50	0	6
Smart Dogs!, Jumbo, Fat-Free (1)	80	0	3
Original, Fat-Free (1)	45	0	2
Smart Franks Deli Style Dogs (1) 2 oz	110	4.5	5
Smart Ground: Original, ⅓ cup, 55g	70	0	7
Taco & Burrito, ⅓ cup, 55g	70	0	7
Smart Links: Brats, German Style (1)	120	7	5
Country Breakfast Style (2) 2 oz	100	3.5	5
Old World Italian Style (1) 2 oz	110	4.5	5
Smart Menu Strips: Chick'n, 3 oz	80	0	5
Steak-Style, 3 oz	80	0	5

Marie Callender's (Cont)

Complete Dinners: *Per Serving*

	C	F	Cb
Beef Pot Roast	330	10	32
Beef Stroganoff	420	18	40
Beef Tips in Mushroom Sce, 13.6 oz	360	12	35
Chicken Fried Beef Steak	540	28	51
Chicken Parmigiana, 1 dinner	650	29	66
Country Fried Chick. & Gvy, 1 din.	670	37	58
Fish w. Mac & Cheese	450	16	53
Golden Battered Fish Fillet	450	16	53
Grilled Chkn & Mashed Pot., 15 oz	450	17	39
Herb Rstd Chicken & Mashed Pot.	530	35	20
Homestyle BBQ Chicken, 14¾ oz	590	28	44
Meatloaf & Gravy w. Mashed Pot.	560	31	39
Pork Chop, 1 dinner	590	33	50
Salisbury Steak & Gravy, 14 oz	400	16	38
Sweet & Sour Chicken, 1 dinner	620	20	90
Pot Pies: Beef	530	32	43
Chicken (10 oz); Turkey, 1 cup	670	41	56
One Dish Classics:			
Cheesy Chicken Breast & Rice	470	19	44
Country Beef Stew w. Cornbread	440	16	52
Fettucini Alfredo, 14 oz	870	51	76
Fettuccini w. Chicken/Broc., 13 oz	630	37	43
Macaroni & Cheese, 8 oz	350	15	36
Meat Lasagna, 8 oz	240	9	24
Crockpot Meals: Turkey & Veges	170	6	21
Chunky Chicken & Noodles	220	10	18
Hearty Beef Vege Soup	130	3	16
Homestyle Chicken Noodle Soup	120	3.5	13
Old Fashioned Beef & Veges	150	4.5	14

Michael Angelo's

	C	F	Cb
Entrees: Chicken Parmesan	260	10	25
Eggplant Parmesan, 6 oz	285	19	23
Fettuccine Alfredo	280	8	40
Manicotti w. Sauce	230	12	11
Sausage & Pepper & Onion	230	7	31
Spaghetti & Meatballs, 15.25 oz	230	9	26
Bowls: Angel Hair & Shrimp, 6 oz	200	6	28
Angel Hair Pasta Pomodoro, 7 oz	200	5	34
Chicken Milano Pasta, 6 oz	290	11	30
Chkn Rosemary Pasta; Saus., 6 oz	250	8	30
Lasagna: Chicken, 8 oz	290	7	37
Four Cheese, 8 oz	400	22	28
Meat Lasagna, 8 oz	290	10	26
Vegetable, 8 oz	230	7	23
Snacks: Four Chse Calzone (1)	360	13	50
Meatball Calzone (1), 5 oz	390	15	45
Mini Calzone (1), avg. 0.7 oz	60	2.5	8

Morningstar Farms

	C	F	Cb
Breakfast Pattie, 1 patty	80	3	3
Burgers: *Made with Organic Soy*			
Classic Burger	150	7	10
Tex Mex Burger	120	1.5	17
Vegan Burger; Veggie Medley, avg.	100	2	8
Zesty Tomato Basil Burger	120	6	7
Thai Burger	100	3.5	7
Grillers: Veggie Burger	130	6	5
Prime Veggie Burger	170	9	4
Vegan	100	2.5	7
Patties: Parmesan Ranch	170	7	17
Breaded Veggie Patties	150	6	16
Poultry: *Made with Organic Soy*			
Buffalo Wings (5)	200	9	18
Chik'n Nuggets (4)	190	7	18
Okara Pattie	120	5	6
Roasted Herb Chicken	150	4	22
Veggie Corn Dogs (1)	170	6	22
Entrees: Lentil Rice Loaf, 1" slice	160	7	16
Nine Bean Loaf, 1" slice	150	7	15
Recipe Crumbles: Grillers, ⅔ cup	90	2.5	5
Sausage Style, ⅔ cup	80	2.5	5

Ore-Ida

	C	F	Cb
Bagel Bites: *Per 4 Pieces (3 oz)*			
Three Cheese, 4 pieces	200	6	28
Cheese, Sausage, Pepperoni	200	6	29
Spicy Nacho; Nacho Cheese	240	10	26

Quorn (Vegetarian)

	C	F	Cb
Garlic & Herb Ckn-Style Cutlets (1)	190	8	20
Gruyer Cutlet	260	15	23
Meat-free Dogs (1), 1.5 oz	80	4	8
Meat-free Links (2), 1.6 oz	90	2	9
Meat-free Meatballs (4), 2.4 oz	110	3	7
Naked Cutlets (1), 2.4 oz	80	2.5	5
Nuggets, 3-4 pieces, 3 oz	190	10	17
Patties (1), 2.6 oz	140	7	13
Tenders, 1 cup, 3 oz	90	2	8
Turkey Style Roast, 3 oz	90	1.5	9

Rosina/Celentano

	C	F	Cb
Entree: *Per Serving*			
Cheese Ravioli, 4 pces	230	3.5	36
Eggplant Parmigiana, 10 oz	460	29	38
Manicotti, 7 oz	420	14	53
Ravioli Stuffed Cheese, Mini, 4 oz	220	2.5	36
Stuffed Shell: 6.5 oz	320	12	36
Light Broccoli, 10 oz	330	5	54

Safeway Select

	C	F	Cb
Gourmet Club Meals: *Per Serving*			
Cha Siu Bao, 1 bau, 3 oz	210	4.5	34
Enchiladas	210	8	25
Low Fat Turkey Lasagna, 1 cup	230	3	36
Macaroni & Cheese	350	19	32
Meat Lasagna, 1 cup	270	7	34
Tamale Bake, 1 cup	290	16	25
6 Vegetable Lasagna, 1 cup	310	17	27
St. Louis Ribs (2), 125g	370	23	17
Stir Fry: Chicken Fajita	130	3	14
Shrimp & Vegetable	120	0	20
Teriyaki Beef	170	4	24
Gourmet Club Eating Right: *Per ½ Package*			
Burgundy Beef Stew	250	9	38
Cashew Chicken, 16 oz	330	5	53
Chicken Lettuce Wraps, 2 oz	80	3.5	8
Chicken Penne Pasta	280	8	34
Chicken Tamales Verde	220	9	25
Creamy Broccoli Beef	290	7	40
Ginger Chicken	350	6	49
Meatloaf Dinner	230	6	31
Orange Glazed Chicken	350	5	56
Shrimp Lo Mein, 10 oz	290	6	41

SeaPak

	C	F	Cb
Coconut Shrimp, 4 pces	270	17	19
Jumbo Butterfly Shrimp, 4 pces	210	10	20
Popcorn Shrimp, 15 pces, 3 oz	210	10	20
Shrimp Scampi, 8 pces	330	29	2
Shrimp Tempura, 4 pieces	240	8	35

Seeds of Change

	C	F	Cb
Per Bowl (11 oz)			
Creamy Spinach Lasagna	340	10	40
Ginger Stir Fry	260	3	47
Penne Marinara	300	8	40
Seven Grain Pilaf	310	9	46
Spicy Peanut Noodles	350	9	51
Spicy Yucatan Frijoles	340	5	54
Teriyaki Stir-Fried Rice	310	2	49
Vegetarian Chicken Teriyaki	300	3.5	47

Stouffer's

	C	F	Cb
Homestyle Dinners: *Per Serving*			
Chicken Fettucini, 16.75 oz	610	33	55
Country Fried Beef Steak, 16 oz	520	33	52
Grilled Lime Chicken, 14 oz	490	14	66
Meatloaf, 17 oz	590	32	43
Monterey Chicken, 14.25 oz	500	17	58
Roast Turkey Breast, 16 oz	390	13	48
Slow Roasted Beef, 14 oz	320	15	27

Stouffer's (Cont)

Entrees:	C	F	Cb
Stroganoff, 9.75 oz	380	17	34
Breaded Boneless Pork Cutlet	370	21	31
Creamed Chipped Beef	140	8	9
Grilled Teriyaki Chicken	300	3.5	45
Chicken a la King	410	14	53
Fish Fillet w. Mac Cheese, 9 oz	420	18	45
Lasagna w. Meat Sce, 10½ oz	350	11	38
Macaroni & Beef w. Tomatoes	330	11	38
Macaroni & Cheese, 1 cup, 8 oz	350	17	34
Salisbury Steak, 16 oz	470	24	45
Spaghetti w. Meat Sauce	360	12	45
Stuffed Pepper, 10 oz	220	10	22
Swedish Meatballs w. Pasta	500	25	40
Tuna Noodle Casserole	370	17	35
Turkey Tetrazzini	380	20	32
Family Style Recipes: *Per Serving*			
Grandma's Chkn & Vege Bake	360	15	36
Lasagna w. Meat Sce, 1 cup	270	10	30
Macaroni & Cheese, 1 cup	350	17	34
Italian Style: Chkn Ravioli, 8.2 oz	360	14	40
Cheese Stuffed Rigatoni, 8.2 oz	460	20	52
Italian Sausage Stuffed Rigatoni	390	15	44
Skillets: *Per Bowl*			
Broccoli & Beef; Garlic Chkn, avg.	330	6	46
Chicken Alfredo	410	11	49
Chicken & Pasta	340	7	42
Chicken & Veges	360	9	43
Homestyle Beef	300	11	32
Teriyaki Chicken, 12.5 oz	310	4.5	44
Steak Teriyaki	310	5	49
Yankee Pot Roast	300	8	39
Corner Bistro: Paninis, average	355	17	31
Chicken Carbonara, 12 oz	530	22	50
Garlic/Rosemary Chicken, 12 oz	420	17	42
Monterey Chicken, 12 oz	500	23	46
Seafood Scampi, 14 oz	410	11	57
Sesame Chicken, 12½ oz	510	15	72

Swanson

	C	F	Cb
Hungry Man Dinners: Meatloaf	680	37	61
Boneless Pork Rib	920	35	71
Boneless White Meat Fried Chkn	710	29	86
Buffalo Chicken Strips	920	35	71
Classic Fried Chicken	960	45	91
Hearty Breakfast	450	27	35
Mexican Style Fiesta	870	38	113
Rotisserie Chicken	690	35	48
Salisbury Steak	490	18	55
Turkey Breast	660	27	81
Hungry Man XXL: Backyard BBQ	860	48	62
Roasted Carved Turkey Dinner	820	36	84
Southern Fried Boneless Chicken	760	16	84

Swanson (Cont)

Pot Pies:	C	F	Cb
Flaky Crust Chicken/Turkey	320	17	31
American Recipe: Salisbury Steak	500	26	48
Boneless White Meat Fried Chkn	520	22	75
Breaded Fish Fillet, 10 oz	510	23	57
Chicken Strips w. Fries	640	30	80
Classic Fried Chicken, 11½ oz	770	37	72
Turkey Breast w. Stuffing & Gravy	380	17	40

TGI Friday's

	C	F	Cb
Buffalo Wings (3)	150	10	2
Honey BBQ Wings (3)	150	9	6
Mozzarella Sticks & Sce, 1 Serve	110	6	10
Popcorn Chicken, 3 pces, 2.6 oz	250	8	29
Potato Skins, Ched. & Bacon, 2	210	12	20
Quesadilla Rolls: Chicken (2)	250	12	26
Steak (2)	230	10	26
Sides: Spinach Dip, 2 Tbsp, 1 oz	45	3.5	2

Trader Joe's

Meals: *Per Serving*	C	F	Cb
Asian Style Chkn Stir Fry w. Sce, 8 oz	90	1	30
BBQ Chicken Teriyaki, 1 cup	150	3.5	11
Chicken Chow Mein, ⅓ pkg, 6.75 oz	240	2	45
Chicken Fried Rice, 1 cup, 5 oz	200	3.5	33
Chicken Marsala, 1 pkg, 11 oz	320	6	34
Citrus Glazed Chicken, 8 oz	270	5	40
Mandarin Orange Chicken, 1 cup	270	10	23
Rice Bowls, average, 11 oz bowl	350	2	62
Shrimp Stir Fry, 6.4 oz	70	0.5	6
Swt & Sr Shrimp w. Rice, ⅓ pkg 7.4 oz	190	0	39
Turkey Saus. Stromboli, ¼ loaf, 4.5 oz	250	7	31
Pies: Shepherds Pie, ½ pie, 8 oz	190	3.5	23
Spinach Pie, ¼ pie, 6 oz	240	4	37
Quiche: Broccoli & Cheddar, 6 oz	460	30	32
Mexicaine, 6 oz	500	34	31
Spinach & Mushroom, 6 oz	460	26	38

For Complete Nutritional Data ~ see CalorieKing.com

Tyson

Meal Kits: Beef Fajita (1)	C	F	Cb
Beef Fajita (1)	140	4	17
Chicken Fajita (1)	130	3.5	17
Chicken Fried Rice, 2½ cups	440	6	69
Chicken Quesadilla (1)	250	10	26
Chicken Stir Fry, 2¾ cups	430	4.5	73
Meals: Buffalo Hot Wings, 4 pieces	220	15	1
Chicken Bites, 13 pieces	270	18	15
Chicken Brst Fillets, breaded (1)	240	9	20

Tyson (Cont)

	C	F	Cb
Meals: Chkn Brst Nuggets, 5 pces	280	16	21
Chicken Breast Strips, 3 oz	120	3.5	1
Chicken Breast Tenderloins, 1 pce	150	7	12
Country Fried Steak, 1 piece	310	23	15
Crispy Chicken Strips, 2 pces	200	10	13
Fajita Style Chicken Strips, 3 oz	110	4	1
Fun Nuggets, 5 pieces	280	18	16
Honey Barbecue Wings, 3 pces	250	15	13
Honey Chicken Brst Tenders, 5 pce	220	13	13
Popcorn Chicken, 9 pces	200	8	17
Southern Style Chkn Brst Patties (1)	240	18	13
Steak Fingers, 2 pces	250	18	14

Van De Kamp's

	C	F	Cb
Butterfly Shrimp, 7 pces, 4 oz	270	13	26
Crispy Battered Halibut, 3 fillets	240	14	22
Crispy Fish Tenders, 4 pces, 4 oz	210	10	22
Crispy Fish Portions, 1 pce	150	8	14
Popcorn Shrimp, 20 pces, 4 oz	260	11	30
Fish Sticks, Breaded, 6 stix, 4 oz	260	13	23
Battered Fillets, 2.6 oz fillet	130	6	11
Crunchy Fish Fillets, 1 pce, 2.6 oz	230	13	18
Crisp & Healthy, Breaded (2), 1.8 oz	170	2.5	25

Weight Watchers

Smart Ones Bistro Selections: Per Meal

	C	F	Cb
Chicken Fettucini	340	8	42
Chicken Parmesan	290	5	35
Chkn Tenderloins w. Barbecue Sce	240	4.5	34
Fajita Chicken Supreme	260	7	32
Glazed Chicken	260	2.5	45
Golden Baked Garlic Chicken	270	5	42
Grilled Mandarin Chicken	280	4.5	42
Meatloaf w. Mashed Potatoes	260	8	22
Oven Roasted Chicken	260	6	37
Roasted Chicken w. Sour Cream	180	4	20
Southwest Style Adobo Chicken	310	10	36
Stuffed Turkey Breast	290	6	42
Thai Style Chicken & Rice Noodles	260	4	43

Smart Ones Entrees: Per Meal

	C	F	Cb
Angel Hair Marinara	230	1.5	41
Broccoli & Cheddar Roasted Pot.	220	6	34
Chicken Enchiladas Suiza	310	8	45
Honey Dijon Chicken	220	3.5	38
Lasagna Bolognese	270	4	43
Lemon Herb Chicken Piccata	250	5	33
Macaroni & Cheese	270	2	52
Radiatore Romano	290	7	43
Roast Turkey Medallions	220	1.5	38

Weight Watchers (Cont)

	C	F	Cb
Smart Ones Entrees (Cont):			
Salisbury Steak	260	7	26
Santa Fe Style Rice & Beans	310	7	51
Spaghetti Bolognese; 3 Chse Mac	310	6	48
Spaghetti Marinara	300	4.5	54
Spicy Szechuan Style Vege & Chkn	240	5	36
Traditional Lasagna w. Meat Sce	300	6	43
Tuna Noodle Gratin	250	4.5	37
High Protein, avg. all varieties	210	8	12
Smart Ones Bowls: Per Bowl			
Southwestern Style Chicken	230	3.5	33
Teriyaki Chicken & Vegetable	270	3	46
Smartwiches, avg. all, 127g	270	6	40

For Complete Nutritional Data ~ see CalorieKing.com

White Castle

	C	F	Cb
Cheese Burger, Microwaveable, 1 pkg, 3.7 oz	320	18	26
Hamburgers, 1 pkg (2 sandwiches)	280	14	26

Worthington/Loma Linda

	C	F	Cb
Bolono, 3 slices, 2 oz	80	3	3
Chik-Nuggets, 5 pieces	250	15	14
Chicken Roll, ⅜ slice, 1.9 oz	90	4.5	2
Chicken Slices, 3 slices, 2 oz	90	4.5	2
ChikSticks, 1 pce, 1.6 oz	100	6	4
Corn Dogs (1)	150	4	22
Corned Beef Slices, 3 slices, 2 oz	140	9	5
Dinner Roast, ¾" slice	180	11	6
Fillets, 2 pieces, 2.9 oz	180	9	8
Fried Chik'n w. Gravy, 2 pieces	150	10	5
FriPats, 1 pattie, 2¼ oz	130	6	5
Golden Croquettes, 4 pieces, 2.9 oz	210	11	14
Leanies, 1 link, 1.4 oz	100	7	2
Meatless Smoked Beef, 3 slices	130	7	7
Prosage: Links, 2 links, 1.6 oz	80	3	3
Patties, 1.3 oz Pattie	80	3	3
Salami, 3 slices, 2 oz	120	7	3
Smkd Turkey Slices, 3 slices	140	9	4
Stakelets, 2.5 oz piece	150	7	7
Stripples, 2 strips	60	4.5	2
Swiss Steak, 1 piece	130	6	9
Tuno (tuna substitute), ½ cup	90	6	3
Wham Vege Slices, 2 slices	110	7	3

Zatarain's

	C	F	Cb
Blackened Chicken Alfredo, 10.5 oz	535	30	44
Jambalaya seasoned w. Chicken w. Sausage	360	8	53
	390	12	58
Red Beans & Rice w. Sausage	565	19	76

Frozen Pizzas	C	F	Cb
Amy's: *Per ⅓ Pizza*			
Cheese; Spinach; Pesto, avg.	310	12	38
Cheese Pesto (Whole Wheat Crust)	360	18	37
Cheese Pizza (Rice Crust) ⅓ pizza	300	14	31
Mushroom & Olive	250	9	33
Roasted Vegetable	270	9	42
California Pizza Kitchen			
Large: Five Cheese & Tomato, ⅙	320	15	29
BBQ Chicken, ⅙ pizza	290	9	33
Small: BBQ/Thai Chkn, average, ⅓	290	10	33
Five Cheese & Tomato, ⅓	320	15	29
Crispy Thin Crust: Sicilian, ⅓ pizza	310	14	30
Margherita, ⅓ pizza	300	13	31
Other varieties, avg., ⅓ pizza	290	12	30
Celeste			
Pizza For One: Cheese, 1 pizza	360	14	42
Deluxe; Pepperoni; Chseburger	410	21	42
Original/Zesty Four Cheese, avg.	400	18	41
Sausage & Pepperoni; Suprema	470	26	44
Zesty Chicken Supreme	340	15	39
Di Giorno			
Rising Crust (Large): *Per ⅙ Pizza*			
Four Cheese	310	11	40
Other varieties, average	355	16	40
Rising Crust (Small): Supreme, ⅓	320	14	35
Four Cheese	350	14	41
Pepperoni/Supreme	370	16	40
Deep Dish: Three Meat, ⅙ pizza	310	15	32
Supreme, ⅙ pizza	320	15	33
Pepperoni, ⅙ pizza	340	18	32
Cheese Stuffed Crust: Supreme, ⅙	350	14	35
Four Cheese, ⅕ pizza	360	14	41
Pepperoni, ⅕ pizza	370	16	40
Three Meat Pizza ⅙ pizza	340	16	34
Half & Half: *Per ⅙ Large Pizza*			
Pepperoni/Cheese: Pepperoni	390	18	40
Cheese	310	11	40
Microwave: 3 Meat, ½ pizza	420	19	44
4 Cheese, ½ pizza	370	15	44
Pepperoni; Supreme, avg., ½	390	18	44
Thin Crispy Crust: *Per ⅕ Large Pizza*			
Four Meat	320	13	37
Grilled Chicken/Tom./Spinach, ⅛	260	8	33
Other varieties, average, ⅛	305	12	34
Ellio's (McCain)			
9 Slice Pizza: All Cheezy, 1 slice	160	5	23
Cheese; Pepperoni, avg., 1 slice	160	5	20
27 Slice Pizza: Cheese, 1 slice	150	3	21
Pepperoni, 1 slice	160	5	20

	C	F	Cb
Essensia *(Albertson's)*			
5 Cheese, ⅙ pizza	320	11	42
3 Meat, ⅙ pizza	360	15	41
Supreme, ⅛ pizza	270	11	31
Freschetta			
Hand Tossed (Large): 4 Chse, ⅕	390	14	47
4 Meat, ⅙ pizza	350	15	40
Pepperoni, ⅙ pizza	340	14	40
Canadian Bacon Pineapple, ⅕	340	9	49
Supreme, ⅙ pizza	350	15	38
Vegetable Primavera, ⅙ pizza	310	11	40
Brick Oven 8": BBQ Chicken, ⅓ pizza	280	11	30
Ham & Mushroom, ½ pizza	325	11	39
Potato, Bacon & Cheese, ½ pizza	395	17	43
Thai Chicken, ⅓ pizza	300	14	27
Italian Style Pepperoni, ¼ pizza	410	21	38
Sauce Stuffed Crust: 4 Chse, ⅕ pizza	340	12	43
Sausage & Pepperoni, ⅕ pizza	370	16	43
Pepperoni, ⅕ pizza	360	15	43
8" Hand Tossed, Pepperoni, ⅕	460	19	51
12" Ultra Thin: Supreme, 3 slices	350	19	27
5 Cheese; Pepperoni, 3 slices	330	17	25
Healthy Choice: *Per Pizza (6 oz)*			
French Bread Pizza: Pepperoni	360	5	56
Supreme; Vegetable, avg.	325	5	50
Cafe Selections Pizza: Four Chse	370	3	58
Gourmet Supreme	360	4	56
Italian Style Pepperoni	370	4.5	58
Jeno's: *Per Pizza (7 oz)*			
Crispy & Tasty: Cheese	440	21	47
Pepperoni; Supreme; Comb., avg.	490	25	50
Three Meat; Sausage, average	480	24	49
Heaven's Bistro: *Per ⅓ Pizza*			
Chicken w. BBQ Sauce	270	2	48
Grilled Vegetable	230	1	42
Pepperoni; Sausage, average	250	3	42
Lean Cuisine			
French Bread Pizza: Cheese, 6 oz	370	7	50
Deluxe, 6 oz	310	9	44
Pepperoni, 5.25 oz	300	7	44
Casual Eating: Deluxe, 6 oz	370	9	55
BBQ Chkn; Margherita, avg., 6 oz	320	9	46
Four Cheese, 6 oz	400	9	59
Rstd Garlic; Mushroom, avg., 6 oz	285	7	39
Roasted Vegetable, 6 oz	330	5	58
Pizza Fit 'n Free			
7" Pizza, 7 oz	250	0	43

Frozen Pizzas (Cont)

Ralph's	C	F	Cb
Pizza Pals: *Per Pizza*			
Cheese; Hamburger, averagw	410	12	57
Taco Supreme	380	12	47
Other varieties, average	455	17	58
Self Rising Crust: 4 Cheese, ⅙	300	8	45
Pepperoni, ⅙ pizza	390	16	45
Other varieties, avg., ⅙ pizza	355	14	45
Red Baron			
Classic (Large): 4 Cheese, ¼ pizza	410	19	40
Pepperoni, ⅕ pizza	330	16	32
Other varieties, average, ⅕ pizza	350	18	33
Deep Dish Pan Style:			
4 Cheese, ⅓ pizza	380	17	41
Pepperoni; Meat Trio, avg., ⅓ pizza	400	20	41
Supreme, ⅓ pizza	420	20	43
Deep Dish Singles: 4 Cheese, 1	430	30	44
Pepperoni, 1 pizza	450	22	45
Other varieties, average, 1 pizza	420	21	43
French Bread Pizzas: Supreme (1)	360	15	42
5 Cheese & Garlic (1)	410	22	39
Pepperoni; 3 Meat, average	360	15	42
Microwaveable Classic: 4 Chse (1)	740	39	62
Supreme, 1 pizza	760	42	64
Other varieties, avg. (1)	795	46	62
Pizzeria Style: *Per ⅙ Pizza*			
4 Cheese; Pepperoni, avg.	350	14	40
Special Deluxe; Supreme, avg.	370	16	41
Thin Crust: *Per ¼ Pizza*			
Mozzarella Tomato Basil	270	13	27
Five Cheese; Meat Trio, avg.	310	16	27
Pepperoni varieties, average	360	20	27
Reggio's			
Individual Pizza: Cheese (1)	250	8	33
Pepperoni, 1 pizza	290	13	33
Sausage & Mushroom (1)	280	10	34
Dinner Size: Cheese, ¼ pizza	330	12	41
Pepperoni & Sausage, ¼ pizza	400	18	41
Sausage; Supreme, ¼, avg.	380	16	41
Stop & Shop			
Single Serving, Cheese, 1	390	19	42
9 Slices, Cheese, 2 slices	350	10	49
Stouffer's			
French Bread Pizzas: Deluxe, 1 pce	430	21	44
Cheese, 1 piece (½ pkg)	360	15	43
Extra Cheese, 1 piece	400	18	44
Pepperoni, 1 piece	410	20	43

Tombstone	C	F	Cb
Original Pizza, 12 inch: *Per Serving*			
Extra Cheese, ¼ pizza	340	15	37
Pepperoni, ¼ pizza	380	20	37
Sausage & Pepperoni, ¼ pizza	370	17	37
Supreme, ⅕ pizza	300	14	31
Light Pizza, Vegetable, ⅕ pizza	230	6	31
Half & Half Pepperoni & Cheese:			
Pepperoni, ⅕ pizza	410	21	37
Cheese, ¼ pizza	330	16	31
Deep Dish Individual:			
Cheese (1)	420	17	50
Pepperoni (1)	460	22	50
Supreme (1)	440	20	51
Thin Crust: 3 Cheese, ¼ pizza	330	18	30
Harvest Wheat Supreme, ¼	260	10	29
Brick Oven Style: Cheese, ⅓ pizza	350	15	38
Other varieties, average, ¼	310	16	29
Tony's			
Original: Cheese, ⅓ pizza	370	15	42
Pepperoni, ⅓ pizza	400	19	42
Sausage & Pepperoni, ⅓ pizza	430	21	42
Supreme, ⅓ pizza	420	20	43
Thin Crust: Cheese, ⅓ pizza	340	15	36
Sausage &/Pepperoni, ⅓ pizza	390	19	32
Supreme, ⅓ pizza	360	19	34
Deep Dish (Individual)**:** Cheese (1)	390	16	47
Pepperoni (1)	480	24	48
Totino's			
Crisp Crust Party Pizza: *Per ½ Pizza*			
Cheese	320	15	34
Pepperoni; Supreme	380	22	34
Trader Joe's: *Per ⅓ Pizza*			
4 Cheese	350	14	42
Formaggio di Capra	360	17	37
Pizza Mascarpene	340	15	45
Vegetarian	300	11	43
Verdi (Safeway Select)			
Self-Rising Crust (Large): *Per ⅙ Pizza*			
Meat Magnifico	350	15	41
4 Cheese	310	11	41
Other varieties, average	365	16	41
Thin Crispy Crust: Supreme, ⅕	360	16	38
Four Cheese, ⅕ pizza	310	11	37
Pepperoni, ⅕ pizza	315	16	37
Weight Watchers (Smart Ones): *Per Pizza*			
Deluxe	360	9	52
Four Cheese	390	10	56
Pepperoni	390	11	50
Veggie Ultimate	330	6	54

Canned & Packaged Meals

	C	F	Cb
Annies Homegrown: *Per Cup (Prepared)*			
Arthur Mac & Cheese	370	14	50
Beef Stroganoff	320	13	24
Cheeseburger Macaroni	350	13	27
Cheesy Lasagna	280	9	26
Penne Pasta w. Alfredo Sauce	360	13	49
Shells & Cheddar	290	5	49
B & M: *Per ½ Cup (4½ oz)*			
Baked Beans: Original	170	2	31
Barbeque	190	0.5	39
Brown Raisin Bread, ½" slice, 2 oz	130	0.5	29
Banquet			
Homestyle Bakes: *Per Serving (Prepared)*			
Beef Stew & Biscuits, ⅔ cup	300	8	43
Chicken & Dumplings, 7.8 oz	260	8	33
Creamy Cheesy Chicken Alfredo	400	22	36
Country Chicken, Potato, Biscuits	380	15	49
Creamy Chkn & Biscuits, 7.4 oz	350	18	39
Betty Crocker			
Casserole Potatoes, prep., avg.	150	5	22
Complete Meals: *Per Serving (⅕ Pkg)*			
Chicken & Buttermilk Biscuits	280	11	37
Chicken Fettuccini Alfredo	240	9	31
Homestyle Chkn & Dumplings	240	9	34
Lasagna Pasta Bake	250	3	46
Stroganoff	200	4.5	30
Three Cheese Chicken	260	10	33
Hamburger Helper: *Per Cup (Prep. as Directed)*			
Bacon Cheeseburger	380	15	38
Cheeseburger Macaroni	340	15	27
Cheesy Enchilada; Quesadilla	360	13	40
Cheesy Hashbrown	400	19	39
Chili Macaroni	290	11	29
Other varieties, average	320	15	27
Tuna Helper: *Per Serving (Prep. as Directed)*			
Creamy Parmesan	260	8	33
Other varieties, average	290	11	35
Chicken Helper: *Per Cup (Prep. as Directed)*			
Cheesy Chicken Enchilada	320	7	40
Chicken Fried Rice	260	9	25
Fettuccini Alfredo	280	8	27
Chicken Teriyaki	290	6	36
Cookbook Favorites: *Per Cup (Prep. as Directed)*			
Chicken Con Queso & Mexican Rice	340	17	24
Creamy Basil Parm. Chicken & Pasta	340	14	29
Fettuccine Alfredo	340	16	27
Garlic & Herb Chicken Penne	240	7	21

Betty Crocker (Cont)	C	F	Cb
Mashed Potatoes: *Per Serving (Prepared)*			
Potato Buds, ⅓ cup	160	8	19
Other varieties, average, ½ cup	160	8	20
Side Dishes/Casseroles: *Per Serving (Prepared)*			
Au Gratin; Cheesy Scalloped, ½ cup	150	6	22
Scalloped Potatoes, ⅔ cup	130	4	20
Three Cheese Potatoes, ⅔ cup	130	4	22
Deluxe Potatoes: *Per ½ Cup (Prepared)*			
Cheesy Cheddar Au Gratin	180	9	22
Loaded Au Gratin	140	4.5	23
Three Cheese Mashed Pot. Bake	190	9	24
Slow Cooker Helper: *Per Cup (Prepared)*			
Beef Stew, 1 cup	200	5	24
Beef Stroganoff	250	8	28
Pot Roast	290	12	28
Chicken & Dumpling	250	6	27
Suddenly Salad: *Prepared As Direcrted*			
Caesar, ½ cup dry	250	10	34
Classic, ⅔ cup	240	8	37
Ranch & Bacon, ¾ cup	330	20	31
Bowl Appetit: *Per Bowl*			
Pasta Alfredo	360	11	53
Three Cheese Rotini	360	10	55
Cheddar Broccoli Rice	290	7	51
Bush's Best: *Per ½ Cup*			
Chili Beans	120	1	20
Dark Red Kidney Beans, ½ cup	130	1	21
Frijoles Negras, ½ cup	100	0.5	20
Frijoles Pintos, ½ cup	110	0	19
Garbanzo Beans/Chick Peas, ½ c.	130	2	22
Refried Beans: Traditional	150	3	24
Fat Free	130	0	24
Baked Beans: Vegetarian	130	0	29
Other flavors, average	145	1	30
Campbell's: *Per Cup (8 fl.oz)*			
Chunky Chili: Roadhouse; Firehouse	220	8	25
Tantalizin Turkey	180	2.5	25
Pork & Beans in Tomato Sauce	140	1.5	25
Spaghetti O's Original	180	1	37
Spaghetti O's Meatballs	240	8	32
Sliced Franks	230	10	27
Supper Bakes: *Per ⅙ Box (Prepared as Directed)*			
Cheesy Chicken	170	4	27
Creamy Stroganoff	190	4	31
Garlic Chicken w. Pasta	230	1	44
Herb Chicken w. Rice	190	1	40
Lemon Chicken w. Rice	200	1	43
Savory Pork Chops	160	1	31
Southwestern Style Chicken	150	1	32
Trad. Roast Chicken w. Stuffing	160	3	29

Canned & Packaged Meals (Cont)

Chef Boyardee	C	F	Cb
Beefaroni, all types, 1 cup	260	10	33
Mini Bites (14.5 oz Can): *Per Cup*			
Mini Beef Ravioli w. Meatballs	280	13	31
Mini Pasta Shells w. Meatballs	260	10	32
Mini Spaghetti w. Meatballs	250	10	30
Jumbo (15 oz Can): *Per Cup*			
99% Fat Free: Beef Ravioli	170	1.5	37
Cheese Ravioli	240	2.5	45
Lasagna	270	10	36
Mini Ravioli	250	9	35
Spaghetti w. Jumbo Meatballs	270	12	28
Overstuffed Ital. Sausage Ravioli	240	4.5	40
Microwaveable Cups: *Per Cup*			
Beef Ravioli	220	7	32
Macaroni & Cheese	190	6	26
Mini Bites Spaghetti Rings	220	8	29
Spaghetti & Meatballs	200	8	23
Rice w. Chicken/Vegetables	230	9	30
Microwaveable Big Bowls: *Per ½ Bowl*			
Beefaroni	250	9	31
Mini Ravioli	240	8	33
Ravioli	220	7	32
Twistaroni: Cheesy Nacho, 1 cup	230	6	36
Chili Cheese Dog, 1 cup	220	6	32
Tomato & Beef, 1 cup	250	6	40
Dinner Kits: *Per Serving*			
Cheese Pizza	250	4	45
Lasagna	340	8	54
Spaghetti & Meatballs	300	8	45

Dennison's Chili (15 oz Can): *Per Cup*	C	F	Cb
Chili Con Carne With Beans:			
Original; Hot, 1 cup, avg.	360	14	35
Chunky	300	10	32
99% Fat Free: Beef Chili w. Beans	210	2	29
Turkey Chili w. Beans	210	3	29

Dinty Moore (Hormel Foods)	C	F	Cb
1½ lb Can: Beef Stew, 1 cup	180	8	17
7½ oz Can: Beef Stew, 1 cup	180	8	17
American Classics: *Per Microwave Bowl (10 oz)*			
Beef Stew	250	11	22
Noodles & Chicken	250	8	28
Microwave Cup: Beef Stew, 1 cup	160	7	16
Chicken & Dumplings	200	6	26
Other varieties, average	180	8	17

Dr. McDougall's: *Per 10 oz*	C	F	Cb
Ramen Noodles	150	0.5	29
Rice Pilaf	130	0.5	26

Eden Soy (Vegetarian): *Per ½ Cup (4½ oz)*	C	F	Cb
Baked Beans w. Sorghum, Mustard	150	0	27
Black Eyed Peas	90	1	16
Black Soybeans	120	6	8
Refried Black/Pinto/Kid. Beans, avg.	95	1	17
Other varieties, average	125	0	21

Fantastic: *Per Cup*	C	F	Cb
3-Bean Chili	180	4	28
Spanish Paella	280	5	55
Tuscan Mushroom Risotto	310	7	50
Rice Noodles: Pad Thai, 7.8 oz	400	11	59
Ginger Shiitake, 7.8 oz	340	10	58

Farmhouse	C	F	Cb
Pasta: *Per ¾ Cup*			
Chicken Pasta	370	15	49
Creamy Garlic	420	20	49
Herb & Butter	430	20	48
White Cheddar Pasta	380	14	50
Rice: *Per ⅓ Cup (Prepared as Directed)*			
Chicken Rice	220	3	42
Long Grain & Wild Herb Butter	220	4	41
Other varieties, average	200	3	41

French's Fried Onions	C	F	Cb
Regular or Cheese:			
2 Tbsp, ¼ oz	45	3.5	3
¼ cup, ½ oz	90	7	6
1 cup, 2 oz	360	28	24

Health Valley (Vegetarian)	C	F	Cb
Fat-Free Beans & Chili:			
Vegetarian/Chili, 1 cup	160	1	30
Turkey w. Chili Beans, 1 cup	220	3	34
Other varieties, ½ cup	80	0	15
Meal Cups, average all varieties	140	1	27

Heinz	C	F	Cb
Vegetarian Beans, ½ cup	140	0.5	27

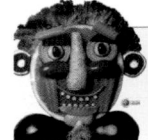

Eat at least 5 servings of fruit and vegetables every day . . . and Enjoy Better Health!

Hormel: *Per Cup*	C	F	Cb
Kid's Kitchen: Beans & Wieners	320	13	37
Cheesy Mac 'N Cheese	350	19	28
Mini Beef Ravioli	250	6	38
Noodle Rings & Chicken	140	4	18
Chili (15 oz Can): *Per Cup*			
With Beans: Homestyle Chili	350	20	28
Reg./Hot/Chunky, average	260	7	33
Turkey (99% Fat Free)	200	3	26
Vegetarian (99% Fat Free)	200	1	38
Less Sodium Without Beans:			
Hot/Chili, 1 cup	210	9	17
Chunky No Beans	210	8	19
Turkey No Beans	190	3	16
Tamales (15 oz Can), 2 Tamales	140	7	15
Hungry Jack Potatoes			
Instant Potato Flakes, ⅓ cup	80	0	18
Hunt's			
Manwich Sloppy Joe, ¼ cup	30	0	7
Knorr Lipton			
Asian Sides: *Per Cup (Prepared as Directed)*			
Beef Lo Mein; Thai Sesame, avg.	280	9	42
Chicken Fried/Teriyaki Rice	240	1.5	50
Teriyaki Noodles	300	6	49
Cajun Sides: *Per Cup (Prepared)*			
Garlic Butter Rice	310	9	49
New Orleans Style Chicken	290	6	51
Dirty Rice	300	6.5	50
Red Beans & Rice	340	6.5	62
Fiesta Sides: *Per Cup (Prepared as Directed)*			
Taco Rice	300	6	52
Smoked Chipotle Rice	260	6.5	55
Nacho Pasta	280	7.5	44
Pasta Sides: *Per Cup (Prepared as Directed)*			
Alfredo; Parmesan	320	12	43
Butter; Stroganoff	270	8	43
Rice Sides: *Per Cup (Prepared)*			
Cheddar Broccoli	310	7.5	50
Creamy Chicken	320	10	49
Herb & Butter	300	9	46
Other varieites, average	300	10	48
Whole Grain Sides: *Per Cup*			
Alfredo	300	11	39
Sesame Chicken	300	9	51
Other varieties, avg.	270	7	45
Kraft			
Minute White Rice, ¾ cup	160	1.5	34
Minute Brown Rice, ⅔ cup	170	1.5	34
It's Pasta Anytime Meals: *Per Package*			
Fettuccine w. Classic Alfredo Sce	580	22	74

Kraft (Cont)	C	F	Cb
Dinners: *Per Serving (Prepared as Directed)*			
Macaroni & Cheese: Orig., ⅓ box	320	6	44
Scooby-Doo Spirals	410	19	47
Mac & Chse: Crazy Noodles, ½ box	410	18	48
Thick'n Creamy, ⅓ box	380	16	50
Easy Mac, avg. all varieties., 1 pch	240	6	40
Deluxe: Orig.; Sharp Chedd., ¼ box	320	10	44
Rotini White Cheese Sce, ½ box	390	15	48
Pasta Salads Gourmet Favorites,			
Asian Sesame, 1 cup	250	10	32
Velveeta Shells & Cheese, ⅓ box	360	13	46
Velveeta Cheesy Potatoes: *Per ½ Cup (Prepared)*			
Au Gratin Potatoes	190	7	26
Bacon Scalloped Potatoes	200	8	26
Mashed Potatoes	200	12	21
La Choy			
Beef Chow Mein, 1 cup	90	2	11
Chicken Chow Mein, 1 cup	100	3	10
Beef Pepper Oriental, 1 cup	100	2	12
Chop Suey Vegetables, ½ cup	15	0	3
Chow Mein Noodles, ½ cup	130	5	19
Lightlife			
Tempeh: Flax; Soy, avg., 4 oz	220	9	16
Fakin' Bacon Strips, 3 sl., 2 oz	100	3	10
Garden Veggie, 4 oz	200	10	17
Three Grain; Wild Rice, avg., 4 oz	230	9	21
Grilles Patty: Lemon (1) 2.7 oz	130	7	8
Tamari (1) 2.7 oz	100	4	10
Light Burgers Patty (1) 3 oz	120	1.5	11
Smart Bacon, 2 slices, 22g	45	2	1
Smart Deli: Country Ham Style, 4 sl.	90	0	5
Old World Bologna Style, 4 sl., 2 oz	60	0	0
Pepperoni Slices, 13 slices, 1 oz	45	0	3
Roast Turkey Style, 4 slices, 2 oz	80	0	4
Three Peppercorn Pastrami Style, 4 sl.	60	0	1
Maruchan			
Ramen Noodles: Beef/Chicken/Shrimp Flavors,			
½ block, 1½ oz	190	8	26
Noodles: Instant Wanton,			
Hot & Sour, 1 pkg	200	12	20
Chicken, 1 pkg	210	13	18
Fried Cup Beef, 1 packet, 2.2 oz	290	12	38
Morningstar Farms			
Kaffree Roma, 1 rounded tsp, 2g	10	0	2
Vegetarian Tuno, ⅓ cup, dr., 2 oz	80	2	2
Vegetarian Chili, 1 cup, 8 oz	180	1.5	25

	C	F	Cb
Near East			
Couscous: *Per Cup (Prepared)*			
Original Plain	230	2	46
Parmesan; Rst Garlic & Oil, avg.	220	4	41
Toasted Pine Nut	230	6	38
Other varieties, avg.	220	5	39
Whole Grain Blends: *Per ⅓ Cup (Prepared)*			
Chicken & Herbs w. Brown Rice	280	6	52
Roasted Garlic w. Brown Rice	220	5	41
Roasted Pecan & Garlic w. Brown	250	9	38
Wheat Pilaf	210	4	41
Pasta, all types	210	4	40
Falafels, ¼ cup, (2½ patties)	220	14	18
Rice Pilaf: *Per Cup (Prepared)*			
Long Grain; Wild Rice; Garlic Herb	220	4	43
Spanish Mix	310	8	54
Tabouli Mix, Wheat Salad	120	3	23
Toasted Almond Mix	230	6	40
Other varieties, average	260	5	42
Nissin			
Cup Noodles, all types, avg.	300	13	38
Chow Mein: Garlic Shrimp, ½ pkg	280	14	32
Chicken Flavor, ½ pkg	240	9	34
Souper Meal, average, ½ pkg	270	10	38
Noodle Chef			
Delecta Bowl: *Per Bowl*			
Tomato Penne	380	4	74
Pizza Mac & Cheese	370	4	70
Nutritious Living: *Per Tray*			
Hi Low: Beef Stew	170	5	8
Chicken Vegetable Parmesan	160	4	13
Tuna Noodle Casserole	200	7	14
Turkey Chili w. Beans	180	6	13
Other varieties, average	180	5	13
Old El Paso			
Dinner Kits: *Per Serving (Prepared)*			
Soft Taco, 82g	380	10	33
Enchilada Bake, ¼ pkg	370	13	33
Fajita (2), 84g	320	12	34
Hard Taco (2)	290	16	18
Shells, Taco Sce, Seasoning (2)	160	6	23
Soft Taco (2)	350	16	31
Taco Dinner (2)	290	16	9
Side Dishes: Chili Beans, 1 cup	240	11	19
Mexe/Pinto Beans, ½ cup	110	0.5	19
Boxed: Chsy Mexican Rice, ⅓ pkt	290	6	55
Spanish Rice, ⅓ pkt	280	4.5	55
Skillet Meal: Cheesy Rice/Beef, 1 c.	250	8	37
Crunchy Enchilada Rice/Chkn, 1 c.	210	4	35

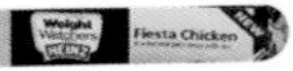

	C	F	Cb
Old El Paso (Cont)			
Refried Beans: Regular, ½ cup	100	0.5	17
w. Green Chilies, ½ cup	100	0.5	19
Vegetarian, ½ cup	100	1	17
Fat Free varieties, ½ cup	100	0	18
Pasta Roni: *Per Cup (Prepared)*			
Angel Hair Pasta varieties, avg.	310	13	41
Fettuccine Alfredo	440	25	47
Chicken (flavor)	300	12	39
Chicken; Shells & White Cheddar	290	12	38
Chicken & Broccoli	360	15	49
Homestyle Deluxe: Four Cheese	390	17	50
Parmesano	370	16	49
World Flavors: *Per Cup (Prepared)*			
Asian Garlic Chicken	280	11	39
Butter Herb Italiana	300	12	40
Chicken Quesadilla	310	13	40
Rice-A-Roni: *Per Cup (Prepared)*			
Beef; Herb & Butter; Rice Pilaf, avg.	310	9	53
Broccoli Au Gratin	360	17	46
Chicken	310	9	51
⅓ Less Salt	270	5	51
Chicken & Broccoli	220	5	40
Chicken & Garlic	250	8	41
Fried Rice	320	11	50
Spanish Rice	260	7	44
(Reduced Fat Recipe: If only 1 Tbsp fat is used instead of 2 Tbsp, deduct 35 calories and 4g fat.)			
Express: *Per Cup (prepared)*			
Asian Fried Rice	280	6	51
Golden Chicken	270	6	51
Other varieties, average	270	6	50
Savory Whole Grains: *Per Cup (Prepared)*			
Chicken & Herb	260	8	41
Roasted Garlic Italiano	270	9	41
Spanish	250	8	42
Rosarita			
Refried Beans: *Per ½ Cup*			
Traditional; Vegetarian; Spicy	120	2	18
Low-Fat Black Bean	90	0.5	18
Fat-Free varieties	100	0	18
Shedd's			
Country Crock Side Dishes			
Mashed Potatoes: Homestyle, ⅔ cup	190	9	23
Garlic, ⅔ cup, 5 oz	170	7	23
Cheddar Mashed Potato, ⅔ cup	200	10	24
Chicken Rice w. Herbs, 1 cup	210	3.5	42
Elbow Macaroni & Cheese, 1 cup	380	17	40

Simply Asia	C	F	Cb
Noodle & Sauce Meal Kits: *Per Cup (Prepared)*			
Chili Garlic	330	5	62
Roasted Peanut	385	14	55
Sesame Teriyaki	285	1	60
Other varieties, average	305	5	58
Noodle Bowls: *Per ½ Package (4 oz)*			
Roasted Peanut	275	12	37
Sesame Teriyaki	200	2	40
Soy Ginger; Spicy Kung Pao, avg.	215	5	39
Quick Noodles: *Per Tray*			
Pad Thai	660	9	133
Szechwan Garlic Chow Mein	650	12	121
Other varieties, average	630	8	126
Take Out Noodle Boxes: *Per ½ Box (5.3 oz)*			
Honey Teriyaki	380	3	73
Pad Thai	390	3	79
Roasted Peanut	410	7	71
Sweet & Sour	370	2	75
Other varieties, average	390	5	71
Stagg Chili			
14.3 oz Box: *Per Cup (8.7 oz)*			
Chili w. Beans: Classic/Dynamite	330	17	28
Country/Laredo	320	16	29
Fiesta Grille	240	9	25
Ranch House Chicken	290	9	32
Rio Blanco Chicken	250	12	19
No Beans: Steakhouse/Double	330	21	16
99% Fat Free: Veg. Gdn/4 Bean	200	1	37
Turkey Ranchers/Silvarado Beef	230	3	33
S & W: *Per ½ Cup*			
Baked Beans, avg. all types	145	0.5	28
Caribbean Black Beans	90	0	19
Kidney Beans	100	0.5	23
Red Beans Louisiana Style	80	0	20
San Antonio; Santa Fe Beans	90	0.5	21
White Beans	80	0.5	19
Taco Bell: *Per ⅓ Cup*			
Home Originals: Refried Beans	120	1	20
Fat Free Beans w. Green Chilles	100	0	18
Tasty Bite			
Vegetarian Entrees: *Per ½ Package*			
Agra Peas & Greens	140	10	9
Bengal Lentils	160	8	16
Bombay Potatoes	105	4	13
Jaipur Vegetables	170	11	10
Jodhpur Lentils	105	4	12
Kashmir Spinach	135	8	8
Madras Lentils	125	5	14
Punjab Eggplant	145	9	13

Tasty Bite (Cont)	C	F	Cb
Ready Meals: *Per Package (w. Rice)*			
Peas Paneer	425	15	54
Spinach Dahl	370	9	62
Vegetable Supreme	315	6	55
Thai Kitchen			
Bowls, avg. all types, 1.7 oz	120	2	24
Rice Noodles: *Per Serving*			
Curry Stir Fry, 1 cup	280	4	55
Lemongrass & Chili Stir Fry, 1 cup	270	2.5	55
Pad Thai varieties, ½ package	270	2	53
Savory Garlic, ½ package	230	2.5	47
Thai Peanut, 1 package	230	2.5	47
Thin/Stir Fry/Wide, 2 oz	195	0	46
Toasted Sesame Stir Fry, 1 cup	260	2.5	55
The Spice Hunter: *Per Cup Meal*			
Stuffed Potato: Creamy Butter	140	3	25
Broccoli & Cheddar	170	3	31
Sour Cream & Chives	160	2	31
Quick Hot Pasta: *Per Cup (Prepared)*			
Primavera Pasta	250	3	45
Roasted Peppers & Garlic	225	3	40
Spicy Mediterranean	230	3	44
Tofurky			
Deli Slices, average all	105	3	6
Holiday: Dumplings (2), 4 oz	210	1	45
Tofurky Roast, 4 oz	190	5	10
Tofurky Wild Rice Stuffing, ½ cup	110	2	21
Tofurky Wishstix, ½ piece	10	0	1
Jurky, 4 pieces	100	2	9
Sausages: Beer Brats (1), 3.5 oz	280	16	8
Kielbasa (1), 3.5 oz	240	12	12
Sweet Italian Sausages (1), 3.5 oz	280	13	12
Trader Joe's			
Bean Medley, ½ cup	150	1	26
Turkey Chili w. Beans, 1 cup	230	3	30
Black Bean Chili, 1 cup	230	1.5	37
Chicken Chili w. Beans, 1 cup	290	9	32
Pasta, Shells & White Cheddar, 1 cup	280	6	48
Refried Beans, avg., ½ cup	110	0	20
Organic Beans, avg., ½ cup	140	0	29
Black Beans: Regular, ½ cup	110	0	19
Cuban Style, ½ cup	120	2	20
Potatoes: Mashed Potatoes, ⅔ cup	120	4.5	20
Garlic Mashed Potatoes, ½ cup	150	7	19
Cheddar Cheese Au Gratin, ½ cup	140	5	21
Premium: Beef Stew, 1 cup	240	11	21
Chicken Stew, 1 cup	230	14	16
Tuna Helper: *See Betty Crocker, Page 71*			

Canned & Packaged Meals (Cont.)

	C	**F**	**Cb**

Uncle Ben's

Flavorful Rice: *Per Cup (Prepared w. Margarine)*

	C	F	Cb
Average all varieties	280	10	44

Country Inn: *Per Cup (Prepared w/out Margarine)*

Broccoli Rice Au Gratin	200	2	43
Other varieties, avg.	200	1	43

Ready Rice: *Per ½ Pouch (Prepared)*

Buttery Rice	190	4.5	47
Roasted Chicken	230	4	41
Whole Grain Brown	220	4	41

Valley Fresh

Chicken: *Per 2 oz*

White & Dark Chunk	80	2	0
Premium Chunk White	70	1	2
Turkey, Premium Chunk White, ¼ can	80	1.5	0

Van Camps

Pork & Beans, ½ cup	110	1	23
Original Baked Beans, ½ cup	140	1	30
Beanie Weanie Original, 7¾ oz	230	8	29
Baked Beans: w. Ground Beef, 1 c.	370	7	57
w. Chicken, 1 cup	360	2	62
Spanish Rice, 1 cup	180	3	37

White Wave (Vegetarian)

Seitan: Chicken w. Broth, 5 oz

Chicken w. Broth, 5 oz	110	2	4
Traditional, 5 oz	90	1	3

Tofu Town: *Per ½ Container*

Grilled Tenders: Havana Black Bean	210	8	18
Light Tamari, 5 oz	120	7	15
Mediterranean Tahini, 5 oz	240	13	16
Sesame Ginger Teriyaki, 5 oz	240	9	24

Soy Milks & Yogurts: *See Pages 27, 30*

Tofu: *See Page 77*

Worthington/Loma Linda (Vegetarian)

Big Franks: 1 link, 1.8 oz	110	6	3
Low-fat, 1 link, 1.8 oz	80	2.5	3
Chili, 1 cup, 8 oz	280	10	25
Choplets, 2 slices, 3.2 oz	90	1	4
Diced Chik, 2 oz	50	0	2
Dinner Cuts, 2 slices, 3.2 oz	90	1	4
FriChik, 2 pces, 3.1 oz	140	8	3
Linketts, (1), 1¼ oz	70	4	1
Little Links, 2 links, 1.6 oz	90	5	3
Low-Fat Veja-Links (1), 1 oz	45	1.5	3
Multigrain Cutlets, 2 sl., 2¾ oz	100	1	5
Prime Stakes (1) 3.2 oz	120	8	7
Redi-Burger, ⅝" slice, 3 oz	120	2.5	7
Saucettes, 4 pces, 3 oz	90	6	1
Super Links (1) 1.6 oz	110	8	2
Tender Bits, 6 pieces, 3 oz	120	4	7
Tender Rounds, 8 pieces, 2¾ oz	120	4.5	6
Turkee Slices, 3 sl., 3.3 oz	180	12	5

Worthington/Loma Linda (Cont)

Vege-Burger, ¼ cup, 2 oz	60	0.5	2
Vege-Links (1), 1 oz	50	3	1
Vegetable Skallops, ½ cup, 3 oz	90	1	4
Vegetarian Burger, ¼ cup, 1.9 oz	70	1.5	3

Yves Veggie Cuisine (Vegetarian)

Breakfast: Brkfast Links (2) 1.8 oz	70	2	3
Breakfast Patties (1) 2 oz	80	2	4
Canadian Veg. Bacon, 3 slices	80	0.5	1
Burgers: Prima Veggie (1) 2.6 oz	120	5	8
Garden Vege Patties (1) 3 oz	90	1.5	9
Bistro Veggie (1)	140	6	9
Veggie Chick'n Burger (1) 2.6 oz	100	3	5
Dogs: Jumbo Veggie Dog (1) 2.6 oz	90	1	5
Hot & Spicy Chili/Good (1) 1.8 oz	70	1.5	2
Veggie/Tofu Dog, avg. (1)	80	5	2
Veggie Deli Slices: Bologna, 2 oz	80	2	2
Ham, 2 oz	100	2	5
Pizza Pepperoni, 1.7 oz (48g)	70	1	4
Salami, 2 oz	80	0	4
Veggie Turkey, 2 oz (62g)	100	1.5	5
Veggie Ground Round: Orig., Ital.	60	0.5	5
Neatballs, 2.1 oz	90	2	5
Mexican, ⅓ cup, 1.93 oz	90	2.5	5
Veggie Entrees: Chili, 10.5 oz	240	1	37
Lasagne, 10.5 oz	240	1	37
Thai Lemongrass Veggie Chicken	330	9	49
Veggie Penne, 300g pkg	220	1.5	36

Zatarain's: *Pasta Dinner Mix (Prepared)*

Gumbo, 1 cup	110	1	23
Jumbalaya, 1 cup	130	1	27

Ready To Serve Complete Meals: *Per Pkg (6½ oz)*

Dirty Rice w. Pork	360	12	52
Jambalaya w. Sausage	350	12	48

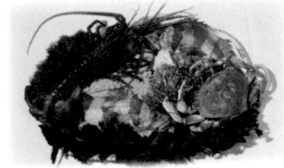

Soybean Products

	C	F	Cb
Cheeses (Soy): *See Page 44*			
Miso Paste, average, 1 Tbsp, ¼ oz	35	1	5
Miso Soup (dry mix), average			
1 Tbsp., dry mix	35	1	5
1 cup, prepared	35	1	5
Natto, ½ cup, 3 oz	160	7	14
Okara (Tofu fiber residue), ½ c., 2 oz	47	1	8
Tempeh: 1 piece, 3 oz	180	8	12
Fried, 3 oz	250	14	14
Seitan *(White Wave)*, Trad., 3 oz	90	1	3
Soybean Protein (TVP), 1 oz	100	0.5	9
Soy Bean Paste, 1 tsp	10	0	2
Soy Beans: *See Page 149*			
Soy Drinks: *See Page 27*			
White Wave: *See Page 76*			

Tofu ~ Packaged

	C	F	Cb
Tofu Stir Fried, average all, 4 oz	120	8	3
Azumaya Tofu: Soft (Silken), 3.2 oz	40	2	1
Soft, Light (Silken), 3.2 oz	40	1	3
Firm; Extra Firm, 2.8 oz	70	4	2
Light Extra Firm, 2.8 oz	60	2	3
Seasoned Tofu, 3 oz	90	5	3
House Foods			
Premium Tofu: Soft (Silken), 3 oz	50	2.5	2
Medium Firm (Regular), 3 oz	60	3	1
Firm, 3 oz	70	3.5	2
Extra Firm, 3 oz	80	4	1

Tofu ~ Packaged (Cont)

	C	F	Cb
House Foods (Cont)			
Organic Tofu: Firm, 3 oz	60	3	0
Extra Firm, 3 oz	90	4.5	0
House Tofu: Tokusen Kinugoshi, 3 oz	90	4	3
Sukui/Soon (Extra Soft), 3 oz	45	2	2
Yaki Tofu: Yaki (Broiled), 3 oz	90	5	2
Tofu Steak: Original, 4.8 oz	80	9	0
Garlic & Pepper, 4.8 oz	80	9	1
Chili & Onion, 4.8 oz	70	8	4
Mori-Nu Tofu (Silken):			
Soft, 3 oz, 1" slice	45	2.5	2
Firm, 3 oz, 1" slice	50	2.5	2
Enriched Firm, 3 oz, 1" slice	70	2.5	6
Extra Firm, 3 oz, 1" slice	45	1.5	2
Organic, 3 oz, 1" slice	60	2.5	2
Lite: Firm, 3 oz, 1" slice	30	0.5	1
Extra Firm, 3 oz, 1" slice	35	0.5	1
Seasoned Tofu: *Per 3 oz*			
Japanese Miso	60	2.5	3
Chinese Spice	50	2	3
Nasoya Tofu: Soft, ⅕ pkg, 2.8 oz	60	3	1
Silken, 3.2 oz	45	2	2
Firm, ⅕ pkg, 3.2 oz	70	3	2
Extra Firm, ⅕ pkg, 2.8 oz	80	4	2
Super Firm, cubed, ⅕ pkg, 2.8 oz	100	5	3
Chinese 5 Spice, ¼ pkg, 3 oz	90	5	3
White Wave: Baked Tofu, 1 square	90	5	2
Soft/Firm Tofu, ⅕ block	110	6	3
Reduced Fat, ⅕ block	90	4	4
Firm, 3 oz	100	6	3

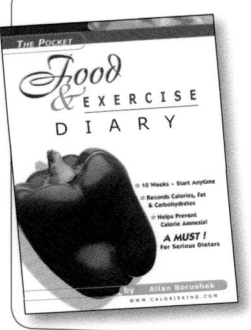
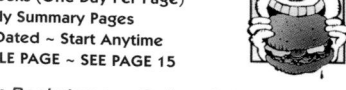

Soups

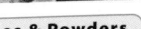

Homemade & Restaurant

Restaurant & Take-Out
Per 8 fl.oz

	C	F	Cb
Bean Medley	200	3	34
Beef Consomme	30	0	2
Borscht (w. Cream)	130	8	14
Bouillabaisse	400	15	10
Chicken & Corn	290	14	20
Chicken & Wild Rice	80	4	9
Chicken Consomme	50	0	2
Chicken Curry	180	8	18
Chicken Jambalaya	160	7	8
Chicken Noodle	80	2	12
w. Chicken	160	4	12
Chicken Soup	80	2	6
Chili with Beans	250	12	25
Clam Chowder	240	15	17
Corn & Crab	120	3	18
Corn Chowder	180	8	16
Cream of Broccoli	200	12	20
Cream of Potato	150	6.5	17
Cream of Mushroom	200	13	15
Creamy Pumpkin	210	10	26
Fish Chowder	220	15	6
French Onion	420	15	25
Gazpacho	50	0	5
Lentil Soup	250	9	28
Lobster Bisque	320	15	10
Matzo Ball (w. 1 large ball)	180	7	24
Minestrone	125	2.5	20
Mulligatawny	300	15	8
Pea & Ham	240	10	25
Potato & Bacon	170	7	19
Shark Fin Soup	100	4	8
Spicy Shrimp Soup, 1 bowl	160	7	10
Split Pea Soup	180	2.5	30
Vegetable (Fat Free)	75	0	18
Vegetable Beef	80	2	10
Vichyssoise	200	9	15
Watercress	90	4	13

Other Soups: *See International & Fast-Foods Sections*

(Arby's, Au Bon Pain, Boston Market, Dunkin' Donuts, Denny's, Schlotzsky's, Sizzler, Souplantation, Sweet Tomatoes, Zoup!)

Homemade Soups: Calculate calories, fat and carbohydrates from ingredients.

Bouillon Cubes & Powders

	C	F	Cb
Bouillon Cubes: *Average all Types*			
Regular, 1 cube	8	0	1
Low Sodium (LiteLine)	12	0	1
Powders: Average, 1 tsp	8	0	1
Herb-Ox: Instant Broth & Seasoning,			
Beef, 1 envelope	5	0	0.5
Chicken; Vegetarian	10	0	2
Herbs, Spices: 1 tsp	5	0	1
Soup Oyster Crackers			
40 small/3 large, ½ oz	60	2	8

Amy's (Organic)

Per Cup (½ Can)

	C	F	Cb
Alphabet (Fat-Free)	80	0	16
Black Bean Vegetable	130	1.5	25
Butternut Squash	100	2.5	20
Chunky Tomato Bisque	120	3.5	21
Chunky Vegetable	60	0	15
Corn Chowder	190	10	25
Cream of Mushroom, ¾ cup, (½ can)	140	9	13
Cream of Tomato	100	2	17
Lentil	150	4.5	19
Minestrone	90	1.5	17
No Chicken Noodle	90	3	12
Pasta & 3 Bean	130	5	19
Potato Leek	180	10	21
Split Pea (Fat-Free)	100	0	19
Vegetable Barley	70	1	13
Other varieties, average	145	4	23

'Light in Sodium' Range *(50% less sodium),*
(Calories/Fat/Carb ~ Same as Regular Range)

Andersen's *Per Cup*

	C	F	Cb
Lentil	110	2	19
Split Pea	130	0	24
Split Pea w. Bacon	140	1	23
Tomato	130	3.5	22

Baxters

Per Cup (Prepared as Directed)

	C	F	Cb
Cream of Asparagus	160	10	15
Cream of Scottish Smoked Salmon	150	8	16
French Onion	70	0	15
Stilton Cheese & White Port	210	15	13
Vichyssoise	210	15	16

Bean Cuisine | C | F | Cb

Per Cup (Prepared as Directed)

	C	F	Cb
13 Bean Boullabaisse; Lentil, avg.	220	0	17
Island Black Bean	210	0	17
Santa Fe Corn Chowder	160	0	18
White Bean Provencal	250	1	32

Bear Creek *Per Cup*

	C	F	Cb
Cheddar Potato	180	5	30
Chicken Noodle	120	1	22
Clam Chowder	140	3.5	25
Creamy Potato	150	3	27
Hot & Spicy	90	1.5	17
Split Pea	110	1.5	20
Other varieties, average	110	0.5	22

Bookbinders

	C	F	Cb
Lobster Bisque, ½ cup	100	4	10
Manhattan Clam Chowder, ½ cup	60	0	10

Campbell's

Classic Red & White: *Per ½ Cup*

	C	F	Cb
Bean w. Bacon; Fiesta Chili Beef, avg.	170	4	25
Beef Noodle	70	2.5	9
Beef w. Veges/Barley; Minestrone, avg.	90	1.5	15
Black Bean	110	1.5	18
Cheddar Cheese	100	4.5	12
Chicken & Dumplings	80	3	10
Chicken Won Ton	60	1	8
Cream of Asparagus	110	7	9
Cream of Broccoli	90	3.5	12
Cream of Chicken & Mushroom	80	6	7
Cream of Mushroom	100	6	9
Cream of Onion	100	6	10
Cream of Potato	90	2	15
Cream of Shrimp	90	6	8
Creamy Chicken Noodle	120	7	11
French Onion	45	1.5	6
Green Pea	180	3	28
Hearty Vegetable w. Pasta	90	0.5	19
Manhattan Clam Chowder	70	0.5	12
New England Clam Chowder	90	2.5	13
Old Fashioned Vegetable	80	1.5	14
Split Pea w. Ham & Bacon	180	3.5	27
Tomato	90	0	20
Tomato Bisque	130	3.5	23
Vegetable	100	0.5	20

Healthy Request: *Per ½ Cup*

	C	F	Cb
Chicken Rice	70	1.5	13
Vegetable Beef	90	1	15
Other varieties, average	90	1.5	18

Campbell's (Cont) | C | F | Cb

	C	F	Cb
98% Fat Free, prep., avg., ½ cup	70	2	10

Chunky: *Per Cup*

	C	F	Cb
Baked Potatoes w. Bacon Bits	170	7	21
Clam Chowder Manhattan	120	3.5	19
Classic Chicken Noodle	60	1.5	8
Grilled Chicken & Sausage Gumbo	140	2.5	21
Hearty Veges w. Pasta	120	2	23
Tomato Cheese Ravioli	160	3	27

Select: *Per Cup (8 fl.oz)*

	C	F	Cb
Beef w. Portabello Mushr. & Rice	110	1	13
Beef w. Roasted Barley	130	1	22
Chicken & Pasta w. Roasted Garlic	100	1	18
Chicken Vegetable	110	0.5	19
Chicken w. Egg Noodles	110	1.5	14
Creamy Chicken Alfredo	180	7	18
Creamy Potato w. Roasted Garlic	180	10	20
Fiesta Vegetable	120	0.5	24
Honey Roasted Chkn w. Potatoes	110	1	19
Italian Style Wedding	110	2.5	16
Minestrone; Tom. Garden; Vege	100	0.5	20
New England Clam Chowder	220	14	16
Rosemary Chkn w. Rstd Potatoes	110	1	17
Savory Lentil	140	0.5	27
Split Pea w. Ham	160	1	29
Tomato w. Rstd Garlic & Herbs	120	0.5	28
Other varieties, average	100	0.5	17

Soup at Hand: *Per Container*

	C	F	Cb
Chicken varieties, average	70	2	11
Creamy Mushroom	120	7	10
Creamy Tomato	190	4	34
Mexican Style Fiesta	150	5	21
New England Clam Chowder	120	6	13
Pizza Soup	140	1	27
Vegetable Beef	60	1	10
Velvety Potato	160	7	21

Soup is an excellent filler as part of a meal, or as a snack.

- *Add lots of veggies, and beans (for extra protein & fiber)*
- *Avoid Noodle Cups (high in fat)*
- *If using low-fat soup mixes, add extra microwaved veges, tofu or canned beans*

Soups (Cont)

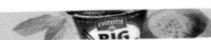

Dr McDougall's C F Cb

Per Serving (Mix)

	C	F	Cb
Split Pea w. Barley, 1.9 oz	190	1	35
Tortilla Soup w. Baked Chips. 1.8 oz	190	1.5	37
Vegetarian Vegetable, 1.5 oz	150	0.5	29
Asian Big Cups: *Per Serving*			
Hot & Sour w. Noodles, 1.9 oz	160	0.5	17
Miso Soup w. Noodles, 1.9 oz	90	0.5	17
Pad Thai/Ramen, avg., 2 oz	100	0.5	21
Western Big Cups: *Per Serving*			
Black Bean & Lime, 3.4 oz	170	1	30
Minestrone & Pasta, 2.3 oz	100	0.5	20
Split Pea w. Barley, 2.5 oz	120	0.5	21
Tamale/Tortilla w. Baked Chips, avg.	100	1	17

Fantastic Cup Soups

	C	F	Cb
Big Soup Noodle Bowls: *Per Serving (½ Pkg)*			
Hot & Sour	130	2	22
Italian Tomato Noodle	130	1	26
Mandarin Broccoli	110	0	20
Miso w. Tofu	100	1	19
Sesame Miso	90	1	17
Spicy Thai Noodle Soup	110	1	22
Spring Vegetable	90	0	19
Big Soup Ramen Noodle, average all varieties,			
½ container, prepared as directed	105	1	20
Big Soup Vegetarian: *Per ½ Container (Prep'd as Directed)*			
Beef Noodle	100	0	21
Cha Cha Chilli	220	2	37
Chicken Noodle	90	0.5	19
Corn & Potato Chowder	130	10	26
Country Lentil; Five Bean	180	1.5	32
Couscous with Lentils Bean	170	1	35
Creamy Broccoli Cheddar	130	2.5	21
Jumpin' Black Bean	230	1.5	41
Minestrone	140	1.5	27
Split Pea	160	1	28
Vegetable Barley	120	0.5	27
Simmer Soup: *Per ¼ Cup*			
Creamy Potato; Split Pea, avg.	130	1.5	21
Vegetable Barley	120	0	26
Soup & Dip Recipe Mix: Average all varieties,			
1 cup, prepared as directed	20	0	5

Health Valley C F Cb

Per Cup

	C	F	Cb
Broths: Beef Flavored, Fat-Free	10	0	0
Chicken: Fat-Free	20	0	0
Low-Fat	35	1.5	0
Organic	25	1	2
Vegetable, Fat-Free	20	0	5
Fat-Free Soup: 5 Bean Vegetable	140	0	32
Black Bean & Vegetable	110	0	24
Italian Minestrone	90	0	21
Lentil & Carrots	100	0	25
Split Pea & Carrots	110	0	17
Other varieties, average	80	0	17
Organic Soup: Black Bean	130	1	25
Lentil	100	1	21
Minestrone	110	0	17
Mushroom Barley	70	0	17
Potato & Leek	70	0	15
Split Pea	110	0	23
Tomato	80	0	18
Vegetable	80	0	18
Soup Cup: *Per ½ Cup*			
Corn Chowder w. Tomatoes	100	0	21
Fat Free: Pasta Italiano	140	0	31
Pasta Parmesan	100	0	20
Spicy Black Bean w. Couscous	130	0	29
Zesty Black Bean w. Rice	100	0	22

Healthy Choice

Per Cup

	C	F	Cb
Bean & Ham	170	2.5	29
Beef and Potato; Chicken w. Pasta	110	1	19
Chicken & Dumplings; Vege Beef	140	3	19
Chicken w. Rice Soup	90	3	12
Country Vegetable	100	0.5	22
Creamy Tomato	100	1.5	22
Fiesta Chicken	100	2	17
Garden Vegetable	120	1	25
Hearty Chicken	120	2	20
New England Clam Chowder	110	1.5	21
Roasted Italian Chicken/ w. Garlic	120	2	21
Split Pea and Ham	170	2.5	30
Zesty Gumbo	100	2	16

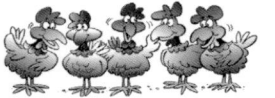

Imagine

C | F | Cb

Per Cup

	C	F	Cb
No Chicken/Vegetable Broth	20	0	2
Free Range Chicken Broth	10	0	1
Organic Creamy: Broccoli	60	1.5	10
Butternut Squash	90	2	18
Crab/Lobster Bisque, avg.	130	5	16
Portobello Mushroom	80	3	10
Potato Leek; Sweet Corn, avg.	115	3	19
Sweet Potato	110	1.5	23
Tomato	80	1	15
Asian Broths: *Per Cup*			
Californian Miso Broth	35	1	5
Free Range Chicken	20	0	2
Soy Ginger Noodle	40	0	10

Knorr

	C	F	Cb
Recipe Classics: *Dry Mix*			
Cream of Spinach, 2 Tbsp	60	1.5	10
French Onion, 2 Tbsp	45	1	9
Leek Soup, 2 Tbsp	60	1	11
Spring Vegetable, 2 Tbsp, 0.3 oz	25	0	6
Tomato w. Basil, 3 Tbsp, 0.7 oz	70	1	15
Vegetable, 2 Tbsp, 0.6 oz	30	0	6
Bouillon Cubes: *Per ½ Cube (1 Cup, Prepared)*			
Beef; Chicken, average	20	1.5	0.5

Lipton

	C	F	Cb
Cup-a-Soup: *Per Envelope*			
Cream of Chicken	70	2	12
Chicken Noodle	50	1	8
Carb Options: Onion, 1 envelope	15	0	1
Mushroom, 1 envelope	10	0	1
Recipe Secrets: *Per Serving (Dry Mix)*			
Beefy Onion, 1 Tbsp	25	0.5	5
Onion, 1 Tbsp	20	0	4
Onion Mushroom, 1⅔ Tbsp	35	0	7
Savory Herb w. Garlic, 1 Tbsp	25	0	6
Soup Secrets: *Per Cup (Prepared)*			
Noodle Soup	60	0.5	9
Chicken Noodle	80	2	11

Manischewitz

	C	F	Cb
Condensed: *Per ½ Cup (Unprepared)*			
Chicken	15	0	2
Chicken w. Kreplach	35	1	5
Chicken w. Matzo Balls	80	3.5	9
Quart Jars: *Per 8 fl.oz (Prepared)*			
Borscht w. Beets	90	0	21
Borscht Low Calorie	25	0	6

Manischewitz (Cont)

C | F | Cb

	C	F	Cb
Ready To Serve: Matzo Ball Soup	110	5	13
Matzo Balls in Broth	215	9	27
Dry Mixes: *Per Cup*			
Matzo Ball & Soup Mix	40	0.5	9
Split Pea Cello	150	0.5	26
Vegetable Soup Cello	120	0	22

Maruchan

Per Cup

	C	F	Cb
Instant Lunch, avg. all flavors	290	12	38
Ramen flavors, ½ pkt, 1½ oz	190	8	26

Miso Cup (Edward & Sons)

Per Cup (Prepared as Directed)

	C	F	Cb
Original; Golden Seaweed	30	1	3
Traditional	35	1	4
Reduced Sodium	25	1	3

Nile Spice

Per Cup

	C	F	Cb
Black Bean; Lentil	170	1.5	36
Cheddar Broccoli	130	3	20
Chicken Flavored Vegetable	110	1.5	21
Country Mushroom	140	2.5	26
Minestrone	140	1	30
Red Beans & Rice	170	1	35
Split Pea	200	1	35
Couscous: Parmesan	200	3	34
Other varieties, average	190	2	36

Pacific Foods

Per Cup

	C	F	Cb
Chicken Broth	10	0	1
Natural, Beef Broth	20	0	1
Organic: French Onion	35	0	6
Creamy Butternut Squash	90	2	17
Creamy Tomato	100	2	16
Roasted Red Pepper & Tomato	110	2	16
Vegetable Broth	15	0	3
Hearty Soups: Chicken Tortilla	140	2	18
Other varieties, average	120	1.5	16

Pritikin

Per Cup

	C	F	Cb
Fat Free Chicken Broth	5	0	0
Hearty Vegetable	80	0	15
Split Pea	130	0.5	23
Vegetarian Vegetable	80	0	17

Soups (Cont)

Progresso

	C	F	Cb
Vegetable Classic: *Per Cup*			
French Onion	50	1.5	8
Green Split Pea	70	3	28
Garden Vegetable	90	0	20
Hearty Tomato	110	1	23
Lentil; Tomato Basil, avg.	150	2	28
Minestrone	110	2	19
Tomato Rotini	140	1	29
Vegetable	80	0.5	16
Traditional: *Per Cup*			
Manhattan Clam Chowder	110	2	17
New England Clam Chowder	190	10	20
Potato Broccoli & Cheese Chowder	220	13	19
Beef Barley	150	4	19
Chkn Herb Dumpling; Minestrone	120	3.5	16
Italian-Style Wedding; Chickarina, avg.	130	5	15
Southwestern Style Chicken	120	7.5	19
Split Pea w/ Ham	150	1	25
Southwestern Corn Chowder	190	7	28
Other varieties, average	100	2	14
Rich & Hearty: *Per Cup*			
Chicken & Homestyle Noodles	110	2.5	14
Chicken Pot Pie Style	170	6	21
Creamy Chicken Wild Rice	150	8	13
New England Clam Chowder	190	9	22
Savory Beef Barley Vegetable	140	1	22
Slow Cooked Vegetable Beef	120	1	20
Steak & Homestyle Noodles	120	3	16
Steak & Sauteed Mushrooms	110	2	18
Other varieties, average	130	1.5	19
Microwaveable Bowl: *Per Bowl*			
Chicken & Wild Rice/Noodle, avg.	90	1.5	12
Minestroni Soup	110	2	19
Vegetable Soup	80	0.5	17
Carb Monitor: *Per Cup*			
Chicken Cheese Enchilada	190	13	7
Chicken Vegetable	70	2	7
Tuscan Style Meatball	110	6	8

Safeway Select

Signature Soups: *Per Cup (8.6 oz)*	C	F	Cb
Baked Potato; Craving Crab, avg.	420	33	20
Broccoli & Cheesy Cheddar	280	21	14
Chkn Noodle; Harvest Vege Beef, avg.	130	3.5	13
Clam Chowder, all varieties	330	24	19
Fajita Chicken & Corn Chowder	350	23	25
Golden Split Pea	200	3	31
Savory Chicken & Wild Rice	170	6	20
Stompin' Steakhouse Chili	260	8	23
Tuscan Tomato & Basil Bisque	310	26	17

Simply Asia

Noodle Bowls: *Per Bowl*	C	F	Cb
Miso Tofu	420	3.5	82
Sesame Chicken	430	4.5	82
Spring Vegetable	420	2.5	84
Szechwan Hot & Sour	480	7	88
Soy Mushroom & Ginger	60	0	8
Soy Savory Onion; Szechwan Garlic	70	0	10
Other varieties, average	270	3	56

Spice Hunter

Per Bowl (10 oz)			
Chicken Noodle	150	3	24
Chicken Vegetable	160	1	31
Creamy Thai Noodle	200	5	31
Split Pea	240	1.5	43

Swanson

Per Cup			
100% Fat Free Chicken Broth	15	0	1
Beef Broth	15	0	0
Chicken Broth	10	0.5	1
Vegetable Broth	15	0	3

Tabatchnick

Per ½ Container			
Barley Mushroom; Wild Rice, avg.	80	1	17
Black Bean	230	2.5	39
Broccoli & Cheese	200	12	15
Chicken w. Dumplings	150	6	19
Corn Chowder	130	4.5	21
Cream of Broccoli	130	5	18
Cream of Mushroom/Spinach, avg.	95	5	11
Creamed Spinach	40	1	7
Lentil	160	0	29
Macaroni & Cheese	250	8	34
Minestrone; Vegetable, avg.	100	1.5	18
New England Potato	110	5	17
New York Chicken	70	1	13
Old Fashioned Potato; Cabbage, avg.	100	1.5	21
Onion	60	1.5	11
Pea	140	0	24
Salmon Chowder	80	1.5	15
Seafood Chowder	130	6	15
Southwest Bean	220	5	35
Tomato Rice	110	3.5	18
Yankee Bean	180	1.5	33
Vegetarian Chili	180	3.5	28
No Salt: Mushroom	80	1	17
Pea	140	0	34
Vegetable	90	1.5	17

Thai Kitchen

C F Cb

7 oz Can: *Per Serving*

	C	F	Cb
Coconut Ginger	190	15	11
Hot & Sour	40	0.5	7

Instant Rice Noodle: *Per Package (Prep. as Directed)*

Bangkok Curry; Thai Ginger	190	3.5	37
Garlic & Vege; Spring Onion	190	3	37
Lemongrass & Chili	190	3.5	37

Rice Noodle Soup Bowls: *Per ½ Bowl*

Hot & Sour	110	2.5	23
Lemongrass & Chili	110	1.5	23
Thai Ginger	120	2	23

Trader Joe's

Per Cup

	C	F	Cb
Barley w. Vegetables	110	3	19
Black Bean	130	1.5	25
Chicken Broth	15	0.5	0
Chicken Noodle	90	1	14
Chunky Minestrone	110	2.5	19
Creamy Corn Chowder	170	6	22
Lentil w. Vegetables	140	3	21
Organic Lentil Vegetable	130	3.5	19
Rich Onion	90	3.5	12
Spicy Black Bean	230	3	41
Split Pea, Low Fat	140	1	26
Condensed: Clam Chowder	160	4	22

Vermont Country Soup

Per Cup

Chicken Noodle; Cream of Potato	290	16	31
Chicken Pomodoro	150	6	17
Country Vegetable	90	1	20
New England Clam Chowder	320	23	23
Tuscan Minestrone	120	1.5	22

Walnut Acres

Per Cup

Autumn Harvest	100	2	19
Country Corn Chowder	150	3	28
Cuban Black Bean	150	1	30
Four Bean Chili	140	1.5	28
Ginger Carrot	100	1	22
Classic Minestrone	100	0	22
Mediterranean Lentil	130	0	26
Savory Tomato	120	2	23

Westbrae Natural

C F Cb

Canned: *Per Cup (Unless Indicated)*

	C	F	Cb
Alabama; Mediterranean Lentil, avg.	140	0	26
New York UnChicken Noodle	60	1	10
Old World Split Pea	150	0	28
Santa Fe Vegetable	160	0	31
Other varieties, average	125	0	25

Condensed: *Per ¾ Cup (Prepared as Directed)*

California UnChicken Broth	15	0.5	2
Monte Carlo Creamy Mushroom	70	3	10
Tuscany Tomato	70	0	16

Wolfgang Puck's

Per Cup

	C	F	Cb
Original: Chicken & Dumplings	220	13	17
Chicken & Egg Noodles	130	5	13
Creamy Roast Chkn w. Wild Rice	200	13	13
Hearty Vegetable Beef	130	3.5	17
New England Clam Chowder	210	12	19
Beef Barley	120	3.5	17
Old World Minestrone	180	6	24
Roast Chicken & Vegetables	180	6	22
Rst Chicken w. Pasta & Mushroom	140	5	15
Signature Recipe: Chicken Tortilla	140	5	17
Beef Burgundy w. Egg Noodles	130	5	12
Chkn Dijon w. Herbed Rice	150	6	15
Crmy Clam Chowder w. Shrimp	160	7	19
Thick Country Vegetable	120	6	25
Other varieties, average	145	6	16
Organic Soup: Classic Minestrone	110	3.5	17
Classic Tomato w. Basil	140	7	19
Old Fashioned Potato	140	7	18
Spicy Bean	160	0.5	30

Wylers

	C	F	Cb
Dry Mix: Mrs Grass Onion, 10g	30	0	6
Homestyle Vegetable, 12g	35	0	7

Mrs Grass Hearty Soup Mix: *Per Cup*

Chicken Noodle	70	1	13
Beef Vegetable	90	0.5	18

Herbs & Spices

Herbs & Spices

	C	F	Cb
Per Teaspoon: Average all types	5	0	1
All Purpose, 1 tsp	0	0	0
Allspice, ground	5	0	1
Chili Powder	8	0	1
Cinnamon, ground	6	0	2
Curry Powder	6	0	1
Garlic Powder	9	0	2
Nutmeg, ground	12	0	1
Onion Powder	7	0	2
Parsley, dried	4	0	1
Pepper, black/red/white, avg.	6	0	1
Saffron	2	0	0
Salt Free Blends, 1 tsp	0	0	0
Tumeric, ground	8	0	1
Seeds: Fenugreek	12	1	2
Mustard, Poppyseed	15	1	1
Other types, average	7	0	1

Seasonings & Flavorings

	C	F	Cb
Accent Flavor Enhancer, 1 tsp	0	0	0
Angostura Bitters, 1 tsp	12	0	3
Bacon Bits, average, 1 Tbsp	35	2	2
Bacon Chips *(Durkee),* 1 Tbsp, 7 g	30	1	2
Bac-Os (Betty Crocker), 1½ Tbsp, 7g	30	1.5	2
Bragg Liquid Aminos, 1 tsp	5	0	0
Butter Buds, 1 tsp	5	0	2
Garlic Bread Sprinkle, 1 tsp	8	0.5	1
Garlic Salt, 1 tsp	20	0	0
Italian Seasoning, 1 tsp	4	0	1
Lemon Pepper Seasoning, 1 tsp	7	0	1
Meat Tenderizer, avg., 1 tsp	7	0	1
Molly McButter, 1 tsp	5	1	1
Mrs Dash Blends, 1 tsp	0	0	0
Salad Crunchies *(McCormick),* 1 tsp	10	0.5	2
Salt: Regular, Sea Salt, Lite Salt	0	0	0
Seasoning Mixes, avg., ¼ pkg	70	1	9
Taco Seasoning, avg., ¼ pkg	30	0.5	4
Old El Paso: Chili Season. Mix, 1 T.	8	0.5	1.5
Cheesy Taco Season. Mix, 1 Tbsp	10	0.5	2
Taco/Burrito Seasoning Mix, 2 tsp	15	0	4
Fajita Seasoning Mix, 1 tsp	10	0	3
Vegit Seasoning Mix, 1 tsp	2	0	0

Condiments, Sauces

	C	F	Cb
Average of Brands & Homemade			
Apple Sauce: *Also see Page 146*			
Sweetened, ¼ cup, 2½ oz	55	0	13
Unsweetened, ¼ cup, 2 oz	25	0	7
Barbecue Sauce, ¼ cup, average	45	1	9
Bearnaise Sauce, ¼ cup, 2½ oz	190	19	5
Buffalo Wing Sce: Honey Mustard, 1 T.	40	3	3
Average other varieties, 1 Tbsp	25	2	2
Catsup (Ketchup), regular, 1 Tbsp	15	0	4
Cheese, h/made, ¼ cup, 2½ oz	150	10	12
Chef-Mate, Hot Dog	15	0.5	2
Chili Sauce: *Heinz,* 1 Tbsp, ½ oz	20	0	4.5
Chef-Mate, Hot Dog, 1 Tbsp	15	0.5	2
Del Monte, 1 Tbsp, ½ oz	20	0	5
Cocktail Sauce, ¼ cup	110	0	15
Sugar Free *(Walden Farms)* 1 Tbsp	0	0	0
Cranberry, all types, ¼ c., 2½ oz	110	0	27
Demi Glaze Gold, 2 tsp	30	0.5	3
Honey Mustard *(French's)* 1 tsp	5	0	1
Horseradish: 1 tsp	2	0	0
Kraft, 1 tsp	20	1.5	0
Ketchup: Regular, 1 Tbsp, ½ oz	15	0	4
Heinz One-Carb, 1 Tbsp	5	0	1
Mushroom Sauce, ½ cup, 2 oz	50	2	5
Mustard, average, 1 tsp	5	0	0.5
Pesto Sauce, ¼ cup, 2 oz	90	5	8
Pizza Sauce, cnd., ¼ cup, 2 oz	30	0	6
Seafood Cocktail Sce, ¼ cup	60	0	15
Soy Sauce: All types, avg., 1 Tbsp	10	0	1
Kikkoman Lite Soy, 1 Tbsp	10	0	1
Sour Cream Sce, ½ cup	250	15	22
Spaghetti Sce, ½ cup, 4½ oz	135	6	19
Steak Sauce: *A1,* 1 Tbsp, ½ oz	15	0	3
Lea & Perrins, 1 Tbsp, ½ oz	25	0	5
Carb Well (A1) 1 Tbsp, ½ oz	5	0	1
Str'berry Puree Sce: Unsweet., 2 T.	9	0	2
Sweet & Sour Sauce:			
Chef-Mate, 1 Tbsp, ½ oz	20	0.5	4
Contadina, 1 Tbsp	40	1	8
La Choy, 2 Tbsp, 34g	60	0	14
Tabasco Sauce, 1 tsp	2	0	0
Taco Sauce, average, 2 Tbsp, 1 oz	10	0	1
Tartar Sauce: *Heinz,* 2 Tbsp, 1 oz	120	11	4
America's Choice, 2 Tbsp, 1 oz	160	17	1
Hellman's: Regular, 2 Tbsp, 1 oz	80	7	4
McCormick, Fat-Free, 2 Tbsp, 1 oz	35	0	6
Teriyaki Sauce *(Kikkoman)*1 T., ½ oz	15	0	3
Vinegar, White or Wine, 2 Tbsp	4	0	1
White Sauce, ½ cup, 5 oz	130	7	10
Worcestershire Sauce, 1 tsp	5	0	1

Pickles & Relish | C | F | Cb |

Average All Brands

	C	F	Cb
Bread & Butter Pickles, 4 sl., 1 oz	25	0	6
Chutney, 2 Tbsp, 1¼ oz	50	0	11
Dill Pickle:			
Slices, 4 slices, 1 oz	4	0	1
1 large,			
(3¾"x 1¼" diam.), 2¼ oz	12	0	3
Extra lrg (4"x 1¾" diam.), 5 oz	30	0	6
Halves: Small, 1 oz	3	0	0.5
Large, 2½ oz	8	0	2
Sweet, small, ½ oz	22	0	6
Gherkins, sweet, 1 med., 1 oz	30	0	7
Green Chilies, chopped, 2 Tbsp	5	0	1
Horseradish, 1 Tbsp	10	0	2
Jalapenos, pickled, 2 whole, 2 oz	10	0.5	2
Jalapeno Relish, 1 Tbsp, ½ oz	5	0	1
Mustard, avg. all brands, 1 tsp	5	0	0.5
Peppers, Hot/Mild (1), 1.6 oz	20	0	4
Pickled: Beets, ½ cup, 4 oz	75	0	19
Onions, 1 medium, ¾ oz	10	0	2
Cocktail Onion, 1 onion	2	0	0
Red Cabbage, ½ cup, 3 oz	65	0	15
Pickles: Sweet, 2 Tbsp, 1 oz	35	0	0
Large (3"x ¾ diam.), 1¼ oz	40	0	10
Pickle in a Pouch, 1 large	12	0	3
Relishes: Sandwich Spread, 1 tsp	20	1	5
Cranberry-Orange, 1 Tbsp	30	0	7
Hot Dog *(Heinz)*, 1 Tbsp, ½ oz	17	0	3
Sweet Pickle, 1 Tbsp, ½ oz	20	0	5
Sauerkraut, ½ cup, 3½ oz	25	0	5
Sweet Cauliflower, 1 oz	35	0	8

Salsa

Average all Types: Per 2 Tablespoons

	C	F	Cb
Regular, no oil, 2 Tbsp	15	0	3.5
Homemade w. Oil, 2 Tbsp	40	3	8
Kaukauna, 2 Tbsp, 1 oz	15	0	3
La Victoria, 2 Tbsp, 1 oz	10	0	2
Old El Paso, 1 Tbsp, 1 oz	10	0	2
Wild Oats, 2 Tbsp, 1 oz	20	0	4

Gravy | C | F | Cb |

Homemade Gravy:	C	F	Cb
Thin, little fat, 2 Tbsp, 1 oz	20	1	3
Thick, 2 Tbsp, 1¼ oz	50	2	9
¼ cup, 2½ oz	100	4	18
Franco-American (Canned)			
Beef; Turkey Gravy, 2 oz	25	0.5	3
Chicken Gravy, ¼ cup, 2 oz	40	4	4
Pillsbury (Gravy Mixes)			
Brown; Homestyle, ¼ cup, 2 oz	15	0	3
Chicken, as prep., ¼ cup, 2 oz	20	0	4

Gravy-In-Jars-Homestyle

	C	F	Cb
Boston Market, ¼ cup, 2 oz	40	2.5	3
Franco-American (In Jars):			
99% Fat Free, ¼ cup, 2 oz	20	0	4
Heinz, reg., all types, ¼ c., 2 oz	25	1	3
Fat Free Roast Turkey, ¼ c., 2 oz	10	0	2
Vons, all types, ¼ c., 2 oz	20	0.5	4

Tomato Products | C | F | Cb |

Whole/Chopped/Crushed/Diced	C	F	Cb
1 cup, 8½ oz	50	0	10
In Aspic, ½ cup	50	0	12
w. Green Chili, 1 cup, 8½ oz	60	0	16
Stewed, ½ cup, 1.7 oz	40	1.5	6.5
Wedges in Tom Juice, 1 cup	70	0.5	18
Salsa, average, 1 Tbsp	15	0	3.5
Tomato Ketchup:			
Regular, 1 Tbsp, ½ oz	15	0	4
One-Carb *(Heinz)*, 1 Tbsp, ½ oz	5	0	1
Tomato Paste, 2 Tbsp, 1 oz	25	0	6
Regular, ¾ cup, 6 oz	140	1	32
Tomato Puree, ½ cup, 4½ oz	50	0	10
Tomato Sauce:			
Regular, ½ cup, 4.4 oz	50	0	11
Spanish Style, ½ cup, 4.3 oz	40	0	9
w. Mushrooms, ½ cup, 4.3 oz	45	0	10
w. Onions, ½ cup, 4.3 oz	50	0	12
Tomato Seasoning, 3 tsp	20	0	4
Sundried Tomatoes:			
Natural, 5-6 pces, 0.4 oz	22	0	5
In Oil, drained, 6 pces, ½ oz	40	2.5	4

Sauces ~ Pasta, Cooking

HEINZ **CLASSICO**

Brands | C | F | Cb

A-1

Steak & Marinades Sauce: *Per Tablespoon (½ oz)*

	C	F	Cb
Bold & Spicy; Teriyaki; New York	20	0	5
Carb Wel	5	0	1
Chicago	20	1	2
Jamaican Jerk	25	0.5	5
New Orleans Cajun	25	0	5
Steak Sauce	15	0	3

Barilla: *Per ½ Cup*

	C	F	Cb
Green & Black Olives; Garden Vege	90	4	12
Roasted Garlic & Onion	60	1.5	11
Other varieties, average	70	2.5	12

Bertolli/Five Brothers: *Per ½ Cup*

	C	F	Cb
Creamy Alfredo	200	18	6
Italian Sausage	100	3	15
Olive Oil & Garlic	90	3	14
Olive w. Sundried Tomato	100	4	13
Marinara; Rst Red Pepper, average	80	2	13
Traditional Basil Pesto	270	27	4

Buitoni

Pasta Sauce: *Per Serving*

	C	F	Cb
Alfredo, ¼ cup	140	11	5
Light Alfredo, ¼ cup	80	5	5
Marinara, ½ cup	80	3	10
Roasted Garlic Marinara, ½ cup	60	1.5	10
Tomato Herb Parmesan, ½ cup	130	8	10
Bruschetta Sauce, avg., 2 Tbsp	30	2	2

Carb Options: *Per Serving*

	C	F	Cb
Alfredo, ¼ cup	110	10	4
Barbeque varieties, 2 Tbsp	10	0	3
Double Cheddar, ¼ cup	90	8	2
Garden Style, ½ cup	80	4.5	7
Hickory Barbecue, 2 Tbsp	10	0	3
Marinades: Italian Garlic, 1 Tbsp	0	0	0
Steak, 1 Tbsp	5	0	1

Catelli

	C	F	Cb
Garden Select Pizza Sauce, 1 fl.oz	15	0.5	2.5
Meat Sauce, ½ cup, 4 oz	85	2.5	11

Garden Select 6 Vege Recipe Sauce: *Per ½ Cup*

	C	F	Cb
Parmesan & Romano	80	2.5	12
Thick & Chunky, Tomato Basil Blast	70	1.5	12
Other varieties, avg.	80	1.5	13

Cento: *Per Serving (½ Cup)*

Sauces: Passata Tomatoes

	C	F	Cb
Passata Tomatoes	40	0	8
Pasta, all natural	50	3	3
Pizza, fully prepared	25	0	5
Tomato: Arrabbiata; Vodka	70	3	6
Marinara; Puttanesca	115	9	6
White Clam	165	13	5

Classico: *Per ½ Cup Unless Indicated*

	C	F	Cb
Homestyle Meat Selections Sce, ½ c.	125	5	14

Signature Recipes Sauce: *Per Serving*

	C	F	Cb
Alfredo varieties, avg., ¼ cup	110	10	3
Cabernet Marinara w. Herbs, ½ cup	60	2	10
Fire Roasted Tomato & Garlic, ½ cup	50	0.5	10
Florentine Spinach & Cheese, ½ cup	80	5	6
Mushrooms & Ripe Olives, ½ cup	60	1	11
Pesto, Sun-Dried Tomato, ¼ cup	90	5	8
Pesto, Traditional Basil, ¼ cup	230	21	6
Rstd Chicken w. Parm. & Garlic, ½ c.	90	2	13
Spicy Red Pepper, ½ cup	60	1.5	7
Spicy Tomato & Pesto, ½ cup	90	4	11
Sun-Dried Tomato, ½ cup	80	3	11

Traditional Favorites Sauce: *Per ½ Cup*

	C	F	Cb
Four Cheese	90	5	10
Italian Sausage w. Peppers & Onions	90	2	13
Roasted Garlic; Triple Mushr., avg.	80	3	11
Other varieties, average	70	1	12

Contadina

Pizza Sauce: Flavored w. Pepperoni

	C	F	Cb
Flavored w. Pepperoni	35	1	5
Original; Four Cheese, avg.	30	0.5	6
Cooking Sauce: Sweet & Sour, 1 T.	40	1	8
Tomato Sauce, avg., ¼ cup	20	0	4

Del Monte

Spaghetti Sauces: *Per ½ Cup*

	C	F	Cb
w. Four Cheeses	70	1.5	15
w. Meat/Mushrooms, average	60	1	14
Other varieties, avg.	75	1	16
Chunky Sauce: Garlic & Herb	60	1.5	11
Italian Herb	60	1	12
Sloppy Joe Sauce, Original, ¼ cup	50	0	11

Dominick's: *Per ½ Cup*

All Natural: Garl. & Onion; Marinara

	C	F	Cb
Garl. & Onion; Marinara	80	4	10
Mushr. & Olive; Tomato & Basil	80	1	8
Italian Classics: Four Cheese	80	2.5	12
Portabella Mushroom	60	2	9
Puttanesca	70	3	8
Spicy Roasted Garlic	70	2	10
Sun Ripened Tomatoes	80	4	8
Tomato Basil	50	1	8

Brands (Cont)

	C	F	Cb
Enrico's			
Sicilian	80	2.5	13
Traditional Italian Style, 3.5 oz	60	1.5	12
Mushroom Onion, ½ cup, 4.4 oz	70	1.5	13
Other varieties, ½ cup, 4.4 oz	60	1	12
Emiril's			
Pasta Sauces: Per ½ Cup			
Homestyle Marinara	90	4	11
Kicked Up Tomato; Rstd Gaaahlic	70	3	9
Puttanesca	80	5	9
Roasted Red Pepper	60	3	7
Vodka Sauce	130	8	13
French's Grill & Glaze			
Honey Mustard, 2 Tbsp	90	1	18
Healthy Choice: Per ½ Cup			
Garlic & Herbs	60	0	13
Traditional Pasta Sauce	60	0	13
Super Chunky: Vege Primavera	60	0	13
Tomato, Mushroom Garlic	45	0	10
Heinz: Per 1 Tbsp (Approx. ½ oz)			
Barbecue Sauces, all flavors	35	0	9
Chili Sauce, 1 Tbsp	20	0	5
Horseradish Sauce, 1 Tbsp	75	6	2
Mustard: Pourable/Mild, 1 Tbsp	10	0.5	0
Spicy Brown	15	1	1
Seafood Cocktail Sauce	60	0	15
Steak Sauce 57	30	0	4
Tartar Sauce, 1 Tbsp	70	7	1
Tomato Ketchup	20	0	5
Worcestershire Sauce, 1 Tbsp	10	0	1
Hunt's			
BBQ Sauce: Original, 2 Tbsp	60	0	15
Hickory & Brown Sugar, 2 T.	60	0	15
Manwich Sloppy Joe Sce, ¼ cup	30	0	6
Family Favorites, avg., 2 oz	30	0	6
Spaghetti Sauce: Per ⅙ Can (26.5 oz)			
Traditional, 4.4 oz	50	0	10
Meat Sauce, 4.4 oz	60	0	11
Light Sauce, 4.4 oz	45	0	9
KC Masterpiece: Per Tablespoon			
Marinades: Garlic & Herb	30	1	5
Honey & Teriyaki	40	0.5	9
Original BBQ	60	0	15
Knorr			
Classic Sauce: Per 2 Tbsp (Prepared)			
Bearnaise	20	0	4
Hollandaise	20	0	4
Classic Gravy, avg., ¼ cup, prepared	25	0	4

	C	F	Cb
Kraft			
CarbWell Sauce, 2 Tbsp	15	0	3
Sauce: Cocktail, 1 Tbsp	30	0.3	6
Horseradish, 1 tsp	20	1.5	1
Sandwich Spread & Burger, 1 T.	45	3.5	3
Sweet 'n Sour, 1 Tbsp	30	0	7
Tartar: 1 Tbsp	70	6	4
Lemon & Herb, 1 Tbsp	75	8	0.5
Fat-Free Tartar, 1 Tbsp	12	0	3
Barbecue Sauces: Average, 2 T.	50	0.5	10
Las Palmas			
Red Chile Sauce, ¼ cup, 2 oz	20	0.5	2
Enchilada Sauces: Green Chile	25	1.5	3
Hot/Original, ¼ cup, 2 oz	15	0.5	2
Lawry's 30 Minute Marinade: Per Tbsp			
Caribbean Jerk	25	0	5
Lemon Pepper	10	0	2
Mesquite	5	0	1
Thai Ginger; Herb & Garlic	10	0	2
Other varieties, average	20	0	3.5
Packet Seasonings: Per 2 teaspoons (Dry)			
Fajitas; Taco, average	10	0	3
Average other flavors	20	0	4
McCormick Sauce Mixes			
Golden Dipt Marinade: Per Tablespoon (Dry)			
Cajun Style	60	4.5	2
Garlic Herb	50	5	1
Ginger Teriyaki	60	3	5
Honey Mustard	25	0	4
Honey Soy	30	0	7
Lemon Herb	80	8	0
Lemon Pepper	25	2	1
Mesquite; White Wine, avg.	10	0.5	1
Grill Mates Grilling Sauces: Per 2 Tablespoons			
Hickory BBQ	80	0.5	17
Mesquite; Teriyaki, avg.	60	0.5	12
Montreal Steak	35	0	7
Grill Mates Marinades, avg., 2 Tbsp	60	0	15
Pasta Sauce Mixes: Per Serving (Dry)			
Creamy Garlic Alfredo, 2 Tbsp	90	6	4
Four Cheese Italian, 1 ⅓ Tbsp	40	1.5	5
Italian Style Spaghetti, 1 ⅓ Tbsp	35	0	7
Pesto Pasta, 2 tsps	10	0	2
Thick & Zesty Spaghetti, 1 Tbsp	25	0	6
Tomato Basil, 1 teaspoon	25	0	5
Finishing Sauce: Per ¼ Cup (Prepared)			
Creamy Mushroom	70	5	3
Honey Mustard	120	1	25
Red Burgundy Wine for Beef; Rst Beef	30	1	3
Roasted Chicken Gravy w. Herbs	50	2.5	4

Sauces ~ Pasta, Cooking (Cont)

HEINZ CLASSICO

Brands (Cont)

	C	F	Cb
Mr Yoshida's			
Original Gourmet, 2 Tbsp, 30ml	90	0	20
Hawaiian Sweet & Sour, 2 Tbsp	70	0	18
Muir Glen: *Per ½ Cup (125g)*			
Organic Pasta Sauce:			
Mushr. Marinara; Portobello Mushr.	50	0	11
Other varieties, average	50	1	11
Newman's Own: *Per ½ Cup*			
Bombolina (Tomato & Basil)	90	4.5	13
Five Cheese	80	3	10
Fra Diavolo	70	3	10
Marinara; Sockarooni	70	2	12
Roasted Garlic & Peppers	70	2.5	11
Vodka	110	5	11
Old El Paso			
Enchilada Sauce: Green Chile, ¼ cup	20	1	3
Other varieties, ¼ cup	25	1	3
Sauce Mixes, 2 teaspoons, 4g	10	0	2
Picante Sauce, all varieties, 2 Tbsp	10	0	2
Taco Sauce, all varieties, 1 Tbsp	5	0	1
Salsas: Make Mine Medium, 2 Tbsp	10	0	2
Wild for Mild, 2 Tbsp	10	0	2
Thick N' Chunky varieties, 2 Tbsp	10	0	3
Pace: *Per 2 Tbsp*			
Picante Sauce	10	0	2
Chunky Salsa, average all types	10	0	2
Salsa Con Queso	90	6	6
Prego: *Per ½ Cup*			
Pasta Sauce: Marinara	100	5	11
Diced Onion & Garlic	120	4.5	18
Flavored w. Meat	130	5	19
Italian Sauasge & Garlic	120	5	16
Mini Meatball	150	6	20
Mushroom & Garlic	110	2	20
Mushroom Parmesan	130	3.5	22
Organic varieties, average	90	2.5	14
Roasted Garlic Parmesan	100	1	20
Three Chse; Tom. Basil & Garlic, avg.	90	1.5	17
Other varieties, average	120	3.5	19
Chunky Garden: Combination	90	1.5	17
Mushroom Supreme	120	4	19
Other varieties, average	110	3.5	17
Hearty Meat: Three Meat Supreme	170	10	13
Other varieties, average	160	8	15

	C	F	Cb
Premier Japan (Organic)			
Garlic/Ginger/Wasabi Tamari, 1 T.	10	0	2
Thai Soynut, 1 Tbsp	25	2	2
Ragu: *Per ½ Cup (Unless Indicated)*			
Pizza Quick Sauce: *Per ¼ Cup*			
Traditional	40	2	4
Homemade Style	30	1	4
Thick & Zesty	40	1.5	5
Cheese Creations: *Per ¼ Cup*			
Classic Alfredo	110	10	3
Double Cheddar	100	9	3
Light Parmesan Alfredo	70	5	3
Chunky Gardenstyle: *Per ½ Cup*			
Mushroom & Green Pepper	100	3	16
Other varieties, average	110	3	18
Light varieties, average	50	0	10
Old World Style: Marinara	80	4.5	11
Meat Sauce	80	4	7
Mushroom; Traditional	70	3	8
Organic: Garden Veggie	80	2.5	12
Cheese; Traditional	80	3	11
Rich & Meaty: Classic Italian Style	150	10	9
Mama's Meat Sauce	130	8	8
Sausage, Peppers & Onions	155	10	8.5
Robusto!: 7-Herb Tomato	80	3.5	9
Chopped Tom., Olive Oil & Garlic	95	5	10
Parmesan & Romano	90	3.5	10
Sauteed Beef, Onion & Garlic	90	5	9
Sauteed Onion & Garlic	80	4	9
Rainforest Organic			
Ginger Curry, 1 Tbsp	15	1	2
Papaya Pepper, 1 Tbsp	0	0	0
Rinaldi: *Per ½ Cup*			
3-Cheese	90	2	15
Original; Meat/Mushroom, avg.	80	3	12
Other varieties, average	70	2.5	12
S & W: *Per Tablespoon*			
Teriyaki, Light/Marinade	20	0	4
Safeway			
Salsa: *Per 2 Tablespoons*			
Chipotle Salsa; Sthwest Salsa, avg.	15	0	3
Peach P'apple Salsa; Salsa Verde, avg.	20	0	4
Sauce: *Per 2 Tablespoons*			
Fiesta Fajita; Rstd Tomato, avg.	15	0	2
Garlic Lovers	10	0	3
Mild Enchilada	20	0	4

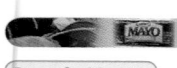

Brands (Cont)

	C	F	Cb
Seeds of Change: Per ½ Cup			
Tomato Basil Sauce	50	0.5	9
Traditional Marinara Sauce	60	3.5	9
	60	3.5	6
Steel's Gourmet Sauce			
Barbeque Sce, 2 Tbsp	15	0	2
Cocktail Sce w. Dill & Lemon, 4 Tbsp	30	0	5
Rocky Mountain Ketchup, 1 oz	10	0	0
Spiced Cranberry Sce, 5 Tbsp	20	0	4.5
Sweet & Spicy, 1 Tbsp	35	2	2
The Wizard's (Organic)			
Hot Stuff, 1 Teaspoon	0	0	0
Vegetarian Worcestershire, 1 tsp	2	0	0.5
Troy's Sauces (Organic)			
Ginger Sauce, 1 Tbsp	10	0	1
Peanut Sauce, 1 Tbsp	25	1.5	2
Timpone's: Per ½ Cup			
Spaghetti Sauce: Classic	50	2.5	8
Family Recipe	80	3	7
Mom's	70	3	7
Tree of Life: Per ¼ Cup			
Tomato	50	2	9
Fat-Free Classic Tomato	40	0	9
Fat-Free Sweet Pepper	35	0	8
Verdi (Vons/Safeway): Per ½ Cup			
Arrabbiata	70	8	10
Four Cheese	70	3	10
Garlic & Basil	70	4	10
Marinara	60	2	10
Mushroom & Onion	60	3	6
Spicy Red Bell Pepper	50	1	9
Sundried Tomato & Olive	60	3	6
Vodka	130	10	9
Walnut Acres: Per ½ Cup (125g)			
Organic Pasta Sauce, average	50	1	9
Wild Oats: Per 2 Tablespoons (1 oz)			
Grilling Marinade: Wasabi	40	4	1
Asian Sesame	45	4.5	1
Ginger Teriyaki	30	3	1
Pasta Sauce: Funghi, ½ cup	100	3.5	4
Marinara, ½ cup	100	9	6
Norma, ½ cup	140	12	6
Puttanesca, ½ cup	120	12	8
Salsa, avg., 2 Tbsp	15	0	3

Quick Guide

Mayonnaise	C	F	Cb
Regular			
Average All Brands, 1 Tbsp	100	11	0
Bestfoods, Kraft, 1 Tbsp	100	11	0
½ cup, 4 oz	800	88	0
Light/Reduced Fat			
Kraft, 1 Tbsp	45	3.5	2
Best Foods, 1 Tbsp	45	4.5	0.5
½ cup, 4 oz	360	36	7
Hain, Safflower Oil, 1 Tbsp	100	11	0
Hellman's, 1 Tbsp	45	4.5	0.5
Spectrum: Canola Mayo, 1 Tbsp	100	11	0
Light Canola Mayo Eggless, 1 Tbsp	35	3.5	0
Fat Free			
Kraft: 1 Tbsp	10	0	2
½ cup, 4 oz	80	0	16
Smart Beat, 1 Tbsp	10	0	3
Sugar Free: Dukes Mayo, 1 Tbsp	100	12	0
Mayonnaise Style Dressing			
BAMA Dressing, 1 Tbsp, ½ oz	50	4	3
Best Foods Sandwich Spread, 1 T.	60	5	2
Gourmayo (French's), 1 Tbsp, ½ oz	50	5	2
Miracle Whip Salad Dressing:			
Regular, 1 Tbsp, ½ oz	40	3.5	2
Light, 1 Tbsp, ½ oz	30	2	3
Free, 1 Tbsp, ½ oz	15	0	2
Nayonaise (Nasoya)			
(Tofu Base/Dairy Free/Eggless)			
Regular, 1 Tbsp, ½ oz	35	3.5	1
Fat-Free, 1 Tbsp, ½ oz	10	0	2

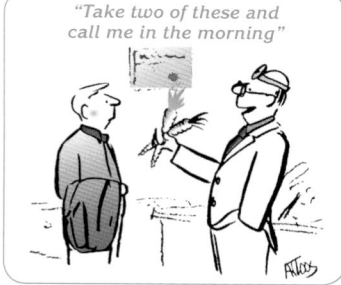

"Take two of these and call me in the morning"

89

Salad Dressings

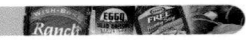

Quick Guide

Salad Dressings
Average All Brands
Per 2 Tbsp (Approx 1 fl.oz)

	C	F	Cb
Balsamic Vinaigrette: Reg., 1 oz	90	9	3
Light, 2 Tbsp, 1 oz	45	4	2
Fat Free, 2 Tbsp, 1 oz	25	0	6
Blue Cheese: Regular, 2 Tbsp, 1 oz	150	16	2
Regular, ¼ cup, 2 oz	300	32	4
Light, 2 Tbsp, 1 oz	30	1	4
Caesar: Regular, 2 Tbsp, 1 oz	155	17	1
Regular, ¼ cup, 2 oz	310	34	2
Light, 2 Tbsp, 1 oz	70	8	5
Coleslaw: Regular, 2 Tbsp, 1 oz	125	11	8
Regular, ¼ cup, 2 oz	245	21	15
Light, 2 Tbsp, 1 oz	110	7	14
French/Italian: Regular, 1 oz	150	14	5
Regular, ¼ cup, 2 oz	290	28	10
Light, 2 Tbsp, 1 oz	65	4	9
Fat/Oil-Free, 2 Tbsp, 1 oz	40	0	10
Ranch: Regular, 2 Tbsp, 1 oz	145	16	2
Regular, ¼ cup, 2 oz	290	31	4
Light, 2 Tbsp, 1 oz	80	3	7
Fat-Free, 2 Tbsp, 1 oz	50	0.5	11
Thousand Island: Regular, 1 oz	120	11	5
Regular, ¼ cup, 2 oz	230	22	9
Light, 2 Tbsp, 1 oz	60	4	7
Fat-Free, 2 Tbsp, 1 oz	40	0.5	10

Brands ~ Salad Dressings
Per 2 Tbsp (Approx 1 fl.oz)

	C	F	Cb
Annie's Naturals			
Cowgirl Ranch, 2 Tbsp	120	11	3
French; Goddess, avg.	90	9	3
Organic: Buttermilk	70	7	1
No-Fat Yogurt	20	0	3
Red Wine & Olive Oil	160	17	1
Thousand Island	90	7	5
Roasted Red Pepper	70	6	3
Shiitake & Sesame	120	13	1
Tuscany Italian	80	7	5
Vinaigrette:			
Balsamic; Cilantro & Lime, 2 T.	100	10	3
Low-Fat: Honey Mustard	45	2	6
Gingerly	40	2	4
Raspberry	35	1.5	5
Bernstein's			
Creamy Caesar, 2 Tbsp	120	13	1
Fat-Free Cheese & Garlic Italian	10	0	2
Italian	110	12	1
Olive Oil Vinaigrette	90	9	3
Restaurant Recipe Italian	120	12	1
Other varieties, avg., 2 Tbsp	110	11	2
Light Fantastic: Cheese Fantastico	25	1.5	3
Roasted Garlic Balsamic	45	3.5	3
Best Foods			
Dijonnaise, 1 tsp	5	0	1
Mayonnaise: Reduced Fat, 2 Tbsp	40	4	4
Light, average., all varieties	90	9	1
Real Mayonnaise, average	90	10	0
w. Lime Juice, 2 Tbsp	180	20	0
Bob's Famous			
Blue Cheese, Lite, 2 tbsp	80	8	1
Ranch Country, 2 Tbsp	150	16	1
Roquefort; Blue Chse	140	15	1
Thousand Island	140	14	4
Brianna's			
Blue Cheese, 2 Tbsp	120	11	5
Blush Vintage	120	7	14
French Vinaigrette, 2 Tbsp	180	19	1
New American	160	17	6
Rich Santa Fe Blend	25	0	5
Zesty French	150	15	4
Other varieties, avg.	155	14	8

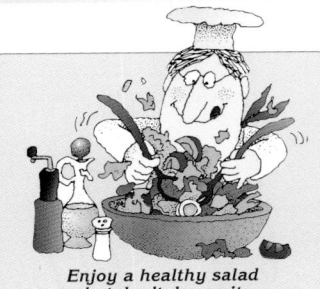

*Enjoy a healthy salad
but don't drown it
in high-fat salad dressings.
Use 'light' dressing to halve
the fat and calories.*

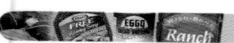

Per 2 Tbsp (Approx 1 fl.oz)	C	F	Cb
Carb Options: Italian	70	8	0
Ranch	150	17	0
Cardini's			
Caesar, 2 Tbsp	160	17	1
Fat-Free Caesar	40	0	9
Light Caesar	80	7	5
Honey Mustard	140	13	5
Parmesan Ranch	150	15	2
Poppyseed w. Shallots	160	14	8
Southwest Caesar	140	14	3
Vintage White Wine	110	12	1
Other varieties, avg.	125	13	1
El Torito: Cilantro Pepita Caesar	140	14	1
Emeril's: *Per 2 Tbsp*			
House Herb Viniagrette	100	10	1
Kicked Up French	80	5	8
Girard's: *Per 2 Tbsp*			
Blue Cheese Vinaigrette	100	10	3
Caesar	140	15	1
Lite Caesar	70	8	5
Champagne	150	16	1
Lite Champagne	60	5	2
Chinese Chicken Salad	120	11	6
Greek Feta Vinaigrette	110	11	1
Olde Venice Italian	120	13	2
Shiitake Chardonnay	100	9	4
Spinach Salad	70	2	4
Fat-Free: Balsamic/Red Wine, avg.	25	0	6
Caesar	40	0	9
Raspberry	50	0	13
Hidden Valley: *Per 2 Tbsp*			
Regular Ranch: Italian Ranch	140	14	2
Old-Fashioned Buttermilk Ranch	140	14	2
Spicy Ranch	150	16	2
Bacon Ranch	140	14	1
Cracked Peppercorn Ranch	120	12	2
Cole Slaw	150	15	5
Light, Original Ranch	80	7	3
Fat-Free, Original Ranch	30	0	6

Ken's Steak House Dressings: *Per 2 Tbsp*	C	F	Cb
Balsamic & Basil Vinaigrette	110	12	1
Chunky Blue Cheese	140	16	1
Country French	150	12	10
Creamy Caesar	160	18	0
Peppercorn Ranch	180	19	1
Ranch	140	15	2
Italian w. Aged Romano	110	12	1
Thousand Island	140	13	4
Lite: Caesar/Olive Oil Vinaigrette, avg.	70	6	3
Ranch	80	6	6
Kraft			
Regular Dressings: *Per 2 Tbsp*			
Honey Dijon	110	10	6
Coleslaw	110	9	7
Creamy Italian	110	11	2
Creamy French	160	15	5
Roka Brand Blue Cheese	130	13	2
Thousand Island, avg.	120	10	5
Kraft Free (Fat-Free): Italian	15	0	4
Caesar Italian	50	0	10
Carb Well: Classic Caesar, 2 Tbsp	110	11	0
Italian	20	1.5	0
Ranch	60	6	0
Roka Blue Cheese	120	13	0
Light: Buttermilk Ranch	60	6	0
Italian, 2 Tbsp	20	1.5	0
Light Done Right!: Italian	40	3	3
Ranch	60	6	0
Other varieties, avg.	80	4.5	9
Special Collection: Caesar Italian	100	10	2
Balsamic Vinaigrette	90	8	4
Sweet Honey Catalina; Poppyseed	130	11	8
Other varieties, avg.	60	5	1
Seven Seas, all varieties	90	9	2
Kroger			
Poppy Seed	200	8	32
Real Mayonnaise	100	11	0
Zesty Italian	90	9	3
Lite: Zesty Italian	35	2	4
Ranch	70	6	3
Fat-Free, avg., 2 Tbsp	30	0	8

Salad Dressings (Cont)

Salad Dressings (Cont)

Per 2 Tbsp (Approx 1 fl.oz)

	C	F	Cb
Litehouse: Caesar	130	13	2
Chunky Bleu Cheese	150	16	1
Coleslaw	100	8	8
Jalapeno Ranch	120	12	1
Lite Bleu Cheese	70	6	2
Other varieties, avg.	120	12	2

Maple Grove: *Per 2 Tbsp (1 fl.oz)*

	C	F	Cb
Balsamic Vinaigrette	50	3	5
Regular: Honey Mustard	120	9	9
Sweet & Sour	110	7	12
Fat Free: Balsamic Vinaigrette	35	0	9
Caesar Vinaigrette; Greek, avg.	10	0	3
Dijon; Poppyseed, avg.	40	0	10
Other varieties, avg.	25	0	6
Low Carb: Dijon	70	8	1
Balsamic; Raspberry Vinaigrette	5	0	1
Lite: Caesar	40	4.5	5
Honey Mustard	80	5	9

Marie's: *Per 2 Tbsp*

	C	F	Cb
1000 Island	160	15	4
Blue Cheese	170	19	0
Caesar	170	19	1
Honey Mustard	140	12	6
Poppy Seed	150	13	8
Ranch (15.5 fl.oz ctn), 2 Tbsp	170	19	1
Premium: Spinach Salad, 2 Tbsp	70	1.5	2
Italian Cheese Blend	180	20	12

Nasoya: *Per 2 Tbsp*

	C	F	Cb
Vegi-Dressing (Tofu Base/Dairy Free):			
Thousand Island	60	5	2
Other flavors	65	7	1
Nayonaise: Regular, 2 Tbsp, 1 oz	70	7	2
Fat-Free, 2 Tbsp, 1 oz	20	0	4

Newman's Own: *Per 2 Tbsp*

	C	F	Cb
Balsamic Vinaigrette, 2 Tbsp	90	9	3
Caesar; Olive Oil & Vinegar	150	16	1
Family Recipe Italian	120	13	1
Parmesan Italiano	140	14	2
Ranch	140	15	2
Two Thousand Island	140	14	4
Lighten Up: Light Italian	60	6	1
Light Raspberry & Walnut	70	5	7
Light Balsamic Vinaigrette	45	4	2

San-J: *Per 2 Tbsp*

	C	F	Cb
Tamari Peanut, 2 Tbsp	70	2.5	8
Tamari Sesame	45	2	5
Tamari Vinaigrette	45	3	4
Fat-Free, Tamari Mustard	25	0	5

S & W: *Per 2 Tbsp (1 oz)*

	C	F	Cb
Light: Italian	35	0	8
Red/White Wine; Raspberry Blush	40	0	10

Seeds of Change: *Per 2 Tbsp (1 oz)*

	C	F	Cb
Balsamic/Greek Feta Vinaigrette	60	4.5	5
Italian Herb Vinaigrette	60	4.5	5

Spectrum

	C	F	Cb
Fat Free: Creamy Dill/Garlic	25	0	4
Sweet On. & Garlic; Tstd Sesame	15	0	3
Low-Fat: Honey Dijon	35	2	4
Zesty Italian	30	2	1
Organic: Greek Goddess, 2Tbsp	110	11	2
Balsamic Vinaigrette	80	8	3
Provencal Garlic Lovers	50	5	2
Rocky Mountain Ranch	130	14	1

Steel's (Sugar-Free)

	C	F	Cb
Honey Mustard, 2 Tbsp	95	7	2
Sweet Ginger Lime, 2 Tbsp	75	7	1

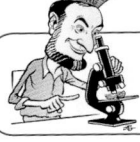

*F*or full nutritional data and product updates
check the database of the author's website
www.CalorieKing.com

Salad Dressings (Cont)

Per 2 Tbsp (Approx 1 fl.oz)   **C** **F** **Cb**

Subway Select: *Per 2 Tbsp (1 oz)*

	C	F	Cb
Premium Collection: Fat-Free Italian	35	0	7
Ranch	100	11	0.5
Atkins Sweet as Honey Mstd, 2 T.	100	11	0.5

T. Marzetti's: *Per 2 Tbsp (1 oz)*

	C	F	Cb
Asiago Peppercorn	160	16	1
Asian Ginger	120	12	4
Baja Ranch	150	15	2
Buffalo Blue Cheese	140	15	1
Chunky Blue Cheese	150	15	2
Honey Balsamic	120	11	5
Original Slaw	170	16	6
Ranch	160	17	2

Toby's: *Per 2 Tbsp (1 oz)*

	C	F	Cb
All varieties, average	120	12	1.5

Walden Farms

	C	F	Cb
Fat-Free, Calorie Free Range, 2 Tbsp	0	0	0

Wild Oats: *Per 2 Tbsp (1 oz)*

	C	F	Cb
Balsamic Vinaigrette	100	10	2
Caesar Style	100	10	2
Ranch	110	11	2
Sesame Goddess	100	10	2
Soy Ginger	50	5	3
Tuscany Italian	100	11	0.5

Per 2 Tbsp (Approx 1 fl.oz)   **C** **F** **Cb**

Wishbone

	C	F	Cb
Regular: 5 Cheese Italian	120	10	6
Chunky Blue Cheese	150	15	2
Creamy Caesar	170	18	1
French: Deluxe French	120	11	5
Sweet 'N Spicy	100	12	6
Italian: Regular	90	8	3
House Italian	100	10	3
Robusto Italian	90	8	3
Ranch: Original	160	13	2
w. Garlic/Spring Onion	130	14	2
Red Wine; Balsamic Vinaigrette	50	5	3
Russian, regular	120	6	14
Thousand Island	130	12	5
Fat-Free: Chunky Blue Cheese	35	0	5
Italian	20	0	4
Ranch	30	0	7
Dressing & Marinades: Asian	70	5	6
Balsamic Olive Oil & Herbs	50	5	3
Lemon Garlic & Herb	70	5	5
Tangy Honey Mustard	80	6	7
Ranch Up!	140	15	2
Just 2 Good!: Blue Cheese	50	2	6
Classic/Creamy Caesar; Ranch	50	2	7
Country Italian; Italian	30	1.5	7
Parmesan Peppercorn Ranch	50	2	7
Thousand Island	50	2	9
Salad Spritzers: All flavors, 10 sprays (¼ fl.oz) for 1 cup salad	10	1	1

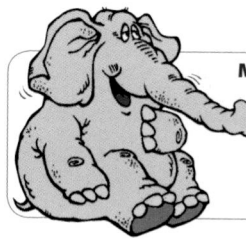

MINIMAL EXERCISES FOR LAZY SLIMMERS

1. After finishing a set meal, place both hands on edge of table and P-U-S-H back hard!

2. Shake your head vigorously from side to side, every time you are offered a second helping of rich food.

Breakfast Cereals

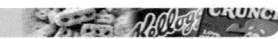

Quick Guide

Cooked Cereals

	C	F	Cb
Buckwheat Groats, roasted:			
Dry, ½ cup, 3 oz	285	2	62
Cooked, 1 cup, 6 oz	155	1	34
Bulgur: Dry, ½ cup, 2½ oz	240	1	53
Cooked, 1 cup, 6½ oz	150	0.5	34
Corn/Hominy Grits:			
Dry, ¼ cup, 1.4 oz	145	0.5	31
3 Tbsp, 1 oz	110	0.5	23
Cooked, ¾ cup, 6½ oz	110	0.5	23
Instant, 1 pkt, 0.8 oz	80	0.5	18
w. Imitation Bacon Bits, 1 oz	100	0.5	22
Cream of Rice, ckd ¾ cup, 6½ oz	95	0	20
Cream of Wheat:			
Regular, ckd, ¾ cup, 6½ oz	100	0.5	21
Quick, ckd, ¾ cup, 6½ oz	95	0.5	20
Instant, ckd, ¾ cup, 6½ oz	110	0.5	24
Farina: Cooked, ¾ cup, 6 oz	85	0	18
Millet, dry, ¼ cup, 1¾ oz	190	2	36
Oat Bran: Raw, ⅓ cup, 1 oz	70	2	19
Cooked, ½ cup, 3¾ oz	45	1	13
Oatmeal: Dry, ⅓ cup, 1 oz	110	2	19
Regular, ckd, ¾ cup, 6 oz	110	2	19
1 cup, 8 oz	145	3	25
Instant: Regular, avg., 1 oz	100	2	18
Flavored, average, 1½ oz	150	2	32
Wheat Hearts, 1 oz dry, ¾ c. ckd	110	1	21

Brans, Wheatgerm, Add-Ons

	C	F	Cb
Bran: Wheat, unprocessed,			
1 Tbsp, 3g	10	0	2
Rice Bran: Raw, 1 Tbsp, 5g	15	1	2.5
¼ cup, 1 oz	90	6	14
Oat Bran: Raw, 1 Tbsp, 5g	15	0.5	3.5
⅓ cup, 1 oz	70	2	19
Wheat Germ: Raw. 1 Tbsp, ¼ oz	25	1	3.5
¼ cup, 1 oz	105	3	15
Fruit: Dried, average, 1 oz	80	0	21
Banana, ½ medium	50	0	14
Prunes in Syrup (5), 3 oz	90	0	24
Honey, 1 Tbsp, ¾ oz	65	0	17
Lecithin Granules, 1 Tbsp, 10g	55	4	0.5
Nuts, Almonds (6), ¼ oz	40	4	1.5
Bee Pollen Granules, 1 T., 8g	25	1	2
Psyllium Husks, 1 Tbsp, 5g	20	0	4

Hot/Cooked Cereals ~ Brands

Per Serving	C	F	Cb
Albers Grits, ¼ cup, 1.4 oz	140	0.5	31
Bobs Red Mill-10 Grain, ¼ c., 40g	180	2.5	35
Country Choice Oats, 1 pouch, avg.	110	2	19
Dr McDougall's			
Oatmeal: 4 Grains, 2.2 oz	220	2	44
Barley, all varieties, 2.5 cup	270	3	51
Wheat, 2.4 oz	220	2.5	44
Eat Well Be Well			
Instant Oatmeal, all varieties, 1.2 oz	120	2	23
Erewhon: Barley Plus, ¼ c., 1.7 oz	170	1	37
Brown Rice Crm, ¼ cup, 1.6 oz	170	1	36
Instant Oatmeal, 1.2 oz pkg, avg.	140	2	26
McCann's Instant Irish Oatmeal			
Apple & Cinnamon, 1.23 oz	130	1.5	27
Maple & Brown Sugar, 1.5 oz	160	2	32
Original, 1 oz pkg	100	1.5	18
Steel Cut Oats, ¼ cup, 1.4 oz	150	2	27
Mother's Oat Bran, ½ cup, 1.4 oz	150	3	25
Nabisco: Cream of Rice, ¼ c., 46g	170	0	38
Cream of Wheat: Orig., 3T., 1 oz	120	0	25
Maple Brown Sugar, 1.2 oz pkg	120	0	27
Malt-O-Meal: Orig., 3T., 1.2 oz	120	0.5	26
Maple Brown Sugar, ¼ cup	170	0	37
Natures Path: Apple Cinn.1.7 oz	190	2	38
Average other varieties	200	4	35
Quaker: Oatbran, ½ cup, 1.4 oz	150	3	25
Brown Sugar, 1.9 oz ctn	200	2.5	42
Honey Nut, 1.5 oz	170	3.5	31
Multigrain, ½ cup, 1.4 oz	130	1	29
Old Fashioned Oats, ½ cup, 1.4 oz	150	3	27
Sun Country Quick Oats, ½ c.,1.4 oz	150	3	27
Grits: Reg. all types, 1 pkg, avg.	130	0.5	31
Instant, all types, 1 pkg, 1 oz	100	1	22
Instant Oatmeal: *Per Package*			
Oatmeal Regular, 1 oz	100	2	19
Bakery Favorites, avg., 1½ oz	160	2	33
Breakfast Blast, avg. all flavors	155	2.5	32
Fruit and Cream, avg. all flavors	140	2.5	26
Nutrition for Workers, avg. all flav.	165	2.5	33
Oatmeal Express, avg. all flavors	205	3	42
Supreme, avg. all flavors	160	3	32
Silver Palate Oatmeal, ⅓ c., 40g	160	3	26
Uncle Sam Oatmeal, 1.2 oz	130	3	24

Quick Guide

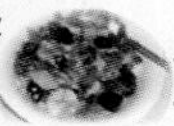

Cold Cereals
Average All Brands

	C	F	Cb
Bran Flakes, ¾ c., 1 oz	95	0.5	24
Corn Flakes, 1 c., 1 oz	100	0	24
Granola, ¼ c., 1 oz	150	9.5	16
Oat Bran Cereal, ½ cup, 1½ oz	145	3	25
Puffed Rice, 1 cup, ½ oz	55	0	12
Puffed Wheat, 1 cup, ½ oz	45	0	10
Raisin Bran, ½ cup, 1 oz	85	0.5	20
Rice Crisps, 1 cup, 1 oz	110	0.5	24
Shredded Wheat, 1 bisc., 1 oz	85	0.5	20
Sugar-frosted Flakes, ¾ c, 1 oz	115	0	28
Wheat Flakes, ¾ cup, 1 oz	105	1	23

Breakfast Bars: See Page 137

Ready-To-Eat Cereal

	C	F	Cb
Arrowhead Mills			
Amaranth, 1 c., 1.2 oz	140	2	26
Bran Flakes, 1 cup, 1 oz	110	1	22
Corn Flakes, 1 cup, 1.2 oz	120	0	27
Kamut Flakes, 1 cup, 1.1 oz	120	1	25
Maple Buckwheat Flake, 1 c., 1½ oz	170	1	35
Multi Grain Flakes, 1 cup, 1½ oz	170	2	33
Nature O's, 1 cup, 1.1 oz	130	2	25
Oat Bran Flakes, 1 cup, 1.2 oz	140	2.5	24
Perfect Harvest, 1 cup, 1.2 oz	140	2	25
Puffed Corn/Rice, avg., 1 c., 0.6 oz	60	1	12
Puffed Kamut, 1 cup, ½ oz	50	1	11
Puffed Millet/Wheat, 1 cup, 0.6 oz	60	0.5	11
Rice Flakes, 1 cup, 1.7 oz	180	1	40
Shredded Wheat, 1 cup, 1.7 oz	190	1	38
Spelt Flakes, 1 cup, 1.1 oz	120	1	24
Atkins			
Morning Start: Blueberry, ½ cup	90	2	12
Crunchy Almond Crisp, ½ cup	90	2	10
Triple Berry, ½ cup	90	2	10
Back to Nature			
Flax and Fiber Crunch, ¾ cup, 1.8 oz	180	2.5	37
Granola, avg., ½ cup, 1.8 oz	170	3	34
Hi Fiber Multibran, ¾ cup, 1.7 oz	140	1	40
Hi Protein Crunch, ¾ cup, 1.7 oz	170	1.5	28
Muesli, ¾ cup, 2.3 oz	230	4	48

	C	F	Cb
Barbara's Bakery			
Alpen Original, ⅔ cup, 1.9 oz	200	3	41
Breakfast O's, 1 cup, 1¼ oz	120	2	22
Brown Rice Crisps; Corn Flakes, 1 c.	110	0.5	25
Crispy Wheats/Soy Essence, ¾ cup	110	0.5	25
Fruity Punch; Puffins, ¾ cup, 1 oz	120	0.5	26
Grain Shop, ¾ cup, 1½ oz	120	1	36
Honey Crunch 'n Oats, ¾ cup, 1 oz	115	1	24
Shredded Oats, 1¼ cup, 2 oz	220	2.5	46
Shred. Spoonfuls; Toasted O's, ¾ cup	120	1.5	24
Shredded Wheat, 2 bisc., 1.4 oz	140	1	31
Wild Puffs Caramel, ¾ cup, 1.1 oz	110	1	25
Breadshop			
Cranberry Crunch Muesli, 1 cup	200	3	44
Granola: Triple Berry Cr., ⅔ cup	220	7	36
Other varieties, avg., ½ cup	220	7.5	32
Cascadian Farms			
Honey Nut O's, 1 cup, 1 oz	120	2	24
Multi-Grain Squares, ¾ c., 1 oz	110	1	25
Oats & Honey Granola, ⅔ c., 2 oz	230	6	42
Wheat Crunch, ¾ cup, 1 oz	110	1	25
Purely O's, 1 cup, 1.1oz	110	2	22
Hearty Morning, ¾ cup, 1.9 oz	200	3	43
Raisin Bran, 1 cup, 1.9 oz	180	1	43
Dr McDougall's: Muesli, 1½ cup	160	2	31
Eat Well Be Well			
Apple Cinnamon, ¾ cup, 1 oz	115	2	23
Vanilla Almond, ¾ cup, 1 oz	115	2	23
Whole Grain & Almond, ¾ cup, 1 oz	115	2	23
Ener-G			
Crumbles, ¼ cup, 1.1 oz	100	3	16
Granola Mix, ⅓ cup, 1.8 oz	260	16	20
Rice Bran, ½ cup, 2.4 oz	220	14	20
Rice Nuts, 1 cup, 3½ oz	380	2.5	84
Erewhon			
Aztec, 1 cup, 1 oz	110	0	26
Corn Flakes, 1¼ cups, 2 oz	210	2.5	45
Crispy Brown Rice: 1 cup, 1 oz	110	0	25
w. Mixed Berries, 1 cup, 1 oz	120	0.5	27
Gluten Free, 1 cup, 1 oz	110	0	25
No Salt Added, 1 cup, 1 oz	110	0	25
Kamut Flakes, ⅔ cup, 1.2 oz	110	0	25
Raisin Bran, 1 cup, 1.8 oz	170	1	40
Rice Twice, ¾ cup, 1 oz	120	0	26

Breakfast Cereals (Cont)

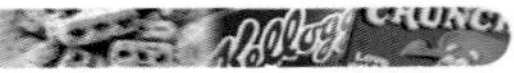

Ready-To-Eat (Cont)

General Mills (Big G)	C	F	Cb
Basic 4, 1 cup, 1.9 oz	200	3	42
Boo Berry, 1 cup, 1 oz	120	1	26
Cheerios: Regular, 1 cup, 1 oz	110	2	22
Apple Cinnamon, ¾ c., 1 oz	120	1.5	25
Berry Burst, all types, 1 c., 1 oz	110	1.5	24
Frosted; Team, avg., 1 cup, 1 oz	120	1	25
Honey Nut, 1 cup, 1 oz	110	1.5	22
Multi-Grain, 1 cup, 1 oz	110	1	24
Chex: Corn, 1 cup, 1 oz	105	0.5	25
Frosted Mini Chex, ¾ cup, 1 oz	110	0.5	26
Honey Nut, ¾ cup, 1 oz	120	0.5	26
Multi-Bran, 1 cup, 2 oz	190	1.5	46
Rice, 1¼ cup, 1 oz	120	0.5	26
Wheat, 1 cup, 1.7 oz	180	1	40
Cinnamon Tst Crunch, ¾ c., 1 oz	130	3.5	24
Cocoa Puffs, 1 cup, 1 oz	120	1.5	26
Cookie Crisp; Count Choc, 1 c., 1 oz	120	1.5	26
Country Corn Flakes, 1 cup, 1.1 oz	110	0.5	25
Fiber One, ½ cup, 1 oz	60	1	14
Fiber One Honey Clusters, 1¼ cup	170	1	47
French Toast Crunch, ¾ c., 1 oz	120	1.5	26
Golden Grahams, ¾ cup, 1 oz	120	1	25
Honey Nut Clusters, 1 cup, 2 oz	210	2.5	45
Kix: 1⅓ cup, 1 oz	120	1	25
Berry Berry, ¾ cup, 1 oz	120	1.5	26
Lucky Charms, avg., 1 cup, 1 oz	120	1	25
Oatmeal Crisp: Almond, 1 c., 2 oz	220	4.5	42
Apple Cinamon, 1 cup, 2 oz	210	2	45
Peanut Butter Toast Crunch, ¾ cup	130	3.5	23
Raisin Nut Bran, 1¼ cups, 2 oz	200	2.5	44
Reese's Puffs, ¾ cup, 1 oz	130	3.5	23
Total: w. Strawberries, 1 cup, 1.8 oz	180	1	42
Honey Clusters, ¾ cup, 1.7 oz	170	1.5	38
Raisin Bran, 1 cup, 2 oz	170	1	42
Vanilla Yogurt, 1 cup, 1.8 oz	190	3.5	43
Whole Grain, ¾ cup, 1 oz	100	0.5	23
Trix, avg., 1 cup, 1 oz	120	1	26
Wheaties, 1 cup, 1 oz	110	1	24

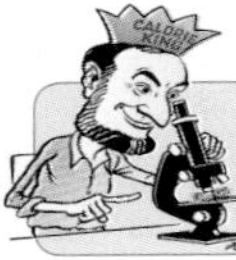

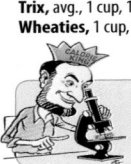

For Extra Listings and Nutritional Data
~ See Author's Website
www.CalorieKing.com

Health Valley	C	F	Cb
Amaranth Flakes, ¾ cup, 1 oz	100	0	24
Blue Corn Flakes, ¾ cup, 1.1 oz	100	0	24
Cranberry Crunch, ¾ cup, 1.8 oz	200	3	41
Crunch-Ems!, avg., 1 cup, 1 oz	110	0	27
Crunches & Flakes, ¾ cup, 1.8 oz	110	0	27
Empower, 1 cup, 2 oz	200	3	42
Fiber 7, Multigrain Flakes, ¾ cup, 1 oz	110	0	27
Golden Flax, serving, ¾ cup, 1.8 oz	190	3	38
Granola, ⅔ cup, 2 oz	180	1	43
Healthy Fiber Flakes, ¾ cup, 1.1 oz	100	0	23
Heart Wise, 1 cup, 55g	200	3	36
Oat Bran Flakes: ¾ cup, 1 oz	100	2	19
w. Raisins, ¾ cup, 1 oz	100	0	23
Oat Bran O's, ¾ cup, 1 oz	100	0	23
Raisin Bran Flakes, 1 ¼ cup, 2 oz	190	0	47
Real Oat Bran Alm. Crunch, ½ cup	200	3	34
Soy Flakes, Raisin, 1 cup, 2 oz	190	1	39
Heartland Natural Cereal			
Granola Cereal: Original, ½ cup	300	11	41
Low-Fat Raisin, ½ cup	205	3	4
Kashi			
7 Whole Grain: Flakes, 1 cup, 1.7 oz	180	1	41
Honey Puff, 1 cup, 1.1 oz	120	1	25
Nuggets, ½ cup, 2 oz	210	1.5	47
Pilaf, ½ cup, cooked	170	3	30
Puffs, 1 cup, ½ oz	70	0.5	15
GoLEAN: 1 cup, 1.8 oz	140	1	30
Crunch!, 1 cup, 1.8 oz	190	3	36
Good Friends: 1 cup, 1.8 oz	170	2	43
Cinna-Raisin Crunch, 1 c., 1.7 oz	170	1.5	41
Heart to Heart: ¾ cup, 1.2 oz	110	1.5	25
Oatmeal: Apple Cinn., 1.5 oz pkg	160	2	33
Golden Brown Maple, 1.5 oz pkg	160	2	33
Raisin Spice, 1.5 oz pkg	150	2	33
Kashi Medley, ¾ cup, 1.1 oz	120	1	26
Mighty Bites: Cinn., 1 cup, 1.1 oz	120	1.5	23
Honey Crunch Cereal, 1 cup, 33g	110	1.5	23
Organic Promise:			
Autumn Wheat, 1 cup, 1.9 oz	190	1	45
Cinnamon Harvest, 1 cup, 1.9 oz	190	1	44
Cranberry Sunshine, 1 cup, 1 oz	110	1	26
Strawberry Fields, 1 cup, 1.1 oz	120	0	28

Ready-To-Eat (Cont)

	C	F	Cb
Kellogg's			
All-Bran: Bran Buds, ⅓ cup, 1.1 oz	70	1	24
Extra Fiber, ½ cup, 0.9 oz	50	1	20
Original, ½ cup, 1 oz	80	1	23
Yogurt Bites, 1¼ cups, 2 oz	190	3	44
Apple Jacks, 1 cup, 1.2 oz	130	0.5	30
Scooby-Doo! Berry Bones, 1 cup	130	1	28
Cinnamon Krunchers, ¾ cup, 1 oz	130	3.5	23
Complete Oat Bran Flakes, ¾ cup	110	1	23
Complete Wheat Bran Flakes, ¾ cup	90	0.5	23
Corn Flakes: Original, 1 cup, 1 oz	100	0	24
w. Real Bananas, ¾ cup, 1 oz	110	2	22
Corn Pops, 1 cup, 1 oz	120	0	28
Cracklin' Oat Bran, ¾ cup, 1.8 oz	200	7	35
Crispix, Original, 1 cup, 1 oz	110	0.5	25
Crunch: Cran-Vanilla, 1¼ cups	200	1	47
Raisin Bran, 1 cup, 1.9 oz	190	1	45
Toasted Honey, 1¼ cups, 2 oz	220	1.5	50
Crunchy Blends: Just Right, ¾ cup	200	2	43
Low-Fat Granola: w. Raisins, ⅔ cup	230	3	49
no Raisins, ½ cup	190	2.5	43
Mueslix, ⅔ cup, 2 oz	200	3	40
Froot Loops: Original, 1 cup, 1.1 oz	120	1	27
Marshmallow, 1.1 oz	120	1	27
Frosted Flakes, ¾ cup, 1 oz	120	0	28
Fruit Harvest: Banana Berry ¾ cup	120	2	25
Other varieties, average	110	0	26
Honey Smacks, ¾ cup, 1 oz	100	0.5	24
Mini Swirlz Cinnamon Bun, 1 cup	120	2	25
Mini-Wheats: Frosted Big Bite (5)	180	1	41
Frosted Bite Size (24), 2.1 oz	200	1	48
Frosted Vanilla Creme (24), 1.8 oz	180	1	43
Nutri-Grain Bars: See Page 137			
Product 19, 1 cup, 1 oz	100	0	25
Raisin Bran: Regular, 1 cup	190	1.5	45
Rice Krispies: Original, 1¼ cup	120	0	29
Berry, 1 cup, 1.1 oz	120	0	27
Frosted, ¾ cup, 1.1 oz	110	0	27
Cocoa; Treats, avg., ¾ cup, 1.1 oz	120	1.5	26
Smart Start: Antioxidants, 1 cup	190	0.5	43
Healthy Heart, 1 ¼ cup, 2.1 oz	230	2	49
Soy Protein, 1 cup, 2 oz	200	1.5	40
Smorz, 1 cup, 1.1 oz	120	2	25
Special K: Original 1 cup, 1.1 oz	110	0	22
Fruit & Yogurt, ¾ cup, 1.1 oz	120	1	27
Low Carb Lifestyle, ¾ cup, 1 oz	100	3	14
Red Berries, 1 cup, 1.1 oz	110	0	25
Vanilla Almond, ¾ cup	110	1.5	25

	C	F	Cb
Malt-O-Meal			
Apple Zings, 1 cup, 1.1 oz	130	1	30
Balance ¾ cup, 1.1 oz	120	1	26
Cinnamon Toasters, ¾ c., 1 oz	130	3.5	24
Coco Roos/Dyno-Bites, ¾ c., 1 oz	120	1	26
Frosted Flakes, ¾ cup, 1.1 oz	120	0	28
Frosted Mini Spooners, 1 c., 1.9 oz	190	1	45
Golden Puffs, ¾ cup, 1 oz	100	0	24
Mateys/Toasty O's, avg., 1 cup, 1 oz	110	1	25
Mother's			
Cinnamon Oat Crunch, 1 cup. 2.1 oz	230	3	48
Cocoa Bumpers, 1 cup, 1.2 oz	120	0.5	29
Groovy Grahams, ¾ cup	100	0.5	24
Honey Round-Ups, ¾ cup	110	0.5	25
Peanut Butter Bumpers, 1 cup, 1.2 oz	130	2.5	26
Toasted Oat Bran, ¾ cup, 1.1 oz	120	1.5	24
Nature's Path			
Corn Flakes, all types, ¾ cup, 1 oz	110	0	24
Eight Grain, ⅔ cup, 1 oz	100	1	23
Flax Plus Multigrain, ¾ cup, 1 oz	100	1.5	22
Heritage, all types, ¾ cup, 1 oz	100	1	23
Honeyed Raisin Bran, ¾ cup, 1 oz	180	1	43
Multigr. Oatbran Flakes, ⅔ cup, 1 oz	100	1	24
Toaster Pastries (1), 52g	210	4.5	40
Granola: Ginger Zing; Hemp, 1 oz	145	6	20
Heritage Muesli w. Raspberry, 1 oz	125	3	22
Pumpkin Flax Plus, ½ cup, 1 oz	140	6	19
Average, other varieties	125	3	22
Kamut Puffs, 1 cup, ½ oz	50	0	11
Kamut Crisp Flakes, ¾ cup, 1 oz	100	0	24
Power Breakfast, 1 cup, 2 oz	190	2.5	40
Spelt Flakes, ¾ cup, 1 oz	80	0.5	20
New England Natural Bakers			
Muesli, ½ cup, 2.1 oz	220	5	40
Granola: Almond Raisin Crisp, ½ c.	220	9	36
Apple Sunrise, ½ cup	210	7	34
Berry Good, ⅔ cup, 2.1 oz	250	6	44
Grateful Date, ½ cup, 1.7 oz	210	7	33
Honey Crunch; Pecan, ½ cup	295	13	37
Low-Fat Granola, ½ cup, 1.7 oz	200	2.5	41
Maple Almond Date, ½ cup	280	11	37
Save The Forest: Chocolate Mix	175	10	18
Fruit & Nut Mix, ½ cup, 2.1 oz	270	12	35
Nut Granola, ½ cup, 2.1 oz	270	12	35
Granola: Absolutely Nuts, ⅔ cup	220	9	30
Raspberry Razzmatazz, ¾ cup	255	9	37

Breakfast Cereals (Cont)

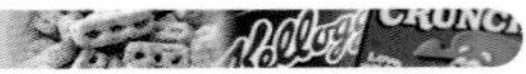

Ready-To-Eat (Cont)

	C	F	Cb
New Morning			
Cocoa Crispy Rice, ¾ cup, 1 oz	120	0.5	26
Cocomotion, ¾ cup, 1 oz	100	0.5	22
Fruit-e-O's, Organic, 1 cup, 1 oz	120	1.5	25
Oatios: Apple Cinn., Organic, 1 c., 1 oz	120	1	18
Honey Almond, 1 cup, 1 oz	120	1	17
Oatios, Original, 1 cup, 1 oz	110	2	22
Nutritious Living			
Hi-Lo, all types, ½ cup, 1 oz	90	1.5	11
40-30-30 Honey Almd, ¾ c.,1.4 oz	150	5	17
Post			
100% Bran, ⅓ cup, 1 oz	80	1	22
Alpha Bits, 1 cup, 1 oz	110	2	22
Bran Flakes, ¾ cup, 1 oz	100	0	24
Carb Well: Cinnamon Crunch, 1 oz	110	2	14
Golden Crunch, 1 oz	110	1	14
Cocoa Pebbles, 1 oz	110	1.5	26
Fruit & Bran, 1 cup, 2 oz	210	3	42
Fruity Pebbles, 1¼ cup, 1 oz	110	1	24
Golden Crisp, ½ cup, 1 oz	115	0	26
Grape-Nuts, ½ cup, 2 oz	195	1	46
Grape-Nuts Flakes, ½ cup, 1 oz	110	1	24
Grape-Nuts O's, cup, 1 oz	110	0	25
Honey Bunches of Oats, ¾ c., 1 oz	115	1.5	24
Honey-Comb Strawb. Blasted, 1 cup	120	1	26
Hulk w. Marshmallow Bits, 1 cup	110	0	27
Oreo O's w. M'mallow Bits, ¾ c., 1 oz	115	2	23
Raisin Bran, ⅔ cup, 2 oz	185	1	44
Selects: Banana Nut Crunch, ½ c.	250	6	44
Blueberry Morning, 1 cup, 2 oz	220	3	45
Cranberry Almond Crunch, 2 oz	220	3	44
Maple Pecan Crunch, ¾ cup, 2 oz	240	6.5	44
Great Grains: Crunchy Pecan, ⅔ c.	225	6	38
Raisins Dates Pecans, ⅔ c.	215	4.5	39
Shredded Wheat: Frosted, 1.8 oz	180	1	43
Honey Nut, 1 cup, 1.8 oz	200	1.5	43
Original, 1 cup, 1.6 oz	155	1	36
Shredded Wheat & Bran, 2 oz	195	1.5	46
Toasties Corn Flakes, 1 cup, 1 oz	105	0	24
Waffle Crisp, 1 cup, 1 oz	115	2.5	24
Quaker			
Oat Bran, ½ cup	150	3	25
100% Natural Granola: ½ cup	225	9	31
Low-Fat, ⅔ cup	225	3	44
w. Raisins, ½ cup	210	3	44
Captain Crunch: Regular, ¾ c., 1 oz	110	1.5	23
Crunch Berries, ¾ cup, 1 oz	100	1.5	22
Peanut Butter, 1 oz	110	2.5	21

Quaker (Cont)	C	F	Cb
Crunchy Corn Bran, 1 cup, 1 oz	90	2.5	23
Honey Graham Oh's, ¾ cup	110	2	23
Life, all types, ¾ cup, 1.1 oz	120	1.5	26

Instant Oatmeal: *See Page 94*

Bars: *See Page 140*

	C	F	Cb
Sweet Home Farm			
Honey Nut Granola, ½ cup, 1.9 oz	220	7	34
Low-Fat Granola, ½ cup, 1.9 oz	195	3	38
Maple Pecan Crisp, 1 cup, 1.9 oz	225	7	36
Trader Joe's			
10 & 10 Cereal, ¾ cup, 1.7 oz	170	3	31
Banana Nut Clusters, 1 cup, 1.9 oz	240	8	40
Cornflakes, 1 cup, 1.1 oz	110	0	26
Cranberry Almd Clusters, 1 c., 2 oz	220	5	40
Crunch: Cherry Almond, 1 c., 2 oz	210	5	39
Van. Almd/Maple Pecan, 1 c., 2 oz	220	6	38
Essentials, 1 cup, 2 oz	170	3	37
Flakes n'Fruit, 1 cup, 1.1 oz	120	0.5	25
Frosted Flakes, ¾ cup, 1 oz	110	0	27
Golden Flax Cereal, ¾ cup, 1.7 oz	190	3	38
High Fiber Cereal, ⅔ cup, 1.1 oz	90	1	25
Honey Nut O's, ¾ cup, 1 oz	120	1.5	24
Joe's O's, 1 cup, 1 oz	110	2	22
More & Less Apple Cinn., ⅔ cup	100	1.5	12
Morning Lite, 1 cup, 1.4 oz	140	2	31
Muesli Cereal Blend, ¾ cup, 2 oz	200	1.5	42
Oat Bran Flakes, avg., 1 cup	200	1.5	45
Raisin Bran, 1 cup, 1.9 oz	170	1	44
Shred. Wheats, Bite Size, 1 c., 1.7 oz	200	1	42
Soy Granola, 1 cup, 1.9 oz	220	3	39
Touch of Honey, ⅔ cup, 1 oz	120	1.5	25
Triple Berry O's, ¾ cup, 1 oz	110	1	25
Toasted Oatmeal Flakes, ¾ c., 1.1 oz	110	1	23
Very Berry Clusters, 1 cup, 1.9 oz	200	4.5	36
Uncle Sam			
Cereal w. Real Mixed Berries, 1 cup	220	4.5	39
w. Flaxseed, 1 cup, 1.9 oz	190	5	38
Weetabix: 2 biscuits, 1.3 oz	130	1	26
Weight Watchers			
Banana Almond Medley, ¾ cup	170	3	31
Cinnamon Cluster Crunch, ¾ cup	150	1	32
Flakes'n Fiber, ½ cup, 1.1 oz	90	2	17
Honey Almond Crisp, ¾ cup, 1½ oz	150	2.5	31
Puffed Vanilla Wheat, 1 cup, 1.1 oz	100	2	20

Grains & Flours | C | F | Cb

Per ½ Cup (8 level Tbsp)

	C	F	Cb
Amaranth Flour, ½ cup, 3½ oz	365	6.5	65
Arrowroot Flour, ½ cup, 2¼ oz	230	0	56
Barley: Regular, ½ cup, 3¼ oz	325	2	67
Pearled, raw, 3½ oz	350	1	78
Flakes, ¼ cup	80	0.5	18
Buckwheat: Regular, ½ cup, 3 oz	290	3	61
Groats: Roasted, dry, ½ c., 2.9 oz	285	2	62
Roasted, cooked, 3½ oz	80	0.5	17
Flour, whole-groat, ½ cup, 2 oz	200	2	42
Bulgur: Dry, ½ cup, 2½ oz	240	1	53
Cooked, ½ cup, 3.2 oz	75	0.5	17
Carob Flour, ½ cup, 1.8 oz	115	0.5	46
Corn Kernels avg., cooked, ½ cup	80	0.5	18
Corn Bran, ½ cup, 1.4 oz	85	0.5	32
Corn Flour/Masa, ½ cup, 2 oz	210	2	44
Corn Grits: Dry, ½ cup, 2¾ oz	290	1	62
Cooked, ½ cup, 4¼ oz	70	0.5	15
Corn Germ, toasted, ½ cup, 4 oz	100	1.5	21
Cornmeal: Average all Types,			
3 Tbsp, 1 oz	100	0.5	22
½ cup, 2½ oz	250	1	54
Mixes: same as above	230	1	48
Made Up, ½ cup, 4.8 oz	95	0.5	20
Cornstarch: 1 Tbsp, 8g	30	0	7
½ cup, 2¼ oz	245	0	58
Couscous, Dry, 1 oz (yield 3 oz ckd)	110	0	22
1 cup cooked, 5½ oz	175	0	37
Farina: Dry, ½ cup, 3 oz	315	0.5	66
Cooked, ½ cup, 4.1 oz	55	0	12
Flaxseed: Seeds, 1 Tbsp, 8g	45	3.5	2
Ground, 2 Tbsp, 8g	60	4.5	4
Garbanzo (Chick Pea), ½ c., 1.6 oz	180	3	26
Kuzu Root Starch, 1 Tbsp, 10g	35	0	9
Matzo Meal, ½ cup, 2.2 oz	230	0.5	48
Millet: Raw, ½ cup, 3½ oz	380	4	73
Cooked, ½ cup, 3 oz	105	1	21
Oat Bran: Raw, ⅓cup, 1.1 oz	75	2	21
Cooked, ½ cup, 3¾ oz	45	1	13
Oats, rolled/oatmeal:			
Dry/Groats, ½ cup, 1.5 oz	160	3	28
Cooked, ½ cup, 4.2 oz	75	1	13
Polenta: *See Cornmeal*			
Potato Flour, ½ cup, 2.8 oz	285	0.5	67
Psyllium Husks, 1 Tbsp (5g)	20	0	4
Quinoa: Dry ½ cup, 3 oz	320	5	58
Cooked, ½ cup, 3¾ oz	255	4	47

Grains & Flours (Cont)

Per ½ Cup (8 level Tbsp)

	C	F	Cb
Rice Bran, ½ cup, 2 oz	185	12	30
Rice Flour, ½ cup, 2¾ oz	290	2	63
Rice Polish, ½ cup, 3½ oz	340	0.5	78
Rye Flour: Dark, ½ cup, 2.3 oz	210	2	44
Medium, ½ cup, 1.8 oz	180	1	40
Light, ½ cup, 1.8 oz	190	1	41
Rye Grain: ½ cup, 3 oz	285	2	59
Flakes, ¼ cup, 1 oz	100	0.5	21
Semolina, ½ cup, 3 oz	300	1	61
Sorghum, ½ cup, 3.4 oz	325	3	72
Soybean Flakes, ½ cup, 1½ oz	235	10	17
Soy Flour:			
Defatted, 1 cup, 3½ oz	330	1	38
Low-Fat, 1 cup, 3 oz	325	6	33
Full-Fat, 1 cup, 3 oz	365	17	29
Soy Meal, defatted, 1 cup, 4.3 oz	410	3	49
Spelt Flour, ½ cup, 2 oz	200	2	48
Tapioca, pearl: Dry, ½ c., 2.7 oz	270	0	67
3 Tbsp, 1 oz	100	0	25
Teff (Seed) Flour, 2 oz	200	1	40
Tortilla Flour Mix, ½ cup, 2 oz	225	2	44
Triticale: ½ cup, 3.4 oz	325	2	70
Flour, whole-grain, ½ cup, 2.3 oz	220	1	47
Wheat Bran, unproc., ½ c., 1 oz	60	1	18
Wheat Flakes, ½ cup, 1½ oz	140	1	28
Wheat Germ: Raw, ¼ cup, 1 oz	105	3	15
Toasted, ¼ cup, 1 oz	110	3	14
Wheat Flour:			
White, All Purpose/Self-Rising,			
1 level Tbsp, 0.6 oz	60	0	13
½ cup, 2.1 oz	220	0.5	46
1 cup, 4.4 oz	455	1.5	95
Whole Wheat, 1 cup, 4.2 oz	410	2.5	87

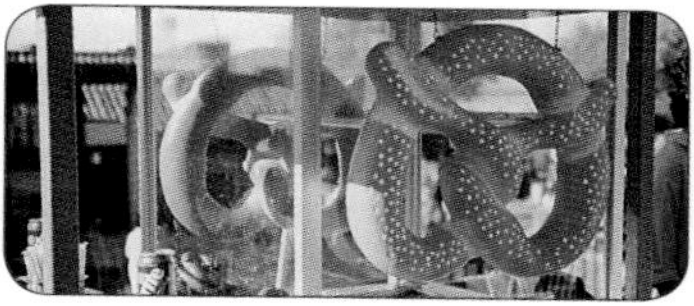

Rice

White Rice

	C	F	Cb
Raw: Short/Med. Grain, 1 c., 7 oz	700	1	155
Long Grain, 1 cup, 6½ oz	675	1	148
Glutinous, 1 cup, 6½ oz	685	1	150
Cooked Rice (Boiled/Steamed):			
Short/Medium Grain:			
½ cup, 3¼ oz	120	0	27
1 cup (½ Pint), 6½ oz	240	0.5	54
2 cups (1 Pint), 13 oz	480	1	108
Long Grain: ½ cup, 2¾ oz	100	0	22
1 cup, 5½ oz	200	0.5	44
Glutinous/Sticky, ckd 1 c., 6 oz	170	0.5	36
Parboiled, cooked, ½ cup, 3 oz	90	0	20
Precook./Instant: Dry,½ c., 3½ oz	370	0	80
Cooked, ½ cup, 3 oz	90	0	20
Wild Rice: Raw, 1 cup, 5½ oz	570	2	120
Cooked, 1 cup, 5¾ oz	165	0.5	35

Brown Rice

	C	F	Cb
Average of Short or Long Grain			
Raw/Dry: ½ cup, 3¼ oz	340	2.5	72
1 cup, 6½ oz	685	5.5	143
Cooked: ½ cup, 3½ oz	110	1	23
1 cup, 7 oz	220	1.5	46

Rice Dishes

	C	F	Cb
Chinese Fried Rice:			
½ cup, 2½ oz	160	5	21
1 cup, 5 oz (½ Pint)	280	9	42
2 cups, 10 oz (1 Pint)	565	18	84
Mexican Rice: 1 cup	500	12	90
Taco John's, 1 serving (6 oz)	240	8	36
Taco Time, 1 serving (4 oz)	160	2	30
Rice-A-Roni: See Page 74			
Rice Pilaf: Restaurant, 1 cup	270	7.5	43
O'Charley's, 1 order	220	6	38
Rice w. Raisins/Pinenuts, 1 cup	400	11	60
Risotto, 1 cup	420	12	70
Saffron Rice (Koo Koo Roo),4 oz	175	7	25
Spanish Rice: 1 cup	390	9	72
El Pollo Loco, 4 oz	160	1	33
Taco Cabana, 4 oz	180	5	30
Sticky Rice (Koo Koo Roo), 5 oz	155	0.5	34
Sushi Rice: 1 Tbsp	25	0	6
1 cup, 5.2 oz	390	0	77
Uncle Ben's: See Page 76			

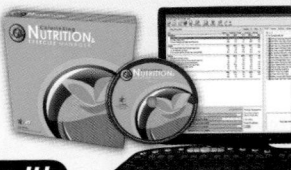

- Macaroni includes all shapes and sizes; (e.g. spaghetti, fettuccini, shells, tubes, ziti, twists, sheets, cannelloni, manicotti, elbows).
- All regular macaroni products have the same cals/fat/carb. on a weight basis.
- 1 oz Dry = approx. 2½ -3 oz cooked.

Dry Spaghetti/Macaroni

	C	F	Cb
1 oz quantity	105	1	21
1lb box/pkg., 16 oz	1685	7	339
Elbows, 1 cup, 3¾ oz	380	2	80
Shells, small, 1 cup, 3¼ oz	330	1.5	69
Spirals, 1 cup, 3 oz	305	1.5	64

Cooked Spaghetti/Macaroni

	C	F	Cb
Plain, All Types (no added fat):			
Firm/Al Dente (8-10 mins.), 1 oz	42	0.5	8.5
Medium (11-13 mins.), 1 oz	37	0.5	7.5
Tender (14-20 mins.), 1 oz	32	0.5	7
(Longer cooking increases water absorbed)			
Spaghetti, ½ cup, 2 ½ oz	90	0.5	18
Medium serving, 1 cup, 5 oz	225	1.5	44
Large (restaurant), 2 c., 10 oz	450	3	88
Elbows/Spirals, 1 cup, 5 oz	220	1.5	43
Small Shells, 1 cup, 4 oz	180	1	36
Protein-fortified: Dry, 1 c., 3⅓ oz	350	2	63
Cooked, 1 cup, 5 oz	230	0.5	45
Spinach/Vegetable: Dry, 1 c., 3 oz	310	1	61
Cooked, 1 cup, 5 oz	180	0.5	38
Whole-wheat: Dry, 1 c., 3¾ oz	365	1.5	79
Cooked, 1 cup, 5 oz	175	1	37

Fresh Pasta (Refrigerated)

	C	F	Cb
Plain/Spinach/Tomato, average:			
As purchased, 4.5 oz	370	3	70
Cooked, 1 cup, 5 oz	185	1.5	35
Home-made, without egg:			
Cooked, 1 cup, 5 oz	175	1	35
Buitoni			
Cut Pasta: Angel Hair, 1¼ cups	230	2.5	43
Fettuccine, 1¼ cups	240	2.5	45
Linguine, 1¼ cups	240	2.5	45
Spinach Fettuccine, 1¼ cups	260	3	45
Ravioletti, Three Cheese, 1 c., 90g	270	5	43

	C	F	Cb
Buitoni (Cont):			
Ravioli: Chkn & Rstd Garlic, 1¼ cup	340	11	47
Chicken Parmesan, 1¼ cups	310	8	45
Classic Beef, 1¼ cup	350	11	47
Four Cheese, 1⅓ cups	330	10	45
Garden Vegetable, 1 cup	250	5	40
Light Four Cheese, 1¼ cups	260	4.5	41
Whole Wheat Four Chse, 1¼ cups	320	14	34
Tortellini: Herb Chkn, 1 cup	340	9	52
Spinach Cheese, 1 cup	320	7	49
Three Cheese, 1 cup	330	8	50
Tortelloni: Chse & Rstd Garlic, 1 c.	270	8	38
Portabello Mushr. & Chse, 1 cup	290	6	49
Other varieties, avg., 1 cup	325	10	47
Pasta Sauces: *See Page 86*			

Noodles

	C	F	Cb
Plain/Egg: Dry, 1 oz	110	1.5	20
1 cup, 1⅓ oz	145	1.5	27
Cooked: 1 oz	40	0.5	7
½ cup, 2¾ oz	110	1.5	20
1 cup, 5½ oz	220	3.5	40
Stir-Fried: 1 cup, 5½ oz	270	9	40
2 cup serving, 11 oz	540	18	80
Yolk Free (Cooked): *Per Cup*			
'No Yolks' *(Foulds)*, 2 oz	210	0.5	41
Passover Gold *(Manischewitz)*	200	0	41
Chinese: Cellophane/Rice, dry, 1 oz	100	0	25
Chow Mein/hard, dry, 1 oz	150	9	16
Ramen Noodles: *See Page 73*			
Japanese: Soba, dry, 1 oz	95	0.5	21
cooked, 1 cup, 4 oz	115	0.5	24
Somen, dry, 1 oz	100	0.5	21
cooked, 1 cup, 6 oz	230	0.5	49
Japanese Style Pan Fried:			
Maruchan's Yaki-Sobu, 5.6 oz cup	260	3	50
Rice Noodles: Dry, 3.5 oz	365	0.5	83
Cooked, 1 cup, 6.2 oz	190	0.5	44
Stir Fry *(Yakisoba)*, 3.5 oz serving	430	6	52
Thai Kitchen: *See Page 75, 83*			
Udon *(Chikara)*, avg., 7.5 oz pkt	250	1	52

Egg Roll Skins/Won Ton

	C	F	Cb
Egg Roll Skins:			
(Golden Dragon) 1 pce, 1 oz	80	0	18
(Wung Hung) 4 skins, 4 oz	300	0	64
Won Ton Wrappers:			
(Nasoya) 8 wrappers, 2.1 oz	160	0.5	31
Egg Roll/Spring Roll Wrapper:			
(Dynasty) 3 wrappers, 2.1 oz	170	1	36

Breads

Note: Most breads have similar calories on a weight basis. However, volume may vary.

For example, 1 oz of bread may equal 1 slice regular bread or 2 slices of a lighter bread.

It is best to weigh bread used and calculate on 1 oz bread = 70 calories.

Quick Guide

Bread

Average All Varieties:	C	F	Cb
Lite slice, ¾ oz	40	0.5	9
Sandwich slice, 1 oz	70	1	12
Standard slice, 1¼ oz	90	1	18
Large slice, 1½ oz	105	1.5	20
Giant slice, 1¾ oz	120	1.5	23
Large/Specialty Bread, 2 oz	150	2	28
1-lb Loaf, 16 oz	1120	16	192

Toast has same calories as bread used.

1 Toasting Slice:			
w. 2 tsp regular spread	140	9	12
w. 2 tsp "light" spread	105	5	12
w. 1 Tbsp regular spread	170	12	12
w. 1 Tbsp "light" spread	120	7	12

Breads

	C	F	Cb
12-Grain, 1½ oz slice	110	1.5	22
Batard (8 oz), thick slice, 2 oz	150	0.5	28
Bran style/Dark, 1 oz slice	70	1	14
Bread w. Soy Isoflavones, 1.2 oz	80	2.5	13
Buttermilk, average, 1½ oz slice	110	1	22
Caraway Rye, 2 oz slice	150	2	28
Challah, ¾ oz slice	85	1.5	17
Chapati, 1 oz	110	3	18
Ciabatta, 1 slice, 2 oz	130	1	26
Corn Bread, average, 1 pce, 3 oz	220	6	37
Cracked Wheat Sourdough, 1½ oz slice	130	0.5	27
Croissants: *See Page 113, 173*			
Crustless Bread, regular slice ¾ oz	40	0.5	8.5
Crusts Only, regular slice, ¼ oz	30	0	7
English Toasting, slice, 2 oz	140	1.5	27
'Enriched' Breads, average, 1 oz sl.	60	1	12
Flax & Sunflower Round, 1.2 oz	90	2	18
Foccacia: Plain, 2 oz portion	150	2.5	28
Cheese & Garlic; Pesto, 2 oz	160	6	21
Tomato & Olive, 2 oz	150	5	21
French Stick/Baguette, 1 oz slice	70	1	15

Breads (Cont)

	C	F	Cb
French Toast, 1 slice, 1.6 oz	140	2	26
Sticks *(Aunt Jemima),* 1 pce, 1 oz	90	2	17
Garlic Bread/Toast:			
Small slice + 1 tsp spread, ¾ oz	80	5	7
Med. slice + 2 tsp spread, 1½ oz	160	10	14
Thick slice + 3 tsp spread, 1.8 oz	220	14	20
Pepperidge Farm, 1 slice, 1.4 oz	160	10	15
Hemp Bread, 1.2 oz	95	2	12
Italian Bread, 2 oz slice	140	1	28
Light Bread, avg., 0.8 oz slice	40	0.5	8
Lower Carb (higher Protein/fiber),			
average all brands, 1 oz	60	1.5	9
MultiGrain, 1 slice, 1.3 oz	60	1.5	17
Nut/Health Nut, 1.35 oz slice	90	1.5	18
Oatmeal/Oatbran Bread, 1½ oz	90	0.5	19
Party Breads *(Pepp. Farm):* Rye, 1 sl.	25	0.5	0.5
Pumpernickel, 1 sl.	25	0.5	4.5
Pita: Average all types,			
Small (4" diam) 1.1 oz	90	0	18
Large (6½" diam) 2 oz	140	1.5	27
Extra Large (9" diam) 4 oz	300	1.5	60
Popovers (1), no butter	130	2	18
Poppyseed (Vienna), 0.8 oz sl.	55	1	10
Pumpernickel, 1.35 oz slice	80	0	15
Cocktail size, 0.4 oz	30	0.5	6
Raisin Bread, 1 oz slice	80	1.5	14
Raisin Walnut, 1 oz slice	70	0.5	15
Roman Meal, 1.1 oz slice	80	1	14
Rye: Average, 1 thin slice, 1 oz	80	1	14
1 thick slice, 2 oz	150	2	25
Cocktail size, 0.4 oz	25	0.5	4
Sandwich Bread, 1 oz slice	70	1	12
Sandwich Pockets, 2 oz	140	1.5	27
Sourdough, 1½ oz slice	120	1	25
Sourdough French, 1 oz	75	0	14
Spelt, 1.6 oz	130	1	26
Sprouted 7-Grain, 1.5 oz slice	110	0.5	18
Squaw, 1.1 oz slice	85	0.5	13
Sweet Hawaiian Bread, 1.3 oz	110	2	19
Tacos/Tortillas: *See Page 104*			
Turkish/Middle Eastern, 1 oz sl.	80	1.5	16
Wheat-Free Breads: Spelt, 1.6 oz	130	1	26
Healthseed Rye, 1.6 oz	90	1	20
Kamut, 1.2 oz	80	2	16
Millet, 1.5 oz	100	1	20

Bread Brands | C | F | Cb

Controlled Carb Gourmet

	C	F	Cb
High Fiber, 1 slice, 1 oz	80	2.5	11
Zero Net Carb Bagel, 1 oz	120	2	14

Ener-G: Gluten-Free Breads

	C	F	Cb
Brown Rice Bread, 1 slice, 1.3 oz	130	6	18
Light Brown Rice, 1 slice, ¾ oz	50	2	7
Corn Loaf, 1 slice, ¾ oz	40	1.5	8
Light Tapioca, 1 slice, ¾ oz	45	1.5	7

Ezekiel

	C	F	Cb
Low Carb: Wheat, 0.8 oz	70	4	4
Savory Herb, 0.8 oz	60	2.5	4
Genesis 1: 29, 0.8 oz	80	2	14

Nature's Path: Per Slice (2 oz)

	C	F	Cb
Manna: Carrot Raisin; Millet Rice	130	0	28
Cinnamon Date	150	0	29
Fruit & Nut	140	1	27
Multigrain	130	0	26
Sun Seed	160	2	29
Whole Rye	150	0	32

Oroweat: Per Slice

	C	F	Cb
100% Whole Wheat, 1.3 oz	100	2	19
Sugar Free Whole Grain, 1 sl., 0.8 oz	50	1	9

Pepperidge Farm: Per Slice

	C	F	Cb
100% Whole Wheat, Thin	70	1	12
Carb Style 7-Grain	60	1.5	8
Cinnamon Swirl	80	1.5	15
Farmhouse Soft	110	2	19
Light Style, average	45	0	9
Raisin Cinnamon Swirl	80	1.5	15

Ralph's, Breakfast Bread: Per Slice (2 oz)

	C	F	Cb
Cranberry Orange, 1 sl., 2 oz	180	4	32
Wild Berry, 1 sl., 2 oz	180	3	33

Sara Lee: Per Slice

	C	F	Cb
Delightful White, 0.8 oz	45	0.5	9
Honey Wheat, 1 oz	80	1	16
Heart Healthy Multi-Grain, 1.4 oz	100	1.5	19

Schwan's: Per Serving

	C	F	Cb
Cheese & Herb Biscuits (1), 34g	110	6	11
Chse Stuffed Bread w. Sauce, 2 oz	160	5	20
Five Chse Garlic French Bread (1), 96g	330	20	26
French Baguette Bread, ¼ loaf, 49g	130	0	25
Garlic Texas Toast, 2 oz	190	10	20
Southern Style Biscuits (1), 2.2 oz	200	10	23

Trader Joe's

	C	F	Cb
Fat-Free Multi-Grain, 1.1 oz	70	0	15
Mom's White, 1.1 oz	90	1	15
Seeded Harvest, 1 oz	65	1	11
Pumpernickel, 1.3 oz	100	0	21

Wonder: Sandwich, 1 slice, 1 oz

	C	F	Cb
Wonder: Sandwich, 1 slice, 1 oz	60	0.5	13
Light Wheat, 1 slice, ¾ oz	40	0.5	9

Bread Rolls & Buns | C | F | Cb

	C	F	Cb
Brown 'n Serve, average, 1 oz	70	1	13
Carb Monitor (Pillsbury), 1.1 oz roll	70	2	11
Ciabatta Roll, 3½ oz	230	4	41
Concha (Mexican Sweet Bread), 3 oz	400	19	50
Dinner Rolls: 1 small, 1 oz	90	1.5	17
1 medium (3" diam), 1½ oz	110	1	23
English Muffins, avg., 2 oz	120	1	25
Frankfurter/Hot Dog: 1¼ oz	110	1.5	21
1½ oz size	130	2	25
French: 1 medium, 1.3 oz	110	1.5	22
1 large, 3 oz	230	2.5	42
Hamburger: Regular, 1½ oz	110	1.5	22
Large, 3 oz	210	3	40
Hoagie/Submarine, 2⅓ oz	160	2	31
Hot Cross Bun, Medium, 1 oz	85	0	19
Kaiser Roll, 2 oz size	200	2.5	35
Onion Roll, 2.4 oz size	180	2.5	34
Parker House Roll, 1 oz size	75	1.5	13
Party Roll, 0.6 oz	45	0.5	9
Sandwich Roll, 2.6 oz size	190	1.5	37
Sourdough Roll, 1¼ oz	110	1	21
Sweet Rolls, 1 oz	100	2	20
w. Icing, average	160	6	20
Wheat Roll: Small, 1.2 oz	100	1	17
Medium, 1¾ oz	130	1.5	23

Breadsticks, Croutons

	C	F	Cb
Breadsticks: Salt Sticks, plain, 1 oz	110	1	20
Fresh baked (1), 2 oz	180	2.5	34
Stella D'oro: Sesame (1)	50	2	7
Original, 1 piece	45	1	7
Croutons: Seasoned, 2 Tbsp, ¼ oz	35	1.5	4
9 small or 6 large, ¼ oz	35	1.5	4
Fat-Free (Pepp. Farm), 2 Tbsp	30	0	5

Bread Products

Bread Crumbs, dry:

	C	F	Cb
Plain or seasoned, 1 oz	110	1.5	20
1 rounded Tbsp, 10g	40	0.5	7
1 cup, 3½ oz	385	5	70
Corn Flake Crumbs, 1.1 oz	120	0	29
Graham Cracker Crumbs, 1 oz	110	2.5	20
Keebler, 3 Tbsp, ½ oz	70	1.5	13
Bread Dough: Frozen, 1 slice, 2 oz	140	2	26
Refrigerated, French, 1" slice	60	1	13
Wheat/White, 1" slice	80	2	14
Coating Mixes: Avg., 2 Tbsp., 1 oz	100	2	20
Stuffing: Average, dry mix, 1 oz	110	1	10
Made-up, ½ cup, 4 oz	180	4	11

Bagels ◆ Tacos ◆ Rice Cakes

Quick Guide

Bagels
	C	F	Cb
Average All Brands			
Plain/Onion:			
1 mini/bagelette, 1 oz	75	0.5	15
1 small bagel, 2 oz	145	1	29
1 medium bagel, 3 oz	230	1.5	45
1 large bagel, 4 oz	285	2	56
Bagel Chips (New York Style),			
4 slices, ¾ oz	100	4.5	12
Pizza Bagel Bites, 4 pces, 3.1 oz	200	6	29
Bagel Bites (Ore-Ida), 4 pces	190	7	25
Bagel Crisps (New York Style), 7 pces	140	6	17

Bagel Brands
	C	F	Cb
Controlled Carb Gourmet			
High Fiber Bagel (1), 2 oz	160	5	22
Individual Wrapped (1), 2 oz	80	6	20
Zero Net Carbs (1), 2 oz	60	1	7
Costco Bakery: Plain, 4 oz	300	1	61
Everything, 4 oz	330	3.5	62
Enjoy Life, all types, 3.2 oz	270	6	50
Lenders: Original, frozen, 2 oz	140	0.5	29
New York, frozen, 3.3 oz	230	1	47
Plain, refrigerated, 2.9 oz	210	1.5	42
Oroweat: Oatmeal, 3.4 oz	270	4	49
Whole Wheat, 3.4 oz	250	1.5	52
Sara Lee: Mini, average, 1.3 oz	100	0.5	21
Toaster Size, all types, 2.2 oz	160	1	34
3.5 oz Size (95g): Plain, 3.4 oz	250	1.5	53
Other flavors, avg., 3.4 oz	260	1	54
Healthy Heart, 3.3 oz	220	1.5	47
4 oz Size: Apple Cinnamon	310	1.5	64
Banana Walnut	350	7	61
Cranberry Orange	310	1.5	64
Western: All flavors, avg., 2 oz	110	0	25
Bagel Sandwiches: See Page 173			
Fast-Foods: See Page 183			

Bagel Sandwiches: See Page 173
Fast-Foods: See Page 183

Bagel Spreads
	C	F	Cb
Cream Cheese:			
Plain: 2 Tbsp, 1 oz	80	8	2
2 oz mini-tub	160	16	4
Reduced Fat: 2 Tbsp, 1 oz	60	5	2
2 oz mini-tub	120	10	4
Flavors: Lox, 1 oz	75	6	1
Raisin Walnut, 1 oz	90	6	8
Strawberry, 1 oz	60	3	7
Sundried Tomato, 1 oz	80	7	2
Vegetable, 1 oz	60	6	1

Rice Cakes
	C	F	Cb
Average All Types/Brands:			
Regular size, 1 cake, 9g	35	0	7.5
Hain, Mini, average, 9 pieces	70	2	12
Lundberg, all types, 15g each	60	0.5	14
Quaker, Large, all flavors, 13g each	50	0	11
Westbrae, 1 cake, 7g	25	0	5

Taco Shells & Tortillas
	C	F	Cb
Tacos: Mini Size (1)	25	1.5	2
Regular size, all types (1)	50	2	7
Super Size (1)	90	4	13
Salad Shell, flour (Del Oro), 1.4 oz	230	17	10
Tortilla (Soft Taco), each	85	2	15
Corn Tortilla: 6", 1 oz each	55	0.5	22
Flour Tortilla: 8", 1.75 oz	145	3	26
Low-Fat	110	1.5	22
Burritos, 1 tortilla, 2.3 oz	190	5	32
Low-Fat	110	1.5	22
Tostada Shells, each	55	3	6
La Tortilla Factory			
Fat Free Flour Tortillas:			
Burrito size, 2.5 oz	120	0.5	34
Soft Taco, 1.8 oz	90	0	24
Low Carb Low-Fat Tortillas:			
Large, 1.26 oz	80	3	19
Original; Flavors, 1.26 oz	50	2	11
Mission Foods			
Tortillas: Per 6" Tortilla			
Flour, 1 oz	80	1.5	13
Low Carb Flour, 1 oz	80	2	12
Low Carb Whole Wheat, 1 oz	80	2	12
White Corn, 0.8 oz	45	0.5	8.5
98% Fat-Free Burrito, 10", 2.4 oz	180	1.5	37

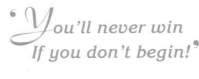

Rev. Dr Robert Schuller

'Inch by inch
Life's a cinch'

'You'll never win
If you don't begin!'

Crispbreads

C F Cb

Per Crispbread/Cracker

	C	F	Cb
Ak-Mak: Sesame, 5 crackers, 1 oz	115	3	19
Finn Crisp: Original, rye, 1	35	0	7
Other types, 1 crispbread	19	0	3
Kavli Norwegian: Thin (3)	50	0	11
Thick, 2 crispbreads	60	0.5	12
Malsovit Meal Wafers, 1	75	4	7
New York Flatbread Crisps, 1	35	0	7
Ry-Krisp: Natural, 1 crispbread	25	0	5
Seasoned, 1 crispbread	30	0	5
Sesame, 1 crispbread	25	1	5
Ryvita: Dark/Light, 1 piece	26	0	4
WASA: Delikatess (1)	25	0	5.5
Fiber (1); Sesam (1)	30	1	5
Original (1)	35	0.2	7.5
Runda (1)	55	1.5	9
Wheat Dore (1)	50	1	9
Westbrae Rice Wafers (7), 15g	50	0	11

Matzos

Manischewitz

	C	F	Cb
Egg 'n Onion Matzo, 1 oz	100	1	23
Grape Matzo, 1 oz each	110	0	25
Mandelin, 9 pieces	35	2	4
Matzo Meal, ½ cup	130	0	28
Matzo Farfel, 1 cup, 2.7 oz	180	0.5	60
Passover Egg Matzos, 1.1 oz	120	0	28
Spelt Matzos (1)	110	1	20
Tim Tam Crackers (10)	130	4	22
Tim Tam Everything (10)	130	5	19
Thin Salted Tea Matzos, 0.9 oz	100	0	22
Unsalted; Whole Wheat, 1 oz	110	0	24
Crackers: Miniatures (12)	110	0.5	25
Passover Egg Matzo (11)	110	0	20

Quick Guide

C F Cb

Crackers

Average All Brands: Per Cracker

	C	F	Cb
Cheese Crackers: Plain, 1" square	5	0	0.5
Small, octagonal	10	0	1
Round (2" diam.)	15	0	1.5
Sandwich (Peanut Butter)	35	1.5	4
Graham, 2½" square, 1 cracker	30	0.5	5
Melba Toast, plain, 1 piece	20	0	4
Oyster & Soup Crackers, ½ oz	60	2	10
(40 small oysters/20 lge hexagons)			
Rice Crackers: 1 small	9	0	2
Rice Snacks, Oriental-Style, ½ oz	70	3.5	7
Saltines, 5 crackers	65	2	11
Snack-type, 1 round cracker	15	0	1.5
Soda Crackers *(Saltine),* 2	25	1	4.5
Water Cracker *(Carr's):* Regular, 1	30	0	7
Small, 1 cracker	15	0	4
Wheat, thin, 1 cracker	9	0.5	1.5
Zwieback Toast, 1 piece	30	0	5

Quick Guide

C F Cb

Cookies

Average All Brands: Per Cookie

	C	F	Cb
Biscotti: Small, 0.5 oz	70	3	10
Regular, 1 oz	140	6.5	18
Chocolate Chip Cookies:			
Small/Thin 0.5 oz	50	2.5	7
Regular, 1 oz	100	5	14
Large, 2.3 oz *(Mrs Fields)*	280	13	40
Jumbo, 4 oz	545	26	76
Oatmeal/Oatmeal Raisin:			
Small/Thin 0.5 oz	65	2.5	10
Regular, 1 oz	130	5	20
Large, 1.7 oz *(Mrs Fields)*	180	7	29
Jumbo, 4 oz	510	20	78
Peanut Butter:			
Small/Thin 0.5 oz	70	3.5	9
Regular, 1 oz	140	7	18
Large, 2.3 oz *(Mrs Fields)*	310	16	34
Jumbo, 4 oz	540	27	67
Low-Fat Cookies			
Choc Chip (Low-Fat), ½ oz (1)	45	1.5	7.5
Oatmeal Raisin (Fat-Free), 1 oz (1)	95	0.5	22
Peanut Butter (Low-Fat), 1 oz (1)	105	5	15

Brands	C	F	Cb
Per Cookie/Cracker (Unless Indicated)			
Archway			
Apple/Date-filled Oatmeal, avg.	95	3	16
Frosty Lemon/Orange	110	4.5	18
Ginger Snaps, Regular/Iced (5)	150	5	23
Molasses (1)	110	3.5	19
Oatmeal	110	4	18
Oatmeal Raisin	100	3	18
Atkins			
Endulge Crisps (1), average	130	10	15
Austin			
Cookies: *Per Package*			
Sandwiches: Lemon OHs!	240	10	35
Vanilla Cremes	160	7	24
Crackers: *Per Package*			
Cheese w. Cheddar Cheese	210	10	26
Cheese w. Cheddar Jack Cheese	200	11	23
Cheese w. Peanut Butter	200	10	23
Crispy w. Cream Cheese & Chives	200	10	24
Dolphins & Friends Cheddar (60)	140	5	24
Sandwiches: Chse & Peanut Butter	170	7	24
Grilled Cheese Flavored	200	10	24
PB & J Flavored	200	10	24
Toasty Crackers w. Peanut Butter	200	10	23
Wheat Crackers w. Cheddar Chse	200	10	24
Zoo Animals (16)	130	2	25
Baker's: *Per Cookie (3 oz)*			
Peanut Butter	320	10	52
Peanut Butter & Jelly	310	9	55
Vegan Peanut But. Choc. Chunk	320	11	53
Other varieties, average	320	6	58
Barbara's Bakery			
Cookies: Fig Bars, avg. (1)	60	0.5	14
Animal Cookies, Vanilla (8)	120	4.5	18
Crisp Cookies (1), average	80	4	9
Snackimals (10), average	120	4	19
Crackers: Cheese Bites (22), 1 oz	120	3	20
Organic Go Go Grahams (8) avg.	130	4	22
Rite Lite Rounds (5), average	60	2	11
Wheatines (4), average	60	1	11
Brent & Sam's			
Cookies: Chocolate Chip (2)	120	6	16
Chocolate Chip Pecan (2)	130	8	14

Carr's	C	F	Cb
Crackers: Table Water (5)	70	1.5	13
Whole Wheat (2)	80	3.5	11
Cookies: Bisc. for Tea (2)	140	6	20
Chococcines (3)	150	9	16
Ginger Lemon Cremes (2)	130	5	20
Hob Nobs (2)	140	6	19
Imperials: Milk Chocolate (2)	140	7	18
Dark Choc (2)	150	7	19
Petites Bijoux (4)	140	5	21
Cookies &			
Cookie Bars: M&M's (1)	170	9	20
Milky Way (1); Snickers (1)	180	11	21
Twix w. Peanut Butter (1)	160	9	17
Twix (1)	180	10	21
Country Choice			
Ginger Snaps (5)	120	5	19
Sandwich Cremes (2), avg.	130	5	19
Soft Baked: Peanut Butter (1)	100	5	13
Avg. other varieties (1)	100	4	16
Vanilla Wafers (7)	120	5	19
Dove			
Cookies: *Per Serving*			
Beyond Chocolate Chunk (1)	110	5	13
Chocolate Walnut Oasis (1)	110	6	13
Chocolate Walnut Rendezvous (1)	110	6	13
Milk Chocolate Moment (3)	160	9	20
Mint Chocolate Serenade (3)	160	8	19
Toffee Chocolate Thrill (3)	160	8	20
Entenmann's			
Soft Baked (1), avg., all flavors	100	5	13
Estee (Fructose Sweetened)			
Chocolate Chip	40	2	5
Coconut Cookies	35	1.5	5
Famous Amos			
Chocolate Chip (4)	150	7	19
Chocolate Chip, Snack Size (4)	160	6	25
Choc Chip & Pecan (4)	150	8	18
Chocolate Creme Sandwich (3)	160	6	25
Oatmeal Choc Chip & Walnut (4)	140	7	18
Oatmeal Raisin (4)	140	6	20
Peanut Butter (4)	160	7	22
Peanut Buter Creme S'wich (3)	160	7	22
Vanilla Creme Sandwich (3)	170	7	25
Low-Fat: Gingersnaps (1 pkg)	200	3	44

Per Cookie/Cracker (Unless Indicated)

Girl Scouts	C	F	Cb
Cookies: Caramel DeLites (2)	140	7	19
All Abouts (2); Cafe Cookies (5)	150	7	20
Cartwheels, Reduced-Fat (5)	140	4	24
Do-Si-Dos (3)	180	9	22
Lemon Coolers (5); Pastry Cremes (3)	130	4.5	22
Peanut Butter Patties (2)	150	8	16
Peanut Butter Sandwich (2)	170	6	24
Samoas (2)	150	8	19
Shortbread (4); Trefoils (4)	130	6	18
Tagalongs (2)	130	9	13
Thanks-A-Lot (2)	150	6	22
Grandma's			
Peanut Butter Sandwich Creme (5)	210	10	28
Rich 'N Chewy, Choc Chip, pkg.	270	12	38
Vanilla Sandwich Creme (5)	210	9	30
Mini Vanilla Bites (9)	150	7	22
Homestyle Big:			
Fudge Chocolate Chip (1)	170	7	27
Oatmeal Raisin (1)	180	6	30
Peanut Butter (1)	200	10	24
Chocolate Chip (1)	190	9	25
Great American Cookies			
Cookies: Original; Pecan (1)	230	12	31
Chewy Pecan Supreme (1)	230	12	31
Chewy Choc. Supreme/Sugar (1)	200	9	29
Double Fudge/ Reese's (1), avg	220	10	33
Oatmeal (1)	230	10	23
Original M&M/Reese's (1)	240	12	32
Peanut Butter/M&M (1), avg	250	13	28
Snickerdodles (1)	240	11	33
White Chunk Macademia (1)	250	14	30
Double Doozies: Original (1)	340	17	46
M&M Big Bite (1)	340	17	46
Brownies: Cheesecake (1)	430	23	54
German Chocolate (1)	420	22	51
Iced Fudge (1)	500	23	71
Iced Fudge Nut (1)	500	27	64
Swirl Cheesecake (1)	440	23.5	56
Cookie Cakes: 16" Cookie (1)	460	22	67
16" M&M Cookie (1)	500	24	73
Heart Shaped (1)	440	21	64
Sliced Cookie Cake, 1 slice	580	27	83
Cakes, avg. 1 slice, ⅛ cake	670	30	95
Brownies: Cheesecake Brownie	400	21	48
Cheesecake Chocolate Swirl	485	25	60
Fudge	495	22	67
Fudge Nut	525	27	63

Hain	C	F	Cb
Cookies: Animal (9), 1 oz	110	2	16
98% Fat-Free, all types (11)	110	0	23
Crackers: Crudites (26)	120	4	21
Mini Munchees (17)	60	0.5	12
Oyster Crackers, Fat-Free (52)	60	1	12
Rich Crackers (11)	130	4.5	21
Soy Munchies (9)	60	2.5	6
Wheatettes (16)	130	3.5	21
Health Valley			
Cookies			
Biscotti Style Low-Fat, 2 cookies	120	3	23
Chocolate Chip Oatmeal (1)	100	4	14
Cookie Cremes Sandwich (2) avg.	125	5	19
Oatmeal Raisin Cookie (1)	90	3.5	14
Peanut Crunch Oatmeal Cookie (1)	100	4	14
Cookie Bars, average	200	7	33
Cafe Creations: Chocolate Chip (1)	100	5	13
Raisin Oatmeal (1)	90	3.5	15
Chunk: Chocolate/Dbl Choc. (1)	120	7	15
White Chocolate (1)	140	7	17
Fat Free, average	100	0	24
Mini: Choc. Chocolate Chip (4)	130	7	16
Other varieties (4)	120	5	16
Crackers			
Original: Amaranth Graham (6)	120	3	22
Oat Bran Graham (6)	120	3	22
Rice Bran (6)	110	3	19
Corn Bread varieties (4)	60	1.5	11
Cracked Pepper; Sesame (1)	60	1.5	10
French Onion (10)	60	1.5	10
Hershey's			
Cookies: Hershey's w. Almonds (2)	150	9	16
Almond Joy Cookies (2)	150	9	17
Reese's Cookies (2)	150	8	17
York Cookies (2)	160	9	17
Joseph's Cookies			
Sugar Free Cookies			
Brownies: Original, 1 ½ oz bag	150	7	26
Pecan Walnut (9 brownies)	100	5	15
Crispy Bite Size: *Per 4 Cookies*			
Chocolate Peanut Butter	95	5	13
Pecan Chocolate Chip	95	5	13
Almond; Chocolate Chip	100	6	13
Chocolate Walnut; Oatmeal Choc	100	6	14
Lemon; Peanut Butter, avg.	95	4	15
Oatmeal; Pecan Shortbread, avg.	100	5	15

Crackers ✦ Cookies (Cont)

Per Cookie/Cracker (Unless indicated)

Keebler	C	F	Cb
Crackers:			
Club: Original (5)	70	3	9
Reduced Fat (5)	70	2.5	12
Grahams: Original (8), 1 oz	130	3.5	22
Low-Fat varieties (8), 1 oz	110	1.5	22
Munch'ems, average (38), 1 oz	140	4.5	22
Toasted, Regular varieties (5)	80	3.5	10
Town House: Original (5)	80	4.5	9
Reduced Fat (6)	60	1.5	11
Wheatables: Reduced Fat (19)	140	4	23
Other varieties, average (17)	140	6	20
Cookies: Chips Deluxe			
Chewy (1)	80	3.5	11
Rainbow (1)	80	4	10
Chocolate Lovers; Coconut (1)	80	4.5	10
Original, 2 oz pkg	300	16	37
Rainbow Mini's 1.4 oz pkg	210	10	27
Country Style Oatmeal (2)	130	6	18
Danish Wedding (4)	130	6	18
E.L. Fudge: Original (2)	140	6	19
Double Stuffed (2)	180	9	23
S'mores Blasted (2), avg	180	9	24
Fudge Shoppe:			
Deluxe Grahams, regular (3)	140	7	17
Fudge Sticks (3), avg.	150	8	19
Fudge Stripes: Regular, avg. (3)	160	8	21
Reduced Fat (3)	130	5	21
Mini's, 1 pkg	210	10	27
Grasshopper (4)	140	7	19
Gripz, avg., 1 pouch	130	5	17
Iced Animal (6)	140	5	22
Sandies Cookies: Reduced-Fat (1)	80	3.5	11
Cookies (1) avg. all flavors	80	5	9
Right Bites, 0.7 oz pouch	100	3	17
Soft Batch (1)	80	3.5	11
Vienna Fingers: Regular (2)	150	7	24
Reduced Fat (2)	140	5	24
Wafers: Golden Vanilla Wafers (8)	140	6	21
Golden Vanilla Minis (18)	150	6	21
Reduced-Fat (8)	130	3.5	25
Vanilla Sugar (4)	160	8	21

Kroger	C	F	Cb
Cookies: Animal Cookies (9)	120	2.5	23
Fig Bars (2)	60	1	2
Fudgie Sticks Wafers (3)	140	8	18
Kid O's (3)	160	6	24
Crackers: Cheddar Crisps (18)	140	6	18
Socialites (12)	140	7	17
Lance			
Nekot: Peanut Butter, 1 pkg	110	11	30
S'Mores, 1 pkg	110	12	31
O Lunch, 1 pkg, avg.	230	10	34
Strawberry Cookies (5)	190	8	27
Crackers: Toasty, 1 pkg	180	9	16
Nipchee, 1 pkg	190	11	22
Toastchee: Original, 1 pkg	220	11	23
Reduced-Fat, 1 pkg	180	7	23
Malt Crackers, 1 pkg	190	10	18
Low Carb Enchantments			
Sugar Free Cookies, avg. (1), 1 oz	140	9	11
Little Debbie			
Fig Bar (1)	160	3	31
Marshmallow Pies, avg. (1)	180	7	28
Marshmallow Treats (1)	100	2.5	18
Nutty Bar (1)	310	18	32
Oatmeal Creme Pies (1)	170	7	26
Chocolate Sugar Wafer (3)	140	7	18
Vanilla Creme Wafer	130	6	19
Crackers: Chse w. P'nut Butter (4)	140	7	15
Toasty w. P'nut Butter (4)	140	7	15
Lu			
Cookies: Marie Lu (3)	160	4.5	27
Le Fondant Wafers (4)	170	10	19
Le Petit Beurre (4)	140	4	26
Le Petit Ecolier, avg. (2)	130	6	17
Shortbread (2)	140	8	16
Pim's: Chocolatier (3)	150	9	17
Orange; Raspberry (2)	100	3	17
Manischewitz			
Matzo Boards: *See Page 105*			
Biscotti: Toffee Crunch Macaroons	50	2.5	7
Cappuccino Chip	70	2.5	10
Chocolate Macaroons, each	45	2	8
Matzo Cracker, Miniatures, each	9	0	2
Tim Tam Crackers: Everything (10)	130	5	19
Original (10)	130	4	22
Whole Wheat Crackers	9	0	2

Per Cookie/Cracker (Unless indicated)

Miss Meringue	C	F	Cb
Chocolettes (10) average	130	3.5	24
Madeleines (2) average	160	9	18
Classiques:	110	0	26
Choc. Chip/Mint Choc. Chip (4)	120	1.5	25
Cappuccino/Rainbow Vanilla (4)	110	0	27
Meringue Minis: Chocolate (13)	110	0	26
Chocolate Chip (12)	130	1.5	26
Mint Chocolate Chip (13)	120	1.5	26
Other varieties (13)	110	0	27
Meringue Minis, Sugar Free (13) avg.	40	0	8

Mrs Fields Cookies: *See Fast-Foods Section*

Mother's	C	F	Cb
Butter Cookies (6)	160	8	21
Checkerboard Wafers (4)	150	9	17
Chocolate Sandwich Creme (3)	170	8	23
Chocolate Chip: Cookies (5)	160	7	21
Chocolate Chip Parade (4)	140	7	19
Cocodas Coconut (2)	160	8	21
Cookie Parade: Animal (4)	150	7	19
Circus Animal (14)	130	4.5	22
Iced Circus (6)	150	7	21
Double Fudge (2)	190	9	26
English Tea/Taffy Sandwich (2)	185	7	28
Iced Lemonade (2)	160	8	22
Peanut Butter Gaucho (2)	190	8	25
Pecan Shortbread (2)	160	9	19
Iced Raisin (2)	170	8	24
Oatmeal Cookies: Regular (2)	130	5	23
Chocolate Chip (2)	160	7	23
Oatmeal Raisin Cookies (5)	150	7	21
Striped Shortbread Cookies (3)	160	7	24
Sugar Cookies (2)	150	7	19
Sugar Free Lemon Creme (3)	160	7	24
Sugared Lemon	75	4	10
Vanilla Cremes (2)	180	7	28
Vanilla Wafers (8)	140	5	22
Bakery Wagon: Macaroons(1)	110	5	15
Peanut Butter (1)	110	6	14
Iced Oatmeal/Lemon (1)	110	4	18
Apple/Rasp. Filled Oatmeal (1)	110	3.5	17
Chocolate Chip Chunk (1)	110	4.5	16
White Chocolate Chip (3)	160	8	22
Double Thick Chocolate Chip (1)	170	8	23
Sugar Free: Chocolate Chip (4)	130	6	18
Checkerboard Wafers (6)	140	9	18
Pecan Shortbread (4)	170	11	17
Chocolate Creme (3)	130	7	23
Peanut Butter (4)	150	9	19
Oatmeal (4)	120	5	19

Murray SugarFree Cookies	C	F	Cb
Choc Chip & Pecan (3)	160	10	18
Double Fudge (3)	140	6	23
Fudge-Dipped Wafer: Vanilla (4)	140	10	19
Shortbread (5)	140	7	17
Gingersnaps (7)	130	5	24
Lemon/Choc Cremes (3)	130	7	18
Lemon Wafers (4)	130	8	20
Oatmeal (3)	150	7	21
Peanut Butter (3)	160	10	18
Shortbread (8)	140	6	21
Shortbread Pecan (3)	170	11	18
Vanilla Sugar Wafers (4)	130	10	20

Nabisco	C	F	Cb
Cookies: *Per Serving*			
Cameo Creme Sandwich (2)	130	5	21
Chips Ahoy!: Chocolate Chewy (2)	120	6	17
Chocolate Chip (3)	160	8	21
Mini Chocolate Chip Bite-Size (5)	170	8	24
Snak Saks (5)	150	8	21
Peanut Butter (1)	80	4	9
Reduced-Fat (3)	140	5	23
Soft Baked Chunky Choc. (1)	120	5	19
White Fudge Chunky (2)	80	4	11
w. 100% Whole Grain (1)	150	8	22
Ginger Snaps (4)	120	2.5	23
Lorna Doone (4)	150	7	19
Mallomars (2)	120	5	17
Morelianas, 1 oz	130	5	19
Newtons: Fig Newtons (2)	110	2	22
100% Whole Grain (2)	110	2	22
Fat-Free (2)	100	0	22
Snack Pack To Go! (2)	90	0	22
Raspberry (2); Strawberry (2)	100	1.5	22
Nilla Wafers: (8)	140	6	21
Reduced-Fat (8)	120	2	24
Nutter Butter: Bites (10)	170	7	24
Peanut Creme Patties (5)	160	9	17
Real Peanut Butter Sandwich (1)	90	4.5	12
Sandwich (2)	130	6	19
Sandwich Bites (10)	140	6	21
Wafers: Chocolate Stix, 1 oz	140	8	18
Chocolate Stix Bars (2)	210	11	26
Social Tea Biscuits (6)	120	4	20
Oreo: Original, 3 cookies	160	7	24
Snack pkg, 2 oz	270	12	40
Reduced-Fat, 3 cookies	150	4.5	26
Choc. Creme; Coffee'n Creme (3)	170	7	24
Double Delight: Mint'n creme (2)	140	7	20
P'nut Butter & Choc Creme (2)	140	6	20
Double Stuf, 2 cookies	140	7	20
Fudge-Covered, 1 cookie	100	5	13
Handi-Snacks (1), 1 oz	130	5	21
Mini Oreo: 9 pieces, 1 oz	140	6	21
Snack Pack, 1.2 oz (35g)	170	7	25
Uh-Oh!, 3 cookies	170	7	24
100 Calorie Packs (1) 4.8 oz	100	2	20

Crackers • Cookies (Cont)

Per Cookie/Cracker (Unless Indicated)

Nabisco (Cont):	C	F	Cb
Teddy Grahams:			
Chocolatey Chip, Mini (53)	140	4.5	22
Cinnamon Snacks (24)	130	4	23
Honey Mini, Snak Saks (30)	130	4	23
Chocolate; Honey Snack (24), avg.	160	5	26
100 Calorie Packs: Cheese Nips	100	3	15
Chips Ahoy! 1 pkg	100	3	18
Fruit Snacks, 1 pkg	100	0	24
Oreo (Thin Crisps), 1 pkg	100	2	20
Wheat Thins, 1 pkg	100	3	16
Crackers: *Per Serving*			
Barnum's Animals (10)	130	4	23
Cheese Nips Chips: Bold Cheddar (13)	140	5	20
Cheese Nips:			
Cheddar: Packs-2-Go!, 1.2 oz	170	7	22
Bag (29), 1 oz	150	7	18
Chips, avg. (13)	140	5	20
Four Cheese, 1 oz bag	150	7	18
Mini Go-Pak (53), 1 oz	150	6	19
Reduced-Fat (31) avg.	130	4.5	20
Cheddar (31), 30g	130	3.5	21
The Fairly Odd Parents, 1 oz	140	6	19
Flavor Originals:			
Better Cheddars (22)	160	8	19
Chicken in a Biskit (12)	160	8	18
Sociables Baked Savory (7)	70	3.5	9
Vegetable Thins (11)	160	9	18
Honey Maid:			
Grahams: Avg. (8)	130	3	24
Sticks (14), avg.	130	3	25
Low-Fat (8), avg.	120	1.5	26
Snack Bars: Regular (1)	150	6	24
Soft Baked varieties (1), avg.	150	4	27
Premium Saltine: Fat-Free (5)	60	0	12
Low Sodium (5)	60	1.5	11
Multigrain (5)	60	1.5	10
Original (5)	60	1.5	11
Unsalted Tops (5)	60	1.5	11
Premium, Soup & Oyster (22)	60	1.5	11
Wheat Thins: Big (11)	150	6	23
Harvest (13)	130	3.5	23
Honey; Low Sodium (16)	150	6	21
Multi-Grain (17)	130	4.5	22
Original, Packs-2-Go, 35g	170	7	23
Original (16), 31g	150	6	21
100 Calorie Packs	100	3	16
Ranch (14), 29g	140	6	19
Reduced-Fat (16), 29g	130	4	21
Toasted Chips: Multi-Grain (12)	120	4	20
Veggie (11), 28g	120	4	20
Wheatsworth, Stone Ground Wheat (5)	80	3.5	10
Zwieback, 8g	35	1	6

Per Cookie/Cracker (Unless Indicated)

Newman's Own Organics	C	F	Cb
Alphabet Cookies (10) avg.	120	3	22
Champion Chip: Chocolate Chip (4)	160	7	21
Expresso Chocolate Chip (4)	150	7	21
Wheat-Free & Dairy-Free (4)	160	8	21
Other varieties, avg.	160	8	21
Fig Newman's: Fat-Free, 2 bars	120	0	28
Low-Fat, 2 bars	140	2	28
Wheat/Dairy-Free, 2 bars	120	1.5	20
Newman-O's: Original (2)	130	4.5	20
Choc. Creme (2); Mint Creme (2)	130	4.5	20
Ginger-O's (2)	120	4.5	19
Tops & Bottoms (6)	120	3	21
Wheat-Free & Dairy-Free (2)	130	4.5	21

Peek Freans			
Assorted Creme (2)	140	6	19
Nice Biscuits (2)	160	6	25
Shortcake (2)	140	7	18

Pepperidge Farm			
Cookies			
Choc Chunk:			
Chocolate Dipped Nantucket (1)	150	8	20
Dark Choc. Pecan Chesapeake (1)	140	8	15
Milk Choc.: Cashew Stowe (1)	130	6	17
Macadamia Nut Sausalito (1)	140	8	16
White Choc. Macadamia (1)	130	6	17
Other varieties, avg. (1)	140	7	18
Chocolate Delight: Rialto (1)	100	3.5	16
Other varieties, avg. (1)	180	9	21
Collection: Ginger Family (4)	160	5	26
Other varieties, avg. (2)	135	7	17
Distinctive Milano: Milk Choc. (3)	170	9	21
Other varieties, avg. (3)	130	7	16
Distinctive: Brussels (3)	150	7	20
Brussels Mint (3)	190	10	22
Chessman (3)	120	5	18
Choc Bottomed Chessman (3)	170	7	23
Geneva (3)	160	9	19
Lido (1)	90	5	10
Raspberry Chantilly (2)	120	3	23
Other varieties, avg. (3)	140	5	22
Homestyle: Gingerman (4)	130	4	21
Shortbread (2)	140	7	16
Sugar (3)	140	6	20

Per Cookie/Cracker (Unless Indicated)

Pepperidge Farm (Cont)	C	F	Cb
Cookies (Cont)			
Mini: Chessmen (9)	140	6	21
Brussels (3)	190	10	22
Milano (6); Mint Milano (6) avg.	160	8	18
Nantucket Dark Choc. Chunk (4)	150	8	20
Soft Baked Cookies (1) avg.	140	5	22
Sugar-Free Cookies (3) avg.	170	9	22
Crackers			
Entertaining Collection (4)	70	2.5	10
Goldfish Crisps (37) average	150	7	17
Goldfish Flavor Blasted (51) avg.	150	7	19
Goldfish Mini Sandwich (11) avg.	140	6	18
Goldfish, Original (55)	150	6	20
Snack Sticks: Three Cheese (25)	150	6	20
Pumpernickel (15)	120	1.5	22
Sesame (12)	140	6	20
Perfect Bite Cookies			
Chocolate Chip; Peanut Butter (3)	80	4.5	13
Lemon (3); Oatmeal (3), avg.	80	4	13
Pirouline: 3 rolls, average, 1 oz	150	8	18
Ritz			
Crackers: Original, ½ oz	80	4	10
Reduced-Fat, ½ oz	70	2	11
Assortment, ½ oz	80	4	10
Dinosaurs, 1 oz	130	3.5	22
Garlic Butter, ½ oz	80	4	10
Mini Bite Size Original, 1.3 oz pkg	190	9	23
Peanut Butter, 1.4 oz pkg	190	9	24
Real Cheese, 1.4 oz pkg	200	11	22
Sticks, 1 oz	150	7	19
Top'ems, ½ oz	70	3	10
Whole Wheat, ½ oz	70	2.5	11
100 Calorie Snack Mix, 1 pkg, 22g	100	3	16
Ritz Bits Sandwiches: Cheese, 1 oz	150	9	16
Cheese Go-Pak (12) 1 oz	175	9	16
Cheese Packs 2 Go!, 1.5 oz	220	13	24
Graham S'mores, 1 oz	150	6	22
Peanut Butter/& Jelly, 1 oz	140	8	16
Peanut Butter Packs 2 Go!, 1.2 oz	170	10	20
Real Cheese, 1 oz	150	9	16
Ritz Chips: Original, 1 oz	130	4.5	21
Cheddar; Sour Crm & Onion, 1 oz	130	6	19
Santa Fe Farms			
Fat Free, average (4)	80	0	18

Snackwell's (Nabisco)	C	F	Cb
Creme Sandwich (2) 1 oz	110	3	20
Creme Sandwich, Packs To Go!, 1 pkg	210	5	38
Devil's Food Cake, Fat-Free (1) ½ oz	50	0	12
Lemon Creme Sandwich Sugar Free (3)	130	6	24
Shortbread Sugar Free (3) 1 oz	130	5	21
Sorbee			
Sugar Free: Animal (10)	100	3	21
Chocolate Chip; Choc. Fudge (1)	110	6	15
Oatmeal (1)	110	4	16
Peanut Butter (1)	110	7	13
South Beach Diet (Kraft)			
Cookies: Peanut Butter, 1 pkg	100	5	15
Oatmeal Chocolate Chip, 1 pkg	100	5	16
Crackers, Whole Wheat, 1 pkg	100	3.5	16
Stella D'Oro			
Almond Delight, 1 oz	160	8	18
Almond Toast (3)	115	2.5	21
Anginetti, 1 oz	130	3.5	22
Anisette Sponge Low-Fat (2)	95	1	19
Anisette Toast Low-Fat (3)	125	1	27
Biscotti, average, ¾ oz	95	4	13
Breakfast Treats: Chocolate Cookie (1)	90	3	15
Original (1)	90	3	15
Original Mini (1)	120	3.5	21
Viennese Cinnamon (1)	90	2.5	14
Coffee Treats: Almond Toast, 1 oz	110	2.5	19
Angel Wings, 1 oz	170	12	14
Anisette Sponge (2)	90	1	14
Anisette Toast, 1.1 oz	130	1	27
Banana Walnut Toast, 1 oz	100	2	19
Blueberry; Cinn. Toast, 1 oz	100	1	20
Roman Egg Biscuits, 1.1 oz	130	4	21
Continental Cookie Collection, 1 oz	130	4.5	20
Egg Jumbo, 1.1 oz	120	1.5	26
Lady Stella Assortment, 1 oz	130	4.5	20
Margherite (2)	130	4.5	20
Margherite Mini, 1.1 oz	150	5	24
Swiss Fudge (2) 1.1 oz	170	9	22
Striels			
Wafers: Chocolate (3)	160	9	19
Vanilla (3)	170	11	18
Kedem Tea Biscuits, all flavors (2)	32	1	6

Crackers ♦ Cookies (Cont) ♦ Refrigerated

Per Cookie/Cracker (Unless Indicated)	C	F	Cb
Sunshine			
Heads & Tails, 1 pkt, 1.5 oz	210	9	28
Hi-Ho Crackers, avg. (1)	15	0.5	2
Krispy: Original; Whole Wheat (1)	10	0.3	2
Oyster & Soup, 16 crackers	60	1	11
Unsalted Tops (1)	10	0.1	1
Trader Joe's			
All Butter Shortbread:			
w. Apricot/Raspberry Filling (2)	145	8	17
w. Chocolate Filling (2)	130	7	15
Brownie Bites (3)	130	6	18
Caramel Cashew Cookies	140	7	16
Cinnamon Grahams (2½ squares)	120	4	18
Chocolate: Almond Laceys (2)	170	12	16
Chip Dunkers (2)	160	7	21
Coated Choc. Chip Dunkers (2)	190	9	24
Coconut Macaroon (3)	160	10	18
Crispy Crunchy varieties (12)	150	8	13
Ginger Animal (7)	120	2	25
Lemon Crisp (5)	120	4	19
Meringues: Cappuccino (4)	110	0	26
Chocolate (4)	120	1.5	25
Fat Free (5)	110	0	27
Soft Lady Fingers (5)	100	1.5	20
Southern Style Pecan (4)	150	9	15
Swiss Almond Crunch (6)	140	8	14
Triple Ginger Snaps (6)	140	5	21
Way More Chocolate Chips (3)	160	11	14
Triscuit			
Baked Whole Wheat Crackers: Per Serving			
Original (15) 1 oz	120	4.5	19
Thin Crisps, Original (15) 1 oz	130	5	21
Reduced-Fat (8) 1 oz	120	3	21
Cheddar (6); Rstd Garlic (8)	120	4.5	19
Deli-Style Rye (8) 1 oz	135	5	21
Garden Herb; Rosemary (6) 1 oz	120	4	20
Low Sodium, 1 oz	130	5	19
Wild Oats			
Ginger Snaps (5)	140	5	21
Crunchy Peanut Butter (5)	150	8	16
Oatmeal Raisin (5)	130	5	21
Sandwich Cremes, avg., (3)	185	7	28
Water Crackers (4)	60	1	12
Assorted Crackers (2)	70	2	11
Zesta			
Crackers: Whole Wheat (5)	60	1.5	11
Fat Free, 5 crackers	60	0	13
Original, 5 crackers	60	1.5	11
Red. Sodium; Unsalted Tops (5)	60	1.5	11
Soup & Oyster, 51 crackers	70	3	10

Thaw, Bake & Serve

	C	F	Cb
Grands! Biscuits (Pillsbury): Per Biscuit			
Extra Rich	210	10	26
Butter Tastin'; Buttermilk, avg.	190	10	24
Reduced Fat	170	6	26
Flaky; Homestyle; Southern Style	190	9	24
Kroger			
Refrigerated Cookies			
Deluxe Oatmeal Cranberry Walnut (1)	170	8	21
Deluxe Moose Tracks (1)	170	9	22
Caramel Caribou (1)	180	9	21
Pillsbury Cookies: Per 1 oz			
Refrigerated Cookie Dough			
Big Deluxe Classics:			
Oatmeal Raisin (1)	180	7	26
Peanut Butter Cup (1)	190	9	24
White Chunk Macadamia Nut (1)	200	11	24
Other varieties (1)	200	10	25
Ready To Bake: Sugar-Free (1)	90	4	16
Chocolate Chip w. Walnuts (1)	120	7	14
Chocolate Chunk Chip (1)	120	6	15
Mini Bites Chocolate Chip (4)	120	6	15
Peanut Butter w. Reese's Pces (1)	120	5	15
S'mores (1); Choc. Candy (1)	120	5	16
Shape Sugar Cookie (2)	140	7	17
Sugar Cookie (1)	120	6	15
Refrigerated Dough: Per 1½" Ball of Dough (1 oz)			
Chocolate Chip/Chunk /Dble Choc	130	7	17
Oatmeal Choc. Chip; Sugar, avg.	130	6	17
Peanut Butter	120	5	17
Toll House (Nestlé)			
Refrigerated Dough			
Chocolate Chip (1)	120	6	15
Chocolate Chunk/Chunk (1)	120	6	15
Fudgy Brownie (1)	190	9	26
Jumbo Chocolate Chip (1)	200	10	26
Mini Chocolate Chip (2)	120	6	15
Walnut Chocolate Chip (1)	70	5	15
Other varieties, avg. (1)	110	5	15
Ultimates Refrigerated Dough			
Chocolate Chip Lovers (1)	180	9	23
Choc. Chips & Chunks w. Pecans (1)	190	10	22
P. Butter Chips & Choc Chunks (1)	180	9	23
Triple Chocolate Decadence (1)	170	8	23
Turtle (1)	180	9	23
White Choc. Macadamia Nut (1)	190	10	22

Cakes, Pastries, Croissants

Ready-to-Eat

Ready-to-Eat	C	F	Cb
Angel Food: Plain, no oil, 2 oz	145	0	33
Plain with oil, 2 oz	145	1	27
w. Cream Frosting	255	7	45
Apple Fritters, 3 oz	360	22	38
Apple Pie: *See Pies/Tarts Page 116*			
Baklava, 1½" square, 1.75 oz	200	10	27
Banana w. Butter Cream, 2 oz	230	9	37
Black Forest, 3 oz (1/12)	345	11	59
Brownie, 3.7 oz	430	21	61
Bundt, 3 oz (1/10)	270	12	36
Carrot Cake: Plain, 3 oz	300	16	37
w. Cream Cheese Frosting	400	22	48
Cheesecake: Small serving, 3 oz	235	13	26
Large serving, 5 oz	395	21	44
w. Low-Fat Cheese/Fruit, 3 oz	170	4	28
Cheesecake Factory: See Fast-Foods Section			
Denny's Cheesecake, 1 slice, ⅙	580	38	51
Cherry Cobbler, 4 oz	240	8	4
Chocolate Cake: Plain, 2 oz	200	9	30
w. Chocolate Frosting, 3 oz	290	12	44
& Cream Filling, 2.2 oz	270	12	38
Chocolate Meringue, ⅙ pie	320	13	48
Churros, 1 stick, 1½ oz	125	5	18
Cinnamon Crumb Cake, 2½ oz	260	9	40
Cinnamon Roll, 3.7 oz	430	21	55
Coffee Cake, 2 oz	180	6	30
Concha: Small, 2.1 oz	240	9	33
Large (5" diameter), 5½ oz	615	23	85
Cream Cheese Crumb, 2 oz	200	9	25
Cream Puff (custard fill), 4.6 oz	335	20	30
Creme Horns, each, 3 oz	210	5	36
Croissants: *See Next Column*			
Cupcake: Plain, 1½ oz	160	7.5	23
w. Frosting	210	10	30
Danish Pastry: Small, 2½ oz	250	14	25
Large, 5 oz	500	28	50
Date Nut Roll, ½" slice, 1½ oz	180	8	27
Devil's Food, w. Frosting, 2.2 oz	210	12	38
Donut Holes, 1¼" balls, 2 oz (5)	260	15	30
Donuts: *See Page 115*			
Eclair, Choc., Cust. fill, 3½ oz	260	16	24
Fried Twinkie (1)	420	34	45
Fig Bars, average, each	160	3	31
Fruit Cake, Dark/Light, 1½ oz	140	4	26
Fudge Nut Brownie, each, 3½ oz	380	18	54
Funnel Cake (1), 9", 3 oz	380	22	40
Gingerbread: From mix, 3" sq.	210	4	41
Honey Bun, each, 2.7 oz	310	15	39
Jelly Roll, 1/12 roll, 1.8 oz	150	2	32
Key Lime Pie, 4.3 oz	400	25	41
Kolacky, Apricot/Rasp., ½ oz (1)	60	3.5	8
Lady Fingers, 3 oz	310	4.5	59
Lemon Cake, 4 oz piece	440	24	49

Ready-to-Eat (Cont)

Ready-to-Eat (Cont)	C	F	Cb
Lemon Poppy Seed Creme, 1.6 oz	180	9	23
Marble Cake, 1 slice, 4 oz	430	23	50
Mississippi Mud Pie, 4 oz	480	22	67
Mud Cake, 1 piece, 4½ oz	380	20	44
Muffins: *See Next Page*			
Orange Creme (Ring), 3 oz	310	16	39
Pineapple Upside Down, 2½ oz	230	9	36
Peach Melba, 3½ oz	300	8	52
Strawberry Creme, 4.7 oz	400	27	33
Strudel Bites, ¾ oz	60	2.5	9
Pecan Twirls, 1 piece, 1.3 oz	170	7	26
Pecan Pie, 4.3 oz	520	24	70
Pies & Tarts: *See Page 116*			
Pound Cake, 4 oz	440	24	49
Raspberry Rugulah, 1 pce, 1.2 oz	110	9	7
Scones: Blueberry, 2 oz	190	8	29
Choc Scones, 2 oz	210	10	31
Raisin Scones, 2 oz	210	9	31
Sponge: Plain, 2½ oz	220	10	33
w. Cream & Strawberry	390	12	69
w. Chocolate Icing	290	12	45
Raisin Bun, 1 bun, 2 oz	230	11	32
Raspberry Rugulah, 1 piece, 34g	110	9	7
Strudel, fruit, average, 4.4 oz	300	17	32
Sweet Roll, average, 1½ oz	150	6	23
Swiss Rolls, (2)	270	12	38
Tarts: *See Page 116*			
Tiramisu, 4.4 oz	440	22	34
Toaster Strudel, 2 oz	190	10	26
Turnovers, fruit, average, 3 oz	290	15	35

Croissants

Croissants	C	F	Cb
Average All Brands			
Plain/Butter/Cheese: Mini, 1 oz	115	6	13
Small, 1½ oz	170	9	19
Medium, 2 oz	230	12	26
Large, 2½ oz	290	15	32
Extra Large, 3 oz	330	19	37
Sweet Croissants: *(aprox. 3oz)*			
Almond Filled	330	18	39
Chocolate Filled	360	19	43
Au Bon Pain: *See Page 187*			
Burger King: *Croissan'wich, See Page 194*			
Dunkin' Donuts: Plain Croissant	330	18	37
Sara Lee: All Butter, 1½ oz	170	8	20
All Butter Petite, 0.8 oz	115	5.5	13
Starbucks: *See Page 255*			
Croissants Sandwiches: *See Page 173*			

Muffins, Sweet Rolls

Quick Guide C F Cb

Muffins: Ready-To-Eat
Average All Types:

	C	F	Cb
Small, 1 oz	80	3	12
Medium, 2 oz	160	6	24
Large, 3 oz	240	9	36
Extra Large, 4 oz	320	12	48
Giant, 6 oz	480	18	60
Super Size, 8 oz	640	24	96
English Muffin, 2 oz	150	2	29

Brands ~ Ready-To-Eat

	C	F	Cb
Awreys: Blueberry, 2.25 oz	240	12	31
Raisin Bran, 1.5 oz muffin	160	8	21
Controlled Carb Gourmet			
Almond Muffins, 3 oz	210	15	28
Entenmann's: Golden, 2.4 oz	240	12	29
Little Bites, Blueberry, 1 pouch	190	9	27
Henry's Market: Muffins, avg. (1)	460	23	57
Mini Muffins, avg. (1)	80	4	10
Hostess: Mini, 1 pouch, avg.	250	14	27
Fruit Pie/Tart, avg., 4.5 oz	475	20	68
Hearty Muffin: Blueberry, 6 oz	690	42	72
Banana Nut, 6 oz	750	48	72
Muffin Loaf: Blueberry, 3.8 oz	420	19	58
Banana Nut, 3.8 oz	460	24	56
My Favorite Muffin: Plain, 6 oz	660	30	75
Chocolate Chip, 6 oz	635	33	81
Fat Free, avg., 6 oz	325	0	78
Otis Spunkmeyer: *Per Whole Muffin (4 oz)*			
Banana Nut, 4 oz	460	22	58
Cheese Strudel	420	18	62
Wild Blueberry	420	22	52
Our Daily Muffin: Each, 3 oz	140	0.5	31
Ralphs: Banana, 5 oz muffin	730	45	68
Bran & Walnut, 5 oz	590	31	69
Fat Free, 1.65 oz	120	0	27
Sugar Free, avg., 0.8 oz	80	5	10
Starbucks: *See Fast-Foods Section*			
Trader Joe's: Banana, 4 oz	280	12	39
Chocolate Chip, 4 oz	430	17	65
Mini: Blueberry, 0.8 oz	110	6	12
Bran w. Raisin, 0.8 oz	80	3	13
Uncle Wally's: Rich & Moist, 4 oz	390	19	51
All Natural; Gourmet, 4 oz	280	4	28
Fat Free Gourmet, 4 oz	240	0	56
Sugar Free Gourmet, 4 oz	120	2.5	28
Weight Watchers: Blueb., 2.5 oz	180	3	38
Double Chocolate, 2.5 oz	190	4	35
Zen Bakery: Bran Muffin (1)	110	2.5	19
Oat Bran (1)	135	3	23
Blue Raspb. Oat Bran (1) 4.8 oz	270	6	46
Fast-Food Restaurants: *See Page 183*			

Muffin Mixes C F Cb

Prepared: Per Muffin

	C	F	Cb
Archer Farms: Wild Blueberry (1)	230	8	40
Lemon Blueberry (1)	230	8	38
Betty Crocker: Apple Streusel (1)	200	6	34
Blueberry (1)	190	7	27
Choc Chip; Cinnamon Streusel (1)	220	8	30
Water Muffins: Choc Chip (1)	160	5	26
Blueb.; Lemon Poppyseed, avg.	130	3.5	24
Cornbread (1)	180	6	24
Hodgson Mill: Wheat Blueberry (1)	145	1	32
Krusteaz: Fat Free, avg. (1)	140	0	32
Banana Nut; Wildberry (1)	200	10	32
Honey Cornbread (1)	120	3.5	20
Other varieties, avg. (1)	180	4.5	32
Pillsbury: Hot Roll Mix, 1 roll	130	3	21
Just Add Milk Blueb. Muffin (1)	170	5	30
Ultimate: Blueberry Streusel (1)	190	12	35
Choc Fudge Choc Chip (1)	270	13	34
Sunmaid: Honey Raisin Bran (1)	280	9	47
Trader Joe's: Pumpkin Muffin (1)	250	11	35

Sweet Rolls & Buns

Note: Weigh for actual weight as can be 10-50% higher than label weight.

	C	F	Cb
Bon Appetite: Cinn. Roll, 5 oz	580	34	64
Mammoth Cinnamon Roll, 5 oz	560	28	70
Cinnabon: Classic	815	32	117
Caramel Pecanbon, 1 roll	1100	56	141
Minibon, 1 roll	340	13	49
CinnaPretzel	755	6	156
Cinnabon Stix (5) no frosting	380	21	41
Cloverhill Bakery			
Jumbo Honey Bun, 4.75 oz	540	26	70
Entenmann's: Cinn. Roll (½) 2 oz	220	8	34
Hostess: Honey Bun, Glazed, 2.7 oz	310	15	39
Actual weight up to 3.9 oz	440	22	55
Iced/Frosted, 3.5 oz	395	5.5	50
Cinnamon Sweet Roll (1)	205	5.5	35
Little Debbie: Pecan Spinwheels, 1 oz	110	4	16
Honey Buns, 1.76 oz	220	12	26
McDonald's: Cinnamon Bun, 3.7 oz	420	18	57
Deluxe Cinnamon Bun, 5.7 oz	590	24	86
Pillsbury: Cinnamon Roll, 1.5 oz	150	5	23
Sugar Free (1) 1.5 oz	110	3.5	22
Ralph's: Cinnamon Roll, 2.5 oz	290	11	44
Trader Joe's: Cinn. Roll, 2.35 oz	250	7	44
Frosted Cinnamon Bun, 4 oz	400	9	66
Van de Kamp's: Cinn. Roll, 1.1 oz	130	7	16
Zen Bakery: Cinn. Raisin Roll, ½	100	1	21

Quick Guide	**C**	**F**	**Cb**
Donuts			
Average All Brands			
Plain, 1¾ oz	210	12	25
Sugared, 1¾ oz	220	11	27
Glazed, 2 oz	250	12	34
Chocolate Iced, 2 oz	260	14	29

Brands	**C**	**F**	**Cb**
Albertson's			
Donut Holes: Assorted	150	8	18
Powdered Sugar (4) 1.7 oz	180	7	26
Gem Donuts: Plain Cake (3) 1.6 oz	190	12	20
Chocolate (3)	260	16	25
Sticky Donuts, 2.2 oz	230	10	32
Bon Appetite			
Cherry Donuts (1) 2 oz	260	15	30
Mini Donuts: Chocolate (4)	270	16	29
Powdered; Crumb, avg. (4)	240	12	32
Cloverfield			
Donut Holes (4)	260	15	30
Dolly Madison			
Regular, 1¾ oz	270	12	40
Gem varieties, ½ oz each	65	3	8
Powdered Mini, ½ oz each	60	3	8
Dunkin' Donuts			
Apple N' Spice Donut	200	8	29
Blueberry Cake Donut	290	16	35
Boston Kreme Donut	240	9	36
Chocolate Frosted Cake Donut	360	20	40
Chocolate Glazed Cake Donut	290	16	33
Cinnamon Cake Donut	330	20	34
Glazed Cake Donut	350	19	41
Jelly Filled Donut	210	8	32
Kreme Filled (Choc./Vanilla)Donut	270	13	35
Old Fashioned Cake Donut	300	19	28
Powdered Cake Donut	330	19	36
Sugar Raised Donut	170	8	22
Entenmann's			
Dark Choc. Frosted, 2 oz	280	19	28
Frosted Devil's Food, 2.3 oz	320	19	35
Glazed Buttermilk, 2¼ oz	270	14	34
Milk Chocolate Frosted, 2.4 oz	310	19	35
Powdered, 1¾ oz	230	14	25
PopEms (bite size): *Per 4 pieces*			
Glazed (4) 2 oz	240	12	31
Glazed Devil's Food (4) 2 oz	240	11	33
Popettes (bite size), 3 pces, 1.8 oz	240	15	24

Brands (Cont)	**C**	**F**	**Cb**
Hostess			
Cinnamon Sweet Rolls, 4.2 oz	410	11	69
Dunkin Stix (3)	490	25	63
Donut Bites, 1 pouch, 2.3 oz	300	15	38
Regular: Plain, 1.4 oz	160	9	18
Chocolate Frosted, 2 oz	230	13	26
Powdered, 1.7 oz	190	9	25
Old Fashioned Glazed, 2.1 oz	240	11	33
Donettes: Frosted (3) 1.76 oz	220	13	23
Crumb (4) 2 oz	220	9	32
Powdered (4) 2.1 oz	240	12	31
Jewel: Cinnamon Spiced, 2 oz	230	15	24
Krispy Kreme			
Chocolate Glazed Cruller	290	15	37
Chocolate Iced Glazed	250	12	33
Chocolate Iced Kreme Filled	350	20	38
Chocolate Iced w. Sprinkles	260	12	38
Cinnamon Twist	230	9	33
Glazed Cruller	240	14	26
Glazed Kreme Filled	340	20	38
Maple Iced Glazed	240	12	32
New York Cheesecake	320	19	35
Original Glazed	200	12	22
Powdered Cake	280	14	37
Traditional Cake Doughnut	230	13	25
Doughnut Holes, Glazed (5)	200	11	24
Little Debbie			
Donut Sticks, 1.65 oz pkg	230	14	25
Mini Donuts, Frosted (4)	230	13	27
Tastykake			
Cinnamon, 1.8 oz	220	13	25
Mini: Frosted Rich (6)	380	22	42
Cinnamon (4) 1.8 oz	210	10	28
Powdered Sugar (6) 2½ oz	280	13	37
Van De Kamp's			
Plain (1) 1.25 oz	150	9	17
Chocolate (1) 1.4 oz	170	9	22
Powdered (1) 1.5 oz	160	8	22
Crumb (1) 1.6 oz	180	7	26
Old Fashioned Glazed: 2.3 oz	270	12	39
Chocolate, 2.3 oz	300	15	36
Glazed Choc. Donut Holes (4)	250	11	37
Mini Donuts: Powdered (3)	210	11	26
Chocolate (3)	250	15	27
Crumb (3)	200	8	28
Zingers			
Devil's/Vanilla Food, avg. (1)	155	5	26

Pies & Tarts

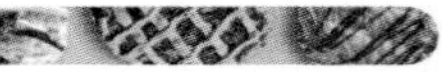

Quick Guide

Pies: *Average All Brands (9")*	C	F	Cb
Apple; Blueberry; Cherry:			
Small, ⅛ pie, 4½ oz	295	14	43
Medium ⅕ pie, 7½ oz	500	23	71
Large, ¼ pie, 9½ oz	640	30	92
Extra Large, ⅓ pie, 12 oz	805	37	116
Whole Pie (9"), 38 oz	2555	119	366
Other Pies: *Per Small Serving (⅙ of 8" Pie)*			
Chocolate Cream Pie	345	22	38
Custard; Coconut Custard	270	14	31
Lemon Chiffon Pie	360	14	50
Lemon Meringue	305	10	53
Pecan Pie	450	21	65
Pumpkin Pie	230	10	30
Strawberry Pie	230	9	37

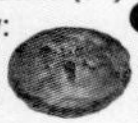

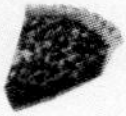

Brands ~ *Per Serving*

	C	F	Cb
Denny's: Apple Pie, 7 oz	470	21	68
Chocolate Peanut Butter, 6 oz	655	39	64
Hostess: Fruit; Cherry, 4.5 oz pie	480	20	68
Lemon, 4.5 oz pie	490	22	69
Long John Silver's: Pecan Pie	370	15	23
Chocolate Cream Pie	310	22	34
Pineapple Cream Pie	290	13	39
Marie Callender's			
Cobbler, avg., ¼ pkg, 4 oz	290	15	36
Mrs Smith's: Peach Cobbler, ⅛ pie	230	10	34
Silk Pies, avg., ⅑ pie	565	40	50
Slices: Apple; Peach, 1 pce	265	13	35
Dutch Apple, 1 piece	240	10	37
Sara Lee			
Pies: French Silk Pie, 1 slice, 4.8 oz	340	21	34
Tangy Lemon Meringue Pie	220	5	41
Tropical Coconut Cream Pie	330	19	37
Cobbler Anytime Pie: Peach, 4 oz	340	17	43
Apple; Blackberry, avg., 4 oz	350	17	48
Oven Fresh Pies (9", 37 oz Box): *Per Slice (4.6 oz)*			
Apple Pie, ⅛	340	16	46
Cherry Pie, ⅛	320	14	44
Mince Pie; Blueberry Pie, ⅛, avg.	370	15	55
Pumpkin Pie, ⅛	260	11	37
Raspberry Pie, ⅛	360	16	50
Southern Sweet Potato Pie, ⅛	280	10	45
Tastykake: Fruit, average	300	11	47
French Apple	320	12	52
Coconut Creme	370	20	42
Lemon Pie	300	14	44
Van de Kamp's			
Pies: Apple; Cherry, avg., ⅙ pie	360	23	36
Pumpkin Pie, ⅙ pie	340	14	48
Pecan; Sweet Potato, ⅙ avg.	390	16	58

Pastry & Pie Crusts

	C	F	Cb
Pie Crust: Baked, 9" diameter shell			
1 Pie Shell, 6½ oz	665	44	60
2-crust Pie, 9", 11¼ oz	1660	109	150
Piecrust Sticks, 8 oz	1180	78	106
Filo Pastry: 4 sheets, 2½ oz	210	2.5	40
Athens: 5 sheets, 2 oz	180	1	37
Mini Dough Shells, 2, 8g	35	2	2
Pepp. Farm, 2 sheets, 1½ oz	120	1	25
Puff *(Pepp.Farm)*, ½ sheet, 4.5 oz	510	33	42
⅙ sheet, 1½ oz	170	11	14
Bake & Fill Shell, 1.7 oz	190	13	16
Pizza Crust, ⅛ whole	80	1	17
Arrowhead Mills, Pie Crust, ⅛, avg.	110	6	14
Bisquick: Baking Mix,			
Original, ⅓ cup, 1½ oz	150	6	26
Heart Smart, ⅓ cup, 1½ oz	140	2.5	27
Betty Crocker, 9", ⅛ shell	110	7	9
Boboli: Thin Pizza Crust, ⅕, 2 oz	170	3.5	28
Original Pizza Crust, ⅛, 1.76 oz	140	2.5	24
8" Mini Pizza Crust, ½	200	5	32
Hershey's *(Keebler)*, Choc Crust, ⅛	100	4.5	14
Keebler: Graham Cracker, ⅛ of 9"	110	5	14
Reduced Fat, ⅛	100	3.5	15
Shortbread Crust, ⅛	100	5	14
Graham Crackers Minis (1)	110	5	15
2 Extra Servings, ⅒ pie	130	6	18
Marie Callendars Deep Dish Pie Shell,			
⅛ pie, 1 oz	140	10	11
Mrs Smith's Deep Dish, 9" (⅛)	130	7	14
Nabisco Oreo, ⅙ of 9" crust	130	7	19
Honey Maid Graham, ⅙, 1 oz	150	8	18
Nilla Pie Crust, ⅙, 1 oz	150	8	18
Orr Brothers, Glaze for Fruit Pie, 3 oz	110	0	27
Pet-Ritz, all types, ⅛, ¾ oz	90	5	11
Pillsbury (All Ready), ⅛ pie, 1 oz	120	8	13
Trader Joe's, Pie Crust, ⅛ pie	190	13	17

Pie Filling (Canned)

Average All Brands	C	F	Cb
Apple: ½ cup, 4¼ oz	125	0	33
21 oz Can	600	0.5	160
Apricot, 2 Tbsp	70	0	17
Blackberry, Cherry, 4 oz	120	0	28
Chocolate, Coconut, 4 oz	140	3	33
Lemon, ½ cup, 4 oz	150	2	33
Mincemeat, 4 oz	190	1	45
Peach, Strawb., Blueberry, ⅓ c., 4 oz	100	0	23
Pumpkin, 4 oz	40	0.5	9
Raisin, 4 oz	130	0	30
Raspberry, Black/Red, ⅓ cup	100	0	25

Cakes, & Pastries – Packaged

Cakes & Pastries

	C	F	Cb
Albertson's Bakery			
Butter Ring Cake, ⅛, 3 oz	310	16	39
Sock it to me Ring Cake, ⅛, 3 oz	290	12	42
Angel Food Bar Cake, ⅕	170	0	38
Cake Slices: *Per Slice (1½ oz)*			
Cinnamon Butter Streusel Creme	190	9	24
Butter Creme Cake	160	5	24
Lemon Creme Cake	180	9	23
Blueberry Creme Cake	170	8	22
Banquet: Cream Pies, avg., ⅓ pie	350	21	39
Bimbo			
Concha, avg., 2.1 oz	240	9	33
Homestyle Pound Cake, 2.6 oz	300	15	37
Pecan Pound Cake, 2.9 oz	330	16	41
Raisin Pound Cake, 2.9 oz	340	16	43
Buon Appetite			
Sliced Cheesecake, 4 oz	440	24	49
Sliced Marble Cake, 4 oz	430	23	50
Sliced Lemon Cake, 4 oz	440	24	49
Sliced Pound Cake, 4 oz	440	24	49
Walnut Brownie, 3.5 oz	380	18	54
Sliced Pound Cake	520	4	49
Cheese Coffee Cake, 2.2 oz	270	15	31
Banana Bread	450	25	49
Claim Jumper: Carrot Cake, 4.6 oz	450	24	54
Choc. Motherload Cake, 5.3 oz	520	27	73
Cheesecake Factory: *See Fast-Foods Section*			
Dolly Madison: Honey Bun, 3.75 oz	440	25	49
Cinnamon Sweet Rolls (1)	210	7	34
Dunkin' Stix, 1 stix	170	9	20
Entenmann's			
All Butter Loaf, ⅙ loaf, 2 oz	220	10	31
Cheese-Filled Crumb Coffee, 2 oz	200	9	25
Chocolate Fudge, ⅙ cake, 3 oz	260	13	39
Coffee Cake: Cheese Topped, ⅑, 2 oz	200	9	26
Bavarian Creme Coffee, ⅛, 2 oz	190	7	30
Gourmet Cinn. Rolls, ½ roll	220	8	34
Louisiana Crunch, ⅑, 3 oz	330	15	47
Pecan Danish Ring, ⅛	250	15	26
Raspberry Danish Twist, ⅛	220	11	28
Muffins/Rolls: *See Page 114*			
Hostess: *Per Cake Unless Indicated*			
Blueberry Danish, 5 oz	490	18	80
Cheese Danish, 5 oz	490	20	74
Cinnamon Streudel Cake (1)	170	6	29
Chocodiles	230	11	36
Cup Cake (1), 1.76 oz	180	6	31

Hostess (Cont)	C	F	Cb
Danish Rollers, 2 rolls, 1.9 oz	200	8	30
Ding Dongs	175	9	24
Fudge Brownie, 3oz	330	12	54
Ho Ho's, each	125	6	17
Pound Cake, 3.2 oz	120	13	45
Raspberry Zinger (1)	160	6	26
Snoballs	170	5	32
Suzy Q , 2 cakes, 4 oz	440	17	70
Twinkies, 1 cake, 1.5 oz	150	4.5	27
Vanilla & Chocolate Zinger (1)	160	5	26
Little Debbie			
Angel Food Cake (1) 1.4 oz	120	0.5	27
Banana Marshmallow Pie (1) 1½ oz	180	6	30
Banana Twins, 2 cakes, 2.2 oz	250	10	38
Boston Crème Rolls (1), 2.2 oz	270	12	40
Brownies (1)	290	13	40
Choc Chip Crème Pie, 1.2 oz	150	6	23
Choc Chip Snack Cake (2), 2.4 oz	300	14	42
Creme-filled Strawb. Cup Cake (1)	210	10	29
Devil Cremes (1) 1.65 oz	200	9	29
Devil Squares, 2 cakes, 2.2 oz	270	12	38
Double Chocolate Rolls, 2 cakes	280	12	41
Fancy Cakes (2)	310	15	43
Frosted Fudge , 1.5 oz cake	190	9	6
Fudge Rounds Cookie (1) 2½ oz	310	12	48
German Chocolate Cookie (1) 1.1 oz	140	7	18
Golden Cremes Cake (1)	150	9	28
Honey Buns, 1.75 oz bun	220	12	26
Marshmallow Pie (1)	180	6	30
Marshmallow Supreme (1)	140	5	22
Oatmeal Creme Pie (1)	170	7	26
Orange Cup Cake (1)	210	10	29
Pecan Spinwheels, 1 roll	100	4	16
Strawberry Shortcake Rolls, 2.1 oz	240	9	39
Swiss Cake Rolls, 2 cakes	270	12	38
Zebra Cakes, 2 cakes, 2.6 oz	330	16	47
Mrs Smith's			
Carrot Cake, ⅙, 2.9 oz	300	16	37
Cinnabon Cinn. Pecan Coffee Cake, ⅙	270	17	25
Nemo's			
Banana Cake, 3 oz	300	12	45
Chocolate Cake, 3 oz	290	12	44
Carrot Cake, 3.6 oz	380	20	46
Red Velvet Cake, 3 oz	290	14	47
Zucchini Cake, 3.6 oz	400	21	47

Cakes & Pastries (Cont)

Pepperidge Farm	C	F	Cb
Turnovers (Frozen): Apple, 3.2 oz	290	15	36
Raspberry, 3.2 oz	290	15	35
3-Layer Cakes: Coconut, ⅛, 2.5 oz	250	11	35
Chocolate Fudge, ⅛ cake, 2.5 oz	250	11	31
Golden, ⅛ cake, 2.5 oz	260	13	34
Fruit Squares: Apple/Blueb./Cherry	210	10	27
Rich's: Mini Eclairs (7)	335	21	32
Mini Creme Puffs (6)	290	24	15

Safeway Select
	C	F	Cb
Molton Chocolate Lava Cake, 4½ oz	440	26	50

Sara Lee (Frozen)
Cheesecake: *Per Slice*	C	F	Cb
Chocolate French, ⅕ cake	430	22	52
Choc. Swirl New York Style, ⅙	470	29	45
French Classic, ⅕ cake	410	25	41
French Strawberry, ⅙ cake	320	14	43
New York Style, ⅙ cake	350	21	35
Original Cream Cherry, ¼ cake	350	12	55
Original Cream Classic, ¼ cake	340	18	38
Original Cream Strawberry, ¼ cake	330	12	49
Cakes: *Per Slice*			
Coffee Butter Streusel, ⅙ cake	190	9	25
Coffee Crumb, ⅛ cake	190	8	30
Coffee Deluxe Cinnamon Rolls			
w. Icing (1)	320	15	41
Coffee Pecan, ⅙ cake	140	13	23
Layer Cakes: *Per ⅛ Whole*			
Layer Coconut, ⅛ cake, 2.8 oz	260	14	33
Layer Double Chocolate, ⅛ cake	260	13	33
Layer Fudge Golden, ⅛ cake	260	13	34
Layer Vanilla, ⅛ cake, 2½ oz	260	14	32
Pound Cakes: *Per ¼ Whole*			
All Butter, 2.6 oz	220	15	34
Free & Light, ¼ cake	200	4	39
Strawberry Swirl, ¼ cake	290	11	44
Bites: *Per Serving*			
Choc. Dipped Orig. Cheesecake (5)	100	7	8
Choc. Dipped Praline Pecan (5)	90	6	8
Triple Choc. Fudge Brownie (1)	90	4	12

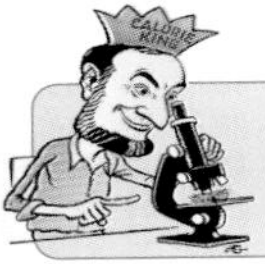

Smart Ones (Weight Watchers)	C	F	Cb
Brownie à la Mode	190	4	33
Carrot Cake (1) 1 oz	80	2.5	16
Chocolate Cake (1) 1 oz	80	3	15
Chocolate Mousse	180	4	28
Chocolate Eclair	140	4	24
Choc. Chip Cookie Dough Sundae	170	3	32
Double Fudge Brownie Parfait	220	3	44
Double Fudge Cake	220	7	35
Key Lime Pie, 3.3 oz	190	4.5	33
Lemon Cake (1) 1 oz	80	2.5	14
Mississippi Mud Pie	160	4	27
New York Style Cheesecake	150	5	21
Tastykake: Chocolate Jnr, 3.3 oz	340	12	55
Creme Filled Koffee Kakes, 3 oz	390	19	51
Koffee Kake Junior, 2.53 oz	280	10	44

Trader Joe's
Bakery: Apricot Tea Loaf 2 oz	C	F	Cb
	160	2	34
Choc Bundt Cake, ½₂ cake	340	21	34
Mini Bundt Cake (1)	190	4	35
Marble Tea Loaf, ⅛, 2 oz	160	2.5	31
Plum Coffee Cake, ⅛, 2 oz	180	6	30
Mini Carrot Cake, 5 oz	400	16	58
Cupcakes: Chocolate, 3.2 oz	430	23	54
Vanilla, 3 oz	400	20	52
Frozen Dessert: Carrot Cake, ⅙, 3 oz	330	17	41
Apple Struesel, ⅓, 4.4 oz	300	17	32
Charlotte Berry Torte, ⅛, 2.8 oz	170	7	22
Chocolate Bahka, 1 roll, 2 oz	170	5	27
Choc Ganache Torte, ⅙, 3½ oz	300	17	34
Choc Lava Cake, 1 mini cake, 3.8 oz	360	23	40
Choc. Peanut Toffee Cake, ¼, 3½ oz	440	29	36
Low-Fat Cranb. Orange Brd, 2 oz	160	2	33
Mango Passion Exotique, ⅙, 1.9 oz	150	8	18
N.Y Deli Cheesecake, ⅙, 5 oz	510	33	46
Old Fashioned Chsecake, ½₂, 4.6 oz	470	29	40
Tiramisu, ⅛, 2.2 oz	220	11	17
Tiramisu Torte, ⅛, 3.2 oz	290	17	33

Van de Kamp's
	C	F	Cb
Angle Food Ring, ⅛ cake	130	0	29
Banana Square Cake, ¼ cake	410	18	60
Bear Claw, 1 pce, 2 oz	250	14	26
Carrot Square Cake, ¼ cake	520	33	54
Cinn. Raisin Danish, 1 pce, 2 oz	230	11	32
Crumb Cake, ⅛ cake, 2.5 oz	330	18	39
Fruit Danish, 1 pce, 2 oz	220	11	28
German Chocolate Cake, ¼ cake	290	16	36

For Extra Listings and Nutritional Data
~ See Author's Website
www.CalorieKing.com

Cakes, Cookies & Dessert Mixes

Made As Directed	C	F	Cb
Arrowhead Mills: *Per Serving (Prep'd)*			
Choc Chip	90	2	16
Cookie (1), avg. all types	90	2	16
Oatmeal Raisin	90	2	16
Wheat Free Brownie, ¹⁄₂₀ pkg	160	7.5	21
Aunt Jemima			
Coffee Cake, ⅛ cake, prep.	180	6	28
Banquet			
Dessert Bakes: *Per Serving (Prep'd)*			
Apple Crisp, ⅙ pkg	220	4	44
Choc. Cherry Decadence, ⅙ pkg	310	5	62
Chocolate Lava Cake, ½ pkg	370	7	73
Cherry Cobbler, ⅙ pkg	250	4	53
Peach Cobbler, ⅙ pkg	240	3.5	51
Betty Crocker			
Cakes (Super Moist): *Per ½ Cake (Prep'd)*			
Butter Recipe Yellow	250	11	35
Chocolate varieties	270	14	33
Cinnamon Swirl	280	11	42
Devil's Food	270	14	33
White	230	10	33
Other flavors, average	270	13	35
Per ⅒ Cake (Prepared): Carrot	350	16	41
Sour Cream	280	12	43
If using No Cholesterol Recipe, deduct 40 cals and 4g fat.			
Other Cakes: Pound Cake, ⅛	260	8	45
Angel Food Cake, ¹⁄₁₂ mix	140	0	32
Gingerbread Cake, ⅛	220	5	39
Pineapple Upside Down, ⅙	390	13	65
Sunkist Lemon Bar (1)	140	4	24
Brownie Mixes: *Per ¹⁄₂₀ Pkg (Prep'd)*			
Chocolate Chunk varieties	180	9	25
Dark Chocolate	170	7	24
Fudge	170	7	22
Low-Fat Fudge Brownie, ¹⁄₁₈	140	2.5	28
Original Supreme	160	5	27
Peanut Butter; Walnut, avg.	180	9	23
Turtle (Caramel & Pecan)	170	9	23
Cookie Mix: *Per 2 Cookies (Prep'd)*			
Rainbow Chocolate Candy	160	7	22
Other varieties, average	170	9	21
Complete Desserts: *Per ⅙ Pkg*			
Apple Crisp	270	6	53
Hot Fudge Cake	440	13	78
Peach Cobbler	290	7	55

Betty Crocker (Cont)	C	F	Cb
Dessert Bars: Almond Joy, ¹⁄₁₂ pkg	200	12	21
Health Toffee Bits, ¹⁄₁₂ pkg	190	9	27
Reeses, ¹⁄₁₅ pkg	180	10	20
Sunkist Lemon, ¹⁄₁₆ pkg	140	4	24
Warm Delights: *Per Bowl*			
Cinnamon Swirl Cake	400	12	70
Fudgy Choc. Chip Cookie	340	11	58
Other varieties, average	365	11	63
Carb Monitor: *Per Serving (Prep'd)*			
Brownie: Choc Chunk, ¹⁄₁₆ pkg	150	9	20
Walnut (1), ¹⁄₁₆ pkg	160	11	20
Cookie, 2 cookies, ¹⁄₁₄ pkg	130	7	18
Muffin (1), ¹⁄₁₂ pkg	160	9	27
Muffin Mix: *See Page 114*			
Dr Oetker: *Per Serving (Prep'd)*			
Chocolate Chip Cookie Mix, ¹⁄₁₂	170	7.5	24
Muffin Mix, ¹⁄₁₂ pkg, average	170	2	30
Simple Organic Cake Mix, ¹⁄₁₂	255	11	32
Duncan Hines			
Angel Food, ¹⁄₁₂ whole	140	0	30
Boston Creme Pie, ⁷⁄₁₂ pkg	420	19	59
Brownie Mix (low-fat recipe)			
¹⁄₁₈ pkg, avg. all types	170	7	25
Choc Molten Lava Cake, ¹⁄₁₂ pkg	310	15	43
Choc Silk Torte, ¹⁄₁₀ pkg	440	18	65
Cookies, all flavors, 1 cookie	65	3	8
Homestyle Cookies, avg. (2)	170	7	24
Hot Fudge Brownie Sundae, ⅑ pkg	350	14	54
Orange Dreamsicle, ¹⁄₁₂ pkg	410	18	57
Moist Deluxe Cake Mix:			
Average, ¹⁄₁₂ pkg, prepared	270	12	36
Lower Fat Recipe, ¹⁄₁₂ pkg, prep.	210	5	37
Ghirardelli: *Per Serving (Prepared)*			
Brownie, ¹⁄₁₆ pkg, avg.	180	8	26
Chocolate Chip Cookie (1)	280	13	38
Jell-O No Bake Cheesecakes: *Prep'd As Directed*			
Cherry/Strawberry, ⅑ pkg	290	10	48
Chips-Ahoy!, ⅙ pkg	360	17	48
Chocolate Silk Dessert, ⅙ pkg	290	14	37
Oreo, ⅙ pkg	370	17	51
Peanut Butter Cup, ⅛ pkg	360	21	41
Real, ⅙ pkg	350	16	48

Frostings ♦ Baking Ingredients

Cakes & Dessert Mixes (Cont)

Made As Directed	C	F	Cb
Krusteaz: Cinn. Crumb Cake, 1"	230	7	38
Lemon/Key Lime Bar, 2" bar	160	3.5	29
Bakery Style Cookie Mix: Per Cookie			
Chocolate Chip, 2½"	140	4.5	19
Fat-Free Fudge Brownie, 2"	120	0	28
Gingerbread, ⅛ cake	210	3.5	41
Snickerdoodle	130	5	20
No Pudge			
Fudge Brownie, 1/12 pkg, prep'd.	120	0	28
Pamela's			
Ultra Chocolate Brownie, 1/16 pkg	170	8	23
Oil Free, 1/16 pkg	110	1.5	24
Robin Hood			
Angel Food Cake, 1/10 cake	160	0	38

Cake Frostings

Betty Crocker	C	F	Cb
Drizzlers, 2½ Tbsp	220	13	26
Rich & Creamy, average, 2 Tbsp	140	7	19
Whipped, all flavors, 3 Tbsp	110	5	15
Easy Flow Icing, 1 tsp	25	1	4
Duncan Hines: Per 2 Tbsp (1.2 oz)			
Creamy Homestyle, avg all flavors	140	6	23
Whipped, avg., 3 Tbsp	160	9	20
Pillsbury: Per 2 Tbsp (approx. ½ Tub)			
Creamy Supreme: Choc Fudge	140	6	21
Classic White	140	5	22
Milk Choc	140	6	21
Vanilla; Vanilla Funfetti	150	6	25
Whipped Supreme, avg all flavors	100	5	14
Decorators, Choc., 1 Tbsp	70	2	11

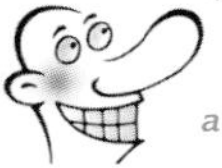

> *In eating, one third of the stomach should be filled with food, one third with drink, and the rest left empty.*
>
> ~ Gitten, the Talmud

Baking Ingredients

	C	F	Cb
Almond Paste:			
(Marzipan), 2 Tbsp	170	7	24
Baking Powder: Regular, 1 tsp	2	0	1
Cream of Tartar, 1 tsp	8	0	2
Baking Mix (Bisquick) :			
Original, ⅓ cup, 1½ oz	160	5	26
Heart Smart, ⅓ cup, 1½ oz	140	2.5	27
Butter/Margarine, ½ cup, 4 oz	810	91	1
Carob Flour, ½ cup	115	0.5	46
Chocolate Baking Bars: Average All Brands			
Unsweetened, 1 oz	140	14	8
Grated, 1 cup, 4½ oz	680	68	36
Semi-sweet, 1 oz	140	9	16
Bitter-sweet/White Baking 1 oz	160	8	20
Chocolate Baking Chips: Average All Brands			
Milk Choc./Semi Sweet 1 oz	160	9	18
¼ cup, 1½ oz	240	12	30
1 cup, 6 oz	960	48	120
Mini Kisses (Hershey), 1 pce	5	0.5	1
M&M's Minis, Nestle Morsels, 1 oz	140	8	18
Reeses Peanut Butter Chips, 1 T.	80	4	8
Cocoa Powder, Baking: Nestle, 1 T.	15	1	3
⅓ cup, 1 oz	80	4	12
Hershey's, 1 Tbsp	20	0.5	3
⅓ cup, 1 oz	115	3.5	21
Coconut, dried: Unsweet., 1 oz	190	18	7
Sweetened/flaked, 1 oz	130	8	15
½ cup, 1.3 oz	195	12	22
Toasted (Baker's), 1 oz	170	13	13
Coconut Cream/Milk: See Page 39			
Cornstarch, 1 Tbsp	30	0	7
Flour, white: 1 Tbsp, 0.6 oz	55	0	12
1 cup, 4.4 oz	455	1	95
Whole Wheat, 1 cup, 4.2 oz	410	2	87
Flavor Extracts: Average All Brands			
Imitation, 1 tsp	10	0	2
Pure Extract, 1 tsp	20	0	4
Almond, Vanilla, 1 tsp	10	0	0.5
Fruit Pectin: Swtnd, ¼ tsp	5	0	1
Unsweetened, ¼ tsp	0	0	0
Gelatin, dry, ¼ oz pkg	25	0	0
Lemon/Orange Peel, ¼ cup	25	0	6
Rennin, 1 pkg (11g)	10	0	2
Sprinkles, all types, 2 Tbsp	120	3	23
Sugar: See Page 123			
Vinegar, avg. all types, 1 oz	5	0	1
Whey, sweet, dry, 1 oz	100	0.5	21
Yeast: Active, dry, ¼ oz pkg	21	0	3
Bakers, compressed, 1 oz	30	0.5	5
Brewers; Torula, 1 oz	80	0.5	11
Fleischmann's, 0.6 oz pkg	0	0	0

Ready-To-Serve

Ready-To-Serve	C	F	Cb
Instant Pudding, Reg., ½ cup	170	4	30
Reduced Calorie: *Estee*	70	0	12
Jell-O, sugar-free, ½ cup	80	2	11
Royal, sugar-free, ½ cup	100	2	17
Dr McDougall's, Rice Pudd., 3 oz	310	1.5	69
Hunt's Snack Pack: *Per 3.5oz Cup*			
Puddin' Cakes: Choc Brownie	180	7	27
German Choc Cake	160	3.5	30
Puddin Pie: Lemon Meringue	130	2.5	20
Apple; Choc Mud	170	7	26
Dessert Favorites, avg. all flavors	140	5	22
Spoonibbles, 3½ oz cup	140	3.5	25
Jell-O			
Pudding Bites, average 1 pouch	90	1.5	18
Pudding & Pie Filling: *Per ¼ Pkg*			
Cook & Serve, average, prep.	100	0	22
Instant, regular, avg.	100	0	25
Fat & Sugar Free, avg.	30	0	8
Pudding Snacks: Fat-Free, 4 oz	100	0	23
Cheesecake Snack, 4 oz	150	4.5	25
Chocolate; Creme Savers, 4 oz	160	5	28
Smoothie Snacks, 4 oz	100	2.5	18
Jewel: Chef's Kitchen			
Rice Pudding, ½ cup, 4.5 oz	230	8	35
Tapioca Pudding, ½ cup, 4.5 oz	170	8	35
Kozy Shack			
Regular flavors, avg., ½ cup	130	3	22
No Sugar Added, avg., ½ cup	90	3	10
Flan: Creme Caramel, ½ cup	150	3.5	27
Mango Sauce, ½ cup	140	4	24
Restaurant Style, ½ cup	190	6	28
Rice Pudding: Original, ½ cup	130	3	22
Cinnamon Raisin, ½ cup	140	3	24
European Style, ½ cup	130	3.5	22
Tapioca, Old Fashioned, ½ cup	130	3	23
Kraft Handi Snacks: *Per Cup (3.5 oz)*			
"Doubles", avg. all flavors	100	1	22
Chocolate Pudding Fat-Free	90	0	21
Rice Pudding	140	6	19
Vanilla Pudding	90	1	20
Kroger: *Per Container*			
Peaches & Cream w. Natural Flav.	180	2.5	36
Whipped Varieties	145	2.5	27
Manischewitz: Choc., ½ cup	110	0.5	26
Passover Gold Noodle, ½ cup	140	2	28
President's Choice			
Key Lime Pie (36 oz), ⅛ pie, 4.5 oz	435	21	56
Mississippi Mud Pie (36 oz), ⅑, 4 oz	405	22	49

Ready-To-Serve (Cont)

Ready-To-Serve (Cont)	C	F	Cb
Swiss Miss Pudding Snacks			
Chocolate, Low-Fat, 4 oz	140	2	27
Chocolate Vanilla Swirl, 4 oz	150	4	26
Creamy Vanilla, 4 oz	140	4.5	23
Milk/Dark Chocolate, 4 oz	160	4	28
Old Fashioned Tapioca, 4 oz	140	3.5	24

Homemade Puddings

Homemade Puddings	C	F	Cb
Apple Tapioca, ½ cup	150	0	32
Bread Pudding, ½ cup	250	8	40
Blancmange, ½ cup	140	5	19
Chocolate, ½ cup	190	6	30
Corn Pudding, ½ cup	135	4	21
Crème Brûlée, ½ cup	400	35	16
Plum Pudding, 2 oz	170	3	32
Rice with Raisins, ½ cup	200	4	38
Sponge Pudding, 3½ oz	340	16	45
Tapioca Cream, ½ cup	110	4	15
Trifle, ½ cup	180	7	26

Custards

Custards	C	F	Cb
Custard Mix: Dry, ⅙ pkg	85	1	17
Prep. w. 2% milk, ½ cup	140	3.5	21
Jello Flan, w. 2% milk, ½ cup	140	2.5	20
Royal-Flan: Prep. w. 2% milk, ½ c.	130	2.5	18
Homemade Custard			
Baked: Plain, ½ cup, 4½ oz	150	7	16
w. skim milk, artif. sweetened	70	3	4
Boiled, ½ cup	165	7	18

Meringues

Meringues	C	F	Cb
Meringue Swirl, ½ oz	50	0	8
Meringue Shell, 1 oz shell	100	0	16

(Add extra calories/fat/carbohydrate for fillings)

Jell-O • Cups • Parfait

Jell-O • Cups • Parfait	C	F	Cb
Gelatin Mix: *Jell-O, Royal ~ Made Up*			
Regular, all flavors, ½ cup	80	0	18
Sugar Free/Low Calorie, ½ cup	8	0	0
Creme Gelatin/Parfait: *Per ½ Cup*			
Ida Mae, ½ cup	60	2	10
Winky: Strawberry (109g)	110	1.5	22
Rainbow (130g)	100	0	24
Reser's, Dessert Parfait (110g)	100	2	19
Mrs Crockett's Kitchen, Str. Parfait	160	4	26
Gel Snacks *(Jell-O):* Regular, 3.5 oz	70	0	17
Sugar Free, 3.2 oz	10	0	1
X-Treme Cups, 2.5 oz	100	0	24
X-Treme Sticks, 2.2 oz	60	0	16

Pancakes & Waffles

Quick Guide   C   F   Cb

Pancakes
Plain: *Average All Types*

	C	F	Cb
Small (3" diam.), ¾ oz	50	2	6
Medium (4" diam.), 1¼ oz	85	3.5	11
Large (5" diam.), 2½ oz	175	7.5	22

Add Extra for Syrups/Butter

	C	F	Cb
Pancake Syrup: Regular, 1 Tbsp	50	0	13
¼ cup, 4 Tbsp	210	0	52
Lite, 1 Tbsp	25	0	6
¼ cup, 4 Tbsp	100	0	26
Butter/Margarine: Regular, 1 T.	100	11	0
Whipped, 1 Tbsp	70	7.5	0

Waffles

	C	F	Cb
Homemade: 7" waffle, 2½ oz	245	13	26
From Mix: 7" waffle, 2½ oz	205	8	28

Frozen Breakfasts

Aunt Jemima

	C	F	Cb
Pancakes: Buttermilk (3)	200	3.5	37
Homestyle (3)	200	3.5	37
Low-Fat (3)	190	2.5	35
Whole Grain (3)	230	6	38
Mini Pancakes (11)	240	4	46
Frozen Breakfasts:			
French Toast, Cinnamon, 2 slices	220	6	34
French Toast, Homestyle, 2 slices	240	6	39
French Toast, Sticks, 5 sticks	330	11	54

Eggo *(Kellogg's)*

	C	F	Cb
French Toast: Toaster Swirlz, set of 4	120	3	20
French Toaster Sticks, avg., (2)	220	6	38
Stuffed French Toaster Sticks (2)	310	7	55
Pancakes: Buttermilk, 3 pancakes	280	9	44
Jungle, 3 pancakes	280	8	46
Nutri-Grain, 3 pancakes	240	7	40
Minis, 11 pancakes	260	8	42

Farm Rich

	C	F	Cb
French Toast Sticks, avg. (5)	300	14	40

Pillsbury

	C	F	Cb
Pancakes: Mini, average, (14)	425	7	88
Chocolate Chip (3)	270	5	50
French Toast Sticks (6)	360	7	69
Dunkables Cinn. Bites/Icing (3)	140	4.5	23
Toaster Strudel, avg. (1)	190	9	26

Krusteaz

	C	F	Cb
Pancakes: Mini (12)	220	2.5	43
Buttermilk (3)	280	4	52
French Toast: Average, 1 slice	115	2.5	18
Sticks, 4 sticks	230	5	41

Restaurant-Style: *See Fast-Foods Section*
Frozen Egg Breakfasts: *See Page 47*

Pancake Brands   C   F   Cb

Atkins:

	C	F	Cb
All-Purpose, 2 tsp. dry mix	30	0	5
Bake Mix, ¼ cup dry mix	80	0.5	8

Aunt Jemima

	C	F	Cb
Buckwheat, 4 x 4" pancakes	170	6	26
Buttermilk, 4 x 4" pancakes	180	6	25
Original Complete, 2 x 4" pancakes	160	1.5	32
Original, 4 x 4" pancakes	250	8	37
Whole Wheat Blend, 3 x 4" pancakes	200	6	29

Betty Crocker Pancake Mixes

	C	F	Cb
Complete Original/Buttermilk, 3	200	2.5	40
Bisquick (Shake 'N Pour), 3	200	3	38
CarbSense: 2 pancakes prep.	320	15	9

Hungry Jack Pancakes
Mixes: *Per ⅓ Cup (Prepared)*

	C	F	Cb
Buttermilk: Complete, 3 x 4"	150	1.5	31
Original, w. 2% Milk, Oil, Egg	250	8	37
w. Skim Milk, Oil, Egg Whites	180	1	37
Extra Lights: Complete (3)	150	2	30
Potato Pancakes, 2 Tbsp mix	70	0	15
Microwave (frozen): Pancakes (3)	270	4.5	51
Krusteaz: No Sugar, prepared,			
3 x 4" pancakes	180	5	23
Northern Pines: 3 x 4" pancakes	380	7	71

Frozen Waffles

Aunt Jemima:

	C	F	Cb
Buttermilk (2)	200	5	33
Homestyle (2); Blueberry (2)	190	5	32
Low-Fat (2)	160	2.5	30

Eggo *(Kelloggs):*

	C	F	Cb
Minis, avg. (3)	250	8	39
Original: Chocolate Chip (2)	210	7	32
Cinnamon Toast (3)	290	10	46
French Vanilla (2)	200	8	27
Other varieties, avg. (2)	190	6	30
Flip Flops, avg. (2)	190	6	29
Homestyle: Original (2)	180	6	27
Lego (2)	190	6	30
Nutri-Grain: Average (2)	170	4.5	27
Low-Fat (2)	140	2.5	28
Special K, 99% Fat-Free (3)	190	1	37
Waf-Fulls (1)	150	5	27
GO-LEAN (Kashi): Average (1)	90	1.5	16
Hungry Jack: Blueberry, 1 waffle	105	4	17
Buttermilk; Homestyle (1)	95	3	15
Nature's Path: Average (1)	120	4	18
Lifestream; Gorilla; Koala, avg.	110	3.5	19
Other varieties, avg. (1)	120	4	17
Pillsbury: Waffles, avg. (1)	90	2.5	15
Waffle Sticks (6) & syrup	340	7	64
Van's: Belgian Original (1)	85	2	15
97% Fat Free (1)	90	1	15
Mini Homestyle (8), avg.	120	4	20

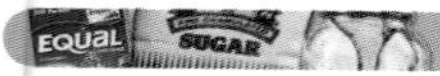

Sugar

	C	F	Cb
White Sugar, granulated:			
1 level teaspoon, 4g	15	0	4
1 heaping teaspoon, 6g	25	0	6.5
1 cube, ½"	24	0	6.5
Single portion, 1 packet	25	0	6.5
1 Tablespoon, 12g	48	0	12
1 ounce, 1 oz	110	0	20
1 cup, 7 oz	770	0	200
1 pound	1760	0	464
Brown Sugar: 1 Tbsp, 13g	50	0	13
1 ounce, 1 oz	109	0	28
1 cup, not packed, 5 oz	540	0	140
1 cup, packed, 7¾ oz	845	0	218
Powdered/Confectioners:			
Sifted, 1 cup, 3½ oz	385	0	98
Unsifted, 1 cup, 4¼ oz	460	0	117
Cinnamon Sugar, 1 tsp	15	0	4
Dextrose, 1¼ tsp	15	0	4
Fructose: Dry, 1 tsp	15	0	4
Liquid, 1 oz	80	0	21
Glucose, 1 oz	110	0	27
Glucose Tablets (1)	20	0	5
Palm Sugar, 3 Tbsp, 12g	45	0	11
Piloncillo (Brown Sugar), 3oz cone	325	0	81
Turbinado Sugar, 2 Tbsp, 1 oz	110	0	27
Unrefined Cane Sugar, 1 oz	110	0	27

Sugar Substitutes

	C	F	Cb
DiabetiSweet, 1 teaspoon	9	0	4
(Carbohydrate as Sugar Alcohol)			
Equal: Tablet/Liquid	0	0	0
Granulated, 1 pkg	4	0	1
Powdered, sachet, 0.04 oz	0	0	0.5
Sugar Lite, 1 tsp	8	0	2
NutraSweet Spoonful, 1 tsp	2	0	0.5
Nutra Taste; Sweet One, 1 pkt	0	0	0
PerfectSweet, 1 tsp	15	0.5	1
Shugr *(Swiss Diet),* 1 tsp	0	0	0
Sorbitol, 1 oz	110	0	27
Splenda: Powder, 1 cup	96	0	24
Sachet, sachet	0	0	0.5
Granular, 1 tsp	5	0	1
Sugar Blend, for Baking, ½ cup	385	0	96
Stevia, 1 pkt	0	0	0
Sugar Twin, 1 pkt	3	0	0
Sugar Substitute, 1 tsp	2	0	0
Sweet 'N Low, 1 pkt	0	0	1
Walgreens Wal-Sweet, 1 pkt	0	0	0
Weight Watchers; Whey Low, 1 tsp	4	0	1

Honey, Jam, Preserves

Average All Brands

	C	F	Cb
Honey: 1 tsp, ¼ oz	22	0	5.5
1 Tbsp, ¾ oz	65	0	17
1 ounce, 1 oz	86	0	23
1 cup, 12 oz	1030	0	269
Single Portion, ½ oz pkg	43	0	11
Jams/Jellies/Marmalade/Preserves:			
Regular, 1 tsp, ¼ oz	18	0	5
1 Tbsp, ¾ oz	65	0	16
1 ounce	90	0	22
Single Portion, ½ oz pkg	38	0	11
Apple/Fruit Butters, 1 T., 0.6 oz	20	0	6
Fruit Spreads: Regular, 1 tsp	16	0	4
Low Sugar, 1 tsp	8	0	2
Low Cal. *(Featherweight),* 1 tsp	8	0	2
Jelly: Regular, average, 1 tsp	18	0	4.5
Imitation, Low Calorie, 1 tsp	4	0	1

Syrups, Molasses

	C	F	Cb
Syrups: *Average All Brands*			
(Corn/Rice/Maple/Pancake/Sundae/Waffle)			
Includes Aunt Jemima, Cary's, Karo, Hershey's,			
Hungry Jack, Log Cabin, Mrs Butterworth's			
Regular/Dark/Light Color:			
1 Tbsp, ½ fl.oz	55	0	14
¼ cup (4 Tbsp)	220	0	55
Single Portion: 1½ oz pkg	170	0	42
Lite: 1 Tbsp	25	0	6
¼ cup (4 Tbsp)	100	0	25
Sugar-Free: *Cary's,* 2 Tbsp, 1 oz	18	0	5
Cozy Cottage, 2 Tbsp, 1 oz	10	0	3
Da Vinci, 2 Tbsp, 1 oz	5	0	1
Honey Cream Syrup, ¼ c., 2 oz	220	0	55
Molasses: Dark/Light: 1 T., ¾ oz	55	0	14
1 cup, 11½ oz	880	0	224
Blackstrap: 1 Tbsp, ¾ oz	47	0	13
1 cup, 11½ oz	750	0	208

Ice Cream Toppings

Average All Types & Brands
(Hershey's, Kraft, Smuckers)

	C	F	Cb
Butterscotch, Caramel, 2 Tbsp	140	1	30
Chocolate: Hot Fudge, 2 Tbsp	140	4	22
Fat Free Chocolate, 2 Tbsp	100	0	23
Pineapple, Strawberry, 2 Tbsp	110	0	28
Smuckers: Guilt-Free/Lite, 2 T.	100	0	24
Magic Shell, 2 Tbsp	210	15	18
Milky Way, 2 Tbsp	130	3.5	24

Candy, Chocolate

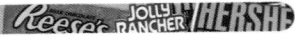

Quick Guide

Chocolate
Average All Brands

Milk Chocolate, regular:	C	F	Cb
Plain/Nuts/Fruit, average, 1 oz	150	10	13
1½ oz Bar	225	15	23
2 oz Bar	300	20	30
4 oz Block	600	40	60
8 oz Block	1200	80	120
1 Pound, 16 oz	2400	160	240
Dark/White Chocolate, 1 oz	150	10	16
Sugar Free *(Hershey's)* 1 pce, 0.3 oz	40	3	5
Chocolate-coated:			
Almonds, 5–6, 1 oz	160	11	14
Clusters, Nut, 3 pces, 1.2 oz	200	18	16
Coffee Beans, 1.4 oz	180	9	22
Creme/Cordial Centers, 1 oz	120	5	20
Fudge, 1 oz	125	4	20
Macadamias, 9 pces, 1.3 oz	220	15	18
Mints, 1 med., ½ oz	55	1	11
Nougat & Caramel, 1 oz	125	5	18
Peanuts, 12 med., 1 oz	145	9	14
Raisins, 28 med., 1 oz	110	4	19
Cooking Chocolate:			
Sweet/Semi-sweet, 1 oz	160	9	18
Chips, 1 Tbsp, ½ oz	70	4	9
Unsweetened, 1 oz	140	15	8
Dipping Choc *(Bakers)*, ½ oz, 1T.	80	5	9
Carob: Plain, 1 oz	150	9	16

Brands & Generic

Per Piece/Serving

	C	F	Cb
Abba Zaba, 2 oz bar	250	5	48
Absolutely Almond, 2.5 oz bar	380	23	40
Aero Bar *(Nestlé)*, 1.45 oz bar	210	13	26
After Dinner Mints, 1 small	25	1.5	3
After Eight Mint *(Nestlé)*, each	35	1	6
Air Head, 1 bar, 15.6g	60	0	15
Allen Wertz: Simply Sugar Free			
Coffee Time (decaf), 4	45	1.5	8
Coffee Toffee, 6	120	3	23
Other types, 4	120	2.5	24
Almond Joy: 1.6 oz bar	235	13	29
King Size, 4 pces, 3.1 oz	450	24	54
Snack, 17g bar	80	4.5	10
Swoops, 1 cup, 1.26 oz	200	12	21
Almond Roca: 3 pces	220	15	17
Sugar Free, 3 pces	150	15	16
Almonds, sugar-coated (15), 40g	175	4	29
Almond Clusters *(Trader Joe's)*, 2 pce, 1.2 oz	210	14	5

Brands & Generic (Cont)

Per Piece/Serving

	C	F	Cb
Altoids *(C & B)*, 10 pces	10	0	2
Amazin' Fruit, 1 bag, 1.9 oz	180	0	41
Andes: Creme de Menthe; Cherry Jubilee			
Choc covered Patty, 1.4 oz	200	13	22
Thins, avg. all flav., (8), 1.4 oz	200	13	22
Anthon Berg: Cognac, each	180	8	25
After Dinner Sweet:			
Marzipan w. Madeira, 1.4 oz	175	7.5	26
Marzipan Brod	120	7	13
Asteroid *(Nestlé)*, 1.9 oz	260	10	40
Atomic Fireball, 1 piece	4	0	1
Baby Ruth: King Size, 3.7 oz bar	480	24	66
2.1 oz bar	280	14	39
Fun size, 2 bars	170	8	24
Minis, 4 bars	200	9	30
Carb Select, 2 bars	180	8	26
Baci *(Perugino)*: 1 pce, ½ oz	75	6	7
Bar, 1.58 oz	230	15	27
Barley Sugar, 1 pce, 0.2 oz	25	0	6
Baskin-Robbins: 3 pce, 0.5 oz	60	1	13
Sugar Free, 4 pces	40	1	15
Big Hunt, 2 oz	230	3	47
Bit-O-Honey, 1.7 oz	180	3.5	38
Chews, 6 pces, 1.4 oz	150	3	32
Blow Pops, each	50	0	14
Bon Bons, 2 pieces	45	0	12
Boston Baked Beans, 11 pces, 15g	70	2.5	10
Brach's: Almond Supremes (11)	220	13	22
Butterscotch Hard (3), 0.6 oz	70	0	17
Caramel Clusters (2), 36g	180	10	20
Choc Bridge Mix (16), 1.3 oz	190	8	26
Circus Peanuts (3), 1.4 oz	160	0	39
Double Dippers (15), 1.4 oz	210	12	23
Golden Butter Toffee (3), 0.6 oz	80	2	15
Malted Milk Balls (15), 1.3 oz	190	7	30
Milk Maid Caramel (4), 1.37 oz	160	4.5	27
Orange Slices (3), 45g	150	0	38
Breath Savers, all types, each	5	0	2
Brite Crackers, 1 bag, 1.5 oz	140	0	32
Bubble Gum: See 'Gum' Page 131			
Buncha Crunch, ⅓ cup, 1.4 oz	180	8	26
Burnt Peanuts, 15 pces, 40g	70	3	10
Butterfinger: 2.1 oz bar	270	11	43
King Size, 3.7 oz bar	480	18	75
Fun size, each	85	3.5	14
Giant, 5 oz	680	32	96
Beast, 140g	640	24	100
On The Go, 4 bars	180	7	29
Mini, each	45	1.5	7
Snack (4) 1.4 oz	180	7	29
Stix, 1 stick, 17g	90	4.5	11

Brands & Generic (Cont)

Per Piece/Serving	C	F	Cb
Butterfinger (Cont):			
Crisp Bar: 1.76 oz bar	250	13	33
King Size, 90g	500	28	62
Minis, 4 pieces	220	11	29
Butterfinger B.B.'s, 1.7 oz bag	220	9	34
Buttermints, 7 pcs, 13g	50	0	12
Butterscotch: 3 pcs	70	0	19
Buttons (Walgreens), 3, 18g	70	0	17
Chips (Hershey's), 1 Tbsp	80	4	10
Discs (Sathers), 3 pcs	70	0	17
Cadbury (Hershey's): Creme Egg (1)	170	6	28
Dairy Milk, 10 pcs, 40g	220	12	24
Mini Eggs, 12 pcs, 40g	190	8	28
Candy Apple, medium, 6.5 oz	280	0	60
Candy Cane, medium, 5", ½ oz	50	0	13
Candy Corn, 1 oz	100	0	26
Candy Jar Mix (Jewel), 3, 17g	70	0	17
Candy Necklaces, 20g each	80	0	20
Caramels: each	40	1	8
Chocolate, each	25	0.2	6
Creams: 3 pcs, 1¼ oz	130	3	23
2.75 oz pkt, 5 pcs, 1½ oz	160	3.5	30
Caramel Nips: 2 pcs	60	1.5	11
Chocolate Parfait, 2 pces	60	2	11
Peanut Butter, 2 pces	60	2	11
Sugar Free Caramel, 2 pces	60	1.5	12
Caramel Popcorn, ⅔ cup	150	6	23
Caramello (Hershey's), 1.6 oz bar	210	10	29
Snack, 0.66 oz	80	4	11
Cadbury: 6 pces	200	9	27
Kingsize, 2.7 oz bar	360	16	49
Certs, Breath Mints, 1 pce	5	0	2
Charleston Chew: 1 bar, 60g	260	7	49
Minis, 2 bars, 24g	110	4	17
Chew-ets Peanut Chews:			
Original, 6 pces, 56g	260	13	25
Chocolate, 6 pces	270	14	34
Chews, 1 roll	120	1	28
Chick O Stick, 2 oz	260	6	44
Chocolate Mints (Hershey's), each	10	0.1	2
Chocolate Parfait Nips, 2 pces	60	2	11
Chuckles Jelly: each	35	0	9
Jujubes (Hershey's), 55 pces, 40g	110	0	28
Chunky Bar (Nestlé): 1.4 oz	190	11	24
King Size, 2½ oz	340	19	43
Giant, 5 oz	680	40	84
Chupa Chups, 1 pce, 0.42 oz	35	0	8
Cinnamon Bears (Walgreens), 5	130	0	34
Cinn. Buttons (Walgreens), 3 pce	70	0	17

Per Piece/Serving	C	F	Cb
Cinnamon Disks (Walmart), 3 pces	70	0	19
Cinnamon Drops (Sathers), 19 pce	150	0	36
Circus Peanuts, 6 pces, 42g	160	0	39
CocoaVia Crunch Bars, 0.7 oz	90	5	11
Coconut Stacks, 8 pieces	260	13	37
Coffee Go Coffee/Cappuccino, ea.	18	0.4	4
Coffee Rio-Gold, each	15	0.5	3
Collard & Bowser, Eng. Toffee (2)	80	4	12
Conversation Hearts (Necco), 1 lge	10	0	4
Cote d'Or: Bouchee, each	130	8	12
Chokotoff, each	210	9	30
Nougatti	150	8	19
Bar & Nuts, 1.3 oz	220	18	12
Cotton Candy, 1 oz	110	0	28
Cough Drops: See Page 131			
Cracker Jack, ½ cup, 1 oz	120	2	23
Creme Savers: See Lifesavers			
Crisped Rice: Almond, 1 bar	130	6	18
Choc Chip, 1 bar	115	4	18
Crows, 12 pieces, 1.5 oz	140	0	35
Crunch: 5 oz bar	680	36	96
King Munch, 2.75 oz bar	380	20	52
1.55 oz bar	220	22	30
Fun size, each	90	4.5	13
King Kong, 3½ oz	480	24	66
w. Caramel, 1.52 oz	200	10	28
King Size, 2.7 oz	370	19	51
Minis, 6 pces, 37g	180	9	25
Pieces, ⅓ cup	180	8	26
White Bar, 1.4 oz bar	220	13	23
Stix, avg., 1 stick	90	6	12
Sugar Free, 4 bars	170	13	21
Dots, 12 dots, 1.5 oz	140	0	35
Double Dip Stick, 1 stick	16	0.5	3
Dove: Promises, 5 pieces, avg	220	13	24
Single: 1 bar, 1.3 oz	200	12	22
Dark Choc, avg., 1.3 oz	190	12	22
w. Caramel, 5 pieces	220	11	24
Milk/Rich Dark Bar, 5 pces	200	12	24
Choc-covered Almonds, 13 pces	215	15	19
Dum Dum Pops (Spangler), 1 pop	25	0	5
Endulge (Atkins): Per Serving			
Caramel Nut Chew Bar, 34g	140	7	14
Peanut Caramel Cluster, 34g	110	6	9
Advantage: Original, avg., 60g	230	10	22
Caramel, avg., 44g	160	8	17
English Toffee, 1 pce	48	3	5
Eda's Sugar Free, all flav., 5, ½ oz	40	0	15

Candy, Chocolate (Cont)

Brands & Generic (Cont)

Per Piece/Serving	C	F	Cb
5th Avenue: 2 oz bar	270	13	35
King Size bar	480	24	60
Snack Size, 0.58 oz	80	4	10
Fanny May: Single Wrapped Pieces			
Mint Meltaway Patty, 3 pcs, 40g	230	15	30
Pixie, 2 pcs, 45g	240	14	26
Trinidad, 1 pce, 42.5g	310	12	25
Fast Break (Reese's): 2 oz bar	270	13	34
King Size	480	24	60
Ferrero Rocher: each	75	5	4
3 pces, 1.3 oz	220	15	17
Fifty 50 Snack Bars:			
Peanut Butter, 2	190	14	17
Almond Choc., 7 pce, 1½ oz	200	17	18
Crunch Choc., 7 pce, 1.1 oz	190	16	19
Dark Choc, 40g	170	14	21
Milk Choc, 3 pce, ½ bar, 43g	190	16	19
Mini Bars, 8 bars, 1 oz	140	9	16
Fluffy Stuff (Charms), 0.6 oz bag	70	0	17
Fondant: Choc-coated, 1.2 oz	120	3	27
Mint, 1 oz	105	0	27
Fran's: Gold Bar, 45g	250	14	17
Gold Bites (Almonds), 23g	120	7	13
Frootsies, 12 pces	140	3	29
Fruit Crystals (Walgreens), 3 pces	70	0	17
Fruit Drops, each	6	0	1
Fruit Gems (Sunkist), 3, 1.2 oz	105	0	25
Fruit Leathers, average, 0.5 oz	45	0	12
Fruit Pastilles, 1 roll, 1.4 oz	100	0	26
Fruit Rolls, 1 roll	70	0	12
Fruit Roll-Ups, ½ oz	50	1	12
Fruit Runts (Walgreens), 12 pces	60	0	14
Fudge: Chocolate/Vanilla (1), 21g	90	5	13
with Nuts (1), 21g	100	6	12
Choco. Marshmallow, 1 oz	120	3	27
w. Nuts, 1 oz	115	3	19
Peanut Butter, 1 oz	115	3	19
Ghirardelli:			
Squares: Dark Choc. (4), 43g	220	17	23
Other varieties (3), 45g	215	12	28
3 oz Bars: Dark Choc., 12 pieces	440	34	46
Other varieties avg., 12 pces	440	28	52
Intense Dark: Twilight, 3 pces	200	17	17
Other varieties, avg., 3 pces	200	15	21
Godiva: Hearts, 7 pieces, 1.4 oz	210	13	23
Bars: Milk/Dark, avg., 1½ oz	230	14	26
Extra Dark 72%, 1½ oz	230	17	18
Sugar Free Bars, avg., 1½ oz	200	15	25
Assorted Chocs: 2 pieces, 31g	160	10	17
Sugar Free, 3 pieces	200	15	23
Bouchee au Chocolate, 2 pces	220	13	23
Chocolate Pretzels, 6 pces, 1.4 oz	200	10	26

Per Piece/Serving	C	F	Cb
Go Lightly: Box Candies, 2-3 pces	220	16	28
Bags: Assorted Taffy, 5 pieces	130	3	36
Vanilla Caramels, 5	150	6	31
Super Free Creme Crunch (4)	150	5	33
Goobers Peanuts, 1 pkg, 1.4 oz	200	13	21
Good & Plenty (Hershey's): 50g	170	0	43
Snack Size, 1 box, 17g	60	0	14
GooGoo Cluster, 1 bar, 1.75 oz	240	11	32
Gum Drops: 1 small, 9g	10	0	7.5
5 pces, 44g	150	0	37
Gummi Bears, 9 bears, 42g	120	0	29
Gummi Novelties (Walgreens), 6	150	0	22
Gummi Savers, 10 pieces	120	0	30
Gummi Sweet Tarts, 1 bug, 1.5 oz	150	0	34
Gummi Watch, 1, 2 oz	105	0	24
Gummi Worms, 8g	25	0	6
Guylian: Milk Choc., 8 squares, 1 oz	120	9	16
Dark Choc., 8 squares, 1 oz	130	9	16
Guylian Twists, 4 pces, 35g	200	3	18
Halvah (Joyvah): Plain, ½ bar, 2 oz	390	25	18
Choc.coated Sesame, ½ bar, 2 oz	380	23	20
Hard Candy: All flavors, 16g	60	0	15
1 regular piece	20	0	5
Heath: Original, 39g	220	12	24
Bites, 15 pces, 39g	210	12	25
King Size, 2.8 oz	430	25	49
Minis, 5 pces	240	14	27
Hershey's:			
Milk Chocolate: 1.55 oz bar	230	13	25
Cookies 'n' Creme, 1.55 oz bar	230	12	26
Snack, 0.6 oz	90	5	10
Kingsize, 2.6 oz bar	400	23	42
7 oz bar, ⅛ bar	200	12	21
w. Almonds, 1.45 oz	220	14	20
w. Almonds King Size	400	24	39
Crisp Bits, 5 squares, 40g	200	10	25
Bites, York (15)	160	3	33
Cacao Reserve:			
Milk Choc. (35% cacao), 1.8 oz	310	22	25
Dark Choc. (65% cacao), 1.8 oz	290	22	23
Candy-Coated Eggs:			
Milk Choc (4), 0.6 oz	90	4	12
w. Almonds (4) 0.6 oz	100	6	9
Extra Dark, avg. all var., 4 pces	210	13	21
Hugs: Regular (1), 4.5g	25	1.5	2.5
Regular (9), 40g	210	12	23
w. Almonds (9), 40g	230	14	21
Kissables: Avg. all var., 39 pces	205	10	28
Snack Size, 13g	65	3	9
Kisses, avg. all var. (1)	25	1.5	3
Miniatures: 5 pces, 1.5 oz	230	13	26
Kisses, 1 bag	420	24	44
Nuggets Snack, 4 pces	215	13	22

Brands & Generic (Cont)

Per Piece/Serving — **C** **F** **Cb**

Hershey's (Cont):

Pot of Gold Chocolate:

	C	F	Cb
Nut Clusters, avg. all, 3 pieces	245	15	24
Nut Assortment, 1.5 oz	140	7	21
Caramel Assortment, 1.5 oz	200	9	28
Creme Assortment, 1.5 oz	170	4	32
Mint Assortment, 1.5 oz	200	10	26
Truffle Assortment, 1.5 oz	200	9	27
Sugar Free Assortment, 1.5 oz	180	16	22
Smart Zone, avg. all varieties, 50g	205	7	22
Snack Barz	115	5	17
Special Dark Choc.: 1.45 oz bar	220	13	24
King Size, 72g	400	22	44
Snack Size, 14g	70	4.5	9
Sticks, avg. all varieties, 11g	60	3	7
Swoops, avg., 1 cup, 1.26 oz	190	11	20
Whoppers, 10 pieces	100	3.5	16
Sugar Free: Choc. Candy (5)	170	13	25
Dark Chocolate Candy (5)	190	15	23
Chocolate w. Almonds (5)	180	14	23
Peanut Butter Cups Minis (5)	170	12	24
York Peppermint Patties, 3 pces	110	45	13
Honeycomb: Plain, 1 oz	115	0	27
Choc-coated, 2 pces	180	7	31
Hot Tamales: 1 box, 60g, 2.1 oz	220	0	55
Sathers, 20 pces, 1.4 oz	150	0	36
Ice Blue Mints (Walgreens), 3, 17g	70	0	17
Jawbreakers (Sathers), 15, 17g	70	0	17
Jellies, 3 medium, 1 oz	130	0	33
Jells Raspberry (Joyva), 3 pces, 44g	160	0	39
Jelly Beans: Small, 22 beans, 1 oz	100	0	24
Regular, 13 beans, 40g	150	0	37
1 bean	10	0	3
Sugar Free, 35 beans	110	0	36
Jumbo, 1 bean	20	0	5
Jewel, 13 beans, 1.4 oz	140	0	36
Sathers/Walgreens, 13 pces	150	0	37
Wonderbeans, 33 beans	100	0	24
Jelly Bellys: each	4	0	1
35 pces, 1.4 oz	140	0	37
Sugar Free Beans/Sours (37), 1.4 oz	120	0	36
Sugar Free Fruit Slices, 8 pces, 1.4 oz	60	0	30
Jelly Rings (Jewel), 5 pces, 42g	120	0	30
Jolly Rancher: Candy (3)	70	0	17
Fruit Chews (6), 1.4 oz	150	1.5	33
Gummies, 10 pces, 39g	120	0	29
Hard Candy (3), 18g	70	0	17
Lollipops, 1 pce, 0.6 oz	60	0	16
Sugar Free, 4 pces, 0.5 oz	35	0	13
Junior Caramels: 13 pces, 42g	190	6	33
Mini, 2 boxes, 24g	110	3	19

Per Piece/Serving — **C** **F** **Cb**

	C	F	Cb
Junior Mints: 52g box	220	4	45
16 pces, 1.4 oz	170	3	35
Juicefuls: Red Raspb., (3), 0.6 oz	60	0	15
Assorted Fruits, 1 pce	20	0	5
Jujubes, all types (55), 40g	110	0	28
Juju Bears, 5 pces	130	0	34
Juju Mix (Sathers), 11 pce, 1½ oz	150	0	36
Jujyfruits, 16 pces, 40g	120	0	32
Kit Kat: 1.5 oz bar	220	11	27
Big Kat, 1.94 oz	290	15	35
Bites, 15 pces, 39g	200	10	25
Caramel Bar (1)	210	10	26
Extra Krispy Bar (1)	240	12	29
King Size, 3 oz bar	440	22	54
Miniature, 5 pces	230	12	27
Multipack/Snack Bar (3), 42g	220	11	27
Triple Choc Snack Bar (1), 14g	75	4	9
White Choc: Bar, 1½ oz	220	12	26
Minis, 5 pces	230	12	27
Krackel: 42g bar	210	11	26
Snack size, 0.6 oz	85	4.5	11
Kraft: Caramels, (5), 40g	160	3.5	30
Kudos: See Page 139			
Lance: Peanut Bar, 1.8 oz pkg	240	14	22
Lemon Drops (3) ½ oz	50	0	14
Sugar Free (Walgreens), 4, 13g	25	0	13
Lemonhead, 10, ½ oz	50	0	14
Licorice: Average all types, 1oz	100	0	25
Bites (Switzer), each	10	0	3
Chews (Panda), each	10	0	3
Tid Bits, each	5	0	1
Twists: Black/Red, avg. 1 pce	35	0	8.5
Sugar Free, 1 pce	13	0	2.5
American Licorice Co.: Laces, 1	35	0	8
Jumbo Rope, 2 pces	140	0	34
Red Bites, 1.4 oz	140	0	33
Snaps, 31 pces, 40g	140	0.5	33
Stick, (1) 0.5 oz	35	0	8.5
Super Red Ropes (1), 66g	240	0	54
Superstring, 1⅓ pces	140	0	34
Vines, 2 pces	70	0	17
Sugar Free Red Twists (7)	90	0	25
Lifesavers: Large size, 1 candy	15	0	3.5
Regular, all flavors, 1 candy	10	0	2.5
1 Roll (14 candies), 1.14 oz	140	0	35
Creme Savers: 3 pces	60	0	11
Sugar Free, 4 pces	35	0	14
Gummi Savers (10), 39g	130	0	30
Fruit Lollipops, 0.4 oz	40	0	10
Peppermint (4)	60	0	15
Fruit Splosion, 10 pces	130	0	30
Sugar-Free Delites: Per Candy			
Orchard Fruits; Summer Blend	7	0	2.5
Butter Toffee; European Collect.	10	1	2.5

Candy, Chocolate (Cont)

Brands & Generic (Cont)

Per Piece/Serving

	C	F	Cb
Lik-m-aid (Nestlé), Wonka Fun Dip, 1 pkg	50	0	13
Lindt: Lindor, Balls, average (3)	75	6	5
Milk Chocolate, 12 pces, 40g	230	16	18
Truffles (3)	220	17	16
Lollipops, each, 11g	45	0	11
Look! Bar, 1.5 oz	190	6	33
M & M's: Plain, 1.7 oz pkg	235	10	34
Milk Chocolate, 1 pce	5	0.1	0.5
20 pces, 0.6 oz	70	3	10
¼ cup, 1.8 oz	255	11	37
Dark Choc.: 3.14 oz pkg	440	20	60
Fun Size, 18g pkg	90	4	13
Almond Choc., 1.3 oz pkg	190	10	22
Crispy, 1.6 oz	225	9	34
Minis, Mega Tube, 1.1 oz tube	150	7	21
Mega: Milk Choc (27), 1.5 oz	210	9	30
Peanut (12), 1.4 oz	210	11	24
Peanut: 1.92 oz pkg	280	14	33
Fun Size, 18g pkg	90	4.5	11
Peanut Butter 1.6 oz pkg	245	14	26
Mamba, 9 pces, 1½ oz	170	2.5	36
Marathon (Snickers) Bar, 1.9 oz	220	7	26
M.Azing: 1 bar, 1.5 oz	230	12	27
Peanut Butter (1), 1.5 oz	230	13	25
Marshmallow Egg, 1 egg, 1 oz	120	3	22
Marshmallows: Firm/Soft, 1 oz	90	0	23
Regular size, 4 pces, 33g	100	0	24
Mini-Marshmallow, ⅔ c., 30g	100	0	24
Choc-coat. Twists (Joyva), each	95	2	10
Fluff, 2 Tbsp, 18 g	60	0	15
Kraft: Mini, ½ cup, 30g	100	0	24
Creme, 2 Tbsp	45	0	11
Jet-Puffed, 5 pces, 30g	100	0	24
Funmallows, ⅔ cup, 30g	100	0	24
Miniature, ⅔ cup, 30g	100	0	24
Marzipan, 2 Tbsp, 39g	160	4	29
Mauna Loa: Choc., 50g	280	19	30
Choc. coated Macadamias 57g	220	15	19
Mexican Hats (7), 38g	120	0	30
Mentos: Regular (1)	10	0	3
Sugar Free (1)	5	0	2.5
Mike & Ike: 1 pkg, 1.1 oz	120	0	28
23 pces, 40g	140	0	36
Milkfulls (Storck), 6 pces, 1.4 oz	170	3	35
Milk Chocolate: See Hershey's			
Milk Duds (Hershey's), 13 pces	180	7	28

Per Piece/Serving

	C	F	Cb
Milky Way: Midnight Bar, 1.75 oz	225	10	33
Regular Bar, 58g	250	10	41
Fun size, 2 bars, 34g	150	6	24
Milky Way To Go, 51g	230	9	36
Miniatures: (5) 43g	205	9	30
Midnight Minis (5), 41g	190	7	29
Pop'ables (3) 39g	180	7	28
Mints: Uncoated, 7 pces	60	0	17
1 small mint (¾" diam.)	4	0	1
1 large mint (1½" diam.)	10	0	2
Mon Cheri (Ferrero), 4 pces, 45g	260	18	21
Mounds: 49g bar	240	13	31
Snack, 0.68 oz	90	5	11
King Size, 3½ bar	490	26	58
Minis, 3 pces, 41g	200	11	24
Mr Goodbar: 48g bar	270	16	27
King Size, 2.6 oz bar	400	24	40
Snack, 17g	80	4.5	10
Bites (25), 40g	230	14	21
Mrs Fields Choc, 2 pieces, 33g	160	8	22
Necco Candy Wafers (40) 57g	220	0	56
Nestle Toll House, 1 pce, 1 oz	120	5	18
Neuhaus, average all types	80	5	7
Newman's Own:			
Caramel Cups 3 pces, 1.2 oz	160	9	21
P'Nut B. Cups (Milk/Dark), 3, 1 pkg	180	12	19
Sweet Dark Choc Bar, 79g	400	26	48
Nibs, all types, 1 pouch, 63g	215	2	49
Nips (Pearson), all flavors, 2, 14g	60	2	11
Nite Bite (Glucose Bar)	100	3.5	15
Nougat, 3 pces, 1 oz	150	2.5	32
Chocolate Covered, 1 oz	125	4	22
Now & Later (Nabisco), 9, 41g	120	1	29
Nutrageous Bar (Reese's): 51g	280	16	27
King Size, 3.4 oz bar	500	30	32
Oh Henry! 2 oz bar	265	13	37
100 Grand: 1.5 oz bar	180	8	29
King Size, 2.8 oz bar	350	14	57
Snack Size, 2 bars, 43g	180	8	30
Orange (Lindt), 5 slices	230	14	23
Orange Slices: Jewel, 3, 42g	140	0	35
Walgreens, 3, 43g	150	0	36
Pastel Mints (Walgreens), 20 pces	60	0	14
Patteez (Sweet n' Low), 4 pces	100	2	19
PayDay Bar: 51g bar	240	11	30
King Size, 3.4 oz bar	480	24	52
Snack Size, 0.7 oz bar	90	5	10
Avalanche, 1.8 oz bar	250	13	29
Avalanche King, 3.1 oz bar	440	24	50
Peanut Bar, 1.6 oz bar	210	14	20
Peanut Butter Cups: See Reese's; Newman's Own			

Brands & Generic (Cont)

Per Piece/Serving	C	F	Cb
Peanut Brittle: 1½ oz	220	15	20
Sugar Free (Judy's), ¾ cup, 1 oz	100	6	2
Peanuts, choc-covered, 15 pces	210	12	23
Pearson's Mint Patties, (5), 38g	150	2.5	31
Pecan Roll, ⅓ bar, 40g	190	10	24
Peppermints, 7 small, 0.5 oz	60	0	15
Brach's, 3 pces	60	0	15
Peppermint Twists (2), 14g	60	0	14
Pez, 1 roll	35	0	9
Planters: Choc. Peanuts (25) 7 oz	220	13	20
Orig. Peanut Bar, 1.6 oz	230	14	22
Hersheys, 2½ oz	390	24	34
Pop'ables: Average, 13 pces, 1½ oz	180	7	29
4.9 oz Package	630	25	101
Poprocks, 9½ g pkg	35	0	9
Positively Pecan, 2.5 oz bar	390	24	38
Pralines: Small, 0.3 oz	38	2	5
1 large piece, 1.4 oz	180	10	24
Pretzels: Choc-covered,			
Minisize (6), 38g	190	9	24
White Choc Bites (23), 40g	200	9	25
Pretzel Flipz (2), 8 pces, 1 oz	130	5	20
Raisinets: 1 pkg, 1.7 oz	205	8	34
King Size, 2.8 oz	330	13	56
Dark Raisinets, ¼ cup, 45g	130	8	32
Raspberry Cream, 2 pces, 36g	155	5	26
Reception Sticks (4)	65	2	12
Red Raspberry Dollars (10)	130	0	31
Reese's			
Peanut Butter Cups: 1½ oz	230	13	24
King size, 2.8 oz	420	24	44
Mini, 5 pces, 39g	210	12	22
Snack size, 1 pce, 21g	110	6	12
Sugar free, 2 pces, avg., 39g	170	12	24
Caramel filled, 1.4 oz	190	10	24
Big Cups: Original, 1.4 oz	210	12	21
w. Nuts: 1.4 oz	220	13	20
King size, 2.8 oz	430	26	41
w. Caramel & Nuts, 1.3 oz	190	10	21
Bites, 16 pces, 40g	220	12	23
Reeses Pieces: 25 pces, 1.6 oz	230	11	28
King size, 3 oz	400	20	46
Reeses Sticks: 1.5 oz	230	13	23
King size, 3 oz	460	26	46
Snack size, 17g	90	5	9
Nutrageous Bar: 1.8 oz bar	280	16	27
King size, 3.4 oz bar	520	30	52
Crispy Crunchy Bar: 1.7 oz bar	260	15	26
King Size, 3.1 oz bar	480	28	48
Fast Break, 2 oz bar	280	14	34
King Size Bar	480	24	60
Swoops, 1 cup, 1.26 oz	190	11	17
Baking Chips, 1 Tbsp, 15g	80	4.5	9

Per Piece/Serving	C	F	Cb
Rice Krispies Treats (Kellogg's):			
1 bar, average all varieties	110	3.5	19
Rice Crunchy Bars, 19g bar	70	0.5	15
Riesen Choc. Chew, 4 pces, 36g	170	6	28
Ritter Sport, w. Hazelnuts (6), 37.5g	210	14	19
Rocky Road, 1.8 oz bar	240	11	34
Robin Eggs, Large (2); Mini (10)	100	3.5	16
Rolo: All types (3), 0.64 oz	85	4	12
Mini Bites, 19 pieces, 1.4 oz	190	9	26
Root Beer Barrels (3) 0.5 oz	70	0	17
Ross Chocolate Bar: White, 1.2 oz	180	13	19
Almond; Crunchy, 1.2 oz	180	13	18
Russell Stover Candy: Creams (1)	65	3	11
Almond Delight, 15 pces	220	18	15
Chocolate Asst., 2 pces	140	6	21
Choc-covered Nuts, 3 pces	230	16	17
Cherry Blimps, 3 pces	170	12	24
Sugar Free: Mint Cremes (3)	190	14	22
Mint Patties, 3 pces	180	11	27
Pecan Delight (2), 1 oz	130	9	5
Cups (3), 1.2 oz	170	13	16
Mint Patties, 3 pces	180	11	27
Salt Water Taffy (Brach's), 5	170	2.5	36
Seashells (Guylian), 1 shell	70	4.5	6
See's Candies: Average all Flavors			
Assorted Candy, 4 pces	210	11	28
Caramels & Chews, 2 pces	175	10	19
Creams, 2 pieces	180	9	24
Little Pops, 4 pieces	55	2	10
Lollypops (1), 20g	80	3	15
Nut Clusters, 3 pieces	225	16	16
Sesame Crunch, 3 pces	80	4	7
Signature Treasures (Nestlé):			
Choc. Creme, 3 pieces, 1.2 oz	170	9	21
Creamy Caramel, 3 pieces, 1.3 oz	170	9	23
Dark Choc Caramel, 3 pieces	160	10	22
Milk Choc Caramel, 3 pieces	170	9	23
Peanut Butter, 3 pieces	180	12	20
Simply Lite, ½ ctn, 36 pieces	130	5	18
Simply Sugar Free: See Allen Wertz			
Sixlets (Hershey), 24 pces	90	3.5	14
Skittles: Sour, 1.8 oz bag	200	2	44
Orig./Trop./Wild Berry. 2.17 oz	250	2.5	54
Fun Size, 1 bag, 15g	60	1	14
King Size, 4 oz bag	440	4.5	102
Large bag (16 oz), ¼ cup, 1.5 oz	170	2	39
Skor Toffee Bar, 1.4 oz	210	12	24
Smarties: Candy Rolls, 1 roll	25	0	6
Giant, 2 pces, 7g	25	0	5
Smores (Hershey), 1.65 oz	240	11	31

Candy, Chocolate (Cont)

Brands & Generic (Cont)

Per Piece/Serving	C	F	Cb
Snickers: 2.07 oz bar	280	14	35
3.7 oz bar	510	24	63
Creme Egg (1), 1.2 oz	170	10	20
King Size, ⅓ bar, 1.2 oz	170	8	21
Miniatures, 4 pieces	170	1	22
Munch Bar, 1.4 oz bar	220	15	18
Pop'ables, 13 pieces, 1½ oz	190	9	24
Cruncher, 1.56 oz	220	11	28
Cruncher To Go, 2.54 oz	350	18	45
Marathon Bar: avg., 1.9 oz bar	210	8	26
King size	440	22	60
Almond, 1.76 oz	230	11	32
Fun Size, 2 bars, 34g	160	8	21
Sno Caps, ¼ cup, 40g	180	8	30
Soft 'N Chewy Butter Toffee, ea.	30	0.5	5
Sorbee: Choc., ½ bar, 40g	200	14	20
Gummie Bears, 16 pces	120	0	30
Peanut Butter, 4 pces	210	15	19
Sour Brite Crawlers, 13 pces	140	0	31
Sour Punch: All types, 2 oz	200	1.5	46
1 straw	20	0	5
Spearmint Leaves: *Jewel,* 5, 40g	140	0	35
Walgreens, 4 pieces, 46g	160	0	39
Spice Drops, 12 pieces, 39g	130	0	33
Spree Candies: Original, 15 pces	50	0	13
Chewy Spree, 8 pces	60	0	18
Starburst: Candy Canes, 0.5 oz	70	0	18
Fruit Chews, each	20	0.4	4
2 oz pkg	240	5	48
Jellybeans, 1.5 oz	160	0	39
Jellybean Egg, 2 oz	200	0	51
Tropical Fruit, 2.07 oz pack	240	5	49
Starlight Mints, 3 pces, 16g	60	0	15
Suckers *(Walgreens),* 1 sucker, 11g	45	0	11
Sugar Babies, 30 pces, 40g	180	1.5	41
Sugar Coated Peanuts, 1 oz	120	8	10
Sunbursts Sunflowers *(Kimmie):*			
Candy Bar Bag, 1.3 oz	145	6.5	21
Coffee Break Tube, 3 oz	330	15	48
Snack Size Bag, 10g	40	2	3.5
Sweet 'N Low: Chews, each	20	0.5	4
Coffee Cremes (1)	40	3	6
Wafer Bars, avg., 3 pieces	140	7	23
Mint Cremes, 3½ pieces	120	9	22
Mint Patteez, 4 pces	100	2	29
Sweet Escapes: *See Hershey's*			
Sweet Tarts *(Nestlé),* 5 pces, ½ oz	50	0	13
Symphony: 1.5 oz bar	230	14	24
Snack: Chocolate (1), 0.6 oz	90	5	10
w. Almds & Toffee (1), .5 oz	230	14	23

Per Piece/Serving	C	F	Cb
Taffy, 1 pce, 23g	80	1	19
Take 5 *(Hershey's):* 1.5 oz bar	210	10	26
King Size, 2.25 oz bar	320	16	38
Marshmallow, 1.3 oz bar	180	9	22
Peanut Butter, 1.5 oz bar	220	11	23
Toffifay, 5 pieces	200	11	25
3 Musketeers: 2.13 oz bar	260	8	46
Fun size, 3 pieces	190	6	34
Miniatures, 7 pieces	170	5	32
Pop'ables (15)	180	6	31
Tang-a-Roos, 1 roll	25	0	6
Terry's Choc Orange, (5), 1.5 oz	230	12	27
Tic Tac, all varieties, each	2	0	0
Toblerone: 50g (1.76 oz) bar	255	15	30
1 bar, 100g (3.5 oz)	510	30	60
⅓ bar, 30g	170	10	20
Mini, 3 pces	200	11	24
Toffees, Regular, 1 oz	160	9	18
Toll House Bars, 1 piece, 1 oz	120	5	18
Tootsie Pops, Mini (3), 24g	90	0	23
Tootsie Roll, 2.25 oz roll	245	2	55
Trolli: Gummies, 18 pieces, 40g	110	0	28
Cherry Bombers, 10 pieces	130	0	31
Truffles: Regular, 1 pce, 12g	60	4	6
Large *(Godiva),* 0.75 oz	110	6.5	12
Extra Large *(J.Schmidt),* 1½ oz	220	13	24
Turtles *(Nestlé):* Avg., each	80	4.5	10
Sugar Free, 3 pieces, 38g	150	11	20
Twists (Sugar Free): Licorice; Strawberry;			
7 twists, 40g	90	0	25
Twix: 2 oz pkg	280	14	37
King Size, 3 oz pkg	405	20	52
Fun Size, 0.5 oz	80	4	10
Twix To Go	480	24	64
Minis, 3 pces, 29g	150	7	19
Caramel, 24g	130	6	16
Peanut Butter To Go	480	28	48
Peanut Butter, 1.8 oz	280	17	28
Twizzlers: Twists, 3 pieces, 38g	130	0.5	30
Bites (17), 40g	140	0.5	31
Pull 'n' Peel Cherry, 62g	210	1	47
Swedish Fish, 51g	180	0	46
Sugar Free, 6 pces	130	1	33
Uno Bar (1), 42g	250	17	22
Velamints Sugar Free, 2 pce	5	0	1
Weight Watchers/Whitmans:			
Butter Cream Caramel, 3 pces	150	8	23
Caramel Medallions, 3 pces	150	9	26
English Toffee Squares, 3 pces	160	10	23
Mint Patties, 3 pces	150	9	26
Peanut Butter Crunch, 4 pces	180	8	31
Pecan Crowns, 3 pces	150	9	22

Brands & Generic (Cont)

Per Piece/Serving

	C	F	Cb
Werther's: Original, 3 pce, 15g	60	1	13
Chewy Caramel (6), 37g	170	5	30
Caramelts (8), 40g	250	18	18
Sugar-Free, 5 pieces	40	1	14
Whatchamacallit Bar, 1.7 oz	240	11	30
King Size, 2.6 oz	370	18	46
Whitman's: Pecan Roll, 2 oz roll	300	20	26
Sampler, 3 pces, 1.4 oz	200	9	28
Assorted; Dark Chocolate, 3 pces	220	12	26
Snoopy Treats, 2 pces	190	10	24
Sucratrol Mint Pattie, 1 oz	120	7	17
Whoppers, 9 pces, 21g	100	3.5	16
Wonka: Wonka Bar (1), 1.3 oz	180	10	25
Laffy Taffy: Orig., 5 bars, 1.5 oz	160	2	36
Stretchy & Tangy, 1½ oz	165	4	33
Nerds, 1 box	240	0	42
Gobstopper: Box, 1.77 oz	650	0	182
Everlasting/Chewy, 9 pces, 15g	50	0	14
Runts Fruit Box, 1.8 oz	210	0	49
Yogurt Candy,			
Coated Raisins, 27 pces, 40g	180	8	28
York Mints: 1.37 oz patty	160	3	32
Snack size, 0.5 oz	55	1	11
Peppermint Patties (3)	160	3	33
King Size (3), 2.86 oz	320	6	66
Sugar Free, Mini (3)	110	4.5	28
Swoops, 1 cup, 1.26 oz	190	11	21
Zachary Old Fashioned Drops, 1 oz	100	0	26
Zagnut, 1.75 oz bar	230	10	31
Zero Bar: 52g	240	9	36
King Size, 3.4 oz	420	16	66
Zingos, 3 pce, 2g	5	0	2

Gum ~ Per Piece

	C	F	Cb
Bazooka, each	15	0	4
Beechies	6	0	1
Big League Chew	10	0	2
Bubble Gum Balls (Hershey's)	5	0	2
Bubble Yum	25	0	6
Sugarless	10	0	3
Candilicious	30	0	2
Carefree (Sugarless/Regular)	5	0	2
Chiclets, 1 piece	5	0	1
Clorets, 1 stick	10	0	2
Dentyne	5	0	0.5
Estee, bubble/regular	5	0	2
Extra (Wrigley's), Sugar-Free (1)	5	0	2
Freshen-Up	10	0	3
Hubba Bubba: Regular	23	0	6
Sugar-free, average	14	0	0.5
Ice Breakers, 12 pieces	0	0	2
Sonic Boom Bubble Gum	15	0	3
Sticklets	7	0	2
Super Bubble	15	0	4
Trident, Original; White	5	0	1
Wrigley's, all flavors	10	0	2

Carob Candy

Per Piece/Serving

	C	F	Cb
Carob: Plain/Natural, 1 oz	160	11	9
Carob Coated: Raisins, 1 oz	130	8	15
Almonds/Peanuts, 1 oz	150	10	14
Malt Balls, 1 oz	135	8	15
Caramels, 1 oz	110	4	18
Dates, 1 oz	125	5	20
Soybeans	145	9	16
Trail/Party Mix, 1 oz	140	9	15
Carob Chips, unsweetened, 1 oz	140	7	19
Carob Bars: Plain/Nut, 1 oz	160	11	13
Fruit & Nut, 1 oz	155	10	13
Mint/Orange, 1 oz	160	11	14
Carafection: Cashew Coconut Crunch,			
½ Bar, (42g) 1.5 oz	250	14	5
Caroby Natural Touch, 3 oz	450	27	36

Cough Drops

	C	F	Cb
Beech Nut, 1 drop	10	0	2
Diabetic Tussin, 1 drop	0	0	0
Halls Defense Vit. C, 1 drop	15	0	4
Halls Fruit Breezers, 1 drop	15	0	4
Halls Menthol Drops, 1 drop	15	0	4
Sugar Free, 1 drop	5	0	4
Halls Plus, 1 drop	20	0	5
Helps Cough, all flavors, 1	15	0	3
Listerine Lozenge (Amer. Chicle)	10	0	2
Luden's Throat Drops, all flavors, 1	10	0	2
Sugar Free, 1	0	0	0
Pine Bros, 1 cough drop	10	0	2
Ricola: Cough Drops, 1 drop	10	0	3
Sugar-Free Lemon Mint, 2 mints	0	0	3
Rite Aid, Menthol Cough, 1 drop	10	0	3
Robitussin: Regular, 1 drop	15	0	3
Honey Cough, 1 drop	40	0	10
Sugar Free Throat, 1 drop	10	0	3
Sunny Cough Vit. C, 1 drop	10	0	3
Rolaids/Sodium Free, 1	5	0	1
Sathers Peppermint Lozenges, 1	15	0	3
Squibb Cough/Throat Loz.'s, 1	10	0	4
Sucrets (Beecham) Lozenges, 1	10	0	3
Wintergreen Loz. (Walgreens), 1	15	0	3
Cough Suppresant Liquids: See Page 142			

Popcorn

Home-Popped Popcorn

	C	F	Cb
Popping Corn Kernels:			
2 Tbsp, 1 oz (makes approx. 3½ cups)	100	1	22
Air-popped (no oil), plain, 1 oz	110	0	22
1 cup (6g)	30	0	6
Oil-popped, plain, 1 oz	140	8	16
1 cup (11g)	55	3	6
Popcorn Oil, 1 Tbsp	120	14	0

Microwave Popcorn

	C	F	Cb
Average All Brands (Popped)			
Butter: Regular, 1 cup	35	2	4
Light, 1 cup	25	1	4
Act II Popcorn:			
Butter, 1 cup, 0.3 oz	30	2	4
5 cups, popped, 1 oz	160	10	18
Light Butter, 1 cup, 0.2 oz	25	1	4
5 cups, popped, 1 oz	110	4.5	19
Butter Lovers,1 cup, 0.3 oz	35	2.5	4
4 cups, 1 oz	170	12	16
Butter Lovers (Reduced Fat), 1 c.	30	1.5	4.5
4.5 cups, 1 oz	130	6	20
American Fare (K-Mart):			
Butter, 1 cup, 0.3 oz	35	2.5	4
3.5 cups, 1 oz	160	9	17
Light Butter, 1 cup, 0.3 oz	25	1	5
3.5 cups, 1 oz	120	3	25
Healthy Choice: Butter, 6 cups	120	3	25
Natural, 6 cups, 1 oz	120	2.5	26
Jolly Time: America's Best, 1 cup	20	0	5
Blast 0 Butter: Regular, 1 cup	45	3	5
Light, 1 cup	30	1.5	4
Healthy Pop, 1 cup	20	0	4
Kettle Mania, 1 cup	45	3	4
Mallow Magic, 1 cup	60	5	5
Newman's Own: Butter, 1 oz	130	5	18
Light Butter Flavor, 3½ cups	120	4	19
Orville Redenbacher's: *Popped*			
Movie Theater Butter, 1 cup	35	2.5	4
4 cups, popped, 1 oz	170	12	16
Light Movie Theater Butter, 1 cup	25	1	4
5 cups, 1 oz	125	5	20
Smart Pop!: Butter, 7 cups	120	2	25
Mini Bags, 6 cups	100	2	24
Tender White, 3½ cups	180	13	14
Pop Secret Popcorn: *Popped*			
94% Fat Free, 6 cups	110	2	23
Jumbo Pop Butter, all types, 4 cups	180	12	17
Light Butter, 6 cups	120	5	20
Movie Theater Butter, 4 cups	180	13	17
One-Step, 4 cups	180	13	17
Other varieties, avg., 4 cups	170	12	17

Bagged Popcorn

	C	F	Cb
Average All Brands (Ready-to-Eat)			
Regular: Plain, ½ oz pkg	80	4	8
1 oz pkg	160	8	16
4 oz pkg	640	32	64
Box (store/airport), 2 oz	320	16	32
Bag (9" high x 5" wide), 3 oz	480	24	48

Brands ~ Bagged Popcorn

	C	F	Cb
Boston's: Fat Free, ⅔ cup, 1 oz	100	0	23
Lite, 2 cup, 1 oz	140	6	19
Gourmet Super Prem., 2 c., 1 oz	160	11	13
40% Less Fat, 2¾ cup, 1 oz	140	6	17
Cracker Jack: Original, ½ c., 1 oz	120	2	23
Fat Free varieties, ¾ cup, 1 oz	110	0	26
Crunch 'N Munch: ½ cup, 1 oz	140	5	22
Buttery Toffee, ⅔ cup, 1 oz	140	5	23
Caramel w. P'nuts, ⅔ cup, 1.2 oz	140	5	22
Fiddle Faddle: Caramel, ¾ c., 1 oz	120	3.5	23
Butter Toffee, ⅔ cup	120	3.5	22
Honey Nut, ½ cup, 1 oz	130	3.5	24
Jay's: Fat Free Caramel Corn, ¾ cup	110	0	26
Korn Krunch: *(Kornfections Treasures):*			
Almond Pecan (Sugar Free), 1 oz	150	8	19
Orville Redenbacher:			
Popcorn Cakes, Minis, avg. (8) ½ oz	65	1	12
Pre-Popped Clusters, ½ cup, 1 oz	130	5	21
Drizzles, avg., ⅔ cup, 1 oz	150	6	23
Savory, avg., 2¾ cups, 1 oz	160	10	16
Poppycock: Pecan Delight, 1 cup	300	14	40
Just Be Nuts!, ¼ cup, 1.3 oz	190	14	15
Wild Oats, all types, 2.5 cup, 1 oz	160	5	21

Movie Theater Popcorn

	C	F	Cb
Small (7 cups): Plain	450	27	30
with Butter	630	47	30
Medium (15 cups): Plain	950	58	92
with Butter	1220	88	92
Large (20 cups): Plain	1280	78	125
with Butter	1630	118	125

Potato Chips, Pretzels, Tortilla Chips

Potato Chips/Crisps

Average All Brands 🅒 🅕 🅒ᵇ

Regular:

	C	F	Cb
Plain or flavored, 1 chip	9	1	1
20 chips, 1 oz pkg	150	10	15
4 oz quantity	600	40	60
Lay's Stax, avg. all, 1 oz	160	10	15
Pringles: 14 crisps, 1 oz	160	11	15
Large, 5.75 oz can	920	63	86
Snack Stack, 23g tub	140	10	12
100 Calorie Pack, 18g tub	100	6	13
Ruffles, 12 chips, 1 oz	160	10	14
Reduced Fat: Pringles, 12 chips, 1 oz	140	7	17
Sun Chips; Terra, average, 1 oz	140	6	18
Low-Fat/Baked, average, 1 oz	120	3	22
Lay's Baked!, 11 chips, 1 oz	110	1.5	23
Ruffles Baked!: 12 chips, 1 oz	120	3	21
Cheddar Sour Crm (15) 1 oz	120	3.5	21
Fat Free: Childer's/Louise's, 1oz	100	0	22
Pringles, 1 oz	70	0	15
Low Carb: Tastemorr, avg., 1 oz	130	5	8

Corn & Tortilla Chips

Average All Brands

	C	F	Cb
Corn Chips: Avg. all types, 1 oz	160	10	15
8 oz bag	1280	80	120
Doritos: (12), avg., 1 oz	140	7	18
Nachos; 4-Cheese, 1 oz	200	8	29
Fritos (Sabritones), 1 oz	155	9	17
Tortilla Chips: Average, 1 oz	140	7	19

(1 oz = approx. 12 chips or 13 strips)

	C	F	Cb
Baked! Tostitos (15) 1 oz	110	1	24
Doritos: 13 chips, 1 oz	140	7	18
Light, 13 chips, 1 oz	100	2	19
Baked! Nacho Cheesier, 1 oz	120	3.5	21
Garden of Eatin', 1 oz	140	6	19
Lay's Kettle, average, 1 oz	150	8	18
Munchies Mix, ¾ cup, 1 oz	130	5	19
Padrino Reduced Fat, 1 oz	130	4	20
Stacy's, Baked, 14 chips, 1 oz	130	4	18
Utz Low-Fat Baked, 8 chips, 1 oz	140	7	19
Wild Oats, 14 chips, 1 oz	140	5	19

Pretzels

Average All Brands 🅒 🅕 🅒ᵇ

Hard Baked Pretzels: *Per Pretzel*

	C	F	Cb
1 oz	110	1	23
Sticks, thin, 2¼" (9/oz), each	12	0	3
Twists, thin, ¼" thick, (5/oz), 1	25	0.2	5
Dutch (2¾"x 2⅝") ½ oz, 1	55	1	11
Sourdough (Shultz), ¾ oz, each	80	0	17
Fat Free Pretzels:			
Snyders (1), avg., 1 oz	100	0	23
Mini (20), 1 oz	110	0	25
Utz Wheels/Nuggets, 1 oz	100	0	22
Rold Gold: Sticks (48), 1 oz	100	0	23
Sourdough Nuggets (12), 1 oz	100	0	23
Sourdough Hards (1), ¾ oz	100	0.5	21
Thins (9), 1 oz	110	1	23
Twists (8), 1 oz	110	1	22
Tiny Twists/Sticks (16), 1 oz	105	1	23
Low Fat Pretzels:			
American Fare Mini Twists, 1oz	110	1	23
Frito-Lay, Rold Gold:			
Butter Checkers, 20 pces, 1 oz	120	1	25
Braided Twists (8), 1 oz	110	1	22
Choc-coated (Snyders), 1 oz	130	6	18
White Choc covered, 7 pces, 1 oz	140	6	19
Yogurt (Wild Oats), 8 pces, 1.4 oz	210	10	27
Soft Pretzels (Twists) average:			
Plain: Regular, 2.5 oz	185	2	36
King Size, 5 oz	370	4	72
Big Cheese, 1.76 oz	130	3	22
Peanut Butter filled (Tr. Joe's) 1 oz	150	8	14

Auntie Anne's: *See Fast-Foods Section*

Frito-Lay Pretzels

	C	F	Cb
Bitesize Twists, 23 pces, 1 oz	140	6	19
Braided Twists, 8 sticks, 1 oz	110	1	22

Snyder's of Hanover Pretzels

	C	F	Cb
Rods (3), 1 oz	120	1	24
Homestyle (15), 1 oz	120	1	25
Nibblers (20), 1 oz	120	0	25
SuperPretzel: Soft Pretzels (1)	160	1	34
Softstix (2)	130	3	22
Soft Pretzel Bites (5)	150	0.5	32
Pretzelfils: Pizza (2)	130	2	21
Pepperjack; Mozzarella, (2), avg.	130	3	20

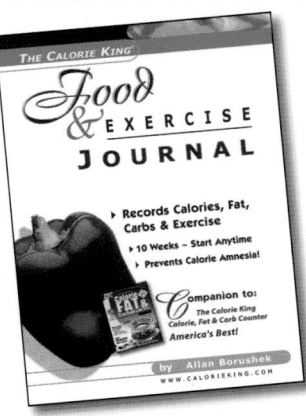
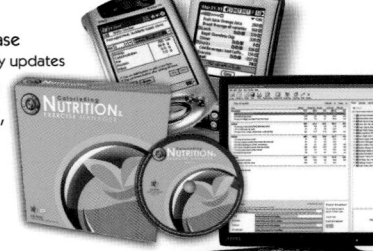

## Snacks	C	F	Cb

Note: Actual weight of packaged snacks is usually 5-10% more than label Net Wt. For accuracy, weigh snack and allow extra calories for any extra weight.

Item	C	F	Cb
Bacon Cheese Crackers, 1 oz	190	10	24
Banana Chips, ¼ cup, 13 chips, 1 oz	150	8	20
Beef Jerky (Lance), average, 1 oz	70	1	4
Beef Sticks (Frito-Lay's) 1 oz	90	7	2
Bugles, Original, 1⅓ cup, 1 oz	160	9	18
Cajun Jerky, 1 strip, ½ oz	55	1	1
Cheddar Lites (Health Valley) 1 oz	120	3	21
Cheese Crackers (Frito-Lay): 1 oz	130	6	18
Cheese Filled, 1 oz	210	11	24
Cheese Curls: 1 cup, 1 oz	150	6	19
Reduced Fat, 1 oz	140	6	18
Cheese Nips (Nabisco), 38, 1 oz	150	6	19
Cheese Puffs: Average, 1 oz	150	8	12
Lite, 1 oz	130	5	19
American Fare, 1¼ cup, 1 oz	150	9	18
Cheese Twists, 1 oz	160	10	13
Cheetos: Regular all flavors, 1 oz	160	10	13
Baked!, cheese flavored, 1 oz	130	5	19
Cheez Balls, 27 balls, 1 oz	170	12	13
Cheez It: White Cheddar, 1 pkt (26)	150	8	18
Original (27)	160	8	18
Reduced Fat (29)	130	4	20
Chex Mix (General Mills):			
Bold Blend; Peanut, ½ cup	140	6	20
Other varieties, avg., ½ cup	135	4.5	22
Churros (Mex. Pastry) 10", 1.2 oz	140	9	12
Cinna Chips (T.J. Cinn.) 3, 1 oz	110	5	15
Combos (Oven Baked):			
Crackers, ⅓ cup, 1 oz	140	6	18
1 cup, 3 oz	420	18	54
Pretzels, ⅓ cup, 1 oz	130	4.5	19
1 cup, 3 oz	390	14	57
Cookies: See Pages 105-112			
Cool Cuts: Carrot & Ranch	60	4	5
Celery & Peanut Butter	170	14	9
Corn Chips: See Page 133			
Corn Crunchies/Spirals, 1 oz	100	1.5	21
Corn Nuts: ⅓ cup, 1 oz	130	4.5	20
1.7 oz bag	220	7.5	34
Corn Puffs: Health Valley, 2 c., 1 oz	120	1.5	25
Pirate's Booty, 1 oz	130	5	18
Wotsits (Walker), 21g, (¾ oz) pkg	110	6.5	11
Dunkin Stixs (Hostess), 3, 4oz	490	25	63
Flavor Twists (Fritos), 1 oz	160	10	16

## Snacks (Cont)	C	F	Cb

Item	C	F	Cb
French's Potato Sticks ¾ c., 1 oz	180	12	16
Funyun's: Onion flavor, 1 oz	140	7	18
Mini, 2 oz	270	13	35
Girlfriend's Booty, 1 oz	120	4.5	8
Goldfish (Pepperidge Farm) 1 oz	140	5	20
Gold-N-Chees (Lance), 1 oz	150	8	17
Handi Snacks (Kraft), avg., 1 pkg	110	5	16
Honey Mustard Onion Pieces			
(Snyder's) 1 pkg, 2 oz	280	14	36
Hot Peanuts (Lays), 3 Tbsp	190	16	6
Jerky (Beef), 1 oz stick	80	1	5
Lance Sandwich:			
Capt. Wafers; Choc-O-Mint, (4)	70	3	9
Sour Dough w. Cheddar, 1 pkg	240	15	23
Other varieties, average, 1 pkg	200	10	22
Munchies (Frito-Lay):			
Classic Mix, ¾ cup, 1 oz	140	7	18
Go Snacks Mini Mix, 2.37 oz can	310	10	48
Kids Mix, ¾ cup, 1 oz	130	4	20
Traditional Mix, ¾ cup, 1 oz	130	5	19
Munchos, 16 pieces, 1 oz	160	10	16
Nabisco: Chips Ahoy, 1.3 oz	160	8	22
Cheese Nips (38), 1 oz	150	6	19
Nutter Butter Bites (10), 35g	170	7	24
Oreo, 1.3 oz	160	7	25
Ritz Bits Go-Pak Cheese (12)	160	9	16
Ritz Bits S'Mores, 1 oz	150	6	22
Mixers, avg., 1 oz	130	4.5	19
Nibblers (Snyder's): Regular (13)	130	3	24
Fat Free (16)	120	0	25
Onion Rings (T.G.I. Friday), 1 oz	140	7	16
Oriental Mix (Rice Snacks), 1 oz	130	4	21
Rice Snacks (Wild Oats) ⅔ c. 1 oz	110	0	25
Oyster Crackers (Sunshine), 1 oz	120	2	22
Party Mix (Cheez-It) ½ c., 1 oz	130	4.5	19
Peanut Butter Nuggets (10), 1 oz	140	6	15
Pirate's Booty w. White Ched., 1 oz	130	5	18
Pita Chips, avg., (9) 1 oz	130	4	18
Popcorn: See Page 132			
Pork Skins/Rind: Baken-ets, 1 oz	160	10	0
Lance, 1 pkg	80	5	0
Potato Chips: See Page 133			
Potato Puffs, 1 oz	110	3	21
Potato Skins (TGI Friday), 1 oz	150	9	17
Potato Sticks (Ralph's), ⅔ c., 1.1oz	170	11	15

Snacks (Cont)	C	F	Cb
Quakes: Caramel Corn (7)	60	0	13
Apple Cinn. (8)	60	0	15
BBQ (10); Ranch (10)	70	2.5	13
Chocolate (7)	60	1	13
Nacho/Cheddar Cheese (9)	70	2.5	11
Sour Cream & Onion (9)	75	2.5	12
Rice Chips, Bar-B-Q/Onion, 1 oz	140	7	18
Sandwich Crackers (Austin): Per Pkg			
Chse Cracker w. Pnut Butter, 1.37 oz	200	10	23
Reduced Fat, 1.26 oz	170	7	24
Chse Cracker w. Cheddar, 1.37 oz	210	10	26
PB & J Cracker Sandwich, 1.37 oz	200	10	24
Santitas (Frito-Lay), 1 oz	130	6	19
Sesame Sticks (Cityfarm), 1 oz	160	11	13
Soy Crisps, avg. 1 oz	105	2	15
Soy Nuts: Dry Roasted, ¼ cup, 1 oz	130	6	9
Choc-coated, 1 oz	140	7	13
Dr Soy Soy Nuts BBQ, 1 oz	150	8	8
Sun Chips (Frito-Lay), 1 oz pkg	140	6	18
TastyKake: Koffee Kake Jnr	280	10	44
Chocolate Jnr	340	12	55
Creme Filled Koffee Kakes (2)	270	13	35
Toast/Cheese Crackers, 1 pkg	220	11	23
Tortilla Chips: See Pages 133			
Tostitos: Regular, average, 1 oz	140	7	19
Light, 1 oz	90	1	20
Trail Mix (Nuts/Seeds/Dried Fruit):			
Regular, 3 Tbsp, 1 oz	150	9	10
Tropical, 3 Tbsp, 1 oz	130	6	17
w. Chocolate Chips, 1 oz	170	9	18
Dr Soy Trail Mix, 1 oz	110	4	12
Turkey Jerky Teriyaki (Oberto), 1 oz	80	1	5
Vegetable Snacks (Snyders), 1 oz	140	7	18
Veggie Chips, 1 oz	120	4	19
Veggie Stix, 1 oz	140	7	18
Wheatables (Keebler): Orig., (17)	140	6	20
Orig., Reduced Fat (19), 1 oz	140	4	23
Honey Wheat (17), 1 oz	140	6	20
Seven Grain (17), 1 oz	140	6	20
Yogurt Raisins (Sun-Maid), 1 oz	130	6	20

Fruit Snacks	C	F	Cb
Betty Crocker: Fruit Gushers, 25g	90	1	20
Fruit by the Foot, 1 roll, 21g	80	1	17
Fruit Roll Ups, 1 roll, 14g	50	1	12
Scooby Doo; G Force, 25g pkg	80	0	21
Kellogg's: Disney Fruit Snacks, 25g	80	0	21
Fruit Streamers, 1 Roll, 0.8 oz	80	1	19
Twistables, 23g	70	0.5	17
Yogos, 23g	90	1.5	18
Nabisco: Fruit Rolls (1), 0.74 oz	80	2	16
CapriSun Juicers, 1 pouch, 26g	80	0	19
Rugrats; Wacky Faces (1)	80	0	18
Blues Clues; Dora the Explorer (1)	60	0	14
100 Calorie Fruit Snacks, 1.1 oz	100	0	24
Sunkist: Fruit Snacks, 1 pouch	90	1	20
Fruit Smoothie Blitze, 1.3 oz	140	1	32

Vending Machines	C	F	Cb
Brownie, frosted (Lance)	320	12	52
Cheese Balls (Lance), 1 oz	170	12	13
Choc Chip Cookies (Nabisco), 40g	190	9	27
Choc Milk, 8 fl.oz	260	9	37
Coca-Cola Classic, 12 fl.oz	150	0	40
Diet Coke, 12 fl.oz	0	0	0
Corn Chips, 1 oz	160	10	15
Hostess Sweet Roll, 2.12 oz	210	7.5	34
Donut, plain, 1¾ oz	230	15	27
Fruit Pie (Hostess), 4½ oz	480	20	68
Granola/Cereal Bars	140	3	26
Hershey's, 1.55 oz bar	240	13	25
Hot Fries (Lance), 1 oz	150	10	15
Kellogg's Rice Krispies Treat	120	4.5	20
Lance Captain's Wafers, 1 pkg	200	10	22
M & M's: Plain, 1.7 oz	240	10	34
Peanuts, 1.7 oz	250	13	30
Milk: Whole, 8 fl.oz	150	8	13
Reduced Fat, 2%, 8 fl.oz	130	5	13
Milky Way, 2 oz	260	10	41
Onion Rings, 1 oz	140	7	16
Orange Juice, 8 fl.oz	110	0	26
Peanuts, roasted (Lance), 1 oz	200	15	6
Popcorn, plain, 1 oz	160	8	16
Pork Skins, 1 oz	160	10	0
Potato Chips, 1 oz	150	10	15
Reduced Fat, 1 oz	140	7	20
Pretzels, 1 oz	110	1	23
Raisins, ½ oz pkg	45	0	11
Reece's Peanut Butter Cups, 1.8 oz	280	17	28
Snickers, 2.1 oz bar	280	14	35
Tortilla Chips, 1 oz	140	7	9

Breakfast Bars ◆ Sports & Diet Bars

Note: Actual weight of bars is usually 5-10% more than label Net Wt. Weigh bar and allow extra calories.

Breakfast Bars

	C	F	Cb
Atkins: Morning Start Bars,			
Crisp, avg., 1.3 oz bar	180	9	14
Cinnamon Bun, 1.4 oz bar	150	7	15
Barbara's Bakery: Multigrain, 1.3 oz	120	1.5	25
Puffins Cereal & Milk Bars, avg.	135	2	24
General Mills: Milk 'n Cereal Bars,			
Cinnamon Toast Crunch, 45g	180	4	33
Peanut Butter Toast Crunch	190	5	33
Other varieties, average	160	4	29
Health Valley Bar, avg., 1.3 oz	130	2	29
Kellogg's			
All-Bran Bar, 1.23 oz	130	3	27
Crunch Bar, avg., 1 oz	110	2	22
Cereal & Milk Bars, avg., 0.8 oz	105	3	17
Smart Start Bars, 1.4 oz	150	2.5	30
Pop Tarts: Sponge Bob Sq. Pants	200	5	35
French Toast, 1 pastry	220	8	35
Fruit/Frosted, avg. all flavors	200	5	37
Low-Fat, all flavors	190	3	39
Pastry Swirls, avg., 2.2 oz	260	11	37
Snak Stix, 1 pastry, 1.8 oz	200	5	36
Yogurt Blasts, 1 pastry	210	6	37
Nature's Path: Crispy Rice, avg.	110	3	20
New England Natural Bakers			
Save the Forest Bars (1)	120	4	19
Nutri-Grain Bars			
Cereal Bars, avg., 1.3 oz	140	3	26
Muffin Bars, avg., 1.6 oz	170	4	31
Yogurt Bars, avg., 1.3 oz	140	3	26
Post, Honey Bunches of Oats Bar	130	3	25
Quaker			
Breakfast Graham Bar (1), avg	130	3.5	22
Fruit & Oatmeal Bites (3) 1 pouch	140	3	27
Fruit & Oatmeal Bars (1), avg.	130	2.5	27
Oatmeal To Go Bars, avg., 2.1 oz	220	4	43
Granola Bars: See Page 140			
Slim-Fast: Optima Bkfast Bars	180	6	22
Low Carb Breakfast Bars, avg.	180	6	19
South Beach Diet (Kraft)			
High Protein Cereal Bars (1), 35g	140	5	15
Special K Cereal Bars, avg., 0.8 oz	90	1.5	18

Other Bars

	C	F	Cb
Per Bar			
AdvantEdge			
Carb Control Crisp Bar	230	7	27
Carb Control Nutrition Bar	200	7	21
Complete Nutrition Bar	210	5	27
Alpen: Per 3.5 oz Bar			
Cereal Bars: Fruit & Nut	395	9	71
Apple & Blackberry w. Yogurt	420	12	73
Fruit & Nut w. Chocolate	430	15	68
Atkins: Endulge (See Page 125)			
Advantage Bar, avg., 2.1 oz	240	11	22
Avid Source (Mission Nutrition)	240	6	22
Balance: Balance Bars, 1.7 oz	200	6	23
Balance Plus Bars, 1.76 oz	200	6	22
Carb Well: Caramel 'n Choc., 1.7 oz	190	8	23
Chocolate Fudge, 1.7 oz	190	6	23
Chocolate Peanut Butter, 1.7 oz	200	8	22
100 Calorie Bar, avg., 1 oz	100	4	14
Gold Crunch Bars, avg., 1.7 oz	210	6	23
Gold Bars, avg., 1.7 oz	210	7	22
Trail Mix Energy Bar, 1.8 oz	210	7	22
Barbara's Bakery Granola, ¾ oz	80	2	14
Bariatrix Proti-Bar: (15g Protein)			
Caramel Nut, 40g	150	4.5	15
Bear Valley: Meal Pack, 3.75 oz	410	12	60
Bumble Bar, average, 1.6 oz	225	12	24
Biochem: Strive, avg., 2.1 oz	190	9	24
Lo Carb Deluxe, 2.5 oz	250	7	23
Sierra, 2.3oz bar	270	10	26
Ultimate Lo Carb, 2.1 oz	210	6	24
Body Smarts: Choc. P'nut Crunch	210	6	34
Yogurt Berry Crunch	200	5	35
Bumble Bar, 1.6 oz	230	15	20
Carb Options, 1.76 oz bar	200	8	17
Carb Solutions: Sugar Free, 1 oz	170	10	17
High Protein: Per Bar (2.1 oz)			
Chocolate Toffee Hazelnut	230	11	21
Other varieties, avg.	250	10	16

Note: Actual weight of bars is usually 5-10% more than label Net Wt. Weigh bar and allow extra calories.

Other Bars (Cont)

Per Bar	C	F	Cb
Carb Watchers: Lean Body, 2.5 oz	290	9	22
CarbWise			
Crisp Bars, avg., 1.76 oz	200	9	24
CarbWise Gold Bar, 1.76 oz	190	7	18
Choc. Peanut Crunch, 2.1 oz	210	10	23
Carbolite			
Choc Almond, 1.75 oz	230	17	25
Choc Crisp Bar, 1.75 oz	250	17	27
Milk/Dairy Choc, avg., 1.75 oz	250	19	28
CarbRite Diet (Doctor's), avg., 2 oz	200	35	23
Champion Nutrition, SnacBar	180	3	24
Cheetah (NutraFig), 2.25 oz bar	210	2	43
Choice, all types, 1.23 oz bar	140	4.5	17
Clif Bars			
Builders Bars, 2.5 oz	270	8	30
Luna Bar, average, 1.5 oz	180	4.5	27
Mojo Bar, average, 1.5 oz	210	8	21
Nectar Bar, average, 1.6 oz	170	6	29
Z Bar, average, 1.26 oz	120	3	22
Designer Whey			
Zanzibar, 3 oz	330	9	34
Gourmet Bars, avg. all flav., 2.7 oz	260	7	7
Detour (Next Proteins), 2.8 oz bar	310	10	30
Dr Soy			
Protein Bar, Lemon, 1.76 oz	170	4	26
Chocolate/Peanut, 1.76 oz	180	4.5	25
Healthy Snacker, avg., 1.7 oz	180	6	28
EAS Advantage Edge			
Carb Control, average, 2.12 oz	200	7	21
Complete Nutrition, 2.12 oz Bar:			
Choc Caramel Chewy	240	8	28
Rocky Road Crisp Bar	210	5	27
EAS Body For Life, avg.	200	7	21

> *Life is what happens to you while you're busy making other plans.*
> ~ John Lennon

Per Bar	C	F	Cb
EAS Myoplex			
Deluxe Nutrition Bar, avg., 3.2 oz	335	9	36
Lite Nutyrition Bar, avg., 1.97 oz	190	4	28
Carb Sense, average, 2.5 oz	255	7	24
Eat Well Be Well			
Rich Velvety Choc, avg., 1.2 oz bar	175	12	16
Elev8 me: Protein & Fruit Trail,			
All Fruit Blend, 2.3 oz bar	210	3	32
Cocoa & Coconut, 2.3 oz	230	6	32
Ensure Healthy Mom (2) 1.4 oz	150	2.5	27
Fi-Bar Nectar Granola Bars, 1 oz	120	2	23
Chewy & Nutty Bar, 1.2 oz	140	4.5	23
GeniSoy: Low Carb Crunch, 1.5 oz	150	4.5	19
Soy Protein Bars, avg., 2.2 oz	235	4.5	33
Glenny's: Light 'n Crispy, ½ oz	60	2.5	9
Slim Carb: Double Fudge, 1.3 oz	130	2.5	19
Other varieties, 1.3 oz	90	4	2
Glucerna: Meal Replacement, 2 oz	220	7	32
Snack Bar, avg., 1.3 oz	140	4	24
GNC ProCrunch: Choc Crisp	260	7	34
Peanut Butter Crunch	260	7	34
Cookies n' Cream; S'Mores	250	4	37
Greens + Bar: + Energy, avg., 2 oz	245	10	33
+ High Protein, avg., 1.6 oz	255	12	22
Health Valley Fruit/Granola, avg.	190	5	29
Henry's Top Vine: Roundup, 1.4oz	165	5	26
Honey Peanutty, 1.4 oz	230	17	10
Hershey's Smart Zone, avg, 50g	200	7	21
High Protein: Peanut Butter, 4 oz	300	6	33
Other varieties, average	335	8	36
HMR Benefit Bar, 1.1 oz	160	5	27
Jay Bar, average, 2 oz	230	10	27
Jenny Craig: Choc/Yogurt, 1.97 oz	220	5	33
Oatmeal Raisin, 1.97 oz	210	3	35
Milk Choc; Lemon Meringue	210	5	32
Joyva Sesame Crunch, 1.1 oz	190	8	15
Joy Ride Bars: See Next Proteins			
Kashi Golean: Bars, avg., 2.7 oz	290	5	48
Crunchy!, avg., 1.76 oz bar	170	4.5	30
Go Lean Roll, avg., 1.9 oz	190	5	28
Kellogg's, Krave Bars, 1.7 oz avg.	200	7	29

Per Bar	C	F	Cb
Kudos: Chocolate Chip	130	5	20
Peanut Butter	130	6	18
M&M's; Snickers, average	100	3	17
Larabar: Apple/Cherry Pie, 1.6 oz	190	9	22
Banana Cookie Dough, 1.8 oz	210	10	24
Lean Body, 76g	280	6	15
Lindora: Chocolate Chip	140	2	15
Other varieties, average	150	4.5	18
Luna Bars: *See Clif Bars*			
Marathon *(Snickers):* Energy, 2 oz	220	7	30
Low Carb, average, 1.7 oz	170	7	19
Protein, average, 2.8 oz	290	8	40
Medifast: Fit! Bar, 1.5 oz	165	4	19
Plus for Diabetics, avg., 1.5 oz	135	4	22
Met-Rx: "Big 100", average, 3.5 oz	360	5	53
Protein Plus, avg., 3 oz	325	8	32
MLO Bio Protein *(BioTech)*, 2.85 oz	300	7	39
Mojo Bars: *See Clif Bars*			
MRM Response, 2.1 oz	200	8	20
Muscle Tech: Nitro-Tech, average	280	7	29
Cookie Bar, 2.7 oz	310	12	25
Oat Bar, 3.4 oz	350	11	40
Myoplex: *See EAS*			
Nabisco, HoneyMaid Bars, 37g	150	4.5	27
Nature Valley Granola Bars			
Chewy w. Yogurt coating, avg, 40g	140	4	26
Crunchy, average, 2 bars, 42g	190	7	30
Heart Healthy: Honey Nut, 40g	160	4	28
Oatmeal Raisin, 40g	150	2	30
Sweet & Salty, avg.,35g	165	8	20
Trail Mix, average, 35g	140	4	26
Nature's Path			
Rebound, 2 oz	190	4	33
Optimum Energy, avg., 1.97 oz	200	3	37
Flax Plus; Hemp Plus, average	170	5	29
Granola: Apricot 'n Nut	180	7	28
Cranberry Soy	170	5	28
New You: Peanut Butter, 1.65 oz	185	5	25
Choc Chip; Lemon Crisp, 1.65 oz	170	3	26

Per Bar	C	F	Cb
Next Proteins: Detour, 2.8 oz	330	10	30
Joy Ride, 2.8 oz	340	12	27
One Way, 3 oz	340	12	29
U-Turn Protein, 2.8 oz	300	8	26
NiteBite (Time-release Glucose Bar)			
Choc. Fudge; P'nut Butter, 25g	100	3.5	15
Nutiva: Hempseed, 1.4 oz	210	14	11
Flax Chocolate, 1.4 oz	200	12	19
NutriSystem Nourish, avg., 1.44 oz	125	3	20
Nutrilite: Protein Bars, average	250	9	22
Meal Replacements, average	220	7	28
XS Power Nutrition, 1.6 oz	185	6	18
Odwalla Energy Bars			
Choc. Chip Peanut/Crunch, avg.	245	7	38
Super Protein	230	4.5	31
Other varieties, avg.	220	3.5	43
One Way Bars: *See Next Proteins*			
Opti-Pro Meal (ABB)	290	5	40
Organic Food Bar, avg., 2.4 oz	300	12	34
Phil's Bar, 50g	200	6	22
Planters CarbWell			
Peanut Butter Crunch, 35g	160	12	16
Caramel Choc Crunch, 38g	180	13	17
PR Bar Ironman, 49.6g	190	6	22
Power Bar: Harvest Dip'd, avg., 2.3 oz	255	5	45
Harvest; Performance, avg, 2.3 oz	250	5	42
Nut Naturals, avg., 1.6 oz	210	10	20
Pria Bars: Average, 1 oz	110	3	17
Carb Select, avg., 1.7 oz	195	8	21
Protein Plus: Average, 2.75 oz	290	5	38
Carb Select, average	270	11	32
Triple Threat, avg., 1.93 oz	210	10	20
Power Crunch, average, 1.3 oz	170	8	8
Premier: Protein Eight, 2.4 oz	260	7	23
Premier Protein Bar, 2.5 oz	280	8	20
Odyssey Bar, avg., 2.8 oz	310	11	29
Twisted Bar, avg., 1.6 oz	190	6	21
Promax: Average, 2.7 oz bar	290	6	40
Triple Layer Bar, 2.5 oz	290	8	34
Protein Complete, avg., 1.97 oz	190	4	18

Granola, Sports & Diet Bars (Cont)

Other Bars (Cont)

Per Bar	C	F	Cb
Prozone Nutrition Bar: 50g	195	6	18
Fruit Snax Bar, 1.4 oz	140	0	23
Pure Protein: *See Worldwide Sport Nutrition*			
Pure Fit, average, 2 oz bar	235	6	27
Quaker Chewy Granola Bars			
Chewy (Regular): Avg. all flavors	120	4	20
Peanut Butter/Chocolate	120	3.5	20
Cookies & Milk, average	120	3.5	20
Dipps: Choc Chip	150	6	21
Peanut Butter	150	7	18
Fruit 'N Crunch, average	160	3.5	31
Trail Mix, average	150	5	24
Wholesome Favorites, avg. 1.2oz	110	2	22
Real Protein, avg., 2.75 oz bar	290	5	28
Resource, OptiSource Mini Bar	90	2.5	10
Revival Soy Bars *(Direct):* Per Bar			
Chocolate Temptation	270	7	32
Apple Cinnamon; Marshm. Krunch	220	3	30
Peanut Butter/Choc Pal, avg.	250	7	29
Smart Carb, average all flavors	235	8	31
Russell Stover: Pecan Delight,			
2 pieces	240	16	22
Pecan Delight Sugar Free, 2 pces	130	9	15
Diabetx : Toffee Square, 1 oz	100	7	14
Pecan Delights, 1 oz	130	9	16
SCAN Diet, 45g	160	2.5	26
Slim-Fast Bars			
High Protein Meal Bars, avg.	195	6.5	20
Optima: Breakfast Bars, avg.	180	6	22
Meal Bars, average	220	5	35
Snack Bars, average	120	4	20
Granola Bars, average	220	6	35
Low Carb Diet: Meal Bars, average	180	6	18
Snacks, average	120	5	18
Original: Brkfst & Lunch Bars, avg.	140	5	20
Meal-On-The-Go, average	220	5	36

Per Bar	C	F	Cb
Skippy Snack Bars, avg., 1.2 oz	170	12	16
SlimWhey, average, 1.1 oz	120	4	14
Solo GI, average, 47g	190	6	23
Spiru-tein *(Nature's Plus),* 1.4 oz	165	4	21
Steel Bar *(ABB),* 2 oz	250	4	36
Strive *(Biochem),* avg., 2.1 oz	230	9	24
The Sports Club/LA:			
Caramel Cr./Choc P'nut (16g prot.)	200	5	22
P'nut Butter Fudge (13g prot.)	185	9	13
Think Thin! Low Carb, avg., 2.1 oz	230	8	23
Energy Bar, 1.23 oz	140	5	20
Green Bar, 1.76 oz	175	5	28
Organic Bar, 1.76 oz	215	10	29
Protein Bar, 2.1 oz	230	8	25
Tiger's Milk: 35g Bar	140	5	19
Peanut Butter varieties	150	7	18
Protein Rich	150	5	18
Tri-O-Plex, avg., 4.2 oz	430	16	45
U-Turn Bars: *See Next Proteins*			
Ultimate Lo Carb: *See Biochem*			
Ultimate Protein Bar, 78g	290	4.5	19
Usana: Fiberg Bar, 48g	100	1.5	23
Nutrition Bar: Wild Berry	150	2.5	23
Peanut Butter Crunch	150	4	20
Vyo-Pro *(AST)* Chocolate, 2.2 oz	200	7	24
Whole Foods			
Ella Bar: Lemon; Huckleberry, 1.7 oz	170	2	29
Other varieties, avg., 1.7 oz	180	4.5	28
Worldwide Sport Nutrition: Pure Protein,			
Country Berry; Choc Chip, 1.76 oz	190	5	19
Chocolate Deluxe, 2.75 oz	270	7	26
Chocolate Peanut Butter, 2.75 oz	300	9	26
Zanzibar *(Designer Whey)* avg.	330	9	34
Zoe Flax & Soy, Choc., 1.8 oz	190	6.5	28
ZonePerfect, average, 1.76 oz	210	7	23

For full nutritional data and product updates
check the food database of the author's
website www.CalorieKing.com

Nuts	C	F	Cb
Per 1 oz Unless Indicated			
Acorns, raw 1 oz	110	7	12
Almonds, Dried/Dry Roasted:			
Whole, 24-28 med., 1 oz	170	15	5.5
½ cup, 2½ oz	420	37	13
Chopped,½ cup, 2¼ oz	380	34	12
Sliced, ½ cup, 1⅔ oz	280	25	9
Choc. coated (5-6), 1 oz	150	10	15
Oil Rstd *(Blue Diamond)*, 1 oz	170	16	5
Honey Roasted, 1 oz	170	14	8
Almond Meal (partially defattened)			
1 cup (not packed), 2¼ oz	260	11	11
Brazil Nuts, 8 medium, 1 oz	185	19	3.5
Cashews, Dry or Oil Roasted:			
14 large/18 med./26 small, 1 oz	165	14	9
½ cup, 2.4 oz	375	31	20
Honey Roasted, 1 oz	165	13	10
Chestnuts, avg. all: Dried, 1 oz	105	1	22
Raw/Fresh, 5-6 nuts, 1 oz	60	0	13
Canned, water chestnuts,			
sliced/whole/drained, 1 oz	30	0	7
Coconut: Flesh, 1 oz	100	10	4
Raw: 1 pce. (2"x2"x½"), 1.6 oz	160	15	7
½ medium (4½" diam.)	700	66	30
Dried (Desiccated):			
Unsweetened, 1 oz	187	18	7
Sweetened: Shredded, 1 oz	140	10	13
Grated, ½ cup, 1.3 oz	185	12	18
Cream (canned), 1 oz	285	26	12
Milk (canned), ½ cup, 4 oz	225	24	3
Water (center liq.), ½ c., 4¼ oz	23	0	4.5
Filberts or Hazelnuts:			
Shelled, 18-20 nuts	180	17	4.5
Chopped, ¼ cup, 1 oz	180	18	5
Ground, ¼ cup, 0.6 oz	120	12	3
Ginkgo Nuts, can., 14 med., 1 oz	32	0.5	6.5
Hickory, 30 small nuts, 1 oz	200	18	5
Macadamia Nuts, shelled:			
Raw, 7 med./14 small, 1 oz	200	21	4
½ cup, 2.3 oz	480	51	10
Dry Roasted, 1 oz	205	22	4
½ cup, 2.4 oz	480	51	9
Choc. coated, 2-3 pces, 1 oz	170	12	14
Mixed Nuts: 18-22 nuts, 1 oz	170	15	7
Planters: Dry Roasted/Honey	170	15	7
Oil Roasted, all types	180	16	7
Sweet Roasts, 26 pces, 1 oz	160	12	10
Nut Toppings: Chopped, 1 T., ¼ cup	40	4	1.5

Per 1 oz Unless Indicated

Peanuts:	C	F	Cb
Raw/Dried: In shell, 1 oz	117	10	3
Shelled, 1 oz	160	14	4.5
Boiled, shelled, ½ cup, 3.1 oz	285	20	19
Roasted: 30 lge./60 sml., 1 oz	165	14	6
1 cup, 5.1 oz	860	76	22
Chopped, 3 Tbsp, 1 oz	165	14	6
Planters: Cocktail, 1 oz	170	14	6
Rich Roasted in Choc., 2½ oz	220	14	19
Roasted in Shell, Salted, 1 oz	160	14	6
Dry Roasted, 1oz	160	13	6
Honey/ & Dry Roasted, 1 oz	160	13	8
Spanish Raw, 1 oz	150	13	6
Spanish Redskin, 1 oz	180	14	5
Sweet N' Crunchy, 1 oz	140	7	16
Pecans: Kernel halves, 1 oz	195	20	4
(20 Jumbo or 31 large halves)			
1 cup halves, 3.8 oz	755	78	15
Chopped, ½ cup, 2 oz	380	39	7.5
Oil Roasted, 15 halves, 1 oz	205	20	4
Honey Roasted, 1 oz	200	21	4
Pilinuts, dried, ¼ cup, 1 oz	215	24	1
Pinenuts, dried, 1 Tbsp, 10g	70	7	1.5
Pistachios: Unshelled, ½ cup, 2 oz	165	14	7
Shelled, ¼ cup, 45 nuts, 1 oz	170	14	8.5
Lance, 1.1 oz package	95	7	4
Sesame Nut Mix: *Planters,* 1 oz	160	13	9
Soy Nuts: Dry Roasted, 1 oz	130	6	9
½ cup, 3 oz	390	18	28
Dr Soy: Choc coated, 1 oz pkg	140	7	13
Flavors, average, 1 oz	150	8	8
Trail Mix *(Planters):* Fruit & Nut, 1 oz	140	9	14
Golden Nut Crunch, 1 oz	160	11	12
Honey Nut & Caramel, 1 oz	160	10	16
Mixed Nuts & Raisins, 1 oz	150	11	10
Nut & Chocolate, 1 oz	160	10	16
Nuts, Seeds & Raisins, 1 oz	160	12	11
Spicy Nuts & Cajun Sticks 1 oz	150	10	13
Sweet & Nutty, 1 oz	150	10	14
Walnuts:			
Black: 15-20 halves, 1 oz	175	17	3
Chopped, ¼ cup, 1.1 oz	195	18	3
English/Persian:			
14 halves, 1 oz	185	18	4
Chopped, ¼ cup, 1 oz	190	19	4
Ground, ¼ cup, 0.7 oz	130	13	3

Seeds ◆ Supplements

Seeds

	C	F	Cb
Alfalfa Seeds, sprouted, ½ c., ½ oz	5	0	1
Caraway, Fennel, 1 tsp	7	0.5	1
Cottonseed Kernels, rst., 1 Tbsp	50	3.5	2
Flax Seeds, 3 Tbsp, 1 oz	140	9	9
Lotus Seeds, dried, 1 c., ½ oz	55	0.5	10
Poppy Seeds, 1 tsp	15	1	1
Pumpkin & Squash Seeds, whole:			
Roasted/Tamari, 1 oz	150	12	4
½ cup, 4 oz	590	48	15
Dried, 142 hulled seeds, 1 oz	155	13	5
Safflower Kernels, dried, 1 oz	150	11	10
Sesame Seeds: Dried, 1 Tbsp, 9g	50	4.5	2
Roasted/Toasted, 1 oz	160	14	7.5
Sunflower Kernels/Seed:			
Dry Roasted, 1 Tbsp, 8g	45	4	2
¼ cup, 1 oz	165	14	7
Oil Roasted, ⅓cup, 1 oz	170	14	6.5
Watermelon, dried, ¼ cup, 1 oz	150	13	4

Quick Guide

Peanut Butter: *Average All Brands*

	C	F	Cb
½ cup, 5 oz	850	70	30
1 level tsp, 6g	35	3	1.5
1 level Tbsp, 0.6 oz (17g)	105	8.5	3.5
2 level Tbsp, 1.2 oz (34g)	210	17	7
1 oz Quantity (28g)	170	14	6
Jif: Reduced Fat, 2 Tbsp	190	12	15
Creamy; Crunchy; Simply, 2 Tbsp	190	16	7
Peanut Butter & Honey, 2 Tbsp	190	15	11
Peter Pan: Plus (Vits/Mins) 2 T., 1.2 oz	190	16	6
Honey Roast, 2 Tbsp, 1.2 oz	190	14	12
Peanut Wonder, 2 Tbsp	100	2.5	13
Smucker's: Honey Swtnd., 2 Tbsp	200	16	9
Goober Grape/Strawb., 2 Tbsp	160	9	16
Skippy: Carb Options, 1 Tbsp	190	8.5	5
Reduced Fat, 2 Tbsp	190	12	15
Squeeze Stix, 1 Tube, 0.9 oz	140	12	5

Other Nut & Seed Butters

	C	F	Cb
Almond Butter, 1 Tbsp, ½ oz	100	10	3.5
Almond Butter Honey Rstd, 1 T.	90	7	5.5
Beanut Butter, 1 Tbsp, ½ oz	90	5.5	7
Cashew Butter, 1 Tbsp, ½ oz	95	8	4.5
Hazelnut Butter, 1 Tbsp, ½ oz	90	10	2.5
Pecan Butter, 1 Tbsp, ½ oz	110	10	2
Pistachio Butter, 1 Tbsp, ½ oz	90	6.5	4.5
Sesame Butter/Tahini, 1 T., ½ oz	90	8	3
Soy Nut Butter, 1 Tbsp, ½ oz	75	5	4
Sunflower Seed Butter, 1 Tbsp	95	8	4
Nutella Hazelnut Spread, 2 Tbsp	200	11	24

Supplements

	C	F	Cb
Aloe Vera Juice, undiluted, 2 fl.oz	5	0	1
Cod Liver Oil, 1 Tbsp	125	13	0
Evening Primrose Oil, capsules, 1	5	0.5	0
Fiber Supplements: Tabs, 1	1	0	0
Metamucil, 1 packet	5	0	1
Regular, 1 rounded Tbsp	34	0	8
Sugar-Free, 1 Tbsp	6	0	1
Fish Oil Capsules, average, 1	10	1	0
Flax Oil: Capsules, 1	10	1	0
Barlean's, 3 softgels	110	11	0
Garlic Tablets/Capsules, each	3	0	1
Lecithin Granules, 1 Tbsp, 10g	55	4	0.5
Protein: Powders, average, 1 oz	100	0.5	0
Tablets, 20 tabs, ½ oz	70	0	0
Seaweed: Dried, 1 oz	85	0.5	22
Soaked, drained, 1 oz	15	0.5	3
Spirulina, 1 tablet	2	0	0.5
Vitamins/Minerals: Tabs/Caps, 1	2	0	0
Vitamin E Capsules, each	5	0.5	0
Viactiv Chews (1)	20	0.5	4
Yeast: Tablets, 2 tabs	4	0	0.5
Flakes, 1 heaping Tbsp, ⅓oz	30	0.5	4
Powder, 1 heaping Tbsp, ½ oz	50	0.5	6

Cough & Pharmaceutical

	C	F	Cb
Cough/Cold Syrups: *Per Tablespoon*			
Regular: w. sugar, 1 Tbsp	35	0	9
w. alcohol, 1 Tbsp	46	0	9
Sugar-Free *(Diabetic Tussin)*, 1 T.	0	0	0
Cough Drops/Lozenges: *See Page 131*			
Antacids: Average, 1 tablet	4	0	1
Liquid, 1 Tbsp	6	0	1
Sudafed Syrup, 1 tsp	14	0	3
Tylenol Liquid: Child, 1 tsp	17	0	4
Extra Strength, 1 tsp	11	0	3

𝒩ut eaters are healthier and live longer say medical researchers.

Nuts are a nutritious source of protein, antioxidants, vitamins, minerals, healthy fats and fiber.

Their fat and fiber content can help to lower blood cholesterol, but watch the quantity if overweight.

Weights As Purchased	C	F	Cb
Acerola, 1 cup, 20 pcs, 3½ oz	30	0	7.5
Apples: Whole, average all varieties,			
1 small (4 per lb), 4 oz	55	0	14
1 medium (3 per lb), 5½ oz	70	0	19
1 large (2 per lb), 8 oz	110	0	29
1 extra large, 11 oz	160	0	43
without skin, 1 medium, 4½ oz	60	0	16
Candy/Caramel Apple, 1 med., 6½ oz	245	4	54
Nut Coated, 1 medium	230	5	46
Apricots: 1 small (12 per lb)	17	0	4
1 medium (8 per lb), 2 oz	25	0	6
1 large (5-6 per lb), 3 oz	40	0	10
Avocado (w/out seed/skin):			
Average, ½ medium, 3½ oz	160	15	8
1 salad slice, ½ oz	25	2	1
Mashed/Puree, 2 Tbsp, 1 oz	50	4.5	2
¼ cup, 2 oz	90	9	5
Californian, ½ medium, 3 oz	160	14	8
Mashed/Puree, ½ c., 4 oz	190	18	10
Florida, ½ medium, 5½ oz	180	15	12
Mashed/Puree, ½ c., 4 oz	140	11	9
½ cup cubed, 3 oz	105	8	7

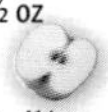

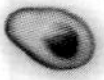

Note: Avocados are nutritious and contain no cholesterol. Fat is mainly monounsaturated and benefits blood cholesterol. Excellent substitute for butter or margarine.

	C	F	Cb
Banana: 1 small (6", 4 per lb), 4 oz	90	0	23
1 medium (7", 3 per lb), 5 oz	105	0	27
1 large (8", 2½ per lb), 7 oz	120	0	30
1 extra large (9"), 9 oz	135	0	35
w/out skin, 1 oz	25	0	6
Berries: (Blueberries/Black/Boysenberries)			
½ cup, 2.5 oz	40	0	10
1 pint, 14 oz	230	1.5	58
Breadfruit, ½ cup, 4 oz	115	0	30
Cactus Pear, 1 fruit, 3½ oz	40	0	9
Cantaloupe: Flesh/no rind, 1 oz	10	0	2
½ small, 20 oz (w. rind/seeds)	195	1	46
½ med., 28 oz (w. rind/seeds)	270	1.5	65
1 slice, 2.5 oz (w/out rind)	25	0	6
1 cup pieces/balls, 5.5 oz	55	0	13
Carambola (Star Fruit), 1 med	30	0	6
Cassava, ⅓ cup, 2½ oz	115	0	27
Cherimoya, 1 cup, 5.5 oz	115	1	27
Cherries: Sweet, 8 fruit, 2 oz	35	0	9
½ lb (30 cherries)	145	0.5	36
Sour, 8 fruit, 2 oz	30	0	7
½ lb (30 cherries)	115	0.5	28
Clementine, 1 med., 2.6 oz	35	0	9

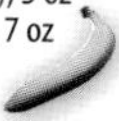

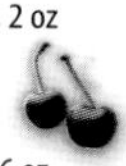

Weights As Purchased	C	F	Cb
Coconut: Fresh,			
1 piece, 2"x2"x ½", 1 oz	100	10	4.5
Shredded, fresh, ½ cup, 1.4 oz	140	13	6
Sweetened, dried, ½ cup, 1.6 oz	235	16	22
Crabapples, ½ cup slices, 2 oz	40	0	11
Cranberries, ½ cup, 2 oz	25	0	6.5
Currants: Per ½ Cup			
European Black, raw, ½ cup, 2 oz	35	0	8
Red & White, raw, ½ cup, 2 oz	30	0	7
Custard Apple, raw, 4 oz	115	1	28
Dates: See Dried Fruits			
Dragon Pearl Fruit, med., 11.6 oz	330	1.5	76
Durian, flesh, 4 oz	165	6	31
Elderberries, ½ cup, 2½ oz	55	0.5	13
Feijoas, 1 medium, 2 oz	30	0.5	5.5
Figs, green/black: 1 med., 2 oz	40	0	10
1 large, 3 oz	60	0	15
Fruit Salad, fresh, average,			
½ cup, 3½ oz	60	0	15
1 cup, 7 oz	120	0	30
Gooseberries, raw, ½ c., 2½ oz	35	0	7
Grapefruit: Average all types,			
½ fruit, 10 oz (6 oz flesh)	55	0	13
1 cup sections w. juice, 8 oz	75	0	18
Grapes: Average, 1 cup, 5½ oz	105	0	28
1 small bunch, 4 oz	80	0	20
1 medium bunch, 7 oz	140	0	36
1 large bunch, 16 oz	315	0	82
Granadilla, flesh, 3½ oz	95	0	23
Groundcherries, ½ cup, 2½ oz	35	0	8
Guava: 1 fruit, 4 oz	80	1	16
½ cup, 3 oz	55	0	12
Honeydew, 1 wedge (⅛ of 7" diam.),			
8 oz (with skin)	80	0	20
1 cup cubes/balls, 6 oz	60	0	14
Honey Murcots, 1 only, 5 oz	45	0	11
Jaboticaba, flesh, 4 oz	75	2	15
Jackfruit, flesh, ⅛ average, 4 oz	105	0	27
Jambos (Brazil Cherry), flesh, 4 oz	35	0	8
Java-Plum, 4 plums, ½ oz	10	0	2
Jujube, 3 oz	65	0	17
Kiwifruit, 1 medium, 2.7 oz	45	0	11
1 large, 3.2 oz	55	0.5	13
Kumquats, 5 medium, 3½ oz	65	1	15
Kiwano, ½ medium, 5 oz	35	0	8
Langsat, Duku, 1 medium, 2 oz	25	0	5
Lemon: 1 medium, 3 oz	25	0	8
1 wedge, 1 oz	5	0	1.5
Peel, 1 Tbsp	4	0	1
Limes, 1 med. (2" diam.), 2.4 oz	20	0	7
Loganberries, froz., ½ cup, 2½ oz	40	0	9

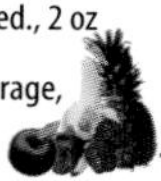

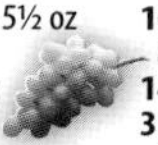

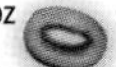

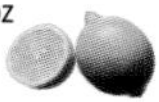

Fresh Fruit (Cont)

Weights As Purchased	C	F	Cb
Longans, 5 fruit, ½ oz	10	0	2.5
Loquats, 4 fruit, 2¼ oz	30	0	8
Lychees, 4 fruit, 2¼ oz	32	0	7
Mamey Apple: 1 whole, 3 lb	430	4	106
¼ fruit (1 cup flesh), 7 oz	100	1	25
Mandarin: 1 small, 3 oz	35	0	9
1 medium, 4 oz	45	0	11
1 large, 5 oz	50	0	13
Mango: Flesh, ½ cup slices, 3 oz	55	0	14
1 whole, medium, 11 oz	205	1	53
Melon, avg, 1 cup, cubes/balls, 6 oz	60	0	14
Monstera Deliciosa (Taxonia), Edible part, 4 oz	50	0	11
Mulberries, 20 fruit, 1 oz	15	0	3
Nashi Fruit (Asian Pear), 1 med., 7 oz	85	0	21
Nectarines: 1 medium, 4 oz	50	0	12
1 large, 5½ oz	70	0	16
Oheloberries, ½ cup, 2½ oz	20	0	5
Olives (Pickled): Green, 10 lrg, 1½ oz	60	6.5	1.5
Ripe, Greek Style, 10 med., 1 oz	70	6	4
Ripe (Black) Californian:			
1 small/medium	5	0	0.2
1 large/extra large	6	0.5	0.5
1 jumbo	7	0.5	0.5
1 colossal	11	1	0.5
1 super colossal	13	1	1
Oranges: Average all varieties,			
1 small, 5 oz (with skin)	45	0	11
1 medium (3" diam.), 7 oz	85	0	21
1 large, 10 oz	130	0	33
Flesh only, 1 cup, 6 oz	85	0	21
Californian Valencia,			
1 medium (2¾" diam.), 6 oz	60	0	14
Californ. Navels (3" diam.), 7 oz	70	0	17
Sunkist Navel, 14 oz	130	0	30
Florida Orange, 1 medium, 7 oz	70	0	17
Peel, 1 Tbsp	0	0	0
Papaya: ½ cup, cubed, 2½ oz	30	0	7
1 medium, (5"x3" diam.), 16 oz	120	0	30
Green (unripe), ½ cup, 3½ oz	20	0	5
Passionfruit, 1 medium, 1¼ oz	35	0	8
PawPaw (see Papaya)			
Peaches: 1 small/donut, 3 oz	30	0	7.5
1 medium (4 per lb), 4 oz	45	0	11
1 large, 6 oz	65	0	16
1 extra large, 10 oz	110	0	27

Weights As Purchased	C	F	Cb
Pears: Bartlett, 1 small, 5 oz	80	0	21
1 medium, 6 oz	95	0	26
1 large, 7½ oz	120	0	32
1 cup slices, 6 oz	95	0	26
Asian, 1 medium, 7 oz	85	0	21
Bosc, 6 oz	95	0	24
D'Anjou, 1 medium, 8 oz	120	0	30
Forelle, 1 medium, 7 oz	90	0	22
Red Pear, 5 oz	85	0	20
Seckel (Wash'ton), 2¼ oz	35	0	9
Pepino, ½ medium, 4 oz	20	0	4
Persimmons: Native, 1 oz	35	0	9
Japanese (2½"d. x 2½"h), 7 oz	120	0	30
Seedless (Maui), 1 md., 5 oz	100	0	25
Pineapple (no skin):			
1 thin slice (½"), 2 oz	27	0	7
1 thick slice (¾"), 3 oz	40	0	10
1 cup, diced, 5½ oz	75	0	19
1 medium, 1½ lb (peeled)	325	0	86
Wedges *(Del Monte)*, 12 oz pkg	195	0	47
Canned: *See Page 146*			
Pitanga, 3 fruit, 1 oz	7	0	1.5
Plaintains, ½ cup slices, 2½ oz	90	0	22
Plums: Average all types,			
Mini/Damson, (1" diam.), ½ oz	7	0	1.5
Small (1¾" diam.), 2.3 oz	30	0	7
Medium (2¼" diam.), 3 oz	45	0	10
Large (2½" diam.), 4 oz	65	0	15
Pluot (plum-apricot), 1 med., 5 oz	80	0	19
Pomegranates, ½ fruit, 2.7 oz	55	0	13
Pummelo, flesh, ½ cup, 3½ oz	35	0	9
Prickly Pears, 1 fruit, 5 oz	40	0	10
Quince, 1 medium, 3½ oz	55	0	14
Rambutan (Rambotang),			
Red/Yellow, 1 medium, 2 oz	15	0	4
Raspberries, ½ cup, 2 oz	30	0	7
Rhubarb, raw, ½ cup, 2 oz	15	0	3
Sapodilla (Chico), 1 med., 7½ oz	140	2	34
Sapotes, ½ medium, 3 oz	150	0.5	38
Satsuma Tangerine, 1 med., 3 oz	45	0	11
Soursop, 1 cup pulp, 8 oz	150	0.5	38
Strawberries: 1 cup, 5½ oz	50	0.5	12
6 medium/3 large, 2 oz	20	0	4
1 pint, 14 oz	115	1	27
Chocolate Dipped, 2 medium	45	2.5	6
Sugar Apples, ½ cup pulp, 4 oz	120	0	30
Tamarillo, 1 medium, 3 oz	20	0	3
Tamarind, 1 fruit (3"x1")	5	0	1.5

Weights as Purchased

	C	F	Cb
Tangelo: 1 small, 4 oz	55	0	13
1 medium, 5 oz	70	0	17
1 large, 7 oz	95	0	24
Tangerine, 1 medium, (2½″ diam.), 4 oz	50	0	13
Tangor, 1 medium, 4 oz	35	0	7
Tomatillos (3), 3½ oz	35	1	6
Tomato: 1 small, 3 oz	15	0	3.5
1 medium, 4.3 oz	22	0	5
1 large, 6.4 oz	33	0	7
1 jumbo (salad/steak), 10 oz	50	0.5	11
Grape, 3 medium	8	0	2
Yellow Tear Drop, 4 medium, 1 oz	8	0	2
Cherry: 1 medium, ½ oz	5	0	1
1 cup, 5.3 oz	27	0	6
Slices (Medium Tomato):			
Thin slice, ½ oz	3	0	0.5
Medium (¼″ thick), ¾ oz	4	0	1
Thick (⅜″), 1 oz	5	0	1
Fried Green Tomato, 1 slice (36g)	70	5.5	4.5
Canned Tomatoes/Products: *See Page 85*			
Tree Tomato (Tamarillo), 3 oz	20	0	5
Ugli Fruit, Tangelo type, 5 oz	40	0	8
Watermelon: Flesh only/no rind, 1 oz	9	0	2
1 cup cubes or balls, 5½ oz	45	0	11
Regular Long Shape:			
1 thick (1″) slice (¼ circle, 4½″ radius)			
9 oz w. rind (5½ oz no rind)	50	0	12
1 thin (½″) slice (¼ circle)	25	0	6
1 thick (1″) slice (½ circle)			
18 oz w. rind	100	1	24
1 whole melon (15″ long, 7½″diam.)			
20 lb w. rind/10lb no rind	1360	7	340
Seedless Round Shape:			
Medium Size (13 lbs, 8¼″ diam.)			
Edible Weight (no rind), 4 lbs	550	3	137
Wedge (⅛ whole melon),			
26 oz (with rind)	70	0.5	17
Flesh only (no rind), 8 oz	70	0.5	17
Wax Jambu (Rose Apple), 2 oz	14	0	3

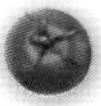

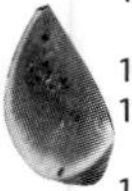

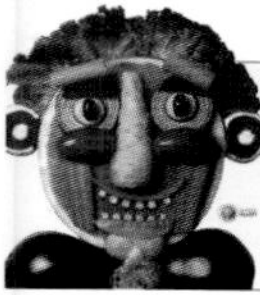

Eat at least 5 servings of fruit and vegetables every day . . . and Enjoy Better Health!

Dried Fruit

	C	F	Cb
Apples, 5 rings, 1 oz	80	0	21
Apricots, 8 halves, 1 oz	65	0	17
Banana Chips, ½ cup, 1½ oz	220	14	24
Banana Flakes, 4 Tbsp, 1 oz	80	0	20
Cranberries, swtn, dr., ⅓ c., 1.4 oz	140	0.5	37
Currants, ¼ cup, 1¼ oz	100	0	27
Dates: 5 medium dates, 1½ oz	120	0	32
Large Calif., 3 dates, 2 oz	170	0	42
½ cup, chopped, 3 oz	255	0	66
Date Crumbles (Bob's Redmill),			
1 oz, ¼ cup	90	0	22
Figs, 3 medium figs, 1 oz	65	0	16
Goji Berries, 3 Tbsp, 1 oz	105	1.5	24
Longans; Lychees, 1 oz	80	0	20
Mango Slices, 5 pieces, 1.3 oz	115	0	27
Mixed Fruit, 1 oz	70	0	18
Papaya Spears, 2 pieces, 1.4 oz	100	0	25
Peaches, 2 halves, 1 oz	60	0	16
Pears, 3 halves, 2 oz	140	0.5	37
Pineapple, 2 pieces, 1.4 oz	130	1	30
Prunes (dried Plums): w. pits, 1 oz	70	0	17
1 Medium (60/lb)	16	0	4
1 Large (50/lb)	22	0	5
1 Extra Large (40/lb)	27	0	6
Without pits, 4 med., 1 oz	70	0	18
Cooked: w. sugar, ½ c, 5 oz	200	0	47
w/out sugar, ½ c, 4½ oz	125	0	30
Raisins: 2 Tbsp, 1 oz package	85	0	22
½ cup, 2.8 oz	245	0.5	64
CinnaRaisins, 1.4 oz pkg	135	0.5	32
Sunsweet: Fruitlings, ⅓ c., 1.5 oz	130	0	31
Plums (5) 1.4 oz	100	0	24

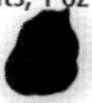

Candied Glacé Fruit

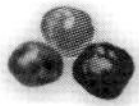

	C	F	Cb
Apricot, 1 medium, 1 oz	100	0	25
Cherry, 3 large, ½ oz	50	0	12
Citron/Fruit Peel, 1 oz	90	0	21
Fig, 1 piece, 1 oz	90	0	21
Ginger, 1 oz	95	0	23
Pineapple, 1 slice, 1¼ oz	120	0	30

Fruit Leather/Rolls

	C	F	Cb
Average All Brands, 1 oz	100	0	24
Fruit By The Foot, (Betty Crocker)			
1 roll, ¾ oz	80	0	17
Fruit Gushers, (Betty Crocker), 1 oz	90	1	20
Fruit Roll-Ups, (Betty Crocker) 1 roll	50	1	12
Stretch Is. Leathers, 2 pces, 1 oz	90	0	24
Other Fruit Confectionery/Snacks/Bars: *Page 137*

Canned/Bottled Fruit ◆ Fruit Snacks

Canned/Bottled Fruit

Solids & Liquids:	C	F	Cb
Per ½ Cup (Approx. 4½ oz)			
Apples, sweetened	70	0	17
Apricots: In water/diet	35	0	9
In juice/lite	60	0	15
In syrup	105	0	27
Black/Blueberries: Heavy syrup	115	0	30
In light syrup	110	0	26
Cherries, pitted: in water	55	0	14
In light syrup	85	0	21
In heavy syrup	110	0	28
In extra heavy syrup	130	0	33
Maraschino (5), 1 oz	50	0	12
Pie, ⅔ cup, 5 oz	60	0	14
Fruit Salad: In water/diet	35	0	9
In juice/Light	60	0	16
In heavy syrup	95	0	25
Gooseberries, Light syrup	90	0	23
Grapefruit: Juice pack	45	0	15
In light syrup	75	0	20
Lychees, ½ cup, 4.5 oz	105	0	26
Mixed Fruit: In water/diet	40	0	10
In fruit juices/light syrup	60	0	15
In heavy syrup	100	0	25
Peaches (halves/slices): In water/diet	30	0	8
In juice/light	50	0	14
In light syrup	70	0	20
drained, ½ peach	40	0	11
In heavy syrup	100	0	26
Pears: In water/diet	35	0	10
In juice/light	60	0	16
In heavy syrup	100	0	26
Pineapple: All types			
In own juice	70	0	17
In heavy syrup	90	0	22
Slices, drained, 2 slices			
In own juice, drained	30	0	7
In heavy syrup, drained	45	0	11
Plums: In water	50	0	14
In juice	75	0	20
In light syrup, 3 plums	85	0	21
In heavy syrup, ½ cup	160	0	41
Prunes: In heavy syrup	120	0	32
In Liqueur, ½ cup, 125g	280	0	70
In Water, ½ cup	135	0	32
Raspberries, in heavy syrup	120	0	30
Strawberries: In water	25	0	7
In heavy syrup	120	0	31
Tropical Fruit Salad: In light syrup	80	0	18
In heavy syrup	95	0	21

Fruit Snack Cups

	C	F	Cb
Deli/Take-Out: Small, 6 oz	70	0	16
Large, 12 oz	140	0	32
Yogurt & Fruit Cup, 15 oz	380	4.5	75
Del Monte Fruit Cups			
Fruit Cups: *Per 4 oz Cup*			
Strawberry Banana	70	0	17
Mandarin Orange Segments	70	0	17
Pineapple Tidbits	70	0	18
Tropical Fruit	70	0	18
Fruit & Gel Cups: *Per 4½ oz Cup*			
Mixed Fruit in Cherry Gel	90	0	23
Peaches in Peach Gel	90	0	22
Lite varieties in Gel, avg.	60	0	14
Carb Clever: *Per ½ Cup (4.2 oz)*			
Fruit Cocktail	40	0	11
Peaches, chunks/slices	30	0	7
Pears, chunks/slices	40	0	10
Pull Top Cans: in 100% Juice, 4 oz	80	0	20
Lite varieties, 4 oz	50	0	13
Dole Fruit Bowls			
4 oz Bowls: Peaches	70	0	17
Mixed Fruit; Tropical Fruit	80	0	19
Pineapple	60	0	16
Fruit n Gel Bowls (4.3 oz): Regular	90	0	22
Reduced Sugar	60	0	16
Mott's: Healthy Harvest, 4 oz cup	50	0	13
Tree Top: Fruit Rocketz, 1 tube	45	0	11
Natural Apple, 1 Pkg., 4 oz	50	0	12
Vons: Mixed Fruit,			
In heavy syrup, 1 cup, 4.5 oz	90	0	22
In lite syrup, 1 cup, 4.5 oz	60	0	13

Apple & Fruit Sauces

	C	F	Cb
Apple Sauce:			
Regular/sweetened, 2 Tbsp, 1.1 oz	23	0	5
4 oz package cup	80	0	20
¼ cup, 2½ oz	55	0	13
Fruit Sauces & Purees:			
Average all fruit types, 2 Tbsp, 1 oz	25	0	6
½ cup, 4 oz	100	0	24
Mott's: Classics, avg. 4 oz	100	0	25
Apple Sauce: Original, 4 oz	70	0	18
Fruit Flavored, avg., 4 oz	90	0	23
Unsweetened, 4 oz	50	0	14
Ocean Spray: *Per ¼ Cup (2 ½ oz)*			
Jellied Cranberry Sauce	110	0	25
Whole Berry Cranberry Sauce	115	0	27

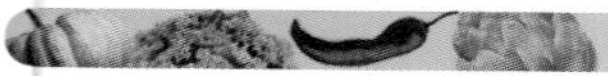

Vegetables

Vegetables	C	F	Cb
Alfalfa Sprouts, ½ cup, ½ oz	5	0	0.5
Artichokes, Globe/French:			
1 medium, 4½ oz	60	0	13
1 large, 5.7 oz	75	0	17
Artichoke Heart *(Fanci Food)*:			
Plain, 1 piece	8	0	1
Marinated, ¼ bottle, 1 oz	25	1.5	2
Asparagus, raw/froz.: 4 med. spears	12	0	2.5
Cuts & Tips *(Del Monte)*, ½ cup, 4.3 oz	20	0	3
Bamboo Shoots, ckd, ½ c, 2 oz	7	0	1
Beans: Green/Snap/String, ½ c., 2 oz	17	0	4
10 beans (4" long), 2 oz	17	0	4
Dried Beans, *average all types: (Kidney, Brown, Haricot, Lima, Mung, Navy, Pinto, Red, White)*			
Raw: 2 Tbsp, 1 oz	95	0.5	18
1 cup, 7 oz	665	3	126
Cooked: 1 oz	35	0	7
½ cup, 3 oz	105	0	21
Bean Sprouts, avg., ½ cup, 2 oz	17	0	3.5
Beets: Raw, 1 beet (2" diam), 3 oz	35	0	8
Cooked, ½ cup, slices, 3 oz	37	0	8.5
1 beet, 2" diam., 1¾ oz	22	0	5
Beet Greens, ckd, ½ c., 2½ oz	20	0	4
Bell Pepper: *See Peppers*			
Bitter Melon/Gourd, 1 c. pces, 1.6 oz	14	0.3	1.5
Black Eyed Peas, ckd, ½ c., 2 oz	100	0.5	18
Bok Choy (Chinese Chard), ckd., 3 oz	10	0	1.5
Breadfruit, ¼ small fruit, 3.4 oz	100	0.2	26
Broadbeans (Fava Beans):			
Green (in pod), raw: 4 pods (3½ oz w. shell; 1.2 oz beans)	30	0	6
1 cup beans (no shell), 4½ oz	110	1	22
Mature Seeds: Raw, 1 c., 5.3 oz	512	2.3	87
Cooked, ½ cup, 3 oz	94	0	17
Broccoflower, ⅕ head, 3½ oz	35	0	7
Broccoli: Raw, chopped, 1 cup, 3 oz	30	0	6
3 Florets, 2½ oz	25	0	5
1 Spear (5" long) 1.1 oz	10	0	2
1 Whole: Medium size, 14 oz	135	1.5	26
Large, 21 oz	203	2	40
1 Head (no stalk), 11 oz	105	1	21
1 Stalk, small (5" long), 5.3 oz	50	0.5	10
Brocco Sprouts, ½ cup, 1 oz	16	0	2
Brussel Sprouts: ckd, ½ cup, 2.8 oz	28	0.5	6
2 Sprouts, 1½ oz	15	0	3
Butterbeans, cooked, ½ cup, 3 oz	90	0	16
Cabbage, All types/colors, average:			
Raw: 1 Leaf, large, 1.2 oz	8	0	2
Shredded, 1 cup, 2½ oz	17	0	4
½ Large Head (7" diam), 22 oz	150	1	35
Cooked, shredded, ½ cup, 2½ oz	17	0.5	3.5
Cactus (Nopal), sliced, 1 cup, 3 oz	14	0	3

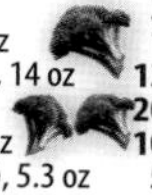

Vegetables (Cont)

Vegetables (Cont)	C	F	Cb
Carrots: Regular thick variety,			
1 small, 4 oz	47	0	11
1 medium, 6 oz	70	0	16
1 large, 8 oz	93	0	22
Chopped, 1 cup, 4½ oz	52	0.3	12
Grated, 1 cup, 4 oz	45	0.3	11
Slices, 1 cup, 4½ oz	50	0.3	12
Sticks (4"), 4, 1½ oz	18	0	4
Long thin variety, 1 medium, 2.2 oz	25	0	6
Baby: Snack size, 3 medium, 1 oz	10	0	2.5
Snack Pack, 3 oz	30	0	7
Cauliflower, Raw: 1 cup (pces), 3½ oz	25	0	5
½ medium head, 10 oz	72	0	15
Cooked, 3 florets, 2 oz	12	0	2
Celeriac, ½ cup, raw, 2¾ oz	33	0	7
Celery: 1 large stalk, 11", 2.2 oz	10	0	2
1 small stalk, 5", ½ oz	2	0	0.5
4 Strips/sticks, ½ oz	4	0	1
Chopped, 1 cup, 3½ oz	14	0	3
Chard (Swiss), ½ cup, ckd, 3 oz	18	0	3.5
Chayote Squash, raw, 1 cup, 4½ oz	22	0	5
Chick Peas (Garbanzo Beans):			
Dry, 1 cup, 7 oz	730	12	121
Cooked, 1 cup, 6 oz	270	4	45
Chicory Greens, 1 cup, 1 oz	7	0	1.5
Chicory/Witloof: *See Endive*			
Chili Peppers: *See Peppers*			
Chinese Long Bean, sliced, 1 c., 3.2 oz	45	0	8
Chives, chopped, 1 Tbsp	1	0	0
Choy Sum, 3 oz	13	0	3
Cilantro (Coriander), 1 Cup	4	0	0.5
Collards, cooked, ½ cup, 3 oz	25	0	5
Corn, yellow/white:			
Raw: Kernels, ½ c., 3 oz	80	0.5	19
Ear (5"x 1¾"), raw, 5½ oz	153	1	37
Cooked: Kernels, ½ c., 3 oz	77	0.5	18
Cob, cooked, dr: Small, 2¼ oz	60	0.5	14
Large ear, 5½ oz	118	1	28
(Also see Frozen & Canned Corn Page 149-150)			
Courgette: *See Zucchini*			
Cress, Garden, raw, ½ cup, 1 oz	8	0	1.5
Cucumber: 1 whole, 11 oz	45	0.5	11
½ cup slices, 2 oz	8	0	2
Mini/Lebanese (1), 3 oz	13	0	3
Daikon Radish, ½ cup, slices, 2 oz	9	0	2
Dandelion Greens, raw, ½ cup, 1 oz	12	0	2.5
Edamame *(Immature green soybeans)*:			
Shelled, ½ cup, 2.6 oz	110	5	8
With shells, 10 pods, 1¼ oz	30	1	3
Eggplant: Raw, ¼ medium, 4 oz	27	0	7
Raw, ½ cup, 1" pieces, 1½ oz	10	0	2.5
1 slice, fried, 1 oz	75	4	10
Endive, Belgian/French: Raw, 1 med. head (6"), 2½ oz	12	0	2.5

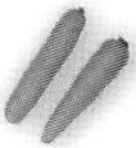

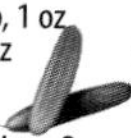

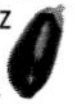

Vegetables (Cont)

	C	F	Cb
Fiddleheads, 3.5 oz	34	0.5	5.5
Fava Beans: *See Broadbeans*			
Fennel, 1 cup, sliced, 3 oz	27	0	6.5
Gai Choy Cabbage, ckd, 1 cup, 6 oz	20	0	3
Gai Lan (Chinese Kale), ckd, 1 cup	36	0.5	7
Garlic, 1 clove	4	0	1
Ginger: ¼ cup slices, 1 oz	20	0	4.5
Crystallized (sugared), 7 pce, 1½ oz	130	0	35
Horseradish, raw, 1 pod, ½ oz	5	0	1
Jerusalem Artichoke, raw, ½ cup	57	0	13
Jicama, raw, sliced, ½ cup, 2¼ oz	23	0	5.5
Kale, 1 cup, chopped, 2½ oz	34	0.5	7
Kohlrabi, ½ cup, cooked, 1¾ oz	17	0	4.5
Lambsquarters, chopped, 1 c., 6.3 oz	60	1.5	9
Leek, cooked, 1 whole, 4½ oz	38	0	9
Lentils, green/brown: Dry, 1 oz	100	0.5	17
Dry, 1 cup, 6¾ oz	678	2	115
Cooked, ½ cup, 3½ oz	115	0.5	20
Lettuce: 1 cup, chop./shred., 2 oz	7	0	1.5
Butterhead, 2 leaves, ½ oz	2	0	0.5
Cos/Romaine, shredded, 1 c., 1.7 oz	10	0	1.5
Iceberg: 1 outer leaf, ½ oz	2	0	0.5
1 medium head, 15-16 oz	75	1	16
Lamb's Lettuce, 2½ oz	15	0	3.5
Lima Beans, baby, ckd,½ c., 3 oz	105	0	20
Lotus Root, 10 slices, ckd, 3 oz	59	0	14
Mung Bean Sprouts, ½ cup, 2 oz	16	0	3
Mushrooms: Raw, 1 medium, 0.6 oz	4	0	0.5
Raw, 1 large, sliced, ¾ oz	5	0	1
Raw, ½ cup pieces, 1¼ oz	8	0	1
Cooked, ½ cup pieces, 2½ oz	22	0.5	4
Mustard Greens, raw, ½ cup, 1 oz	7	0	1.5
Nopal (Cactus): 1 leaf, 4½ oz	20	0	4.5
Sliced, 1 cup, 3 oz	14	0	3
Okra, cooked, ½ cup, slices, 2¾ oz	18	0	3.5
Onions, Raw: 1 small, 2½ oz	29	0	7
1 medium, 4 oz	48	0	11
1 large, 5½ oz	63	0	15
1 jumbo, 16 oz	190	0.5	46
Chopped: Raw, ½ cup, 3 oz	34	0	8
1 Tbsp, 0.4 oz	4	0	1
Slices: 1 cup, 4 oz	48	0	12
1 thin slice, small, 0.4 oz	4	0	1
1 medium slice (⅛"), ½ oz	6	0	1.5
1 large slice (¼"), 1⅓ oz	16	0	4
Dehydrated flakes, ¼ c, ½ oz	50	0	12
Rings, breaded/fried, 2 rings	80	5	9
Scallions, ½ cup, 2 oz	16	0	3.5
Spring, ½ cup, chopped, 2 oz	16	0	3.5
French's Fried Onions: *See Page 72*			
Blossom/Blooming: See Fast-Foods (Chili's/Outback)			

	C	F	Cb
Parsley, chopped, ½ cup, 1 oz	10	0	2
Parsnips: 1 medium, 4 oz	85	0	20
Cooked, ½ cup slices, 2¾ oz	55	0	13
Peas: Raw, Green, ¼ cup, 1½ oz	30	0	5
Raw, with pods, ½ lb	70	0	13
Snow Peas, 10 pods, 1.2 oz	14	0	2.5
Split: Dry, hulled, 1 oz	97	0.5	17
Cooked, 1 cup, 7 oz	230	1	42
Peppers: Sweet, 1 medium, 4.2 oz	28	0	6.5
Bell: 1 medium, 4.2 oz	28	0	6.5
½ cup, chopped, raw, 2½ oz	20	0	4.5
1 ring (3" diam. x ¼" thick)	3	0	0.5
Chili: Green/Red, 1½ oz	18	0	4.5
Habanero, 1 only, 8g	11	0	2
Pigeon Peas, cooked, ½ cup, 3 oz	94	1	17
Pimientos, 3 medium, 3½ oz	25	0	5
Poi, ½ cup, 4.2 oz	134	0	33
Pumpkin: Mashed, ½ cup, 4⅓ oz	25	0	6
Raw, 1" cubes, 1 cup, 4 oz	30	0	7.5
Pumpkin Flowers, 1 cup, 1.2 oz	5	0	1
Purslane: Cooked, ½ c., 2 oz	10	0	2
Raw, 1" cubes, 1 cup, 1.5 oz	7	0	1.5
Potatoes: Raw (with skin)			
1 Baby, Gourmet, 2 oz	45	0	10
1 Small, 6 oz	130	0	30
1 Medium, 7.5 oz	164	0	37
1 Peeled, 4 oz	90	0	20
1 Large, 8 oz	175	0	40
1 Extra large (Russet), 13 oz	284	0	65
1 Jumbo (Russet), 16 oz	350	0.5	80
Baked (no fat); large, 10 oz raw:			
Plain, with skin, 7 oz	185	0.3	42
without skin, 5½ oz	145	0	34
Garlic Potatoes, mashed, 4 oz	128	5	19
w. Skin/Toppings: + 2 tsp fat	270	8	58
+ Sour Cr./Chives, 2 Tbsp	320	6	60
+ Plain Yogurt, 2 Tbsp	260	1	60
+ Grated Cheese, 1 oz	370	9	58
+ Cottage Cheese, 2 oz	315	2	60
Mashed w. milk and fat, ½ c.	120	4.5	18
Hash Browns: w. Butt. Sce, 2½ oz	125	6	17
Homemade, ½ cup, 2¾ oz	207	10	27
Potato Skins: (w. Cheese topping),			
½ whole (8 oz baking), 4 oz	240	13	22
French Fries: Small serve, 2.6 oz	250	13	30
Medium serve, 4 oz	380	20	47
Froz., uncooked, 18 fries, 4 oz	167	5.5	28
Oven-heated, 18 fries, 4 oz	167	5.5	28
Take-Out, 1 cup, 5 oz	440	25	60
McDonald's: Small, 2.6 oz	250	13	30
Medium, 4 oz	380	20	47

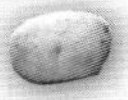

Vegetables (Cont)

	C	F	Cb
Potatoes (Cont)			
Fried, 18 fries, 4 oz	167	5.5	28
Au Gratin, ½ cup, 4.3 oz	162	9	14
Pancakes, 2 small, 2 oz	120	6.5	12
Kugel, 5 oz	300	20	26
Puffs, fried, 4 puffs, 1 oz	53	2.5	8
Scalloped, ½ cup, 4¼ oz	114	5.5	15
Ore-Ida Frozen Potatoes: *See Page 150*			
Potato Salad, ½ cup, 4½ oz	180	10	14
Radicchio, 2 leaves, ½ oz	4	0	1
Shredded, 1 cup, 1½ oz	18	0	3.5
Radish: Avg., 10 only, 1½ oz	7	0	1.5
Oriental, ½ c. slices, 1½ oz	8	0	2
Rutabagas, ckd., ½ c. cubes, 3 oz	33	0	7.5
Salsify, ckd, ½ c. slices, 2½ oz	48	0	11
Sauerkraut, ½ cup, 2½ oz	13	0	3
Seaweed: Average, dried, 1 oz	7	0	2
Soaked, drained, 1 oz	15	0	4
Nori/Laver, dried, 6 sheets, ½ oz	35	0	5
Shallots, chopped, 1 Tbsp, ½ oz	7	0	1.5
Sorrel, raw, ½ cup, 4 oz	23	0.5	4
Soybeans: Mature, dry, 1 oz	118	5.5	9
Dry, ½ cup, 3⅓ oz	387	18	28
Cooked, ½ cup, 3 oz	150	7.5	8.5
(Soy Products/Tofu/Tempeh: See Page 77)			
Spinach: Cooked, ½ cup, 3 oz	20	0	3.5
Raw: 3 leaves/1 cup, 1 oz	7	0	1
1 Bunch, 12 oz	78	1.5	12
Creamed, avg., ½ cup, 4½ oz	187	15	8
Squash: Summer, raw, ½ c., 2¼ oz	10	0	2
Cooked, ½ cup slices, 3 oz	14	0	3.5
Winter, cooked,			
Acorn, ½ cup cubes, 3½ oz	34	0	9
½ medium (10 oz raw wt.)	114	0	30
Butternut, ½ c. cubes, 3½ oz	40	0	10
¼ medium (9 oz raw wt.)	115	0	30
Spaghetti, ½ cup, 1¾ oz	16	0	3.5
Succotash, ckd, ½ cup, 3⅓ oz	110	1	23
Sweetcorn: *See Corn*			
Sweet Potatoes: Cooked with Skin (no fat)			
1 medium, 4 oz	103	0	24
No skin, mashed, ½ c., 5½ oz	125	0	29
Swedes, ½ cup, 2 oz	20	0	4.5
Swiss Chard, ckd, chopped, 1 c., 6 oz	35	0	7
Taro, cooked, ½ cup, 2⅓ oz	94	0	23

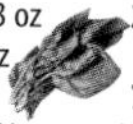

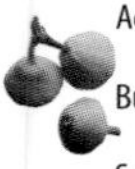

Vegetables (Cont)

	C	F	Cb
Tomatoes: 1 small, raw, 3⅓ oz	15	0	3.5
1 medium, raw, 4½ oz	22	0	5
1 large, raw, 6½ oz	33	0	7
Cooked, ½ cup, 4¼ oz	22	0	5
Fried, 1 small, 3 oz	175	13	12
Also See Fruit: *Page 145*			
Tomatillo, 1 medium, 1.2 oz	10	0	2
Turnips: White, ckd, ½ cup, 2¾ oz	17	0	4
Greens, cooked, ½ cup, 2½ oz	14	0	3
Water Chestnuts: 5-6 nuts, 1 oz	56	0.5	13
½ cup slices, 2¼ oz, raw	60	0	15
Canned, 1 oz	14	0	3.5
Watercress, 10 sprigs, 1 oz	3	0	0.5
Yam: Cooked, ½ cup, 2½ oz	80	0	19
Baked, 1 medium (6") 8 oz	264	0.5	63
1 large (9") 12 oz	395	0.5	94
Yardlong Bean, 1 pod, ½ oz	6	0	1
Yucca Root, ½ cup, 3½ oz	165	0.5	39
Zucchini: 1 medium, 7 oz, raw	30	0.5	6.5
½ cup slices, cooked, 3 oz	14	0	3.5

Frozen Vegetables

	C	F	Cb
Birds Eye			
Broccoli/Corn/Vegetables, ⅔ cup	50	1	9
Chopped Spinach, ⅓ cup, 3 oz	30	0	3
Other varieties, average, 1 cup	30	0	6
Baby: Corn & Vege Blend, ⅔ cup	50	1	9
Broccoli Florets, 1 cup, 3 oz	30	0	4
Corn, Pea & Bean Blend, ¾ cup	70	0.5	13
Sweet Peas, ⅔ cup, 3 oz	70	0	12
Whole Green Beans, 1 cup, 3 oz	35	0	5
Deluxe Vegetables: *Per Cup*			
Sugar Snap Stir Fry, 3½ oz	40	0	7
Broccoli, Cauliflower & Peppers	25	0	3
Broccoli, Carrots & Water Chestnuts	35	0	6
Steam Fresh: *Per Serving*			
Broccoli Cuts, 1 cup	30	0	4
Mixed Veges, ⅔ cup	60	0	12
Super Sweet Corn, ⅔ cup	70	1	14
Stir Fry: *Prepared (Includes Pasta)*			
Asian, 1 cup	60	1	12
Green Bean & Almonds, ¾ cup	80	4	8
Voila! Meals: *See Page 61*			
Green Giant			
Vegetables: Asparagus Cuts, ⅔ c.	20	0	3
Corn: Nibblers, ½ ear, 2.2 oz	70	0.5	14
Extra Sweet Niblets, ⅔ cup	70	1	13
Shoepeg, no sauce, ½ cup	70	1	15
Honey Glazed Carrots, 1 cup	90	3	15
Le Sueur Baby Sweet Peas, ¾ cup	60	0.5	11
Spinach, no sauce, ½ cup, 3½ oz	25	0	3

Vegetables – Frozen, Canned, Bottled

Frozen Vegetables (Cont)

	C	F	Cb
Green Giant (Cont)			
Veges In Cheese & Cream Sauce: *Prepared*			
Alfredo Vegetables, ¾ cup	70	2.5	9
Broccoli, Cauliflower, Carrots, 1 c.	50	1.5	7
Cauliflower & Cheese Sce, ½ cup	60	2.5	6
Creamed Spinach, ½ cup	70	2.5	9
Rice & Vegetables: *Per ½ Pkg (Prepared)*			
Cheesy Rice & Broccoli	135	2.5	25
Rice Medley	140	2	26
Rice Pilaf	115	1.5	22
White & Wild Rice	140	3	25
Ore-Ida (As Purchased):			
French Fries: Country, 18 fries, 3 oz	120	4	19
Crispers 20 pces, 3 oz	210	12	23
Crispy Crunchies, 13 fries, 3 oz	160	8	20
Fast Food Fries, 27 fries, 3 oz	180	7	21
Waffle Fries, 8 fries, 3 oz	160	6	22
Golden Crinkles, 12 pces, 3 oz	130	4	17
Golden Fries, 14 pces, 3 oz	120	2.5	20
Oven Chips, 7 pces, 3 oz	160	7	22
Shoestrings, 32 pces, 3 oz	150	6	19
Steak Fries, 7 fries, 3 oz	120	3	17
Zesties, 12 pces, 3 oz	140	5	22
Hash Browns: Toaster, 2 patties	220	12	25
Potatoes O'Brien, ¾ c., 2 oz	60	0	13
Onion Rings: Gourmet, 3 pces, 3 oz	190	9	24
Onion Ringers, 6 pces, 3.2 oz	220	12	25
Sweet Potatoes: 4 oz	80	0	18
Tater Tots: 9 pces, 3 oz	150	7	22
Mini, 19 pces, 3 oz	190	10	19
Onion, 9 pces, 3 oz	160	7	22
Extra Crispy, 12 pces, 3 oz	145	7	19
Twiced Baked: Potatoes, 1, 5 oz	190	7	26
TGI Friday's			
Potato Skins, avg., 3 pces, 3½ oz	210	11	20
Wild Oats: Tater Bites, 9 pces, 3 oz	150	6	21
Shredded Hash Browns, 1 c., 3 oz	70	0	15
French Fries, 14 pces, 3 oz	110	3	17

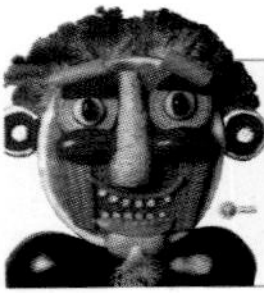

Eat at least 5 servings of fruit and vegetables every day . . . and Enjoy Better Health!

Canned/Bottled

	C	F	Cb
Solids & Liquid			
Artichoke Hearts *(Fanci Foods):*			
Plain, 1 oz (1)	8	0	1
Marinated, ¼ bottle, 1 oz	25	1.5	2
Asparagus, Drained: 3 spears, 2 oz	10	0	1.5
Pieces, ½ cup, 4.3 oz	25	0.5	3
Bamboo Shoots, 1 cup, 4½ oz	25	0	4
Bean Salad, ½ cup, 4⅓ oz, no oil	90	0	20
Beans: Green, ½ cup, 2½ oz	15	0	3
Baked Beans, ½ cup, 4½ oz	120	0.5	27
Butter Beans, ½ cup, 4½ oz	90	0	16
Italian, cut, ½ cup, 4½ oz	30	0	6
Kidney Beans, ½ cup, 3½ oz	105	0.5	19
Lima Beans, ½ cup, 4½ oz	80	0	15
Pinto Beans, ½ cup, 4½ oz	105	1	18
Beets: Sliced, ½ cup, 3 oz	26	0	6
Crinkle/Pickled *(Del Monte)* ½ cup	80	0	20
Carrots: Sliced, ½ cup, 2½ oz	20	0	4
Honey Glazed *(Del Monte)* ½ cup	75	0	18
Corn: Kernels, ½ cup, 4½ oz	80	0.5	18
Creamed style, ½ cup, 4½ oz	92	0.5	23
Garbanzo/Chick Peas, ½ c., 4.2 oz	143	1.5	27
Green Chilis, diced, 2 Tbsp, 1 oz	6	0	1.5
Hearts of Palm (1), 1.2 oz	7	0	1
Mushrooms: ½ cup, 2¾ oz	20	0	4
in Butter Sauce, 2 oz	20	1	2
Onions: Pickled, 1 med., ¾ oz	10	0	2
Cocktail, 1 onion	0	0	0
French's Fried Onions: *See Page 72*			
Peas, ½ cup, 3 oz	60	0.5	10
Peppers: Hot Chili, Jalapeno, (1), 1 oz	6	0	2
Sweet, undrained, 2½ oz	13	0	3
Jalapeno, w. liq., ½ c. chopped	18	0.5	3
Fried, drain, 2 Tbsp, 1 oz	60	5	3
Salsa, average all types, 2 Tbsp	10	0	2
Sauerkraut, undrained, ½ c., 4 oz	27	9	6
Spinach, ½ cup, 3½ oz	25	0.5	3.5
Succotash: w. Cr. Style Corn, ½ c.	100	0.5	23
w. whole kernels, undrained, ½ c.	80	0.5	18
Sweetcorn: *See Corn*			
Sweet Potato: ½ cup, 3½ oz	90	0	24
Tomatoes, Sundr.: Natural, 5-6 pce	22	0	5
In Oil, drained, 6 pces, ½ oz	38	2.5	4
Tomato Products: *See Page 85*			
Vegetables, mixed, ½ cup, 4 oz	45	0	8
Yams: in Light Syrup, ½ cup, 4 oz	105	0	25
Candied, ½ cup, 5 oz	170	0	46
Zucchini in Tom. Sce., ½ c., 4 oz	30	0	8

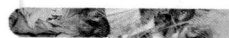

Take-Out Salads & Vegetables

Avg. All Outlets: Per Serving	**C**	**F**	**Cb**
Antipasto Salad, ½ cup	135	8	13
Bean Salad, ½ cup	110	4	17
Bulgur Salad, ½ cup	70	2	12
Caesar Salad, Classic, 1 cup	200	14	15
Side Salad, no Dressing	25	0	6
Carrot Raisin: No Dressing, ½ cup	20	0	5
with Dressing, ½ cup	135	12	6
Chef Salad: Regular, no Dressing	620	37	8
w. 2 oz 1000 Island	860	61	8
Chicken Salad Platter, 6 oz	200	8	12
Coleslaw: Traditional, ½ cup	150	8	18
w. Low Cal Dressing, ½ cup	50	2	8
Corn, Mexican, ½ cup	240	12	33
Cucumber: Non-Oil Dressing, ½ c.	60	0	14
w. Oil Dressing, ½ cup	140	12	8
Eggplant Salad, ½ cup	75	5	7
Fettucini w. veges, ½ cup	135	6	16
Garden Salad, no Dressing, 1 cup	10	0	2
Greek Salad, 1 cup	105	8	7
Greek Vegetables, 1 cup	110	8	6
Lettuce, hearts, ¼ head	15	0	2.5
Lobster Salad Platter, 6 oz	200	8	12
Macaroni Salad, ½ cup, 4 oz	140	6	17
Nicoise, 1 cup	450	32	18
Pasta Salad, ½ cup	200	11	19
Pineapple Coconut Slaw, ½ cup	100	9	4
Potato Salad: Dijon, 3 oz	120	7	13
w. Mayonnaise, ½ cup	215	15	17
Lowfat, ½ cup	110	1.5	21
Rice Salad, ½ cup	150	10	13
Saffron Rice, ½ cup	145	3	26
Spinach Salad, 1 cup	180	13	13
Tabouli, ½ cup	125	7	13
Three Bean Salad, ½ cup	90	4.5	12
Tomato & Mozzarella, ½ cup	180	14	10
Tortellini w. Basil Pesto, ½ cup	150	9	15
Waldorf w. Mayo, ½ cup	110	7	12

Signature Salads: *Per Serving (6 oz)*
(Supplied to Deli's and Institutions)

Antipasto Salad, 6 oz	510	50	4
Artichoke Salad, marinated	400	41	8
California Medley	120	7	15
Cheese Agnolotti	250	8	23
Chicken Salad	420	33	11
Crabmeat Flavored	450	38	20

Take-Out Salads (Cont)

Signature Salads (Cont)	**C**	**F**	**Cb**
Egg Salad	300	23	14
Fresh Button Mushroom	190	16	6
Garden Olive	630	67	3
Ham Salad	400	32	14
Prima Pasta Salad	360	30	18
Seafood Pasta Del Mar	170	10	21
Seafood with Crab & Shrimp	420	34	20
Shrimp Salad	360	32	8
Tuna Salad	450	36	14

Fast-Food Restaurants: *See Page 183*

Fresh Salad Packs

Pre-Packaged (Supermarkets)

Dole: Caesar Kit, 3½ oz	170	15	8
Asian Crunch Kit, 3½ oz	120	6	12
Bacon Lettuce Kit, 3 oz	130	9	8

Regular Salad Packs *(no added dressing):*

Classic Coleslaw, 3 oz	25	0	5
Classic Iceberg, 3 oz	15	0	4
Soy Cheese, 3½ oz	80	6	3

Fresh Mates: *Per ¼ Container*

Broccoli ranch, 1½ cups	230	13	25
Cheddar Bacon Ranch, 1½ c.	370	22	35
Garden Vegetable, 1½ cups	240	14	25
Italian Herb, 1½ cups	270	12	33

Fresh Express
Salad Kits: *Per Serving (Prepared)*

Caesar, ⅓ kit	150	13	8
Caesar w. Light Dress., ⅓ kit	100	7	8
Caesar Supreme, ⅓ kit	170	14	8
Asian, ¼ kit	170	10	17
Taco Fiesta, ⅓ kit	110	8	7

Salad Toppings

	C	**F**	**Cb**
Bacon Bits, average, 1 Tbsp	35	2	2
Chow Mein Noodles, dry, ½ cup	120	7	13
Croutons, 2 Tbsp, 10g	40	1	7
Olives, 5 medium	25	2	0
Potato Chips, 20 chips, 1 oz	150	10	15
Sunflower Seeds, 1 Tbsp, 8 g	45	4	1.5
Tortilla Chips, 12 chips, 1 oz	140	7	19

Fruit & Vegetable Juices/Smoothies

Quick Guide | C | F | Cb

Orange Juice
Average ~ Fresh or Sweetened:

	C	F	Cb
½ Cup, 4 fl.oz	55	0	13
Small Glass, 6 fl.oz	82	0	20
Regular Glass, 8 fl.oz	110	0	26
8¾ fl.oz Box	120	0	28
10 fl.oz Bottle	140	0	32
11½ fl.oz Can	160	0	36
16 fl.oz Bottle	220	0	52
20 fl.oz Bottle	275	0	62
64 fl.oz/½ Gallon	875	0	200

Juices ~ Generic

Average All Brands: Per 8 fl.oz Unless Indicated

	C	F	Cb
Aloe Vera Juice, unsweet., 2 oz	10	0	1
Apple Juice: 8 fl.oz	120	0	30
10 fl.oz Bottle	150	0	38
16 fl.oz	240	0	60
Carrot Juice: Fresh, 6 fl.oz	60	0	14
Sweetened, 6 fl.oz	75	0	17
Cranberry Juice, Cocktail/Blend	140	0	35
Fruit Blends, average, 8 fl.oz	110	0	27
Fruit Nectars, average, 8 fl.oz	140	0	36
Grape Juice, 8 fl.oz	155	0	38
Grapefruit Juice, 8 fl.oz	115	0	27
Lemon/Lime Juice: 1 Tbsp	3	0	1
1 cup, 8 fl.oz	50	0	15
Concentrate, 1 tsp	0	0	0
Noni Juice: Tahitian, 2 Tbsp, 1 fl.oz	5	0	1
Southern Cross Botanicals, 1 fl.oz	6	0	1
Tahiti Traders, 1 fl.oz	20	0	5
Orange Juice, 8 fl.oz	110	0	26
Passion Fruit Juice (Fresh):			
Purple, 1 cup, 8 fl.oz	125	0	34
Yellow, 1 cup, 8 fl.oz	150	0	36
Papaya/Peach Nectar, avg., 8 fl.oz	140	0	36
Pear Nectar, 8 fl.oz	150	0	40
Pineapple Juice, 8 fl.oz	135	0	35
Prune Juice, 8 fl.oz	180	0	45
Strawb./Raspberry Juice, 8 fl.oz	100	0	23
Tangerine Juice, 8 fl.oz	125	0	30
Tomato Juice, 8 fl.oz	40	0	10
Vegetable Juice, 8 fl.oz	50	0	10
Wheat Grass Juice: 1 fl.oz 'Shot'	5	0	1
2 fl.oz 'Shot'	10	0	2

Quick Guide | C | F | Cb

Fruit Smoothies
Average All Brands

	C	F	Cb
Fruit Only: 8 fl.oz	105	0	25
12 fl.oz	160	0	38
16 fl.oz	210	0	50
24 fl.oz	320	0.5	76
Fruit + Nonfat Milk/Soy:			
12 fl.oz	190	0.5	40
16 fl.oz	250	0.5	53
24 fl.oz	380	1	80
Fruit + Nonfat Frozen Yogurt/Sherbet:			
12 fl.oz	210	0.5	47
16 fl.oz	280	0.5	62
24 fl.oz	420	1	94

Juice Brands | C | F | Cb

Per 8 fl.oz Unless Indicated

	C	F	Cb
Apple & Eve			
Naturally Cranberry	130	0	32
Cranberry/Raspberry Apple	120	0	26
Cranberry Grape	140	0	34
Bolthouse			
100% Juices: Carrot, 8 fl.oz	70	0	14
Passionfruit Apple Carrot	120	0	29
Valencia Orange	110	0	24
Vedge	65	0	14
Lemonade: Cranberry	130	0	33
Mango	120	0	30
Prickly Pear Cactus	130	0	34
Fruit Smoothies: *Per 8 fl.oz*			
Berry Boost	110	0	30
C-Boost	150	0	36
Green Goodnesss	140	0	33
Strawberry Banana	125	0	29
Bright & Early *(Minute Maid)*			
Orange Juice (Chilled/Frozen)	110	0	30
Campbell's			
Tomato Juice: 5.5 fl.oz can	30	0	6
11.5 fl.oz	60	0	13
Capri Sun			
Sport, all flavors, 6.75 fl.oz	60	0	16
Big Pouch: *Per 11.2 oz Pouch*			
Iced Tea; Mountain Cooler, avg.	150	0	39
Average other flavors	160	0	42
Clamato			
Tomato Cocktails, average, 8 fl.oz	60	0	11

Juice Brands (Cont)

Per 8 fl.oz Unless Indicated

	C	F	Cb
Crystal Geyser			
Juice Squeeze: *Per Bottle (12 fl.oz)*			
Blackberry Pomegranate	170	0	43
Orange Lime	160	0	40
Ruby Grapefruit	150	0	36
Average other flavors	140	0	32
Dole			
100% Juice, Pineapple, 8 fl.oz	120	0	29
100% Fruit Juice Blends: *Per 6 fl.oz*			
Pine-Orange Banana	75	0	18
Pineapple Orange	100	0	24
Donald Duck			
100% Orange Jce (+Calcium), 8 fl.oz	110	0	27
Eden, Organic Apple, 8 fl.oz	90	0	24
Five Alive *(Minute Maid):* **Frozen Concentrate,**			
made up, 8 fl.oz	120	0	30
Florida's Natural			
Cranberry Apple, 8 fl.oz	120	0	30
Orange Juice, 8 fl.oz	110	0	26
Ruby Red Grapefruit Juice, 8 fl.oz	100	0	24
Fuze: *Per 8 fl.oz*			
Refresh, 8 fl.oz	90	0	24
Slenderize, 8 fl.oz	5	0	0.5
Vitamin Tea	60	0	16
Goya Nectar			
Apricot Nectar, 12 fl.oz	130	0	31
Pear Nectar, 12 fl.oz can	240	0	59
Hain: Carrot Juice w. Lutein	80	0.5	16
Veggie Juice w. Lutein, 8 fl.oz	45	0.5	11
Hansen's: *Per 8 fl.oz Unless Indicated*			
Fruit Juice: Apple varieties	120	0	28
Grape Promegranite	160	0	40
Light Juice Cocktail, avg.	35	0	8
Juice Slam*: Per Box (6.75 fl.oz)*			
Apple	90	0	23
Other varieties, avg.	120	0	29
Smoothies: *Per Can (11.5 fl.oz)*			
Fruit flavors, regular, avg.	175	0	43
Energy Island Blast	170	0	45
Low Carb Smoothie, 11.5 fl.oz	40	0	9
Energy Smoothies: *See Page 159*			
Hawaiian Punch			
Fruit Juicy: Red, 8 fl.oz	120	0	30
Box, 8.45 fl.oz	120	0	30
Red Light, 8 fl.oz	45	0	11
Hawaii's Own			
Frozen Concentrate: *Per 8 fl.oz (Prep'd)*			
Average all varieties	110	0	28

Per 8 fl.oz Unless Indicated

	C	F	Cb
Hi-C Juice Drinks: Average, 8 fl.oz	120	0	32
6.75 fl.oz box, average	100	0	27
Blast, 6 fl.oz pouch	100	0	26
Hood: Apple, 8 fl.oz	120	0	31
Fruit Punch	120	0	30
Orange	120	0	30
Jamba Juice (California): *See Fast-Foods Section*			
Jera's Juice (Boston): *Per 24 fl.oz*			
Berry Blitz	440	2	105
Cape Codder	335	0.5	80
Citrus Burst	320	1.5	75
Mango Passion	290	0	68
Orange Bite; Flu Fighter, avg.	280	1.5	65
Razzle Dazzle	380	1	94
Soy Smoothie (7g protein)	320	3.5	68
Strawberry Smile	345	0.5	84
Triathlete (15g protein)	300	1.5	71
Whey-Out Protein (27g protein)	325	1.5	56
Juicy Juice (Nestle): *Per Box (6.75 fl.oz)*			
Grape	110	0	27
Average other flavors	100	0	24
4.23 fl.oz box, average	60	0	15
Kerns All Nectars			
Canned Juice: *Per Can (11.5 fl.oz)*			
Pear	220	0	54
Pineapple Coconut	280	8	53
Other flavors, average	210	0	52
Kool Aid			
Jammers: Sugar Jammers	10	0	2
Other varieties, 6.75 fl.oz pouch	90	0	24
L & A: Black Cherry, 8 fl.oz	180	0	45
Grape Juice Plus	160	0	40
Mixed Berry	120	0	30
Prune Juice	180	0	41
Average other varieties	140	0	32

"I've worked on vitamins for years and I've discovered that the three most important elements necessary to life are breakfast, lunch and dinner."

153

Fruit & Vegetable Juices (Cont)

Juice Brands (Cont)   **C** **F** **Cb**

Per 8 fl.oz Unless Indicated

Lakewood Organic

	C	F	Cb
Carrot Pineapple, 6 fl.oz	85	0	19
Coconut, 6 fl.oz	90	1.5	20
Cranberry/Lemonade, 8 fl.oz	90	0	22
Mango, 6 fl.oz	80	0	20
Papaya; Pure Carrot, avg., 6 fl.oz	75	0	18
Pure Cranberry, 6 fl.oz	50	0	12
Pure Pineapple, 6 fl.oz	95	0	23
Pure Prune, 8 fl.oz	165	0	40
Pure Pink Grapefruit, 8 fl.oz	90	0	22
Red Tart Cherry, 6 fl.oz	80	0	19
Super Veggie, 6 fl.oz	40	0	9
Average other varieties, 8 fl.oz	105	0	26

Langers: *Per 8 fl.oz*

	C	F	Cb
Apple Juice; White Cranberry avg.	120	0	28
Cranberry/100 Varieties, avg.	140	0	35
Cranberry Berry	135	0	34
Cranberry Grape; White Grape, avg.	150	0	37
Cranberry Raspberry	150	0	36
Low Carb: Apple Juice	60	0	14
Cranberry/Grape	30	0	8

Seasonal Blends: *Per 8 fl.oz*

	C	F	Cb
Summer	125	0	31
Spring; Autumn; Winter	120	0	30

Frozen Concentrate: *Per 8 fl.oz (Prepared)*

	C	F	Cb
Cranberry	150	0	36
Other flavors, average	120	0	30

Malibu Beach: *Per 8 fl.oz*

	C	F	Cb
Teas: Tropical Tea	10	0	3
Beach Peach; Oceanside	10	0	3
Juices: Malibu Mango	10	0	3
Sunset Strawberry; Redondo	10	0	3

Martinellis

Sparkling Juice: *Per 8 fl.oz*

	C	F	Cb
Apple-Cranberry	110	0	27
Apple-Grape	120	0	31
Cider	140	0	35

Mauna Lal Hawaiian: 8 fl.oz   **140   0   32**

Mistic (Mega 24 fl.oz)

	C	F	Cb
Mega 24 fl.oz: Avg. all flavors, 8 fl.oz	120	0	30
24 fl.oz	360	0	90
Tropicals, all flavors, 8 fl.oz	120	0	31
Lemon Tea, 8 fl.oz	90	0	23
Grape Strawberry, 8 fl.oz	130	0	32
Watermelon Kiwi, 8 fl.oz	110	0	28
Peach Beach, 8 fl.oz	0	0	0
Diet Lemon tea, 8 fl.oz	100	0	24

Per 8 fl.oz Unless Indicated

Minute Maid

	C	F	Cb
Orange Juice, Premium, 8 fl.oz	110	0	27
Light Orange Juice	50	0	13
Heart Wise; Kids Plus	110	0	27
Lemonade, all flavors	110	0	30
Premium Blends, avg. all flavors	110	0	27
Simply Orange	105	0	26
Tropical Punches	120	0	32
Juices to Go, avg. all flav., 11.5 fl.oz	160	0	44
Boxed Juices, average, 6.75 fl.oz	90	0	25
Coolers, average, 6.75 fl.oz	100	0	28
Disney, 6.75 fl.oz box	100	0	26
Soft Frozen Lemonade, 12 fl.oz	300	0	77
Frozen Concentrates, 8 fl.oz (Prep'd),			
Average all varieties	105	0	28

Mott's

	C	F	Cb
Apple Juice, 8 fl.oz	120	0	29
Fruit Punch, 10 fl.oz	145	0	36
Grape Apple, 10 fl.oz	180	0	42

100% Fruit Juice Boxes: *Per Box (4.2 fl.oz)*

	C	F	Cb
White Grape	90	0	22
Average other flavors	60	0	15
Juice Paks: All flavors, 6.75 fl.oz	100	0	25
Mini Motts, 4.23 oz	60	0	15
Plus Lite Applejuice, 8 fl.oz	60	0	15

Naked Juice

Just Juices: *Per ½ Bottle (16 fl.oz)*

	C	F	Cb
Apple, 8 fl.oz	120	0	30
Carrot	80	0	13
O-J Orange	110	0	25
Tangerine Scream	110	0	25

Fruit Smoothies: *Per ½ Bottle (16 fl.oz)*

	C	F	Cb
Antioxidants: Berry Blast, 8 fl.oz	120	0	30
Mighty Mango	120	0	30
Pomegrananate varieties, avg.	150	0.5	37
Rainforest Acai	160	1.5	35
Energy: Orange Mango Motion	120	0	30
Strawberry Kiwi Kick	110	0	27
Proteins: Chocolate Karma, 8 fl.oz	190	2.5	31
Protein Zone	250	4	32
Vanilla Chai	190	3	30
Superfoods: Blue Machine, 8 fl.oz	170	0	41
Green Machine	130	0	32
Purple Machine	180	1.5	34
Red Machine	150	2	31
Well Being: Power-C, 8 fl.oz	120	0.5	29
Strawberry Banana-C	140	0	32
Tropical-C	140	0	32

Juice Brands (Cont)	C	F	Cb

Per 8 fl.oz Unless Indicated

Nantucket Nectars
Juice Cocktails: *Per 8 fl.oz*

	C	F	Cb
Carrot Orange Mango	130	0	30
Cranberry	140	0	34
Fruit Punch	130	0	32
Grapeade Guava; Orange Mango	130	0	33
Other varieties, avg.	120	0	30

100% Juice: *Per 8 fl.oz*

	C	F	Cb
Cranberry Raspberry Grape	150	0	38
Grape Juice	160	0	39
Peach Orange	130	0	31
Pineapple Orange Guava	120	0	31
Premium Orange Juice	120	0	27
Other varieties, avg.	100	0	25

Fruit Juice: Apple Cider | 100 | 0 | 25

Squeezed Nectar Teas: *Per Bottle (16 fl.oz)*

	C	F	Cb
Diet Lemon Tea	0	0	1
Original Lemon Tea	90	0	23

NectarFizz, all other varieties, avg. | 90 | 0 | 23
Nectar Lemonades, avg., 8 fl.oz | 130 | 0 | 32

Newman's Own

	C	F	Cb
Lemonade (Reg./Pink), 8 fl.oz	110	0	27

Fruit Juice Cocktail: Gorilla Grape | 140 | 0 | 34

	C	F	Cb
Orange Mango Tango	150	0	37
Razzma Tazz Raspberry	120	0	28

Northland
100% Juice: *Per 8 fl.oz*

	C	F	Cb
Cranb./Peach/Blackberry; Raspb.	140	0	34
Cranberry Grape	140	0	36

Ocean Spray: *Per 8 fl.oz*

	C	F	Cb
Cranberry Juice Cocktail, avg.	130	0	33
100% Cranberry Juice, avg., 8 fl.oz	140	0	35
White Cranberry Juice, avg.	120	0	31

Cranberry Blends: *Per 8 fl.oz*

	C	F	Cb
CranApple; CranTangerine, avg.	140	0	35
CranCherry	130	0	32
CranGrape	140	0	35
CranMango/Raspberry/Strawberry	120	0	30

Light Juice Drinks: *Per 8 fl.oz*

	C	F	Cb
Light Cranberry Drinks	40	0	10
Light Ruby Grapefruit Juice Drink	40	0	10
Diet Juice Drinks, 8 fl.oz	5	0	2

100% Grapefruit Juices: *Per 8 fl.oz*

	C	F	Cb
Ruby Red Grapefruit/Tangerine	120	0	30
White Grapefruit, 8 fl oz	100	0	24

Ruby Grapefruit Juice Drinks: *Per 8 fl.oz*

	C	F	Cb
Ruby Red Grapefruit	120	0	30
Light Ruby Grapefruit	40	0	10

Per 8 fl.oz Unless Indicated

Odwalla

	C	F	Cb
AntioxiDance; Grapefruit, avg	90	0	21
B Berrier; Quencher	120	0	30
Carrot Juice	70	0	15
Carrot, Orange, Apple	100	0	23
Glorious Morning; B Monster	140	0	33
Mo'Beta	150	0	37
Poma Grand, average	160	0	40
Strawberry Lemonade	110	0	28
Super Protein	190	1	35
Wellness Echinacea	150	1	33

Smoothies: Blueberry B Monster | 140 | 0 | 33

	C	F	Cb
C Monster	150	0	36
Blackberry Fruitshake	150	1	36
Mango Tango	150	1	34
Strawberry Banana	130	0	31

Old Orchard: Apple Juice, 8 fl.oz | 120 | 0 | 29
Frozen Concentrate: *Per 8 fl.oz (Prep'd)*

	C	F	Cb
Apple	120	0	29
Other flavors	130	0	31

Orange Julius: Original (Orange, Strawberry),

	C	F	Cb
16 fl.oz	220	1	54
20 fl.oz	270	1	68
32 fl.oz	440	1	108

Other Drinks: See Fast-Foods, Page 229

Pom Wonderful
100% Juice: *Per 8 fl.oz*

	C	F	Cb
Mango	140	0	34
Blueberry; Pomegranate	160	0	39
Cherry	150	0	38
Tangerine	140	0	34

R.W. Knudsen
Fruit Juices: Apple | 120 | 0 | 30

	C	F	Cb
Cranberry Raspberry	130	0	32
Creamed Papaya	40	0	10
Grapefruit; Just Blueberry, avg.	100	0	23
Guava Strawberry	120	0	28
Hibiscus Cooler	90	0	24
Just Concord	160	0	40
Tomato	60	0	14
Other varieties, average	120	0	30

Sparkling Juice, avg., 8 fl.oz | 120 | 0 | 30
Nectars: Coconut | 140 | 5 | 27

	C	F	Cb
Peach	130	0	31
Boysenberry, average	130	0	33

Very Veggie, 8 fl.oz | 50 | 0 | 11
Simply Nutritious: Mega C | 140 | 0 | 34

	C	F	Cb
Average other varieties	125	0	30

Fruit & Vegetable Juices (Cont)

Juice Brands (Cont)   C   F   Cb

Per 8 fl.oz Unless Indicated

	C	F	Cb
Ralphs			
Lemonade (Premium Juice), 8 fl.oz	110	0	29
Orange Juice, 8 fl.oz	120	0	30
Pineapple Juice, 8 fl.oz	130	0	33
ReaLemon - ReaLime (Borden)			
Lemon/Lime Juice (from concentrate)			
1 teaspoon	0	0	0
2 Tbsp, 1 fl.oz	6	0	2
Lemonade, 8 fl.oz	110	0	29
Iced Tea, 8 fl.oz	100	0	25
Half Lemonade/Half Iced Tea, 8 fl.oz	100	0	27
Santa Cruz (Organic)			
Apple Juice; Cider & Spice	120	0	30
Concord Grape; White Grape	160	0	40
Orange Mango	130	0	31
Tropical Blend	140	0	33
Average other varieties	100	0	24
Nectars: Cranberry	110	0	27
Average other varieties	120	0	30
Sodas: *Per 12 fl.oz*			
Cherry	140	0	34
Concord Grape	150	0	36
Cranberry	110	0	27
Lemonade; Champagne Style	100	0	26
Raspberry Lemonade; Apricot	120	0	29
Other varieties	130	0	33
Juice Boxes: *Per 8 fl.oz*			
Lemon	120	0	29
Orange; Grape, average	105	0	25
Tropical Punch	120	0	27
Simply Orange			
Lemonade, 8 fl.oz	120	0	30
Limeade	120	0	31
Orange Juice, all varieties	110	0	26
Snapple			
Fruit Drink Blends, 8 fl.oz	120	0	29
Grapeade; Orangeade 8 fl.oz	120	0	29
Lemonade, all types	110	0	28
Diet: Snapple Apple	15	0	4
Kiwi Strawberry	20	0	5
Avg. other flavors	10	0	2
Snap.E Tom			
Tom. & Chile Cocktail, 11.5 oz can	70	0	15
Stonyfield Farm: *Per Bottle (10 fl.oz)*			
Peach Smoothie	250	3	49
Wildberry; Strawberry Smoothie	250	3	46
Light Smoothies, 10 fl.oz	130	0	41

Per 8 fl.oz Unless Indicated   C   F   Cb

	C	F	Cb
SunnyD			
Baja Juice: *Per 10 fl.oz Bottle*			
Berry	145	0	36
Orange	160	0	39
Red Punch	145	0	36
Strawberry Kiwi	175	0	44
Blends, avg., ½ bottle, 8 fl.oz	80	0	20
Intense Sport, 11 fl.oz bottle	65	0	16
Originals: *Per 8 fl.oz*			
w. Calcium	140	0	35
Fruit Punch	120	0	29
Lemonade; Mango	130	0	31
Reduced Sugar	60	0	15
Smooth Style	130	0	32
Tangy Original Style	120	0	29
Sunsweet			
Prune Juice/w. Pulp, 8 fl.oz	180	0	43
Tampico: Citrus Punch, 1 cup	110	0	25
Mango/Trop. Frt. Punch, 1 cup	110	0	28
Tang			
Pouches, average all flavors (1)	90	0	24
Mix: *Prepared As Directed*			
Regular (2 Tbsp dry), 6 fl.oz	100	0	24
Sugar Free, 8 fl.oz	5	0	0
Trader Joes: *Per 8 fl.oz*			
Refrigerated: Carrot Juice	80	0	13
Ginger Lemonade	110	0	28
Organic Carrots & Greens	80	0	19
Original Lemonade	120	0	30
Strawberry Lemonade	120	0	25
Strawberry Smoothie	130	1.5	30
Other varieties, average	110	0	25
w. Vitamins Added:			
Dairy Free Protein w. Pzazz	150	1	28
Avg. other varieties	130	0	31
100% Juice, all varieties	120	0	30
All Natural Pasteurized: *Per 8 fl.oz*			
Cranberry Harvest	130	0	36
Cranberry; White Grape	140	0	36
Garden Patch; Vege -10	50	0	11
Hawaiian Pineapple	110	0	29
Just Pomegranate; Concord Grape	160	0	40
Lemon Ginger	100	0	25
Mango Lemonade	140	0	30
Mango Passion Fruit Blend	130	0	33
Rio Red Grapefruit	140	0	35
Average other varieties	125	0	30

Juice Brands (Cont)	**C**	**F**	**Cb**

Per 8 fl.oz Unless Indicated

Tree Top

	C	F	Cb
Apple Reserve/Fruit Punch	120	0	30
Apple Berry/Grape	120	0	31
Cider: Apple/Spiced	120	0	32
Cranberry Apple	130	0	32
Fiber Rich: Apple	140	0	35
Apple Apricot/Orange Banana	160	0	37
Grapefruit	105	0	24
Grower's Best, Apple NSA	120	0	29
Island Blends, avg.	105	0	26
Orange	120	0	29
Orange Passionfruit	110	0	26
Orchard Blends	130	0	32
Boxes: Average, 6.8 fl.oz	100	0	26
Frozen Concentrate, prep., 8 fl.oz	120	0	29

Tropicana

	C	F	Cb
Chilled Juices: Grape	150	0	38
Cranberry; Cranberry Cocktail	140	0	34
Orchard Berry/Apple, avg.	115	0	29
Essentials: Fiber, 8 fl.oz	120	0	29
Healthy Heart; Healthy Kids	110	0	26
Immunity Defense; Low Acid	110	0	26
Light'n Healthy varieties	50	0	13
Non-Refrigerated Juice Drinks: *Per 8 fl.oz*			
100% Fruit Punch	140	0	32
100% Grape	155	0	38
100% Orange; Apple; Ruby Red	110	0	27
100% Pineapple Orange	130	0	32
100% Strawberry Orange	140	0	34
Light'n Healthy, average	50	0	14
Pure Premium: Apple, 8 fl.oz	110	0	27
Blends: Orange Tangerine	110	0	25
Other varieties, average	130	0	30
Grapefruit: Golden; Ruby Red	90	0	22
Sweet	130	0	31
Lemonade: Homestyle, 8 fl.oz	110	0	28
Orchard Style	120	0	31
Orange Juice, all varieties	110	0	26
Refrigerated Juice Drinks: *Per 8 fl.oz*			
Berry Punch; Fruit Punch	130	0	32
Fruit Punch	130	0	32
Lemonade	120	0	29
Orangeade; Peach Orchard Punch	130	0	33
Tropical Punch	120	0	31
Light varieties, average	10	0	3
Twisters: Average, 8 fl.oz	120	0	29
20 fl.oz bottle	300	0	74
Light varieties, 8 fl.oz	50	0	12
20 fl.oz bottle	300	0	74
Fruit Smoothies, avg., 11 fl.oz	220	0	54

Per 8 fl.oz Unless Indicated

V8® Juices & Drinks	**C**	**F**	**Cb**
V8 100% Vegetable Juice, 5.5 fl.oz	35	0	7
1 Can, 11.5 fl.oz	70	0	15
V-8 Splash, all flavors, 8 fl.oz	80	0	19
V-8 Splash Smoothies, 8 fl.oz	90	0	20
Diet V-8 Splash, all flavors, 8 fl.oz	10	0	3
Fusian, all flavors, 8 fl.oz	120	0	28

Veryfine

	C	F	Cb
Apple Juice (100%)	110	0	27
Grape Juice (100%) w. Calcium	110	0	25
Orange Juice (100%)	120	0	30

Walnut Acres: *Per 8 fl.oz*

	C	F	Cb
Organic: Apple	110	0	27
Apricot; Raspberry	130	0	32
Cherry	140	0	34
Cranberry	110	0	26
Incredible Vegetable	50	0	12
Other varieties, avg.,	120	0	32

Welch's

	C	F	Cb
100% Red Grape	170	0	44
100% White Grape	160	0	39
100% White Grape Blends, avg.	140	0	35
Tomato Juice, 8 fl.oz	50	0	10
Concentrates: *Per 8 fl.oz Made Up*			
100% Grape	170	0	42
100% White Grape	170	0	41
American White Grape	160	0	39
Apple	120	0	29
Fruit Fantastic	130	0	32
Grape	165	0	41
Wild Berry	145	0	36
Cocktails: *Per 8 fl.oz Made Up*			
Concord Grape	120	0	29
Harvest Blend	140	0	35
Mountain Berry	140	0	34
Orange Pineapple Apple	140	0	35
Strawberry Breeze	130	0	33
Light Cocktails: *Per 8 fl.oz Made Up*			
Grape	70	0	18
White Grape	70	0	18
White Grape, Peach	70	0	18
Sparkling Cocktail, avg., 8 fl.oz	160	0	40

Wild Oats

	C	F	Cb
Down to Earth, average, 8 fl.oz	140	0	34
Beautiful Juices, average, 8 fl.oz	120	0	27

Nutrition/Energy Shakes & Drinks

Nutritional Shakes/Drinks

Per 8 fl.oz Unless Indicated

	C	F	Cb
180 High Energy, 8.2 fl.oz	120	0	33
180 Sport, 8 fl.oz	15	0	3
ABB: Performance,			
Power Drinks, 22 fl.oz	310	0	43
Blue Thunder, 22 fl.oz	300	0	43
Carbo Force, 21 fl.oz	320	0	105
Mass Recovery	380	0	60
Pure Pro Shake, Choc., 12 fl.oz	175	1	6
Weight Gain: Pure Pro, 22 fl.oz	180	0	2
Extreme XXL, 24 fl.oz	1090	0.5	215
AdvantEdge (EAS): *Per Container (11 fl.oz)*			
Essential Energy Drink	190	7	21
Carb Control Ready-to-Drink	100	3	3
Coffee Hour, 11 fl.oz	110	3	3
Complete Nutrition Ready-to-Drink	180	3	29
Airforce, Nutrisoda, 250ml	10	0	1
AllSport, all flavors, 8 fl.oz	60	0	16
AMP Energy Drink, 8.4 fl.oz can	120	0	31
16 fl.oz can	220	0	59
Amway: Trim Advantage, 11.2 oz	140	3	14
XS Energy Drink, 8.4 oz	8	0	0
XS Power Protein Shake, 11 oz	250	3	6
Arizona: Caution Energy, 8.3 oz	130	0	34
Caution Energy Low Carb, 8.3 oz	10	0	3
Rx Energy, 8 oz	120	0	31
Rx Stress, 8 oz	50	0	16
Atkins: Advantage Shake, 11 oz can	170	9	4
Bacchus Energy, 16 fl.oz can	240	0	58
Balanced: Kids Choc., 8 fl.oz	160	3	30
Choc., Strawb.; Van., 11 fl.oz	230	6	31
Bally Total Fitness: Whey Pro, 1 scoop	100	1.5	2
Blast, 8.3 oz	120	0	29
Bariatrix Shakes, 1 serving	100	2	6
Anytime Drinks avg., 8 oz	100	4	3
Proti 15 Drink, avg., 1 pkg	70	0.5	1
Bawls Guarana, 10 fl.oz	120	0	32
Guaranexx Sugar Free, 10 fl.oz	0	0	0
Bliss Energy Drink, 8.4 fl.oz	25	0	5
Blox Energy: Citrus, 8.4 fl.oz	120	0	29
Black Cherry; Orange Rush, 8.4 fl.oz	110	0	26
Blue Sky: Blue Energy, 8.3 fl.oz	110	0	27
Blue Sport, 8 oz	45	0	12
Body for Life (EAS) 11 oz	190	7	20
Body Fuel (w. NutraSweet), 1 scoop	80	0	20
Bookoo Energy, 16 fl.oz can	220	0	54
Boost: Nutritional Energy, 8 fl.oz	240	4	41
Boost High Protein, 8 fl.oz can	240	6	33
Boost Plus, 8 fl.oz	360	14	45
Boost w. Fiber, 8 fl.oz can	240	4	42
Breeze Juice Drink, 8 fl.oz can	160	0	31

Per 8 fl.oz Unless Indicated

	C	F	Cb
Carbolite At Last! Shake, 11 oz can	150	3	8
Carboplex (Unipro) mix, ½ cup, 2 oz	210	0	52
Carnation Instant Breakfast			
Powder: 1 envelope, 1.3 oz	200	1	40
Carb Conscious, 1 envel., 21g	150	1	24
Ready-to-Drink, avg, 11 fl.oz	250	5	40
Celebrity Juice Diet, 4 fl.oz	60	0	14
CeraSport: Liquid, 11 fl.oz	70	0	17
20g package (makes 16 fl.oz)	80	0	19
Champion Lyte, Sports Drink	0	0	0
Champion Nutrition			
Heavywt Gainer 900, 4 sc., 5.4 oz	630	10	101
Ultramet: Regular, 1 pkt, 2.7 oz	280	2	24
Ultramet Lyte, 1 pkt, 2 oz	190	1	17
Ultramet Low Carb, 1 pkt, 2 oz	230	6.5	6
Citrucel Fiber Shake, 1 pkg	50	2	6
Coca-Cola Black 8 fl.oz	45	0	12
Curves Protein Drink (mix):			
Chocolate; Vanilla, 2 scoops	100	1.5	8
made with skim milk, 8 fl.oz	190	1.5	23
Designer Whey Protein 1 scoop	90	1.5	2
e10 Energy Drink, 8.4 fl.oz	5	0	1
EAS ~ *See AdvantEdge/Myoplex*			
Elements: Avg., all varieties	125	0	31
Diet Air/Ice, 8 fl.oz	10	0	2
Endura (Unipro), 2 scoops, 1.3 oz	120	0	30
Ensure: High Protein, 8 oz bottle	230	6	31
Ensure Fiber, 8 fl.oz	250	6	42
Ensure Plus, 8 fl.oz bottle	350	11	50
Ensure Regular, 8 fl.oz	250	6	40
Glucerna, 8 fl.oz can	220	8.5	29
Weight Loss Shake, 11 fl.oz	290	11	39
Healthy Mom, 8 fl.oz	200	3	33
High Calcium, 8 fl.oz	230	6	31
Enterex Diabetic (w/fiber), 8 fl.oz			
Carbohydrates as Maltodextrin	237	9	27
Equaline (Albertson's)			
Advanced, 8 fl.oz	250	6	40
Plus, 8 fl.oz	350	11	50
Fruit2O (Veryfine), 8/16/20 fl.oz	0	0	0
Full Throttle (Coca-Cola), 16 fl.oz	220	0	57
Sugar Free	5	0	0
Fuze: Slenderize, 8 fl.oz	5	0	1
Refresh, 8 fl.oz	90	0	24
Mega Energy, 8 fl.oz	15	0	1
Go Fast Sports, Reg., 11.9 fl.oz	130	0	33
Gatorade: Endurance, 8 fl.oz	50	0	14
Lemonade/Raspb. Lem, 8 fl.oz	50	0	14
Nutrition Shake, 325ml can	370	6	62
Rain; X Factor, 8 fl.oz	50	0	14

Nutritional Shakes/Drinks (Cont)

Per 8 fl.oz Unless Indicated	C	F	Cb
Genisoy: Ultra XT, 1 scoop, 1.4 oz	140	0	20
Protein Powder, 1 scoop, 1.2 oz	130	0	18
Glaceau: Vitamin Water, 8 fl.oz	50	0	13
Smart Water	0	0	0
Glucerna Wt Loss Shakes, 11 oz	290	11	39
GNC Pro Performance:			
Protein 95, 1 scoop	130	1.5	5
Mega MRP: Original, 1 pkt	280	3.5	22
Extreme Choc., 3 scoops	290	3	11
Quick Fuel, 1.9 oz	200	0	50
Hydro Pro, 1.9 oz	190	0	46
Electroaide, 1.2 oz	100	0	25
Kore Energy Drink, 8 oz	120	0	28
HMR: 70 Plus, 1 package	110	0.5	13
500	100	0.5	16
Hansen's: Energade, 8 fl.oz	60	0	16
Energy Original, 8.3 fl.oz Can	140	0	36
Diet Red Energy, 8.3 fl.oz Can	10	0	3
EnergyWater, 8 fl.oz	10	0	3
Rumba, 8 fl.oz	120	0	28
Smoothies: *See Page 153*			
Hollywood Celebrity Diet: ½ cup	125	0	31
24hr/48hr Miracle, 4 oz	100	0	25
Hydra Fuel (Twin Labs)	70	0	17
Impulse Energy Drink, 8.3 oz	110	0	28
invigor8, all types, 8 oz	110	0	27
Isopure Perfect, 1 pkg (88g)	300	0	25
Jarrow: Whey Protein, 1 scoop	100	1	5
Berry High, 1 scoop	20	0	5
Muscle Optimal, 2 scoops	150	2	14
Jones: Energy, 8.4 fl.oz	140	0	32
Whoop Ass, 8.4 fl.oz	110	0	29
Kashi GoLEAN Shakes: Vanilla	220	2.5	38
Chocolate, 325ml can	240	3	38
Powdered, avg., 2 scoops	220	1	32
Knudsen: ReCharge, all flavors	70	0	18
Simply Nutritious, ½ bot., 16 fl.oz	120	0	30
Kombucha, Wonder Drink, 8.5 fl.oz	60	0	16
La Brada Lean Body, 11 oz	200	6	8
Lipovitan EB3, 8.2 fl.oz	110	0	29
Lost Energy Drink, 8.3 fl.oz can	100	0	26
Max Velocity (Albertson's), 8.45 fl.oz	120	0	33
Lite, 8.45 fl.oz	10	0	0
MDX (Mountain Dew)	0	0	0
Met-Rx: Original, 1 pkt	260	3	19
Protein Plus, 3 scoops	210	1.5	3
Ultra, 1 pkt	265	2.5	20
RTD 40, 15 fl.oz can	240	3	13

Per 8 fl.oz Unless Indicated	C	F	Cb
Metabolol: Endurance, 2 scp, 52g	200	5	24
Met, 2 scoops, 66g	200	3	40
Met Max, mix, 2 scoops	230	2.5	11
Creatinine Extreme, 2 scoops	280	0	68
Monster Energy: Assault, 12 fl.oz	100	0	27
Low Carb, 12 fl.oz	10	0	3
Monster Khaos, 8 oz	90	0	21
MRM: Low Carb Protein, 1 scoop	120	2.5	4
Whey Protein Isolate, 1 scoop	115	1.5	1
Whey Pumped, 1 scoop	100	1	5
Muscle Tech Nitro: Meso Tech, 1 pkt	290	4.5	18
Cell Tech Creatine, 2 scoops	320	0	75
Mass Tech Weight Gain, 5 scoops	830	5	150
Extreme Energy Tech, 8.4 oz	0	0	0
Myoplex: Original Shake, 17 fl.oz	310	7	20
Carb Sense Shake, 11 fl.oz	140	3.5	5
Lite (Ready to Drink), 11 fl.oz pkg	190	2.5	20
Powder, 1 pkt, 2.7 oz	270	3	23
Lite Powder, 1 pkt, 2 oz	180	2	19
Naturade: Power Shake, 1 scoop	100	1	10
Protein Booster, avg. ⅓ c. dry	80	1	1
Pure Soy, 2 Scoops (1.3 oz), dry	160	5	21
Ribo-tein, avg., 1 oz scoop	100	0.5	21
Total Soy: Plus, 1 scoop, 1.3 oz	150	2	21
Low Carb Shake, 2 scoops	100	1.5	1
Menopause Relief, 1.1 oz	120	1.5	16
Nature's Best: Isopure	260	0	25
Isopure Endurance, 20 fl.oz	320	0	60
Carbo Power, 16 fl.oz	400	0	100
Zero Carb, 2 scoops, 2.1 oz	160	0	0
Perfect Protein Drink, 11 fl.oz	250	1	42
Nitro Speed, all flavors, 18 fl.oz	110	0	7
Noni: Tahitian/Pacific, 2 Tbsp	10	0	3
Noni Juice, 1 fl.oz	10	0	3
Liquid Hawaiian/Tahiti, 1 Tbsp	30	0	8
Nutrament (Mead Johnson), 12 fl.oz	360	10	52
NuVim, 1 cup, 8 fl.oz	10	0	2
Ny-Tro Pro 40, average	260	1	23
Optifast 800: Powder, 1 serving	160	3	20
Ready-To-Drink, Chocolate	160	3	20
Optimum Pro Complex, 2 scoops	245	2	4
Pedialyte (Abbott)	25	0	6
Pimp Juice Energy, 250ml	140	0	33
Piranha Energy (EAS), 8.4 oz	140	0	33
Pitbull Energy Drink, 1 can	110	0	28
Power Dream (Imagine Foods):			
Java Jolt; Soy High Chai, avg., 11 fl.oz	245	4.5	42
X-Treme Choc, 11 fl.oz	260	5	48
Vanilla Blast, 11 fl.oz	240	5	39

Nutrition/Energy Shakes & Drinks (Cont)

Nutritional Shakes/Drinks (Cont)

Per 8 fl.oz Unless Indicated

	C	F	Cb
Powerade: Regular, 12 fl.oz	90	0	25
20 fl.oz bottle	150	0	43
Light, 8 fl.oz	25	0	7
20 fl.oz bottle	65	0	17
Option, all flavors, 8 fl.oz	10	0	2
PowerBar: Recovery, 1 scoop	90	0	20
Endurance, 1 scoop, 0.7 oz	170	0	42
Power Gel, Chocolate, 1.5 oz	110	0	27
ProBalance, 8.45 fl.oz	300	41	56
Pro-Cal 100 (R-Kane), 1 pkt	105	2	7
Red Bull Energy Drink, 8.3 fl.oz	113	0	28
Sugar-Free, 1 can	10	0	3
Red Devil Energy Drink, 12 fl.oz	160	0	38
Red Jak, Energy Drink, 8 fl.oz	10	0	1
Resource (Novartis): Shake, 6 fl.oz	270	6	45
Shake Plus, 8 fl.oz	480	15	69
Health Shake, 4 fl.oz	200	4	35
Diabetishield, 8 fl.oz	150	0	30
Breeze, 237ml	250	0	54
Benefiber, 1 Tbsp	15	0	4
Revenge Pro (Champ. Nutr.), 1 oz	100	0	20
Pro-Score 100, 2 scoops	225	2	1.5
Revival Soy Mix: Plain Soy, 1 pkg	120	3.5	3
Chocolate Day Dream, 1 pkg	240	2.5	36
Other varieties, avg., 1 pkg	225	2	33
Rhino's Energy Drink, 250ml can	125	0	31
Rite Aid Nutritional, 8 fl.oz	280	7	45
Rockstar: Energy Drink, 8 fl.oz	110	0	29
Diet Energy Drink, 8 fl.oz	10	0	2
Juiced, 16 fl.oz can	180	0	44
Rush Energy Lite, 8 fl.oz	0	0	0
Sav-on Nut'l: Plus, 8 fl.oz	350	11	50
Equaline Advance, 8 oz	250	6	40
High Protein, 8 oz	230	6	31
Scan Diet (Soy-base), 1 scoop	160	3	22
Six Star Body Fuel:			
Advanced Whey Protein, 1 scoop	110	2	2
Advanced Creatinine, 1 scoop	170	0	43
Slim-Fast			
Ready to Drink Shake:			
Original, 10.8 oz	220	3	40
High Protein, 11 oz	190	5	24
Optima Shake, 10.8 oz can	190	6	25
Powder Shake Mix: 1 scoop	100	3	18
w. 8 fl.oz fat-free milk	190	4	30
Snapple: Diet, 8 fl.oz	15	0	4
Diet Tea, 8 fl.oz	0	0	1

Per 8 fl.oz Unless Indicated

	C	F	Cb
SoBe: Power, avg., 8 fl.oz	120	0	30
Fountain, 8 fl.oz	110	0	30
Ice, 8 fl.oz	110	0	31
Synergy, 11.5 oz	120	0	32
Adrenaline Rush,8.3 fl.oz	140	0	37
Juice Elixers, 8 fl.oz	100	0	26
Lean, all flavors, 8 fl.oz	5	0	1
Life, 8 fl.oz	50	0	13
Lizard, avg. all types, 8 fl.oz	120	0	31
No Fear: Regular, 8 fl.oz	130	0	36
Sugar Free	5	0	1
Solaray Soytein (Protein Energy Meal),			
Natural, 1 heaping scoop, 24g	70	0.5	5
Flav., 1 heaping scoop, 32g	90	5	10
Sport Pharma Biomax, 2 scoops	250	3.5	4
Spiru-Tein Powder, 1 scp, avg., 35g	100	1	13
Stacker 2: Protein Water, 19.4 oz	80	0	1
SunnyD Intense Sport, 12 oz	70	0	17
Sweet Success (Nestlé):			
Healthy Shake, 11 fl.oz can	200	3	38
Powderblend, 2 scoops, 32g	180	0	45
Synergy, all flavors, 11½ fl.oz	120	0	32
Tab Energy, 10 fl.oz	5	0	0
The Sports Club/LA, PTS Protein Powder,			
Choc/Mocha/Van., 2 scoops, 1 oz	110	3	5
Total Balance: 9.5 oz can	230	7	25
Drink Mix, avg., 2 scoops	190	6	21
Twin Lab: Ultra Fuel, 16 fl.oz	400	0	100
Energy Fuel, 250ml can	0	0	0
Usana: Nutrimeal, 2 scoops, 43g	230	7	32
SoyaMax, 2 scoops	110	1	1
Walgreens Nutritional Drinks			
Nutritional Drink, 8 oz can	250	6	40
Plus, 8 oz can	350	11	50
Theragran-m, 8 oz	250	6	40
Theragran-m Plus, 8 oz	350	11	50
Weider (Powders):			
Creatine ATP, ½ cup, 1.7 oz	210	0	37
Mass 1000, 1⅓ cups	740	4	146
Ultra Whey Pro, ⅓ cup, 1 oz	110	1.5	4.5
Dynamic:			
Muscle Builder, 2 scps, ½ c., 45g	160	1	22
Weight Gainer, 4 scps, ⅔ c.,85g	450	1	99
Worldwide: Carbo Rush, 20 fl.oz	270	0	88
Pure Protein, 11 fl.oz bottle	170	0.5	9
Rapid Recovery, 20 fl.oz	280	0	33
Thermo 525, 20 fl.oz bottle	5	0	1
Xtreme Trim, 20 fl.oz	25	0	7
Supercharged tea, 20 fl.oz	15	0	4
XS Energy Citrus/Energy, 8.4 fl.oz	8	0	0
Zone Perfect, avg., 8 fl.oz	250	8	27

Quick Guide

Cola Soda Drinks
Average All Brands   **C** **F** **Cb**

Includes *Coca-Cola* and *Pepsi*

	C	F	Cb
8 fl.oz Cup	100	0	25
12 fl.oz Can	150	0	37
16 fl.oz Bottle	200	0	50
20 fl.oz Bottle	250	0	63
24 fl.oz (Pepsi)	300	0	75
1-Liter Bottle (34 fl.oz)	400	0	100
2-Liter Bottle (68 fl.oz)	800	0	200

Other Soda Drinks *(Average All Brands)*

	C	F	Cb
Club Soda, 12 fl.oz	0	0	0
Cream Soda, 12 fl.oz	170	0	42
Diet/Low Cal Drinks, avg., 12 fl.oz	5	0	1
Ginger Ale, 12 fl.oz	120	0	30
Lemon Lime, 12 fl.oz	220	0	55
Orange, 12 fl.oz	180	0	45
Root Beer, 12 fl.oz	165	0	41
Tonic Water, 12 fl.oz	135	0	34
Mineral Water: Plain, 12 fl.oz	0	0	0
Sweetened/flavored, 12 fl.oz	150	0	37
w. Fruit Juice, 12 fl.oz	120	0	30
Soda Water/Seltzer:			
Plain/Diet, 12 fl.oz	0	0	0
Sweetened/flavored, 12 fl.oz	150	0	37
w. Fruit Juice, 12 fl.oz	120	0	30
Soft Frozen Lemonade, 12 fl.oz	300	0	77

Fountain, Movie Theater & Take-Out

Average All Flavors

	C	F	Cb
Small Cup, 12 fl.oz: No Ice	160	0	40
With ⅓ Ice	120	0	30
Regular, 16 fl.oz: No Ice	210	0	53
With ⅓ Ice	160	0	40
Medium, 22 fl.oz: No Ice	290	0	73
With ⅓ Ice	220	0	55
Large, 32 fl.oz: No Ice	420	0	105
With ⅓ Ice	320	0	80

(Note: ⅓ Cup of Ice = ¼ Cup Liquid)

Soda Brands

Per 12 fl.oz Unless Indicated

	C	F	Cb
A&W: Cream Soda	180	0	46
Diet Cream Soda/Root Beer	1	0	0
Root Beer	180	0	46
Albertson's: Max Cola	165	0	44
Lemon Lime	150	0	41
Other flavors, average	170	0	46

Soda Brands (Cont)

Per 12 fl.oz Unless Indicated

	C	F	Cb
Barq's: Root Beer	165	0	44
Floatz, 12 fl.oz	190	0	50
Big Red, 12 fl.oz	150	0	38
Blue Sky: Cola; Orange Cream	160	0	42
Cherry; Raspberry; Root Beer	170	0	44
Grape; Lemon Lime; Dr Becker	140	0	36
Organic, all flavors, avg.	170	0	43
Other varieties, average	150	0	39
Bubble Up, 12 fl.oz	160	0	42
Cactus Cooler, 12 fl.oz	150	0	40
Canada Dry: Club Soda	0	0	0
Ginger Ale, all flavors	140	0	35
Tonic Water	90	0	24
Diet, 12 fl.oz	0	0	0
Clearly Canadian, average	130	0	34
Coca-Cola: *Per 12 fl.oz*			
Classic/Caffeine Free	140	0	39
Diet Coke, all flavors	0	0	0
Cherry Coke/Vanilla Coke	150	0	40
Coca-Cola C2, 12 fl.oz	70	0	18
Coca-Cola Zero	0	0	0
Coca-Cola Blak, 8 fl.oz bottle	45	0	12
Country Time, Lemonade	140	0	35
Crush, all flavors	180	0	49
Diet Rite, Pure Zero	0	0	0
Dr Pepper: Regular	150	0	40
Cherry Vanilla	140	0	39
Diet, all flavors	0	0	0
Fanta, all flavors	110	0	27
Fresca: Regular	4	0	1
Peach Citrus	0	0	0
Fruitopia: *See Page 153*			
GuS, average all flavors	100	0	25
Hansen's: Diet Soda	0	0	0
Natural Orange Mango, 8 fl.oz	160	0	44
Other flavors, average	150	0	44
Hawaiian Punch: Island Citrus	150	0	41
Light	10	0	2
Henry Weinhard's: Root Beer	170	0	43
Cream flavor, average	175	0	42
Hires, Root Beer	160	0	43
IBC: Root Beer	110	0	29
Cherry Limeade	170	0	44
Cream Soda; Black Cherry	180	0	48
Diet Root Beer	0	0	0

Soft Drinks (Cont)

Per 12 fl.oz Unless Indicated	C	F	Cb
Icee: Coca-Cola, 12 fl.oz	105	0	27
Barq's; Minute Maid, 12 fl.oz	195	0	48
Smoothee Lemonade, 12 fl.oz	255	0	64
Jolt Cola, 12 fl.oz	150	0	41
Jones Soda: Cola	170	0	43
Other flavors, average	185	0	46
Diet	0	0	0
Lucozade, 7 fl.oz	136	0	34
Manzanila Sol	160	0	43
MDX Energy Soda (Sugar Free)	0	0	0
Mello Yello: Regular	180	0	45
Diet, 12 fl.oz	5	0	0
Minute Maid: Fruit Punch	170	0	46
Fruit Falls, 6.8 fl.oz pouch	5	0	2
Fruit Punch	170	0	46
Orangeade	160	0	43
Pink Lemonade	150	0	42
Soft Frozen Lemonade, 12 fl.oz	300	0	78
Light flavors	10	0	2
Fruit Juices: See Page 154			
Mountain Dew: Live Wire; Code Red	170	0	45
Diet flavors	0	0	0
Moxie Original Elixir	150	0	37
Mr Pibb, Regular	150	0	37
Mug Root Beer	160	0	43
Natural Brew: Vanilla, Cream	170	0	42
Ginseng Cola, Ginger Ale	170	0	42
Root Beer	180	0	44
Nehi, Royal Crown Peach	195	0	51
Orangina: 10 fl.oz bottle	120	0	45
Rouge, 8 fl.oz	90	0	22
Pepsi: Regular/Blue/Caffeine Free	165	0	41
Diet Pepsi; Jazz	0	0	0
One, 12 fl.oz	1	0	0.5
Twist	160	0	40
Wild Cherry; Vanilla	165	0	43
Perrier, Carbonated Water	0	0	0
Qibla-Gold, 330ml can	185	0	46
RW Knudsen, Spritzers, average	170	0	43
RC Cola: Regular; Cherry	160	0	43
Diet Cola	0	0	0
Reed's, Ginger Brew, avg. all var.	145	0	38
7·UP: Regular	140	0	38
Cherry, Gold	155	0	38
Caffeinated	170	0	46
Diet varieties, 12 fl.oz	0	0	0
7·UP Plus, 12 fl.oz	12	0	3
Safeway: Cola	160	0	44
Cherry Cola	160	0	43
Ditto Lemon Lime	160	0	40
Parker's Cream Soda	170	0	42
Parker's Root Beer	170	0	47
Diet flavors	0	0	0
Santa Cruz, Sparkling, all types	150	0	37

Per 12 fl.oz Unless Indicated	C	F	Cb
Schweppes: Bitter Lemon/Sour	165	0	41
Seltzer	0	0	0
Tonic Water; Ginger Ale	120	0	30
Shasta: Cream Soda	190	0	47
Cherry Cola; Doc Shasta	160	0	40
Club Soda; Diet, all flavors	0	0	0
Fruit Punch, Pineapple; Orange	200	0	50
Ginger Ale	130	0	33
Other flavors, average	170	0	46
Sierra Mist, Lemon Lime	150	0	39
Sprite: Regular	150	0	37
Diet, 12 fl.oz	4	0	1
Tropical Remix	0	0	0
Zero	170	0	46
Squirt, Citrus Burst	150	0	40
Star Ruby (GUS): Valencia Orange	100	0	26
Other flavors	95	0	24
Stewarts: Root Beer	160	0	41
Grape	190	0	48
Key Lime	180	0	46
Sunkist: Orange	190	0	52
Diet Sunkist	0	0	0
Cherry Limeade	170	0	44
Sunny D, 12 fl.oz	180	0	45
Surge, Citrus	170	0	46
TAB, 12 fl.oz	0	0	0
Think!: Cola, 8.4 fl.oz	112	0	29
Sparkling Citrus, 8.4 fl.oz	130	0	31
Thomas Kemper: Root Beer	140	0	34
Other flavors, average	155	0	38
Tropicana Twister, avg., 12 fl.oz	190	0	50
Vault, Zero	5	0	0
Vernor's: Ginger Ale	150	0	37
Diet, 10 fl.oz	0	0	0
Welch's: Soda, 12 fl.oz	190	0	51
Sparkling	180	0	45
Wild Oats, Down to Earth	150	0	37
Wink, 12 fl.oz	195	0	48

Powdered Soft Drink Mix

Per 8 fl.oz (Prep'd)	C	F	Cb
Capri Sun, ½ pkg	25	0	6
Cool Splashers, 8 fl.oz	60	0	16
Country Time: Lemonade	60	0	16
Other flavors, average	85	0	22
Lite	35	0	9
Crystal Light, 8 fl.oz	5	0	1
Flavoraid, ⅛ pkg	2	0	0.5
Kool-Aid: All flavors	70	0	17
Unsweetened, 6 fl.oz	2	0	0.5
Propel, ½ pkg	10	0	3
Tang, 8 fl.oz	40	0	9

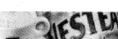

Instant Coffee

	C	**F**	**Cb**
Powder/Granules: Regular or Decaffeinated,			
1 level tsp	2	0	0.5
1 rounded tsp	4	0	1
Ground, 1 Tbsp	5	0	1
Brewed/Percolated, 1 cup, 8 fl.oz	5	0	1
Coffee With Milk/Cream/Creamers:			
Per Cup Coffee (8 fl.oz):			
w. Whole Milk: Dash, 1 Tbsp	10	0.5	1
2 Tbsp, 1 fl.oz	20	1	1.5
w. 2% Milk, 2 Tbsp	15	0.5	1.5
w. 1% Milk, 2 Tbsp	12	0.3	1.5
w. Fat Free Milk, 2 Tbsp	10	0	1.5
w. Half & Half, 2 Tbsp	45	4	1
w. Cream (light coffee), 2 Tbsp	65	6	1
w. *Coffee Mate:* Liquid, reg., 1T.	40	2	5
Liquid Fat Free, 1 Tbsp	15	0	2
Powder, 1 heaping tsp	20	1	2
Sugar ~ Add Extra: 1 heaping tsp	25	0	6
Single portion, 1 package	25	0	6

Flavored Coffee Mixes

Chicory: Instant Coffee, 1 tsp	6	0	1
Coffee Essence, 1 tsp	16	0	4
Caffé D'Vita: Mixes, 3 tsp	65	2.5	10
Sugar Free Mixes, 2 tsp	35	2	3
General Foods: Average, ½ oz	60	3	10
Sugar-free, average, 1 tsp	30	1.5	3
Cappuccino Coolers, ½ oz	60	0	15
Jakada *(Folgers):* Coffee Latte, 3 Tbsp	100	5	14
Cappuccino, 3 tsp	85	2	16
Maxwell House: Cappuccino, 1 pkt	90	2	19
Mocha, sugar-free, 1 envelope	60	3	7
Van., Irish Cream, 1 envelope	90	1	20
Nescafé: Average all flavors	80	0	19

Coffee Substitute Mixes

Roasted Cereal Beverages: (No Caffeine)			
Cafix Instant Beverage, 1 tsp	5	0	1
Kaffree Roma *(Natural Touch)* , 1 tsp	6	0	1
Postum, Instant Hot Beverage, 1 tsp	10	0	3
Revival Soy "Coffee", 1 Tbsp	5	0	1
Teeccino Caffe, 1 tsp	10	0	2

Vending Machine

Cappuccino, 1 cup, 8 fl.oz	70	4	6

Coffee Shops/Restaurants

Per 8 fl.oz Cup (Unless Indicated)	**C**	**F**	**Cb**
Coffee (Regular/Percolated/Filtered)	5	0	1
Americano Drip Coffee, 1 cup	5	0	1
Cafe Au Lait: 1 cup, 8 fl.oz	70	4	6
Nonfat Milk, 1 cup, 8 fl.oz	45	0	7
Caffe Latté:			
8 fl.oz cup: w. Whole Milk	130	7	10
w. 2% Milk	105	3.5	11
w. Nonfat Milk	80	0	12
12 fl.oz: w. Whole Milk	200	11	16
w. Nonfat Milk	120	0	18
16 fl.oz: w. Whole Milk	260	14	21
w. Nonfat Milk	160	0	24
Cafe Mocha (Mochaccino): 1 cup	150	6	20
12 fl.oz	240	10	31
16 fl.oz	300	12	40
Cappuccino:			
8 fl.oz cup: w. Whole Milk	75	4	6
w. 2% Milk	60	2	7
w. Nonfat Milk	50	0	7
12 fl.oz: w. Whole Milk	120	6	10
w. 2% Milk	100	3.5	11
w. Nonfat Milk	80	0	11
16 fl.oz: w. Whole Milk	150	8	13
w. Nonfat Milk	100	0	14
Mocha (with cream):			
8 fl.oz: w. Whole Milk	200	11	21
w. Nonfat Milk	175	6	22
12 fl.oz: Whole Milk	310	17	32
w. Nonfat Milk	260	9	34
Iced Mocha (no cream):			
12 fl.oz: w. Whole Milk	170	6	26
w. Nonfat Milk	130	1.5	27
Espresso: Single (Solo)	5	0	1
Doppio (Double)	10	0	2
Espresso Con Panna,			
(w. dollop whipped cream), solo	80	9	3
Espresso Macchiato, solo	10	0	1
Frappuccino: Tall, 12 fl.oz	200	3	39
Grande, 16 fl.oz	270	4	52
Frappuccino Mocha (w. Cream):			
Tall, 12 fl.oz	310	12	46
Grande, 16 fl.oz	420	16	61
Iced Latte: *Similar to Caffe Latte*			
Starbucks: *See Fast-Foods Section*			

For Complete Nutritional Data ~ See CalorieKing.com

Hot Chocolate ◆ Caffeine Counter

Irish & Liqueur Coffees

	C	F	Cb
Irish Coffee (no sugar)	175	10	0
Liqueur Coffee, avg. all types	200	10	16

Cocoa & Hot Chocolate

	C	F	Cb
Cocoa (8 fl.oz cup): w. Whole Milk	210	14	19
w. Nonfat Milk	80	8	2
Tall (12 fl.oz): w. Whole Milk	300	20	26
w. Nonfat Milk	120	11	5
Hot Chocolate:			
8 fl.oz cup: w. Whole Milk	200	10	25
w. Nonfat Milk	140	2	25
Tall (12 fl.oz): w. Whole Milk	300	15	38
w. Nonfat Milk	210	3	38
Cinnabon, Mocolatta Chill, 16 oz	405	14	55

Coffee Extras

	C	F	Cb
Chocolate (Cocoa) Topping, ½ tsp	10	0	2
Flavored Syrups: Regular, 2 Tbsp	80	0	20
Sugar-free, 2 Tbsp	0	0	0
Half & Half Cream, 2 Tbsp	40	3	3
Light Whipped Cream, 2 Tbsp	30	2	2
Marshmallows, miniature, 2 Tbsp	20	0	5
Hershey's Chocolate Syrup, 2 Tbsp	100	0	24

Bottled Coffee (Chilled)

Ready-To-Drink: *Per Bottle*

	C	F	Cb
Arizona Mocha Latte 10½ fl.oz	130	2	24
Carnation: Malted Milk Vanilla, 3 T.	90	2	15
Chocolate, 3 Tbsp	90	1	18
Kahlúa Cappuccino Shake 15½ fl.oz	195	3	36

Main St Cafe

	C	F	Cb
French Vanilla Ice Latte, 12 fl.oz	190	3	31
Nescafe: Ice Java, avg., 2 Tbsp	80	0	20

Royal Mills: *Per Can*

	C	F	Cb
Hawaiian Kona; Iced, 10.8 oz	125	2	27
Iced Cappuccino, 10.8 oz	165	3	32
Island Mocha, 10.8 oz	220	3.5	42
Kona Blend, 11.5 oz	90	1.5	18

Starbucks: *Per 9.5 fl.oz Bottle*

	C	F	Cb
Frappuccino: Caramel	200	3	37
Coffee	190	3.5	35
Hazelnut; Mocha	200	3.5	37
DoubleShot, 6.5 fl.oz can	140	6	18

Swiss Miss, Caramel Cream Hot Cocoa,

	C	F	Cb
1 packet	110	2.5	21

CAFFEINE COUNTER

Moderate caffeine intake is not harmful to healthy adults. However, frequent large amounts (over 350mg/day) may cause dependency ('caffeinism') and adversely affect health. To be safe, limit caffeine to 200mg/day. Avoid if pregnant; breast feeding; a child under 8; or have heart arrhythmias.

	Caffeine (mg)
Coffee: Instant, Weak, 1 level teaspoon	45
Medium, 1 rounded teaspoon	70
Strong, 1 heaping teaspoon	100
Decaffeinated, 1 round teaspoon	2
Bags *(Folgers)*, 1 bag (6-8 fl.oz)	115
Ground, 1 Tbsp, 6g	60
Bottled (Ready-To-Drink), 9.5 fl.oz	70
Coffee Shop: Brewed, 8 fl.oz	110 - 150
Cappuccino: 1 cup, 8 fl.oz	80
Tall, 12 fl.oz	120
Large, 16 fl.oz	160
Decappuccino (decaffeinated)	5
Espresso: Regular/Solo	80
Double (Doppio) Espresso	160
Iced Coffee, 12 fl.oz	80
Latte, 1 cup, 8 fl.oz	80
Mocha, 8 fl.oz	90
Hot Chocolate, 8 fl.oz	10
Tea (Black/Green): Weak, 1 cup	20
Medium Strength, 1 cup	40
Strong, 1 cup	70
Herbal Tea	0
Iced Tea, Tall Glass/Can, 12 fl.oz	25
Soda Drinks: *Per 12 fl.oz Can*	
Coca-Cola, Pepsi (Reg./Diet)	35
Coca-Cola Blak, 8 fl.oz bottle	45
Diet Coke; TAB; RC Cola (Regular)	45
Dr. Pepper (Reg./Diet)	40
Sunkist Orange Soda; Mr PiBB	40
Jolt Cola; SunDrop	65 - 70
Pepsi One; Mtn Dew; Mellow Yellow; Surge	55
Energy Drinks (w. caffeine): Avg., 8 fl.oz	80
Full Throttle, 16 fl.oz	150
Red Bull (Regular/Sugar Free), 8.3 fl.oz	80
Tilt (Anheuser-Busch), alcoholic, 16 fl.oz	70
Chocolate Bars: Milk Chocolate, 2 oz	12
Dark Chocolate, 2 oz	30
Cocoa/Hot Choc. Mix, 1 oz pkt	5
Chocolate Milk, 1 cup, 8 fl.oz	3
Choc Chip Cookies, 1 medium, 1 oz	3
Chocolate Syrup, 2 Tbsp, 1.4 oz	7

Extensive Caffeine Counter ~ www.CalorieKing.com

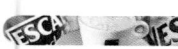

Tea & Iced Tea

Quick Guide

Teas

	C	F	Cb
Regular: Bag, Loose or Instant			
Brewed, 1 cup, 8 fl.oz	1	0	0
(Add extra for sugar/milk)			
Herbal: Average all varieties, 1 cup	1	0	0
Bigelow: Apple Orchard, 1 cup	5	0	1
Other Varieties	2	0	0.5
Celestial Seasonings:			
Bengal Spice; Spearmint	5	0	0.5
Lemon Zinger	4	0	1
Roastaroma	10	0	2
Other varieties	2	0	0.5
Bubble Tea, average, 12 fl.oz	240	0	55
Chai Tea: *Cafe D' Vita,* 2 Tbsp	120	3.5	21
Starbucks: *See Fast-Foods Section*			

Iced Tea

	C	F	Cb
Average All Brands			
Pre-Sweetened: 8 fl.oz	100	0	25
12 fl.oz	150	0	38
16 fl.oz	200	0	50
Unsweetened: 8 fl.oz	2	0	0

Iced Tea Mixes

Per Serving (1 Cup, Made-Up)

	C	F	Cb
4C Instant	90	0	22
Carb Options, 1 cup	0	0	0
Celestial Seasonings Iced Delight	4	0	1
Crystal Light Sugar Free	3	0	1
Lipton: Instant	0	0	0
Instant Lemon/Raspberry	3	0	1
Lemon	55	0	14
Peach/Raspb, Sugar Free	5	0	1
Nestea			
Lemonade Tea, 1⅓ Tbsp	60	0	15
Lemon flavored Iced Tea, 1⅓ Tbsp	60	0	15
Sugar Free Lemon Iced Tea, 2 tsp	5	0	1
Unsweetened Tea, 2 tsp	0	0	0
Concentrate: Green Tea, 2 Tbsp	80	0	17
Lemon Tea, 2 Tbsp	80	0	18
Raspberry, 2 Tbsp	90	0	20

Bottled & Canned Teas

Per 8 fl.oz Unless Indicated

	C	F	Cb
Arizona: Sweet Tea	90	0	23
Green Tea(s)/Asian Plum; Herb	70	0	18
Diet Green/Lemon	0	0	0
Ginseng Tea	60	0	15
Peach/Raspberry	100	0	25
No Carb, all flavors	5	0	2
Brisk: Raspberry, 1 can	95	0	24
Diet	5	0	1
Lemon: 8 fl.oz can	90	0	23
Gold Peak, 1 Bottle, 16.9 fl.oz	170	0	45
Hansen's: Natural Iced Tea, 8 fl.oz	70	0	21
Low Calorie Blueberry/Raspberry	10	0	3
Honest Tea: Green Dragon, 16 fl.oz	60	0	18
Lori's Lemon Tea	0	0	0
Lipton (16 fl.oz Bottle): *Per 8 fl.oz*			
No Lemon	70	0	18
Lemon	90	0	21
Peach; Raspberry	110	0	26
Diet Green Tea	0	0	0
Nantucket: Blueberry Tea, 8 fl.oz	80	0	20
Original Lemon Tea; Half & Half	90	0	23
Diet Lemon Tea	10	0	2
Nestea Iced Tea: Diet Lemon	5	0	1
Lemon/Peach/Raspberry, 8 fl.oz	90	0	23
Green Tea, 1 bottle, 20 fl.oz	210	0	23
Diet Green Tea	0	0	0
Oregon Chai: Herbal Bliss, ½ cup	70	0	18
Nirvana/Kashmir Green, ½ cup	80	0	20
Shasta, 8 fl.oz	80	0	20
Snapple: Reg., sweetened, avg.	105	0	26
Diet/Unsweetened	0	0	0
SoBe: Green/Lemon Tea, 8 fl.oz	90	0	23
20 fl.oz bottle	225	0	57
Ssips *(Johanna Farms),* 8.45 fl.oz	100	0	25
Tazo: Iced Teas, 8 fl.oz	70	0	17
Juiced Teas, 8 fl.oz	85	0	21
Organic Iced Teas, 8 fl.oz	35	0	9
Turkey Hill: Regular, 8 fl.oz	90	0	22
Raspberry Cooler, 8 fl.oz	110	0	28

> "A woman is like a teabag. You never know her strength until she's in hot water."
>
> ~ Eleanor Roosevelt

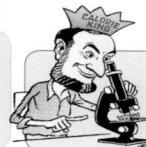

For Extra Listings and Nutritional Data
~ See Author's Website
www.CalorieKing.com

Alcohol Guide

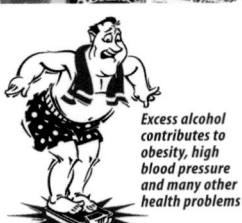

Health Hazards: Excessive alcohol intake contributes to obesity, high blood pressure, stroke, heart and liver disease, some cancers, and even impotence. **Concentration and short-term memory** are reduced as well as sporting performance.

Other alcohol hazards include stomach upsets, menstrual problems, anxiety, headaches, insomnia, work absenteeism, risky behaviors, and social problems.

Excess alcohol contributes to obesity, high blood pressure and many other health problems

Alcohol contributes to obesity through its high calories and by lessening the body's ability to burn fat. Fat storage is promoted, particularly in the belly - a health danger zone. Alcohol can also stimulate the appetite.

Alcohol is potentially more harmful while dieting. Blood sugar levels may drop with resultant tiredness and further impairment of concentration, reflexes and driving skills - and maybe even the dieter's resolve!

LOW RISK ALCOHOL LIMITS

 WOMEN: No more than **1 drink** per day

 MEN: No more than **2 drinks** per day

(At least 2 days a week should be alcohol-free)

1 DRINK CONTAINS 14 GRAMS ALCOHOL
- 12 fl.oz Regular Beer (5% Alc.)
- OR 14 fl.oz Light Beer (4.2% Alc.)
- OR 5 fl.oz Wine (12% Alc.)
- OR 1½ fl.oz Spirits (80 Proof)

Note: You cannot save daily drinks for one occasion. Binge drinking is particularly harmful ~ 4 drinks for males or 3 drinks for females (within 2 hours).

HOW TO CALCULATE ALCOHOL CONTENT

Percent alcohol on label refers to alcohol volume (ml alcohol/100ml).

100ml = 3½ fl. oz

To convert to grams (weight) of alcohol, multiply the percent volume by 0.8 - since 1 ml of alcohol weighs only 0.8 grams.

EXAMPLE
12 fl.oz Can Beer (5% alcohol)
5% alc.volume = 5% of 12 fl.oz
= 0.6 fl.oz
= 18ml alcohol
(1 fl.oz = 30ml)

Weight (18ml x 0.8) = 14.4g alc.

For some people, **safe drinking** will mean no alcohol drinks at all. Even one drink may impair driving skills, particularly if tired; and each drink after the first drink increases breast cancer risk in women by 9%.

It is advisable not to drink at all if you are:
- pregnant, trying to conceive or breastfeeding
- taking medication or have liver or heart disease (unless approved by your doctor or pharmacist)
- planning to drive, use machinery or play sport
- studying or needing to concentrate
- a child or adolescent

Note: Women and adolescents are more prone to alcohol's ill-effects due to their lower body weight, smaller livers and lesser capacity to metabolize alcohol.

Ten Hints to Avoid Harmful Drinking: See Page 172

GOVERNMENT WARNINGS!

(1) According to the Surgeon General, women should not drink alcoholic beverages during pregnancy because of the risk of birth defects.

(2) Consumption of alcoholic beverages impairs your ability to drive a car or operate machinery, and may cause health problems.

Quick Guide

Alc ~ Alcohol (Grams)
Cb ~ Carbohydrate

Beer

Beer Contains Zero Fat

	C	Alc	Cb
Regular Beer (5% Alc. Vol.)			
7 fl.oz Glass	80	8.5	4
12 fl.oz Bottle/Can/Glass	140	14	10
16 fl.oz Bottle/Can	185	19	13
22 fl.oz Bottle	260	25	20
24 fl.oz Can	280	28	20
32 fl.oz Bottle	370	35	28
40 fl.oz Bottle	470	46	35
50 fl.oz Football	590	57	50
Light Beer (4.2% Alc. Vol.)			
7 fl.oz Glass	65	7	4
12 fl.oz Bottle/Can/Glass	110	12	7
16 fl.oz Bottle/Can	145	16	9
22 fl.oz Bottle	200	22	13
24 fl.oz Can	220	24	14
Non-Alcoholic/Near Beer			
(Less than 0.5% alcohol by volume)			
Average All Brands, 12 fl.oz	70	1	14

Beer Brands

Per 12 fl.oz Serving **Alc** ~ Alcohol (Grams)
Percentage alcohol listed below is by volume - not by weight.

	C	Alc	Cb
Amber Ice (5.3% alcohol)	130	15	6
Amstel Light (3.5%)	100	10	5
Anheuser World Select (5%)	165	15	15
Anchor Steam (4.6%)	155	13	16
Arrogant Bastard Ale (7.2%)	190	20	12
Artic Ice (5.3%)	150	15	8
Artic Ice Light (3.9%)	100	11	6
Asahi Super Dry (5.2%)	150	15	11
Aspen Edge Low Carb (4.1%)	95	12	3
Augsburger Bock (4.9%)	170	14	17
Bass (5.51%)	140	16	13
Beck's (5%)	145	14	10
Beck's Light (3.8%)	105	11	6
Big Sky (4.8%)	150	14	12
Big Sky Light (4.5%)	105	13	5
Black Label (5.6%)	155	15	11
Blackhook Porter (4.9%)	160	14	14
Blatz (4.6%)	145	13	13
Blatz LA (2.3%)	75	7	6
Blatz Light (3.9%)	110	11	8
Blonde (4.3%)	140	12	10
Blue Moon: Belgian (5.4%)	170	15	14
Pumpkin Ale (5.8%)	185	16	18
Bud Dry (5%)	130	14	8

Brands (Cont)

Alc ~ Alcohol (Grams)

Beer Contains Zero Fat

	C	Alc	Cb
Bud Light (4.2%)	110	12	7
Bud Ice (5.5%)	150	15	9
Bud Ice Light (4.2%)	110	12	7
Budweiser	145	14	11
Budweiser Select (4.3%)	100	12	3
Busch (4.6%)	135	13	10
Busch Ice (5.9%)	170	16	13
Busch Light (4.2%)	110	12	7
Carling (4.4%)	140	13	10
Carlsberg (5%)	135	13	10
Carta Blanca (4.0%)	125	11	11
Castlemaine XXXX (4.7%)	140	13	9
Colt 45 Malt (5.6%)	160	15	11
Coors Original (5%)	140	14	11
Coors Extra Gold (5%)	145	14	11
Coors Light (4.2%)	105	12	5
Coors Winter Fest (5.6%)	190	16	17
Corona Extra (4.6%)	150	13	13
Corona Light (4.1%)	105	12	5
Dos Equis Lager (5%)	130	14	9
Drop Top Amber Ale (4.8%)	165	13	16
Fosters Lager (4.9%)	135	14	9
George Killian's: Irish Brown (5.2%)	185	15	15
Irish Red (5%)	160	14	13
Goebel (4.1%)	130	11	12
Goebel Light (3.9%)	110	11	8
Grolsch Premium (5%)	140	14	11
Guinness Draught (4.2%)	125	12	10
Guinness Extra Stout (5.8%)	175	17	14
Hamm's (4.7%)	145	13	12
Special Light (4.1%)	110	12	7
Harp (4.5%)	150	12	13
Heineken (5%)	150	14	12
Heineken Special Dark (5.2%)	175	15	16
Heineken Premium Light (3.5%)	100	10	7
Hop Jack Pale Ale (5%)	185	14	14
Hurricane (5.8%)	160	16	10
Icehouse (5.0%)	135	14	8
Icehouse (5.5%)	150	15	9
Jacob Best Ice (5.8%)	160	16	11
Keystone: Premium (4.4%)	110	12	5
Ice (5.9%)	145	16	7
Light (4.2%)	100	12	5
Killarney's Red Larger (5%)	200	14	23
Killain's Irish Red (4.9%)	165	14	14
King Cobra (5.9%)	170	16	12
Kirin Lager (4.9%)	145	14	11
Kirin Light (3.2%)	95	9	7
Labatt's Blue (5%)	145	14	9

Beers ◆ Ales (with Alcohol Counts)

Brands (Cont)

Alc ~ Alcohol (Grams)
Cb ~ Carbohydrate

Beer Contains Zero Fat
Per 12 fl.oz Serving

	C	Alc	Cb
Leinenkugel's: Original (4.6%)	150	13	14
Light (4.1%)	105	11	6
Lone Star: Regular (4.7%)	140	13	12
Light (3.9%)	110	11	8
Lowenbrau Dark/Special (4.9%)	160	14	15
Magic Hat #9 (4.8%)	140	14	12
Magnum Malt Liquor (5.6%)	155	16	10
Meister Brau (4.5%)	130	13	12
Memphis Brown (4.6%)	120	13	6
Michelob: Regular (5%)	155	14	13
Light (4.3%)	135	12	12
Amber Bock (5.2%)	165	15	15
Golden Draft (4.7%)	150	13	14
Golden Draft Light (4.1%)	110	11	7
Honey Larger (4.9%)	175	14	18
Michelob ULTRA (4.1%)	95	12	3
Mickey's Malt Liquor (5.6%)	160	16	11
MGD (5%)	145	14	13
MGD Light (4.5%)	110	13	7
Miller High Life (5%)	145	14	13
Miller High Life Light (4.5%)	110	13	6
Miller Lite (4.5%)	100	13	4
Milwaukee's Best (4.5%)	130	13	12
Milwaukee's Best Ice (5.9%)	145	16	6
Milwaukee's Best Light (4.5%)	100	13	4
Minnesota's Best (4.9%)	140	14	10
Molson Canadian (5%)	150	14	12
Molson Ice (5.6%)	160	14	12
Molson Special Dry (5%)	145	14	10
Moosehead (5%)	125	14	14
Natural Light (4.2%)	95	12	3
Negra Modela (5%)	155	14	14
Newcastle Brown Ale (4.5%)	140	12	13
Northstone Amber Ale (4.9%)	150	14	8
Olde English "800" (5.9%)	160	16	11
Old Milwaukee (4.6%)	145	13	13
Light (3.9%)	110	11	8
Ice (5.9%)	180	16	15
Old Style (4.7%)	140	13	12
Old Style Light (4.2%)	115	12	7
Olympia Gold Light (2.2 %)	70	6	6
Pabst (4.3%)	145	13	12
Pabst Blue Ribbon (4.7%)	145	14	12
Pabst Light (3.9%)	110	11	8
Pabst Extra Light (2.2%)	70	6	6
Pearl Light (2.2%)	70	6	6
Pete's Wicked Ale (5.3%)	175	15	17
Piels (4.3%)	125	12	9
Pilsner Urquell (4.4%)	155	13	16
Red Dog (5%)	150	14	14
Red Hook ESB (5.7%)	180	17	16
Red Hook India Pale Ale (4.7%)	180	13	19
Red Stripe Jamaican Ale (5.0%)	155	14	14
Red Wolf (5.4%)	150	15	10
Rolling Rock (4.5%)	120	13	7
Sam Adams Light (4%)	130	11	10
Samuel Adams (4.6%)	170	13	17
Samuel Adams Lager (4.7%)	180	13	19
Sapporo Draft (3.9%)	135	11	14
Schaefer (4.6%)	145	13	12
Schaefer Light (3.9%)	110	11	8
Schlitz (4.6%)	145	13	12
Schlitz Light (3.9%)	110	11	8
Schmidt's (4.6%)	145	13	13
Schmidt's Light (3.9%)	110	11	8
Sheaf Stout, 5.7%	180	16	17
Sierra Nevada: Pale Ale (5.6%)	200	16	12
Big Foot (9.6%)	295	28	25
Porter (5.6%)	200	16	16
Wheat Beer (4.4%)	150	12	12
Silver Thunder (5.9%)	165	17	11
Skyy Sport (5%)	160	14	15
Sol Cerveza Especial (4%)	125	11	11
Southpaw Light (5%)	125	14	7
St Pauli Girl (5%)	135	14	13
Stella Artois, 5%, 330ml	135	14	9
Stroh's (4.6%)	145	13	12
Stroh's Light (4.0%)	130	12	10
Tecate (4.5%)	155	13	16
Tequiza (4.5%)	130	13	9
The Governator (5.2%)	150	15	11
Warsteiner Verum/Dunkel (5%)	155	14	13
Weinhard's: Pale Ale (4/6%)	150	13	13
Hefeweizen (4.9%)	155	14	13
Wheat Hook (4.8%)	150	14	12
Widmer: Hefeweizen (4.7%)	155	13	16
Zeigenbock Amber (4.4%)	145	12	13

Home-Brewed Beer: Similar to regular beers, according to alcohol content.

Alc ~ Alcohol (Grams) **Cb** ~ Carbohydrate

Non-Alcoholic Brews

	C	Alc	Cb
Less Than 0.5% Alcohol			
Average All Brands (Busch NA, Coors NA, Kaliber, Kingsbury, O'Douls, Old Milwaukee NA, Pabst NA, Stroh's NA, Sharp's, Haake Beck, Texas Select)			
12 fl.oz Can/Bottle	70	1	14
O'Doul's Amber, 12 fl.oz	90	1	18

Cider

Alcoholic Cider: Average, 6% alcohol,			
Dry, 12 fl.oz	130	17	12
Sweet, 12 fl.oz	170	17	15
Hardcore Crisp Hard Cider (6%)	190	17	19
Hornsby's: Draft Cider (6%)	170	17	16
Hard Apple Cider (5.5%)	200	16	27
Woodchuck (5%) Amber, 12 fl.oz	200	15	21
Dark & Dry, 12 fl.oz	180	15	17
Granny Smith, 12 fl.oz	165	15	11
Wyder's: Raspb. (4%), 11.5 fl.oz	140	11	15
Peach (5%) 11.5 fl.oz	150	13	16
Pear (5%), 11.5 fl.oz	130	13	14
22 fl.oz bottle	250	25	28

Quick Guide

Table Wines

	C	Alc	Cb
Average All Varieties (11.5% Alcohol)			
Wine Contains Zero Fat			
4 fl.oz 1 small wine glass			
OR ½ large wine glass	90	11	3
6 fl.oz (¾ large wine glass)	135	16	4
8 fl.oz (1 large wine glass)	180	22	6
½ Carafe/Bottle, 375ml	290	34	10
1 Bottle, 750ml	580	68	20

Table Wines

	C	Alc	Cb
Red: Claret/Burgundy/Chianti, 4 fl.oz	80	11	2
Sparkling Reds, 4 fl.oz	90	11	3
Rose: Medium, 4 fl.oz	80	11	2
White: *Per 4 fl.oz*			
Dry (Chablis/Hock/Riesling)	75	11	1
Zinfandel Sweet			
(Moselle/Sauterne), 4 fl.oz	85	11	2
Sparkling, 4 fl.oz	95	11	4

Table Wines (Cont)

	C	Alc	Cb
Champagne: *Per 4 fl.oz Serving*			
Average 1 glass, 4 fl.oz	85	11	2
w. Orange Jce (3:1 orange)	75	8	4
w. Orange Jce (1:1 orange)	65	5	7
Cold Duck, 4 fl. oz	108	11	8
Mulled Wine *(Gluhwein)*, 4 fl.oz	180	14	20
Non-Alcoholic Wine, avg., 4 fl.oz	50	0	12
Reduced Alcohol Wine (6%):			
Average all types, 4 fl.oz	50	0	12
Sake: Rice Wine (16% alc.), 4 oz	125	15	5

Flavored Wine

	C	Alc	Cb
Average All Brands (6% alcohol)			
(Examples: Arbor Mist, Wild Vines, Boones)			
1 small wine glass, 4 fl.oz	80	6	11
1 large wine glass, 8 fl.oz	160	11	21
1 bottle, 750 ml (25.4 fl.oz)	510	36	67

Dessert Wines

	C	Alc	Cb
Madeira (18% alc), 2 oz	85	9	5
Marsala (18%), 2 oz	110	9	11
Port, Muscatel, (18%), 2 oz	85	9	5
Sherry (18%), 2 oz			
Dry, 1 Sherry glass	65	9	0.5
Sweet/Cream, average	85	9	5
Vermouth: Dry (18%), 2 oz	65	9	0.5
Sweet (15%), 2 oz	85	7	5

Cooking Wine

	C	Alc	Cb
Average All Brands			
Red/White: 2 Tbsp, 1 oz	20	3	1
1 cup, 8 fl.oz	160	22	12
Marsala, 2 Tbsp, 1 oz	35	4	2
Sherry, 2 Tbsp, 1 oz	40	4	2

Cooking with Wine:
For alcohol to evaporate, sufficient heat and cooking time (at least 30 minutes) is required.

Red and white table wines would then contain negligible residual calories.

Sweetened wines (marsala/sherry) would contain 10 calories per 1 fl.oz.

Flambé Desserts: Only surface alcohol is burnt off, so negligible reduction in alcohol or calories.

Liquors ✦ Coolers ✦ Cocktails

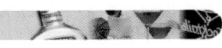

Quick Guide   Alc ~ Alcohol (Grams)

Spirits/Liquors
Includes Bourbon, Brandy, Gin, Rum, Scotch, Tequila, Vodka, Whiskey.
Note: All spirits with same proof (alcohol) have similar calories and zero fat.
Average All Brands

	C	Alc	Cb
80 Proof (40% Alcohol by Volume):			
1 fl.oz	65	9.5	0
1½ fl.oz (1 shot)	100	14	0
3 fl.oz (Double shot)	200	29	0
½ Bottle, 350 ml	810	120	0
1 Bottle, 700 ml	1620	240	0
86 Proof (43% Alc): 1 fl.oz	70	10	0
1½ fl.oz (1 shot)	105	15	0
1 Bottle, 700 ml	1750	250	0
100 Proof (50% Alc): 1½ fl.oz	120	18	0
Shochu (Soju) ~ Izakaya Lounges			
Average all types (20% alc), 2 fl.oz	65	9	0

Chu-Hai Cocktails ~ Next Page
Flavored Spirits ~ Average All Brands
Includes Malibu Rum; Captain Morgan

	C	Alc	Cb
70 Proof (35% Alc): 1½ fl.oz	105	13	1
3 fl.oz (Double shot)	210	26	3

Hard Lemon(ade) & Sodas

	C	Alc	Cb
Doc's Hard Lemon (5%), 12 fl.oz	170	14	17
Henry's Hard L'ade (5%), 12 fl.oz	285	14	46
Hooch Hard (5.2%), 330ml	215	14	32
Hooch Ice (5.7%), 330ml	230	15	32
Mike's Hard Lem. (5.2%): 11.2 fl.oz	240	13	38
16 fl.oz bottle	345	19	54
Mike's Light Lem. (4%), 11.2 fl.oz	120	10	12
Mike's Hard Iced Tea (5%), 11.2 fl.oz	195	13	27
Rick's Spiked (5.2%), 12 fl.oz	250	14	39
Twisted Tea: Half & Half (5%) 12 fl.oz	250	14	37
Hard Iced/Raspberry (5%) 12 fl.oz	220	14	30
Two Dogs (4.2%), 355ml	205	12	30

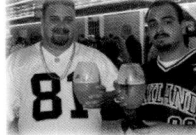

Enjoy a beer but watch the portion size. Those footballs hold 50 fl.oz!

Coolers & Premix Cocktails

Ready-To-Drink
Zero Fat Unless Indicated

	C	Alc	Cb
Arbor Mist: Blenders, all flavors (12.5%), 4 fl.oz	100	11	14
Bacardi: Silver (5%), 12 fl.oz	230	14	33
Silver O³ (5%), 12 fl.oz	230	14	33
Silver Raz (5%), 12 fl.oz	230	14	33
Silver Limon (5%)	230	14	33
Silver Low Carb: Black Cherry (4%)	100	12	3
Apple (4%)	95	11	4.5
Ready to Pour (1.75 liter bottle)			
Bahama Mama (10%), 4 fl.oz	130	13	16
Hurricane (12.5%), 4 fl.oz	144	12	16
Rum Island Ice Tea (12.5%), 4 fl.oz	150	12	16
Bartles & Jaymes			
Malt Based Coolers (3.9% alc): Per 12 fl.oz			
Black Cherry; Classic Original	200	11	30
Exotic Berry, Juicy Peach	210	11	33
Fuzzy Navel; Hard Lemonade	230	11	38
Margarita, Pina Colada	270	11	48
Raspberry Daiquiri	220	11	38
Strawb. Cosmopolitan/Daiquiri	230	11	35
Raspb. Lemonade, Lusc. Blackb.	230	11	38
B-to-the-E (Anheuser-Busch), 10 fl.oz	150	12	17
Cruzan Island Cocktails (5% alc): Per 12 fl.oz			
Jumbie Brew	230	14	32
Mojito	300	14	50
Wazi Koki	285	14	46
Jack Daniels Country Cocktails (5.9%)			
average all flavors, 6.8 fl.oz	170	10	25
Jack Daniels Hard Cola (5%) 12 oz	234	14	34
Jose Cuervo Authentic Margarita (5.9% alc)			
Margarita/ Lime.Strawb. 200ml	180	10	27
Sauza Diablo (5%), 12 fl.oz	260	14	40
Seagram's Coolers (5%)			
Smooth Red/Citrus 12 fl.oz	240	14	35
Skyy Blue (5%), 12 fl.oz	280	14	45
Stolichnaya Citr. (5%), 12 fl.oz	240	14	36
Smirnoff Ice (5%), 330ml	220	13	33
Black Ice (5.5%), 12 fl.oz	240	19	36
TGI Friday's: Per 3 fl.oz			
On The Rocks: Margarita (7.5%)	90	6	14
Long Island Ice Tea (15%)	130	11	14
Mudslide (10%)	200	8	18
Blenders (12.5% alc) Per 3 fl.oz:			
Mudslide (12.5%)	120	8.5	15
Orange Dream (12.5%)	120	8.5	15
Strawberry Shortcake (12.5%)	115	8.5	12
Tilt (Anheuser-Busch) 6.6% alc., 16 fl.oz	390	24	56

Coolers & Premix Cocktails (Cont)

Ready-To-Drink   **C**   **Alc**   **Cb**

The Club *Premix Cocktails (8 oz Can):*
Per 4 oz Serving (½ can)

	C	Alc	Cb
Long Island Ice Tea; Manhattan	220	16	30
Margar.; Screwdriver; Vodka Martini	210	7	40
Mudslide (9g fat)	270	12	41
Pina Colada; Or. Craze; Whisk. Sour	260	10	40
Zima (5.9%), 12 fl.oz	235	15	20

Shooters   **Alc** ~ Alcohol (Grams)

Alabama Slammer	110	14	2
Amaretto Sours	120	6	19
Cranium Meltdown	75	7	2
Duck Fart	85	7	5
Kamakazie	150	20	2
Kool-Aid	160	15	14
Liquid Cocaine	130	13	10
Mud Slide	160	13	17
Fuzzy Navel	120	13	7
Pineapple Bomber	130	11	13
Turbo	110	14	3

Cocktail Mixers

Non Alcoholic ~ No Alcohol Added

Bacardi: *Frozen Concentrate*
(Made Up from 2 fl.oz concentrate)

Margarita, 8 fl.oz	90	0	25
Pina Colada, 8 fl.oz	170	0	35
Strawberry, 8 fl.oz	120	0	35
Baja Bob's (Sugar Free),			
Cocktail/Martini Mix, 4 oz	10	0	2
Daily's Pina Colada, 3 oz	160	0	37
J.Cuervo Margarita, 4 fl.oz	100	0	24
Malibu Beach, all flavors, 8 fl.oz	10	0	3
Mr & Mrs T: Mai Tai, 4.5 fl.oz	140	0	33
Bloody Mary, 8 fl.oz	40	0	9
Margarita, 4 fl.oz	100	0	26
Pina Colada, 4.5 fl.oz	180	0	43
Strawberry Daiquiri, 4 fl.oz	200	0	50
Sweet 'n' Sour, 4 fl.oz	90	0	23
Sauza Margarita, 3 fl.oz	70	0	18
Skyy Cosmo, 4 fl.oz	140	0	36
TGI Fridays: Hurricane, 2.3 fl.oz	60	0	15
Long Island Ice Tea, 3.3 fl.oz	55	0	14
Mudslide, 2.3 fl.oz	120	0	24

Cocktails   **Alc** ~ Alcohol (Grams)

Made to Standard Recipes (Standard Size)
(Main Reference: The New American Bartender's Guide)

Zero Fat Unless Indicated   **C**   **Alc**   **Cb**

	C	Alc	Cb
Bloody Mary	95	10	16
Blue Lady	230	15	16
Blushin' Russian (9g fat)	365	14	47
Bourbon & Soda	130	19	0
Brandy Alexander (10g fat)	300	20	17
Chi Chi (5g fat)	255	14	26
Chu-Hais (w. 2oz Shochu):			
On the Rocks	65	9	0
Aloha (w. 2 oz Juice)	100	9	9
Cherry Blossom (w. 1 oz Ginger Ale)	95	11	5
Geisha House (w. cucumber slice)	70	9	1
Sora (Sky) Martini,			
(w. 1 oz Curacao/Plum Wine)	120	14	4
Chupa Naranjas (w. 1½ oz Tequila)	150	16	8
Collins (with 2 oz Gin)	180	20	11
Cosmopolitan	215	24	12
Daiquiri, average all types	140	19	4
Frozen Daiquiri: no fruit	155	19	6
with fruit (and less Rum)	140	14	10
Gin & Tonic	220	19	22
Grasshopper	280	13	30
Harvey Wallbanger (2 oz Vodka)	200	19	17
Highball (1½ oz Whiskey)	110	14	3
Irish Coffee (contains 5g fat)	175	14	6
Kahlua Mudslide: w.milk (3.5g fat)	150	11	10
w. cream (12.5g fat)	230	11	0
L.A. Sunrise	280	26	21
Lady Killer	165	13	20
London Rock	165	18	10
Long Island Iced Tea (w. 8 oz Cola)	290	22	31
with Diet Cola	190	22	6
Mai Tai (with 2 oz Rum)	220	21	16
Manhattan	130	17	3
Margarita	150	18	4
Martini	135	20	0
Mint Julep	210	29	4
Mojito (with 2 oz Rum)	160	19	6
Pina Colada (contains 12g fat)	325	19	12
Rainbow Room	265	30	14
Screwdriver	160	14	14
Sex On The Beach	240	20	26
Singapore Sling	210	25	9
Spritzer (with 3 oz Wine)	60	8	2
Tequila Sunrise	200	14	25
Tom Collins	210	24	12
Tom & Jerry	170	9	8
Whiskey Sour	150	19	5
White Russian	250	20	16

Liqueurs (with Alcohol Counts)

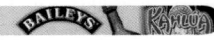

Liqueurs/Cordials

	C	Alc	Cb
Per 1 fl.oz			
Advocaat (36 Proof; 2g fat)	85	4	9
Alizé: Cognac	70	11	2
Gold/Red Passion	105	4.5	11
Amaretto (56 Proof)	110	6	17
Baileys Irish Cream (34 Proof; 5g fat)	95	4	5
Lite (30 Proof; 2g fat)	75	4	7
Benedictine (80 Proof)	90	10	5
Chambord (33 Proof)	105	5	11
Chartreuse (80 Proof)	100	10	7
Cherry Brandy (48 Proof)	80	6	9
Coffee Liqueur (53 Proof)	90	6	11
Cointreau (80 Proof)	100	10	7
Creme de Cacao (54 Proof)	100	6	15
Creme de Menthe (60 Proof)	120	7	14
Curacao (70 Proof)	95	8	6
Drambuie (80 Proof)	105	10	9
Frangelico (48 Proof)	80	6	9
Galliano (80 Proof)	100	10	8
Grand Marnier (80 Proof)	100	10	7
Kahlua (53 Proof)	90	6	11
Kirsch (68 Proof)	80	8	6
Midori (42 Proof), average all types	80	5	11
Ouzo (80 Proof)	105	11	11
Pernod (80 Proof)	75	10	2
Sambuca (84 Proof)	100	10	7
Schnapps (80 Proof)	100	10	7
Southern Comfort (70 Proof)	80	10	3
Starbucks Coffee Liqueur (40 Proof)	80	4	13
Tia Maria (64 Proof)	90	8	9
Triple Sec (60 Proof)	80	7	4

Liqueur Coffee & Hot Drinks

Per Standard Drink			
Liqueur Coffee, avg. all types	200	10	10
Egg Nog	270	10	25
Hot Toddy, w. 2 oz liquor	200	19	17
Irish Coffee, w. 2 Tbsp whip. crm	80	7	4
Mulled Wine (Glühwein), 5 oz	175	14	6

Flavorings/Syrups

Angostura Bitters, ¼ tsp	3	0	0
Ginger Ale, 8 fl.oz	80	0	22
Grenadine/Cassis, 2 Tbsp, 1 oz	70	0	17
Lime/Lemon Juice, 2 Tbsp, 1 oz	10	0	2
Maraschino Cherry, 1 small	8	0	2
Pure Lemon Extract (70%) avg., 1 oz	145	20	0
Sugar Syrup, 2 Tbsp, 1 oz	70	0	17
Sour Mix, 2 Tbsp, 1 oz	10	0	2
Tonic Water, 8 fl.oz	90	0	22
Vanilla Extract, (35%), avg., 1 oz	80	10	3.5

TEN HINTS TO AVOID HARMFUL DRINKING

1. **Add up the alcohol** you typically drink each day and on social occasions. How does this compare with 'low risk' amounts?

2. **Compare the alcohol content** of different drinks and select the lowest. Request half ounces of alcohol in cocktails and mixed drinks. Dilute them and keep topping off with non-alcoholic drinks.

3. **Go easy on 'Light' beers.** At 4% alcohol, on average, they are still high in alcohol compared to regular beer (5% alcohol).

4. **Try low alcohol or non-alcohol** alternatives such as fruit juices and mineral water. Take your own to parties.

5. **Before drinking alcohol,** quench your thirst with water and non-alcoholic drinks - particularly after vigorous exercise or sport.

6. **Slow the rate of drinking.** Chugging or drinking fast is the major cause of illness and death from alcohol poisoning.

7. **Avoid drinking in 'rounds'.**

8. **Have a non-alcoholic 'spacer'** between drinks (e.g. mineral water, orange juice).

9. **Don't drink on an empty stomach.** Food slows the rate of alcohol absorption.

10. **Keep track of the number of drinks** and know when to stop. Stick to a set limit.

Note: • Alcohol can be very dangerous when taken with prescription or street drugs or when you are very tired.

Extra Info: www.CalorieKing.com

"The doctor told him to cut down to just one glass a day."

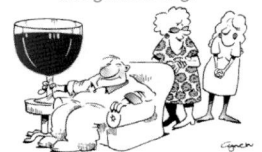

CAFE

Cafeteria-Style Foods

	C	F	Cb
Apple & Cinnamon, 1.23 oz	130	1.5	26
Beef Stroganoff, 5 oz	195	13	7
Beef Stroganoff w. 4 oz noodles	350	14	36
Chicken Lasagna, 1 piece	300	11	32
Chicken Chop Suey w. 4 oz rice	245	4	37
Deep Dish Burrito, 7 oz	265	13	20
Grnd Beef Casserole, 2 scoop, 6 oz	245	13	17
Italian Meat Sce for Spagh., 5 oz	150	9	9
w. 5 oz Spaghetti	350	10	49
Lasagna, 1 piece	275	11	25
Meatloaf, 3 oz	205	13	4
Ranch Beans, 2 scoops, 6 oz	350	11	45
Red Beans & Rice, 7 oz	280	9	37
Scalloped Potato/Ham, 6 scp, 6 oz	160	6	20
Stuffed Shells in Sauce (1)	105	3	17
Swedish Meatballs (3)	205	12	9
Sweet & Sour Pork/Rice, 9 oz	240	3	40
Swiss Steak w/Mushr. Gravy, 6 oz	280	11	4
Tator Tot Casserole, 2 scoops, 6 oz	260	15	20
Tenderloin Tips/Mushr. Gravy, 5 oz	210	13	3
w. 5 oz noodles	395	15	38
Tuna Noodle Casserole, 2 scp, 6 oz	180	6	17
Turkey Tetrazini, 2 scoops, 6 oz	195	7	17
Vegetable Lasagna, 1 piece	250	13	21

Croissants

	C	F	Cb
Unfilled: Medium 1½ oz	180	10	21
Filled: w. Ham (2 oz), Salad	280	14	24
w. Ham (2 oz), Cheese (2 oz)	470	30	20
w. Chick (2 oz) Cheese (2 oz)	470	30	20
w. Turkey/Ham/Chse (2 oz ea.)	580	36	20
Au Bon Pain: Ham & Cheese	340	10	46
Spinach & Cheese	250	9	32

7-Eleven: *Page 246*

Bagels

	C	F	Cb
Plain: Large, 4 oz (no filling)	320	2	65
with 2 oz Cream Cheese	500	27	54
with 2 oz Lox (Smoked Salmon)	400	4	65

Also see Bagels Section: *Page 104*
Fast-Foods Restaurants: *Page 183*
Au Bon Pain: *Page 187*
Bruegger's: *Page 193*
Einstein Bros Bagels: *Page 207*

Sandwiches

	C	F	Cb
No Spreads Unless Indicated			
(Includes 2 Slices Bread ~ 3 oz)			
BLT (5 strips Bacon, 2 Tbsp Mayo)	600	40	46
Breaded Chicken & Salad	540	28	46
Chicken (5 oz) Salad w. Mayo.	580	30	49
Chopped Liver, Egg, Mayo.	630	25	44
Corned Beef (5 oz) w. Mustard	560	28	44
Cream Cheese w. Olives (5 large)	340	14	46
Egg Salad w. Mayonnaise	570	29	49
Egg Salad Club w. Bacon, Mayo.	780	53	49
Grilled Cheese (3 oz)	540	30	44
Ham (5 oz); Cheese (4 oz), Mayo.	910	56	44
Lobster Salad (4 oz) w. Mayo.	530	25	45
Overstuffed Tuna Salad (7 oz)	870	39	75
Philadelphia Cheese Steak S'wich	550	23	42
Reuben (6 oz Beef/Pastrami, 2 oz Cheese,			
2 Tbsp Dressing)	920	60	28
Roast Beef (4 oz) w. Mustard	460	12	45
Roast Pork (4 oz) w. Apple Sauce	500	16	55
Shrimp Salad Club w. Bacon, Mayo.	800	57	48
Sloppy Joe w. Sauce (7 oz)	600	30	45
Steak Sandwich (5 oz cooked)	680	32	41
Triple Cheese (4 oz) Melt	720	45	46
Tuna (5 oz) Salad w. Mayo.	610	30	49
Turkey Breast (5 oz) w. Mayo.	460	18	44
Turkey Breast (5 oz) w. Mustard	360	7	44
Turkey Club w. Bacon, Mayo.	830	38	31
Vegetarian w. Avocado, Cheese	820	49	72

7-Eleven: *Page 246*
Schlotzsky's: *Page 247*
Subway: *Page 258*

Wraps & Roll-Ups

	C	F	Cb
Average All Types			
(Meat/Chicken/Fish/Veges)			
Small size, approx. 9 oz	500	25	48
Regular, approx. 15 oz	830	40	80
Large, approx. 22 oz	1400	70	134

Fast-Foods Restaurants: *Page 183*
Au Bon Pain: *Page 187*
Sonic Drive-In: *Page 252*
Subway: *Page 258*
The Wrap: *Page 263*
WAWA: *Page 267*

Fair & Carnival Foods

Fair & Carnival Foods

	C	F	Cb
Mexican			
Burritos w. Bean/Beef, 17 oz	1100	41	104
Carne Asada, 14.5 oz	820	44	58
Fish Tacos, 1 taco, 5 oz	270	13	31
Nachos w. Cheese, 9" plate	860	59	70
Taco Chicken, 3.3 oz	210	12	16
Tamale (1), 3.5 oz	180	8	21
Taquitos, 5 oz	370	17	43
Greek			
Baklava, 2" square	245	13	32
Falafel, 11.6 oz	660	27	85
Greek Salad, 14 oz	520	48	17
Gyros, 7.5", 12 oz	680	40	55
Spanakopita, 8 oz	200	7.5	23
Italian			
Garlic Bread, ½ loaf, 10 oz	1135	40	147
Pizza Bread Pepperoni, ½ loaf, 12 oz	1115	32	151
Pizza on a Stick, 1 piece	535	28	55
Personal Pizza, 7": Cheese (1)	670	24	80
Pepperoni (1)	795	35	80
Ham & Pineapple (1)	800	31	87
Low Carb			
Beef Patty, wrapped in lettuce, 4 oz	480	33	0
Sandwiches: *Per 7½" Roll*			
Ham, 11 oz	645	39	47
Hot Pastrami, 9 oz	760	17	62
Roast Beef, 11 oz	620	36	46
Philadelphia Cheese Steak, 13 oz	680	36	49
Tuna, 12 oz	830	60	46
Turkey, 11 oz	665	24	65
Veggie, 11 oz	490	23	49
Oriental: Fried Egg Roll, 6 oz	400	19	44
Rice Bowl: Beef, 6" Bowl	880	13	136
Chicken, 6" Bowl	870	15	135
Hamburgers			
⅓ Pound Burger, 7.5 oz	670	41	26
Burger w. Cheese, 6 oz	550	36	25
Hot Dogs/Franks: *With Bun*			
Hot Dog: Regular, (1)	215	14	28
with Chili, 6 oz	450	32	32
with Chili & Cheese, 7.3 oz	500	36	31
⅓ Pound Hot Dog	550	41	31
Foot Long Hot Dog	470	26	41
Corn Dog: Regular, 4 oz	250	14	23
Jumbo, 6 oz	375	21	36
Jumbo Franks w. Bun:			
Bratwurst; Sausage; Kielbasa, avg.	800	60	28

Fair & Carnival Foods (Cont)

	C	F	Cb
Barbeque Items *(Weights with Bone)*:			
Beef Stew over Rice, 2 cups	440	14	61
Chicken, 15 oz	740	24	34
Chili, 1 cup	280	11	24
Corn on the Cob, 8" (1), 16 oz	200	1	42
Pork Ribs, 18 oz	1360	68	21
Smoked Turkey Legs (1), 19 oz	1135	54	0
Potatoes & Fries			
Australian Battered Potato, 12 oz	1290	66	155
Baked Potato, 14 oz	435	0.5	100
Fries: French, 7 oz	560	24	70
Cheese Fries, 10 oz	645	38	62
Chili Fries, 10 oz	700	36	83
Chili/Cheese Fries, 13 oz	745	45	57
Curly Fries, 7 oz	620	30	78
Tasti Chips, 40 chips, 6.5 oz	780	33	117
Sweet Potato, 14 oz	405	0.5	97
Ranch Dip, 3 oz	165	14	9
Finger Foods			
Artichoke: Steamed, 6 pieces	65	0	16
Fried, 9 pieces	250	14	24
Chicken Nuggets (6)	340	17	26
Chicken Strips (4), 4.5 oz	445	21	33
Finger Steaks (2), 4 oz	400	20	26
Mushrooms, Fried, 10-12 pieces	395	26	34
Onion Rings, 3 rings	310	13	40
Onion Flower	1320	72	140
Shrimp, Fried, 10-12 pieces, 5 oz	535	30	36
Sweet Potato Strips, Fried, 4 pces	750	30	106
Zucchini, Fried, 4 slices	620	40	42
Salads/Sides			
Baked Beans, 4 oz	140	2	38
Cole Slaw, 5 oz	350	21	37
Pickle, whole (6")	30	0	8
Potato Salad, 5 oz	290	15	35
Popcorn: Plain, small, 3 oz	450	24	48
Large, 6 oz	900	48	96
Kettle Corn: Small, 5 oz	600	15	110
Large, 10 oz	1200	30	220
Cakes, Donuts, Cookies			
Funnel Cake: Plain	760	44	80
Toppings: Cinn. & Sugar, 2 tsp	30	0	8.5
Apple Cinnamon, 2 oz	85	3	36
Strawberries & Cream, 2 oz	70	0	16
Cinnamon Roll, large	730	24	114
Churros, 1½ oz	150	8	18
Donuts, Jumbo Twist, 7.5 oz	905	49	109

Fair & Carnival Foods (Cont)

Cakes, Donuts, Cookies (Cont)

	C	F	Cb
Fried Snickers, 5 oz	445	29	42
Fried Oreos, 3 cookies	300	10	33
Fried Twinkie, 1	420	34	45
Cotton Candy, 5½ oz bag	625	0	156
Red Rope Licorice, (24"), 2 oz	200	0	46
Cream Puff, 4.3 oz	500	43	22
Puff-on-a-Stick (4), 8.6 oz	995	86	44
Strawberry Crepe, 4.3 oz	280	14	36
Chocolate Dipped Straw, 1 pce	125	7	15
Fudge, 1.5 oz	200	11	25
Twinkie Dog (Sundae)	500	14	89
Key Lime Pie Bar, 6 oz	635	40	59
Cheesecake on a Stick, 6 oz	655	47	56
Cobbler, 5 oz	350	10	62
Soft Pretzel, 4.5 oz	340	2	70
Candied Apple, 7 oz	330	0.5	80

Ice Cream & Frozen Treats

	C	F	Cb
Dippin' Dots Ice Cream: Small, 4 oz	150	7	17
Medium, 8 oz	305	14	35
Large, 16 oz	600	28	70
Snow Cone (includes 3 oz syrup)	270	0	68
Frozen Yogurt in sugar cone, 14 oz	475	2	94
Ice Cream: Small, sugar cone, 10 oz	775	42	83
Large, sugar cone, 14 oz	935	54	96
Sherbet, 8 oz	270	4	59
Frozen Banana, choc cover, 5 oz	240	4	53

Drinks

	C	F	Cb
Lemonade, 18 fl.oz	210	0	52
Orange Julius, 20 fl.oz	490	10	96
Strawberry Julius, 20 fl.oz	430	0	98
Icee, 16 fl.oz	235	0	59
Malt, 16 fl.oz	690	33	85
Slushies, 16 fl.oz	260	0	65
Soft Frozen Lemonade, 12 fl.oz	300	0	78
Smoothies: Berry Flavors, 16 fl.oz	350	1	80

Stadium Foods

Sandwiches

	C	F	Cb
Bacon Burger, 8.3 oz	470	25	34
Cheeseburger, 8.3 oz	450	23	33
Chicken Sandwich: w. Cheese, 8.3 oz	510	29	40
no Cheese, 7.7 oz	460	25	40
w. Bacon, 8.3 oz	530	31	41
Hamburger, 7.8 oz	400	19	33
Polish Sausage Sandwich, 7 oz	565	33	46
Fries, French Fries, 6.4 oz	470	34	39
Fruit Cup, 6 oz	80	0	20

Hot Dogs

	C	F	Cb
Chili Dog, 7.7 oz	520	29	45
Hot Dog, 6.4 oz	465	21	50
Jumbo Dog, 8 oz	440	25	38
Kraut Dog w. Sauerkraut , 7.8 oz	490	27	41
Nachos, 40 chips w. 4 oz cheese	1100	59	132

Individual Pan Pizza (6"): Per 10 oz Pizza

	C	F	Cb
BBQ Chicken	630	24	71
Cheese	630	27	71
Pepperoni	660	30	70

Snacks

	C	F	Cb
Brownie, 2.5" x 4.5"	360	18	44
Cheese Sauce, 1.25 oz	100	8	4
Cheetos, 2.75 oz pkg	440	28	42
Chocolate Chip Cookie, 2.3 oz	280	12	40
Churros, 8", 3 oz	325	15	42
Doritos Nacho, 2.75 oz pkg	390	20	48

King Size Candy:

	C	F	Cb
Butterfinger, 3.75 oz	485	18	75
Nestle Crunch, 2.75 oz	390	21	85
Lays Chips, 2.75 oz pkg	440	28	42
Peanuts in shell, 8 oz	930	80	24
Popcorn: Small (9 cup size)	575	35	56
Large (15 cup size)	950	58	93
Red Vines, 5.5 oz box	560	0	136
Soft Pretzel: Regular, 5.5 oz	490	3.5	101
Giant, 8 oz	710	5	147
Beverages: Orange Juice, 12 fl.oz	180	0	2
Beer: Heineken, 16 fl.oz	200	0	16
Light Miller, 16 fl.oz	165	0	10
Miller Draft, 16 fl.oz	205	0	18
Jack Daniels Punch, 12 fl.oz	235	0	34
Wine, White, 9 fl.oz	190	0	6
Soda (with ½ ice), average: 20 fl.oz	160	0	40
32 fl.oz	260	0	65
Snow Cone, 18 oz (incl. 3 oz syrup)	270	0	68
Starbuck's Frappuccino, 12 fl.oz	195	2.5	39

Restaurant & International Foods

Chinese & Asian Dishes

	C	F	Cb
Appetizers			
Crab Cake, 63g	105	5	0.5
Curried Meat Triangles, 1 pce	150	5	12
Dumplings: Pork, steamed, 1	40	3	4
Pork, fried, 1 dumpling	75	7	4
Vegetable, steamed, 1	25	0.5	4
Egg Rolls, mini, 3 rolls	100	3	11
Rice Paper Roll, 1	80	2	10
Spring Roll: Small, 1½ oz	100	7	10
Medium, 3 oz	200	12	20
Large, 5 oz	350	15	33
Wonton, 1 only	55	3	4
Soup: Clear, 1 bowl	30	1	4
with Noodles	100	3	12
Chicken & Corn	150	8	8
Rice: Plain, 1 cup (½ Pint), 6½ oz	240	0.5	54
2 cups (1 Pint), 13 oz	480	1	108
Fried: 1 cup, 5 oz	320	13	42
Large dish, 16 oz	1010	40	134
Noodles: Chinese Egg, ckd, 1 cup	200	3	42
Entrees & Mains: *Per Whole Dish*			
Beef Satay, 17 oz	760	50	15
Beef in Black Bean Sce, 17 oz	530	33	17
Beef with Broccoli, 16 oz	650	30	31
Chicken & Almonds, 18 oz	685	50	18
Chicken (sliced) & Broccoli	280	12	13
Chop Suey: Chicken, 20 oz	560	37	7
Pork, 20 oz	680	50	12
Chow Mein, Beef/Chicken, 24 oz	940	60	50
Crab Puff/Rangoon, 1 dumpling	80	4.5	7.5
Crispy Fried Chicken, 8 oz	485	33	12
Egg Drop Soup: w. Noodles, 1 cup	120	3	15
w/out Noodles, 1 cup	70	3	3
Egg Foo Yung w. Sauce, 1 cup	225	12	11
Lemon Chicken, 10 oz	580	32	25
Lo Mein (stir-fried)	620	29	61
Moo Shu Chicken, 2 wrapped crepes	430	16	43
Omelet, Chicken/Shrimp, 16 oz	990	82	10
Steamed Whole Fish, ½ Red Snapper	500	11	1
Sweet & Sour: Fish, 20 oz	1160	58	106
Pork, 18 oz	950	50	92
Vegetable Combination, w. oil, 6 oz	250	17	19
Vegetables, Steamed (no oil), 6 oz	120	1	25
Bubble Tea, average, 12 fl oz	240	5	55
Fortune Cookie: each	25	0.5	5

Cajun & Creole

	C	F	Cb
Alligator, 4 oz cooked	160	2	0
Baked Herb Chicken, 1 serving	850	53	2
Bouillabaisse	400	15	10
Cajun Fried Turkey, 1 serving	630	25	0
Cocktail Sauce, 2 Tbsp	30	0	6
Couche-couche, ½ cup	80	0	17
Crawfish Bisque, 1 serving	500	10	10
Crawfish, cooked, 2 oz	45	0.5	0
Creole Jambalaya, 1 serving	550	30	15
Frog's Legs, steamed (2)	45	0	0
Guinea Fowl, flesh, 4 oz, ckd	160	4	0
Hogshead Cheese, ¼ cup	80	5.5	0
Jambalaya, Shrimp & Crabmeat	520	14	12
Red Beans & Rice, 1 serving	400	17	52
Roasted Quail, w. Bacon on Toast	550	25	15
Remoulade Sauce, 2 Tbsp, 1 OZ	110	11	2
Shrimp Creole, 1 serving	450	20	10
Stuffed Smothered Steak,			
w. 1 cup Rice	890	50	50
Turtle, cooked, 3 oz	120	3	0

Cuban

	C	F	Cb
Bl. Beans w. Rice (Moros con Cristianos)	510	22	76
Blk.-eyed Pea Fritters (Bollitos de Carita)	80	5	6
Casserole Corn Tamale	445	20	55
Chkn w. Yellow Rice (Arroz con Pollo)	925	49	87
Cuban Bread (Pan Cubano)	80	1.5	15
Donuts in Syrup (Bunuelos)	170	5	10
with Melado	100	5	10
Grilled Plantains	145	0	40
Gypsy's Arm Cake (Brazo Gitano)	260	18	42
Roast Pork S'wich (Pan con Lechon)	640	30	62
Seasoned Beef w. Olives & Raisins			
(Picadillo)	435	36	10
Shredded Beef (Ropa Vieja)	550	35	10
Taro Root Mash (Pure de Malanga)	315	3	69
Yuca with Citrus Garlic Dressing			
(Yuca con Mojo)	190	9	25

French Foods

	C	F	Cb
Blanquette d'Agneau (Lamb Stew)	800	30	17
Brioche, 1 cake	280	14	34
Bouillabaisse (Fish Stew)	400	15	10
Coq au Vin (Chicken in Wine)	800	30	16
Coquilles St. Jacques, fried, 6 lge.	300	14	2
Crème Brulée, 1 serving	460	40	21

French Foods (Cont)

	C	F	Cb
Creme Caramel (Caramel Custard)	260	10	38
Crepe Suzette, 1x6" crepe w. sauce	220	10	13
Duck a l'Orange	780	35	47
Escargots (Snails), garlic butter (6)	200	10	4
French Stick Bread, 3 slices, 2.2 oz	150	1	35
Frogs Legs, fried, 4 med. pairs	400	20	10
Lamb Noisettes, fried, 2 chops	500	40	1
Mousse au Chocolat	380	15	33
Potage Creme Crecy (Carrot Soup)	360	18	14
Salade Nicoise (Tuna/Oliv./Veg.)	450	13	14
Veal Cordon Bleu (Veal/Ham/Ch)	650	25	18
Vichyssoise (Pot./Leek Soup), 1 c.	200	9	15
Baguette & French Stick: *Page 102, 103*			
Croissants: *Pages 113, 173*			

German

	C	F	Cb
Bavarian Bread Dumpling, 3 small	330	10	28
Beef Goulash with Veges	520	20	46
Black Forest Cake, 1 slice	380	16	30
Bratwurst, grilled, 1 medium, 6 oz	450	37	2
Chicken: Fried, Viennese-style	530	20	28
Livers w. Apple/On., 6 oz	460	28	10
Herring, Pickled: Rollmops, 4 oz	260	16	3
with Sour Cream, 4 oz	310	20	3
Hot Sausage Curry	300	7	6
Kugelhupf Cake, 1 lge slice, 4 oz	400	23	40
Sauerbraten Pork (Pot Roast)	650	35	15
Torte: Linzer (Alm./Raspb. Jam)	430	18	58
Sacher (Choc./Apricot Jam)	260	12	23
Weiner Schnitzel, 1 medium	750	35	38

Greek

	C	F	Cb
Baklava Pastry: Small	240	13	32
Large, 3¾ oz	400	21	45
Calamari, deep fried, 1 cup	300	13	17
Chicken Kebob Plate	345	13	8
Galactobureko, 1 only			
(Filo, Custard, Pastry in Syrup)	360	15	48
Greek Chicken Salad	400	18	9
Gyros, 4 oz	380	33	6
Hummus & Pita, 4 oz	260	12	30
Kataifi, (Filo, Nut, Pastry in Syrup)	350	11	56
Moussaka, 1 serve, 8 oz	350	22	22
Soup: Argolemono (Egg Lemon Soup with Chicken & Rice)	85	6	5
Souvlakia (Lamb), each, 2 oz	120	6	1

Greek (Cont)

	C	F	Cb
Stuffed Tomatoes, 2 only	250	12	17
Taramosalata, 1 Tbsp, ½ oz	40	3	2
Tyropita (Filo/Egg/Cheese Pastry)	350	26	31
Tzatziki (Cucumber/Yog. Dip), 1 T.	20	1	1
Vine Leaves, stuffed, 3 rolls, 6 oz	200	5	13
See Daphne's: *See Fast-Foods Section*			

Hawaiian

	C	F	Cb
Ahi Tuna, grilled (6 oz fillet), no fat	220	2	0
Chicken Long Rice, 1 cup, 7 oz	240	14	12
Gyoza, 1 only	55	2	6
Haupia (Coconut Pudd.), 1 pce (4"x 2½")	120	6	17
Hawaiian Sweet Bread, ½" sl., 2 oz	180	4.5	29
Kalua Chicken, 4 oz	280	16	0
Pork, 4 oz	350	24	0
Kim Chee (pickled cabbage), ½ c., 4 oz	20	0	5
Kulolo (Taro Pudding), 1 slice	125	5	19
Lau Lau: Chicken (1) 7 oz	280	21	3
Pork (1) 7 oz	320	26	5
Loco Moco (rice/burger/egg/gravy)	650	27	63
Lomi Salmon, ¼ cup, 4 oz	20	1	2
Malasadas (Donut), 2 oz	240	13	26
Manapua (Char Siu Pork Bun), 2.3 oz	180	8	25
Poi (mashed ckd taro), 1 c., 8½ oz	270	0.5	65
Poke, avg all types, 3 oz	90	1	0
Portuguese Sausage, 2 oz	180	15	2
Potato Salad, ½ cup, 5 oz	170	10	17
Shave Ice *(Matsumoto)*, all flavors:			
w. Icecream, 1 large	300	4	64
w. Beans, 1 large	290	0	72
Spam Musubi: w. Regular Spam	265	11	34
(4 oz rice+1.3 oz Spam/7-Eleven Hawaii)			
Homemade: w. Lite Spam (50% less fat)	220	5	34
Taro Pancake Mix, ⅓ cup (makes 2)	140	2	26
Plate Lunches:			
Chicken Katsu (9 oz) w. 2 scp Rice	1110	48	108
+ Macaroni Salad, ¾ cup	1360	68	123
or Tossed Salad + Fr. Dress. (2 T.)	1240	61	111
Hamburger (5 oz) w. 2 scoops Rice	710	24	81
Gravy + Macaroni Salad	1135	49	112
MahiMahi (7 oz) w. 2 scoops Rice	650	12	90
+ Macaroni Salad + Tartar Sce	1150	58	109
or Macaroni Salad, no Tartar Sce	935	34	108
or Tossed Salad + Fr. Dress. (3 T.)	815	27	96
or Tossed Salad, no dressing	670	12	93
Teri Beef (5 oz) w. 2 scoops Rice	790	23	94
+ Macaroni Salad, ¾ cup	1095	47	113
or Tossed Salad, no dressing	800	23	95

Indian & Pakistani   C   F   Cb

Per Serving
(Meat dishes allow 4 oz meat/serving)

	C	F	Cb
Aloo Samosa, each	155	12	12
Alu Gosht Kari (Meat/Pot. Curry)	600	40	23
Chicken Korma	500	35	6
Chicken Pilaf (Murgh Biriyani)	700	53	50
Chicken Tikka	260	16	2
Chicken Vindaloo	400	20	8
Chapati/Roti, 7" diam. piece	60	0.5	11
Dal (Lentil Puree): 1 cup, no oil	230	1	37
1 Tbsp Tadka (oil topping)	120	13	0
Dhakla (Lentil Dish), 1" sq., 1 oz	105	5	13
Dhansak, ½ cup	105	3.5	11
Gosht Kari (Meat Curry/Tom./Pot.)	460	25	17
Lamb Pilaf	520	35	40
Lassi (Sweet or Mango), 1 cup, 8 oz	160	4	24
Masala Gosht (Beef/Tom./Gravy)	400	25	18
Mulligatawney Soup, average	300	15	9
Murgh Tikka, 1 cup	300	4	7
Naan Bread, ¼ (8" x 2"), 1 oz	75	2	11
Pappadum, 1 large/2 small	50	3	5
Pesrattu (Lentil Crepe), 9", 2.6 oz	130	5	15
Pork Vindaloo Curry	620	47	3
Rajmah (Kidney Bean Curry), 1 cup	225	5	35
Rogan Josh (Lamb/Yogurt Sce)	500	30	3
Shahi Korma (Braised Lamb)	430	28	3
Tandoori Chicken: Breast	260	13	3
Leg/Thigh portion	300	17	6

Sal Monella Restaurant

"I wonder why business is so bad these days?"

Italian Dishes   C   F   Cb

	C	F	Cb
Baked Ziti: Small	370	27	32
Regular	575	42	49
Breadstick (1), 2 oz	120	2.5	25
Broccoli Fettucine Alfredo, reg.	815	23	125
Bruschetta, 2 slices	380	17	53
Calzones, average, all types	840	34	101
Cannelloni, 1 tube, 6 oz	280	15	18
Cheese Breadstick (1), 2.4 oz	180	8	20
Cheese Ravioli w. Sauce	495	17	65
Chicken Alfredo	775	29	82
Chicken Parmigiana, 11 oz	520	22	16
Fettucine Alfredo: Small	525	15	80
Regular	775	22	119
Meat Lasagne, 16 oz	700	36	60
Meat Ravioli	725	22	102
Minestrone Soup, 1 bowl	110	2	18
Shrimp & Scallop Fettucine	595	16	81
Spaghetti w. Marinara: Small	410	6	74
Regular	600	8	111
Spaghetti w. Meatballs: Small	710	31	80
Regular	1010	42	119
Spaghetti w. Meat Sauce: Small	425	8	74
Regular	625	11	111
Vegetable Primavera	610	8	116

Pizza: *Per Slice*

Thin Crust, *(⅛ Medium, 12"):*

	C	F	Cb
Cheese, Hawaiian	200	8	21
Pepperoni	210	10	21
Sausage	280	16	22
Veggie	180	7	23

Thick/Pan Crust, *(⅛ Large, 14"):*

	C	F	Cb
Cheese, Hawaiian	350	13	40
Pepperoni	380	16	40
Veggie	330	11	41

Personal Pan Pizza, *(6"):*

	C	F	Cb
Hawaiian	600	24	70
Pepperoni	640	29	67
Desserts: Lemon Ice	180	0	45
Gelato: Vanilla (Milk Base), ½ cup	200	15	18
Choc. Hazelnut (Milk), ½ cup	370	29	26
Water Base, ½ cup	100	0	25
Tiramisu, 1 piece, 5 oz	400	29	30

For more listings see Fast-Foods Section.

Restaurant & International Foods

Japanese

	C	F	Cb
Sushi Rice: cooked, 1 Tbsp	25	0	5
1 cup, 5¼ oz	380	3	82
Sushi (Maki) Rolls: *Per Piece*			
Average all types (California Rolls; Crm Cheese w. Crab; Eel; Salmon; Shrimp; Tuna; Yellowtail; Vegetable)			
Small (1⅛" diam. x 1⅛" high), 0.8 oz	25	0.5	3.5
Med. (1¾" diam. x 1¾" high), 1.6 oz	50	1	7
Large (2¼" diam. x ⅞" high), 2 oz	60	1.5	9
Sushi Packs: *Per Pack*			
Average all types: 6 large pces	370	5	55
9 medium pieces	360	6	60
12 small pieces	265	3	45
Futomaki (thick roll), 6 pieces	380	5	72
Hand Roll (Cone) 4 oz	120	2	18
Inari (rice filled soybean pocket), 4 pce	420	2	73
Sushi-Nigiri (fish on rice):			
average all types, 1 piece	70	0.5	12
Sushi Plate: Assorted, 6 pieces	420	3	36
Combination (Sushi & Sushi Rolls)			
2 Sushi + 6 sm. & 3 med. rolls	400	7	72
Sashimi (Sliced Raw Seafood/Beef)			
Ika (Squid), 4 oz	105	2	0
Hamachi (Yellowtail), 4 oz	165	6	0
Maguro (Yellowfin Tuna), 4 oz	120	1	0
Niku (Beef), 5 oz	200	10	0
Saba (Mackerel), 4 oz	160	7	0
Suzuki (Sea Bass), 4 oz	110	0.5	0
Tako (Octopus), 4 oz	95	1	0
Dipping Sauces: Average, 2 Tbsp	30	0	7
Ginger Vinegar Dressing, 2 Tbsp	20	0	5
Edamame (young green soybeans):			
Steamed/Salad (in pods), 4 oz	60	3	5
Boiled beans (no pods), 4 oz	160	7	12
Katsu-don Pork w. Rice	1100	39	141
Miso Soup w. Tofu pces, 1 cup	85	3	11
Seaweed Salad, 1.5 oz	20	2	0
Sukiyaki (Beef/Tofu/Veg.), 8 oz	400	24	32
Tempura (Batter-fried Shrimp & Veges)			
3 large shrimp & veges	320	18	25
1 shrimp only	60	4	3
Teppan Yaki (Steak, Seafood & Veges)			
10 oz serving	470	30	15
Teriyaki: Beef, 4 oz serving	350	25	4
Chicken, 4 oz serving	260	9	7
Salmon, medium, 6 oz serving	270	8	3
Sake Wine (16% alc.), 3 fl.oz	115	0	7
Yakatori, 1 skewer, 2½ oz	140	5	1

Kosher/Deli Foods

	C	F	Cb
Bagel/Bialy, 1 small, 2 oz	160	2	32
Beiglach (Cheese Knish)	350	17	35
Blintzes: Average, 1 only	120	1	25
w. Sour Crm. & Preserves	370	10	30
Borscht: (no cream), 1 cup	85	3	14
Diet/Reduced Cal., 1 cup	30	1	7
Cabbage Roll (meat/rice), 5 oz	170	6	21
Chicken Broth: 1 cup	80	8	0
with vegetables	100	8	0
with noodles	150	9	16
Lowfat, plain, 1 cup	25	1	0
Cholent, 1 med serve, 1 cup	350	16	48
Chopped Liver: 1 serve, 3 oz	110	6	5
with Egg Salad, ¼ cup	100	7	3
Farfel, dry, ½ cup	90	0.5	21
Hallah (Yeast Bread), 1 sl., 1 oz	85	2	14
Gefilte Fish Balls: Reg., medium, 2 oz	55	2	4
with jelled broth	80	2	6
Cocktail size, 1 oz	30	1	2
Sweet, medium, 2 oz	65	2	4
with jelled broth	95	2	9
Herring: Smoked, 2 oz	120	8	0
in Sour Cream, 2 oz	150	10	0
Kasha, cooked, ½ cup	100	0.5	20
Kipfel (Vanilla/Almd. Cookie), 1 pce	60	2	7
Knaidlach ~ See Matzo Balls			
Knish: Kasha/Potato, 1 only	130	4	22
Cheese, 1 only	350	17	35
Kreplach, beef, 1 piece	40	1	6
Kugel, potato/noodle, 1 serve	300	20	25
Latkes (Potato Pancake), 2 oz	200	11	22
3 Latkes w. Sour Cr./Apple Sce	750	25	95
Lochshen: Plain, 1 cup	130	2	26
Pudding, 1 cup	380	13	48
Lox (Smoked Salmon), 2 oz	65	2	0
Mandelbrot (Almond Bread),			
1 slice, ¼" thick	45	2	5
Matzo (See Page 105), 1 oz board	110	0.5	23
Matzo Balls: 2 small, or 1 large, 2"	90	3	12
Extra large ball, 3"	180	6	24
Matzo Ball Soup:			
Cup w. 2 small or 1 large ball	150	5	27
Bowl with Chicken & Noodles	325	13	34
Jerry's Deli, large bowl	560	17	56
New York Cheesecake, 4 oz	350	24	26
Pierogi, potato/cheese, 1 pce	90	4	11
Reuben S'wich w. ½ lb corned beef	920	60	28
Schmaltz (Rend'd chick. fat), 1 T.	90	10	0

Restaurant & International Foods

Korean Food

Food	C	F	Cb
Bibimbab (Vege & Beef on Rice), 1 cup	565	15	89
Bulgogi (Barbeque Beef), 3.5 oz	325	12	15
Galbi (Short Ribs), 16 oz	975	61	16
Gujeolpan (Pancake w. Meat & Vegetables), cup w. 1 pancake	340	11	39
Japchae (Noodle w. Vege & Meat), 1¼ cup	365	19	34
Sides:			
Kimchee (Cabbage Relish), ½ cup	30	0	6
Namool (Assorted Veges) 1 cup	125	6.5	9
Soups: *Per Serving*			
Muguk (Radish & Chive Soup), 6 oz	105	7	6
Samgyetang (Ginseng Chicken Soup)			
no Chicken Skin, 1 cup	520	11	60
w. Chicken Skin, 1 cup	725	35	60
Yuk Gae Jang (Spicy Beef Soup), 1¼ cup	180	13	5

Lebanese/Middle East

Food	C	F	Cb
Baba Ghannouj, 2 Tbsp, 1 oz (Eggplant/Sesame Dip)	70	6	2
Baklava, 1 pastry, 1¾ oz (Pastry, Nuts, Syrup)	245	18	18
Cabbage Rolls, 1 roll, 3 oz (Cabbage Leaf, Meat, Rice)	100	3	12
Cous Cous, 1 serve (Semolina, Milk, Fruit, Nuts)	400	21	43
Felafel (Chick Pea Fritter):			
Fried, 1 medium, 1 oz	60	4	4
Hummus, ¼ cup, 2.2 oz	105	3	5
Fried Kibbi, 1 piece, 3 oz (Wheat, Meat, Pinenuts)	180	8	15
Kafta, 1 skewer, 1½ oz (Ground Lamb Saus. on Skewer)	85	5	2
Kibbeh Naye, 1 cup, 9 oz (Raw Lamb, Bulgur & Spices)	450	18	28
Lebanese Omelet, 1 serving, 4 oz (Egg, Spinach, Pinenuts, Onion)	200	12	13
Pilaf, 1 cup (Rice, Onion, Rais., Apr. Spice)	400	11	60
Shawourma, 1 serve, 4 oz (Spit Roast Beef)	280	15	2
Shish Kabob, 1 stick, 2½ oz	130	7	2
Spinach Pie, 1 piece, 3½ oz	290	21	20
Sweet Almond Sanbusak, 1 pce (Pastry, Almonds, Spices)	200	15	11
Tabouli, 1 serve, 4 oz	170	14	7
Tahini Sauce, avg., 1 Tbsp	90	8	2

Mexican

Food	C	F	Cb
Black Bean Soup, 1 bowl	200	3	34
Bueso Fresco, ¼ cup	80	4.5	1
Burritos (Taco Bell): Bean	370	10	55
Supreme® Beef	440	18	50
Chili, plain, ¼ cup	90	6	8
Chili con Carne: w. Beans, 1 cup	310	17	15
w/out Beans, 1 cup	370	28	10
Chimichangas, Beef, 5 oz	400	19	43
Chorizo Sausage, 2 oz	265	23	0
Churros, 1½ oz	150	8	18
Corn Chips, ½ cup, 1 oz	160	10	17
Costillas Ribs, 6 oz	675	52	0
Enchilada, average	330	10	49
Fajitas, Chicken (Soft)	200	7	20
Guacamole, avg., 2 Tbsp, 1 oz	45	4	2
Horchata: Don Jose, 1 cup, 8 fl. oz	140	4	25
Cacique, 1 pint bottle, 16 fl. oz	320	7	62
Margarita (w. 1½ oz Tequila)	160	0	6
Menudo, ½ cup	55	1.5	10
Nachos: Del Taco, Regular	395	24	40
Macho Nachos	1145	63	113
Taco Bell: BellGrande®	760	43	80
Supreme®	470	26	42
Nachos: with cheese, peppers, 1 portion (6-8 nachos), 7 oz	600	33	60
with cheese, beans, ground beef, peppers, 1 portion (6-8 nachos), 9 oz	570	31	56
Nopal Cactus Salad, 1 serving	130	9	11
Papas Fritas (Fried Potatoes) (1), 6 oz	325	18	40
Piloncillo (Brown Sugar): 1 Tbsp, 13g	50	0	13
Cone, small, 3", 3 oz	325	0	81
Quesadilla, Cheese (Taco Bell)	490	28	39
Refried Beans, ¾ cup, 6 oz	160	3	26
Rice Pudding (Arroz Con Leche), 4 oz	140	3	24
Sopes (Gorditas), 2 oz	120	0	27
Taco (Taco Bell): Regular, Crispy	170	10	13
Ranchero Chicken	270	15	21
Taco Supreme®	220	14	14
Double Decker® Taco	340	14	39
Taco Salad w. Salsa	840	52	85
Taco Sauce, average, ¼ cup	15	0	3
Taco Shell, regular	50	2	8
Tamales, Beef/Chicken, avg, 4.5 oz	250	11	27
Taquitos, Beef & Cheese, 4.5 oz	330	15	36
Tostada (Taco Bell)	250	10	29
Tortilla, Corn, 6" diam.	70	1	14
Tortilla Chips, 1 oz	150	8	18
Extra Listings of Mexican Dishes:			

• **Fast-Foods Section** (Taco Bell, Del Taco)
• **Canned Bean/Chili Products:** See Pages 71-76

Mexican (Cont)

	C	F	Cb
Breads: Bolillos, 1 roll, 3½ oz	240	4	42
Telera, 2 oz	150	1.5	19
Mexican Cornbread, 4" square	210	11	19
French Baguette, 2 oz	140	1.5	26
Cakes, Cookies, Pastries			
Banderilla (Pastry Puff), 1 shell	140	10	8
Bigotes, 7"	570	22	44
Calvos, 2½ oz	320	18	38
Capirotada (Bread Pudding), 10 oz	810	38	107
Cinnamon Cookies, 2	125	8	13
Cocadas, 1 oz	120	6	15
Cortadillo, 1 cookie, 1.9 oz	300	11	48
Concha (All Colors):			
Small (3" diam), 2½ oz	250	8	38
Medium (4" diam), 3½ oz	350	11	53
Large (5" diam), 5½ oz	550	18	84
Cream Puff with Custard, 4¼ oz	255	14	25
Cuerno, 2 oz	200	4.5	34
Cuerno Fine, 2¾ oz	330	17	40
Donus (Donuts), 4", 3½ oz	440	21	58
Elotes, 3½ oz	450	24	51
Empanadas (Average all types):			
Small, 2 oz	230	10	28
Regular, 3 oz	300	14	42
Fiesta Cookie, 2¼ oz	280	8	47
Galletas Mixtas (1), 1 oz	100	2.5	16
Guayaba, 3¼ oz	360	14	53
Jelly Rolls, 3¼ oz	240	4	46
Mantecadites (Almond Shortbread), 4½ oz	670	42	64
Mini Pound Cake, 3 oz	260	12	33
Mini Cupcakes, 1¾ oz	180	8	25
Muffins/Nino Enbuelto, large, 6 oz	465	11	48
Novcias, 2¾ oz	290	9	46
Nuez, 3¼ oz	380	17	52
Ojo De Buey, 4 oz	360	15	55
Orejas Ears, 3 oz	310	15	38
Pan Dulce (Mexican Sweet Bread), 1 bun	330	10	45
Panquecitos, 2½ oz	260	11	36
Piedras, 4 oz	470	15	76
Polvorones, 3 oz	370	18	48
Puerquitos, 5 oz	600	24	88
Rebanadas, 3½ oz	390	18	51
Roles De Canela (Cin. Roll), 4½ oz	490	15	81
Roscas, 2¾ oz	360	18	44
Semitas, 3 oz	300	10	46
Sopapillas (flaky pastry puffs), 1 pce	100	7	10
w. Honey & Cream	200	14	18
Strawberry Crème Roll (⅙), 2½ oz	240	5	45

Extra Food Listings ~ See CalorieKing.com

Polish

	C	F	Cb
Cabbage Rolls w. Sour Cr., 2 sm.	220	10	30
Chicken Casserole w. Mush., 1 cup	520	27	5
Kielbasa (Sausages, Onions, fried), 2 large	350	28	2
Meatballs in Sour Cream, 3 x 1½" balls	300	16	11
Pierogi, Fruit/Veg, 3" ball	80	2	15
Pork Goulash (Pork/Veg. Stew)	550	21	38
Pot Roast with Vegetables	630	21	28

Soul Foods

	C	F	Cb
Breakfast Sausage, fried, 2 patties	250	17	0
Brunswick Stew, 1 cup, 8.5 oz	320	14	19
Cornbread, home-made, 3 oz	200	7.5	28
Fatback, raw, ¼ oz	60	6.5	0
Ham Hock	90	6.5	2
Hog Maw	45	2.5	0
Hominy, cooked, ¾ cup	110	0.5	25
Hush Puppies, 5 pieces	260	12	35
Kale, cooked, ½ cup	20	0.5	4
Opossum	65	3	0
Oxtail	70	3.5	0
Pig Ear, ¼ ear	50	3	0
Pig Foot, ½ foot	70	4.5	0
Pig Tail, ⅓ tail	115	10	0
Poke Salad, cooked, ½ cup	16	0.5	3
Pork Brains	40	2.5	0
Pork Chitterlings, simmered, 3 oz	260	25	0
Pork Cracklings, ½ oz	80	6	0
Pork Neck Bones	65	4	0
Pork Skin, 1 cup	70	4.5	0
Pork Tongue, ⅓ tongue	75	5.5	0
Sousemeat	60	4.5	0
Succotash, ½ cup	80	1	17
Sweet Potato Pie, ⅛ of 9" pie	250	12	34
Tripe, 2 oz	55	2	0
Vienna Sausage, 2 small	90	8	1
small	45	4	0.5

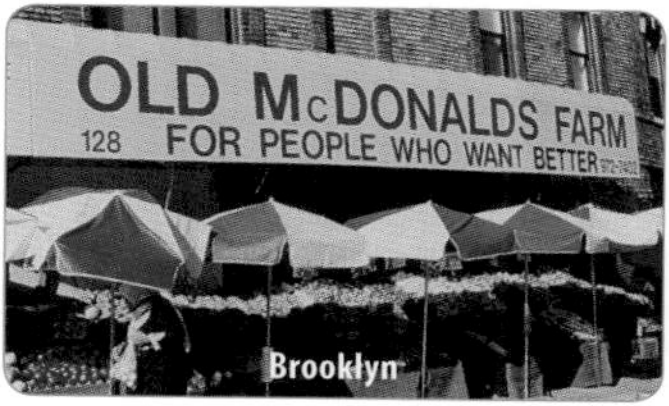
OLD McDONALDS FARM
128 FOR PEOPLE WHO WANT BETTER
Brooklyn

Restaurant & International Foods

Spanish

	C	F	Cb
Arroz Abanda (Fish with Rice)	340	8	31
Arroz Con Pollo (Rice/Chick. Sal)	500	23	50
Clams Marinara, 8 clams	330	16	22
Cochifrito (Lamb w. Lemon/Garlic)	650	25	5
Cochinillo Asado, 2 sl. (Rst Suckling Pig)	300	15	3
Cocido Madrileno (Madrid-Style Boiled Dinner)	450	27	18
Flan de Leche (Caramel Custard)	325	9	52
Fritadera de Ternera (Sauteed Veal)	450	27	2
Gazpacho, 1 bowl	60	0	15
Paella a la Valenciana (Chicken & Shellfish Rice)	900	42	70
Pollo a la Espanola (Chicken)	475	30	4
Ternera al Jerez (Veal w. Sherry)	660	29	6
Zarzuela (Fish & Shellfish Medley)	530	27	40

Thai Foods

	C	F	Cb
Appetizers: Satay Pork, 1 oz	100	4	2
Spring Roll, 1¼ oz	110	6	13
Soups: Tom Yam (Hot & Sour):			
Spicy Shrimp/Seafood, 1 cup	100	4	6
1 bowl	160	7	10
Vegetarian, 1 cup	50	0	11
Curries: Chicken w. Ginger, 1 cup	390	34	4
Thick Red Curry w. Beef, 1 cup	600	50	7
Thai Chicken Curry, 1 cup	340	23	4
Massaman Curry, 1 cup	680	57	8
Green Curry w. Pork, 1 cup	480	44	5
Pad Thai, Large serving, 18 oz	990	38	125
Fish: Steamed w. Spicy Thai Sce	450	8	46
Crispy Fried, 5 oz	290	15	9
Spicy Chicken (w. veges), stir-fry	450	22	14
Spicy Garlic Tofu w. veges, stir-fry	340	18	18
Sticky Thai Rice: Plain 1 cup, 6 oz	170	0.5	36
w. Coconut & Sesame Seeds, 1 cup	880	28	120
Stir-fried Rice Noodles, 1 c., 5½ oz	270	9	45
Stir-fried Vegetables, 1 cup	100	3	18
Salads: Green Papaya Salad	160	0	40
Spicy Prawn, 9 shrimp	170	3	15
Thai Chicken, 1 serving	330	9	17
Thai Beef Salad, 1 serving	260	9	15
Thai Noodle, 1 serving	410	13	45
Satay Chicken & Peanut Sauce:			
1 satay stick	390	24	20
Sauces: Peanut Satay, ½ cup, 4 oz	160	10	13

Vietnamese

	C	F	Cb
Banh Cuon (Steam Rice w. Pork), 1 roll	105	7	8
Bo Nuong (Beef Satay), 2 sticks	265	9	4
Bo Xao Dau Phong (Ginger Beef w.Onion, Fish Sce.)	750	30	10
Ca Chien Gung (Whole Snapper/Ging.)	600	16	6
Canh Chay (Veg./Tofu Soup)	80	3	13
Cari (Curry) Chicken, 1 cup	475	29	16
Cari (Curry) Chicken, w. Rice Noodle, cup curry & cup cooked noodles	660	29	60
Cari (Curry) Chicken, w. Steam Rice, cup curry & cup rice	650	29	55
Cuu Xao Lan (Curried Lamb, Veges in Coconut)	900	40	80
Ga Chien (Crisp Chick + Plum Sce)	900	40	105
Ga Nuong (Chicken Satay + Sce)	240	10	4
Ga Xao Rau (Marinated Chicken Braised w. Veg.)	800	26	100
Gio Lua (Lean Pork Pie), ⅙ of pie	245	12	0
Goi Cuon (Cold Spring Rolls), each	60	1	5
Rau Cai Xao Chay (Stir Fried Vege.)	400	15	65
Thit Bo Vien (Beef Balls), 6 balls	225	14	2
Thit Heo Goi Baup Cai, each (Spicy Cabbage Rolls w. Pork)	200	7	11
Soup: Per Bowl (1½ Cup)			
Bun Bo Hue (Hot & Spicy Soup no Pork Feet	340	9	35
w. Pork Feet	830	45	35
Chicken & Rice Noodle Soup	400	3	55
Pho Bo (Beef Noodle Soup)	410	7	59
Pho Ga (Chicken Noodle Soup)	460	6	58
Pho Tai (Rare Beef & Noodle Soup)	440	7	73
Salad: Per ½ Cup			
Goi Du Du (Green Papaya Salad)	155	3	29
Sauce: Nuoc Cham (Hot Sauce)	5	0	1

Gourmet & Miscellaneous

	C	F	Cb
Ants Eggs/Larvae, 1 Tbsp	20	0	0
Ants, Choc. coated, 3 Tbsp	140	7	2
Bee Maggots, canned, 3 Tbsp	65	2	0
Caviar, black/red, 1 Tbsp	40	3	0
Caterpillars, canned, 2 oz	60	2	0
Frogs Legs, fried, 1 pair (large)	125	7	0
Haggis, boiled, 4 oz	350	24	22
Locusts, roasted, 1 oz	35	1	0
Silkworms, raw, 1 oz	60	2	0
Snails in garlic butter, 6 large	200	10	4
Snake, roasted, 4 oz	160	6	0

Fast-Food Chains & Restaurants

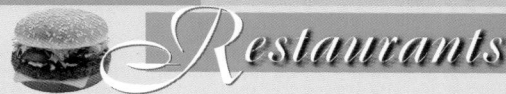

©2006
Allan Borushek
FOR MORE RESTAURANTS
See www.CalorieKing.com

Fast - Foods & *Restaurants*

A&W®

Sandwiches & Burgers	C	F	Cb
Cheeseburger	470	24	40
Cheeseburger Deluxe	510	28	41
Cheeseburger Deluxe Bacon	570	33	41
Cheeseburger Deluxe Double	720	42	46
Cheeseburger Deluxe Double Bacon	800	49	47
Crispy Chicken Sandwich	580	25	57
Grilled Chicken Sandwich	400	13	35
Hamburger	430	22	37
Hamburger Deluxe	460	26	37
Chicken			
Chicken Strips, 3 pces	500	29	32
Hot Dogs: Plain, 3.2 oz	280	17	22
Cheese Dog, 4.4 oz	320	20	25
Coney (Chili), 4.4 oz	310	18	24
Coney (Chili) Chse Dog, 5.4 oz	350	21	27
Fries & Sides: Per Serving			
Fries: French, Regular, 4 oz	310	12	45
French, Large, 5.5 oz	430	16	62
Cheese Fries, 6 oz	390	19	50
Chili Fries, 6 oz	370	16	49
Chili Cheese Fries, 7 oz	400	19	51
Dipping Sauces: Barbeque, 1 oz	40	0	10
Honey Mustard	100	6	12
Sweet and Sour	45	0	12
Poutine, small, 6 oz	420	24	38
Onion Rings, 4 oz	350	17	45
Salads: Coleslaw, Individual	90	6	7
Potato Salad, Individual	160	8	22
Macaroni Salad, Individual	175	9	22
Desserts			
Hot Caramel Sundae	340	9	57
Hot Fudge Sundae	350	11	54
Other Sundaes, avg.	310	8	52
Polar Swirl™: M&M; Oreo, small	720	25	107
Reese's, small	750	31	97
Soft Ice Cream Cone, regular, avg.	250	7	41
Milkshakes & Floats: Per 16 fl.oz			
Chocolate Milkshake	695	29	100
Strawberry Milkshake	670	29	90
Vanilla Milkshake	720	31	97
A&W Root Beer Float	340	5	71
Drinks: Per 20 fl.oz			
A&W Root Beer	295	0	76
Diet A&W Root Beer; Diet Coke	0	0	0
Cola	290	0	74
Sprite	300	0	72

Applebee's®

	C	F	Cb
Appetizers: Onion au Gratin Soup	150	8	12
Tortilla Chicken Melt	480	13	50
Veggie Patch Pizza (10") ⅙ pizza	150	9	12
Entree Meals: Includes Sides/Sauces			
Applebee's Riblets	2025	130	106
Crispy Buttermilk Shrimp	845	34	83
Crispy Orange Chicken Skillet	1710	69	209
Fiesta Lime Chicken	1285	47	156
Grilled Tilapia, w. Rice Pilaf & Mango	320	6	30
Madeira Steak Tips	910	38	82
Teriyaki Steak & Shrimp Skewers	370	7	33
Burger & Sandwiches: No Sides			
Angus Bacon Cheeseburger	940	53	58
Cowboy Burger	1150	62	89
Clubhouse Grill Sandwich	870	39	55
Tango Chicken Sandwich	460	7	48
Roll-Ups: Chicken Fajita, w. Dress.	1130	66	58
Oriental Chicken	710	25	72
Salads			
Pecan Crusted Chicken	1180	65	63
Half serving , no dressing	675	36	44
Shrimp & Spinach	570	41	14
Half serving, no dressing	220	11	10
Sizzling Fajitas: Includes 4 Tortillas			
Average all types	1900	76	174
Tortilla (8"), each, 1.6 oz	145	3	25
Teriyaki Bowls: Steak	1610	45	230
Combo Teriyaki	1440	29	224
Weight Watchers: Complete Dish			
Confetti Chicken	370	7	34
Grilled Shrimp Skewer Salad	210	2	22
Grilled Tilapia w. Mango Salsa	320	6	27
Mesquite Chicken Salad	350	4	42
Onion Soup au Gratin	150	8	10
Sizzling Chicken Skillet	360	4	43
Southwest Cobb Salad	440	8	59
Teriyaki Steak & Shrimp Skewers	370	7	33
Tango Chicken Salad	370	9	38
Tortilla Chicken Melt	480	13	50
Desserts: Per Serving			
Blue Ribbon Brownie			
w. 2 scoops Ice Cream	735	30	105
Chocolate Raspberry Layer	230	3	46
Cheesecake, Berry Lemon	230	7	34
Sizzling Apple Pie w. Ice Cream	1085	56	146
Triple Chocolate Meltdown Cake	725	31	107

Most figures above are author calculations and not intended for clinical use.
For Extra Listings ~ see CalorieKing.com

Arby's®

Breakfast: Per Serving	C	F	Cb
Blueberry Muffin, 3 oz	320	12	49
Biscuit: Plain	275	15	28
Bacon, Egg & Cheese	460	28	30
Chicken	415	23	39
Ham, Egg & Cheese	435	23	31
Sausage, Egg & Cheese	555	38	30
Croissant: Bacon & Egg	335	22	23
Ham & Cheese	275	12	22
Sausage & Egg	435	32	23
French Toastix, no Syrup, 4.3 oz	310	13	44
Sourdough S'wich: Egg & Cheese	390	12	40
Bacon, Egg & Cheese	435	16	40
Sausage, Egg & Cheese	515	27	40
Wraps: Bacon, Egg & Cheese	515	29	50
Sausage, Egg & Cheese	690	45	50

Market Fresh Salads	C	F	Cb
Chicken Club Salad: No Dressing	505	26	32
w. Buttermilk Dressing	830	60	35
Martha's Vineyard, no Almonds	275	8	24
w. Raspb. Vinaigrette, Almonds	550	30	44
Santa Fe: no Dressing, Tortilla Strips	500	23	42
w. Dressing, Tortilla Strips	865	57	94
w. Grilled Chicken	305	11	21

Sandwiches	C	F	Cb
Arby's Melt	300	12	36
BBQ Bacon 'n Jack 2/For	360	16	42
Beef 'n Cheddar	445	21	44
Chicken Naturals:			
Chicken Bacon & Swiss, Crispy	685	33	55
Chicken Bacon & Swiss, Grilled	460	17	38
Chicken Fillet, Crispy	640	33	53
Chicken Fillet, Grilled	415	17	36
Cordon Bleu, Crispy	710	35	52
Cordon Bleu, Grilled	490	19	35
Southwest Chipotle, Crispy	740	41	54
Southwest Chipotle, Grilled	515	25	37
Fish Sandwich	570	26	63
French Dip & Swiss	475	18	38
Roast Beef, Regular	320	14	34
Roast Beef, Super	400	19	40
Sourdough Roast Beef Melt	355	14	40
Subs: French Dip w. Au Jus	450	17	48
Hot Ham & Swiss	500	18	45
Italian	620	33	48
Philly Beef & Swiss	670	35	46
Roast Beef	725	42	46
Turkey Sub	635	30	47

Market Fresh Sandwiches	C	F	Cb
Chicken Salad	770	39	79
Roast Beef & Swiss	775	41	73
Roast Ham & Swiss	705	31	75
Roast Beef Gyro	540	29	49
Roast Turkey & Swiss	725	30	75
Roast Turkey Ranch & Bacon	835	38	75
Ultimate BLT	780	45	75
Wraps: Rst Turkey Ranch & Bacon	700	37	44
Ultimate BLT	650	44	45

Sauces & Condiments	C	F	Cb
Dipping Sauce: BBQ, 1 oz	45	0	11
Bronco Berry, 2 oz	120	0	30
Buffalo Sauce, 2 oz	20	1	3
Cool Ranch Sour Cream, 1 ½ oz	160	16	2
Sauce: Arby's, 1 oz	15	0	4
Cheddar Cheese, ¾ oz	30	2	2
Chipotle Mayo, ½ oz	90	9	0
Horsey Sauce, ½ oz	60	5	3
Italian Sub, 1 oz	125	12	3
Monterey Jack Cheese, ¾ oz	25	2.5	2
Smoky Q, ½ oz	25	0	5
Sour Cream, 2 oz	120	12	2
Spicy Three Pepper, ½ oz	20	1	3
Swiss Cheese, serving, ¾ oz	30	2	3
Tangy Southwest, 2 oz	335	34	5
Dressing: Raspb. Vinaigrette, 2.2 oz	195	13	18
Buttermilk Ranch, 2.2 oz	325	34	4
Light Buttermilk Ranch, 2.2 oz	110	6.5	13
Santa Fe Ranch, 2.2 oz	295	31	4
Sides: Potato Cakes, 2 cakes	245	18	26
Baked Potato: Plain	270	0	63
w. Broccoli & Cheese	535	22	73
w. Butter & Sour Cream	495	24	65
w. Sour Cream	395	12	65
Deluxe	645	32	67
Fries: Curly, small, 3.7 oz	340	20	39
Homestyle, small, 4 oz	300	20	44
Chicken Fingers, 3 pieces	435	21	32
Chicken Tenders, 2 pieces	145	7	10
Jalapeno Bites, no Sauce, 5 bites	305	21	29
Loaded Potato Bites, no Sce, 5 bites	355	22	27
Mozzarella Sticks, no Sce, 4 sticks	425	28	38
Onion Petals, no Sauce, reg., 4 oz	330	22	35
Shakes: Chocolate, reg., 13.2 fl.oz	510	13	83
Other flavors, regular, 13.2 fl.oz	500	13	81

Desserts	C	F	Cb
Apple Turnover w. Icing	375	16	65
Cherry Turnover w. Icing	375	15	65

For Complete Nutritional Data ~ see CalorieKing.com

Arthur Treachers®

Meals: Per Serving	C	F	Cb
Fish N Chips	1540	101	132
Fish Sandwich,	480	23	40
Seafood Sampler	3380	270	226
Shrimp N Chips	2050	123	225
Sides			
Cole Slaw, 5 oz	215	8.5	34
Hush Puppy (2)	275	10	42

Atlanta Bread Company®

Bagels: Per Bagel	C	F	Cb
Asiago Cheese	380	10	53
Cinnamon Crisp	330	2.5	68
Everything	320	3.5	60
Low-Carb Cranberry Walnut	110	3.5	16
Poppy Seed	320	5	57
Sesame	360	9	57
Other varieties, average	270	1.5	54
Sandwiches: No Cheese or Dressing			
ABC Special on French Roll	420	4.5	61
Peanut Butter & Jelly	600	14	99
Roasted Turkey Breast	430	7	61
Tangy Roast Beef	390	4	56
Tuna Salad, 4 oz	360	32	4
Veggie on Nine Grain	340	5	63
Focaccia: Hot Pastrami	460	10	59
Bella Basil on Tom. & Rosemary	660	35	58
California Avocado on Tom. On.	690	40	71
Chicken Salad, 4 oz	280	21	2
Grilled Chse on French Bread	390	11	57
Honey Maple Ham	410	5	63
Paninis: Chicken Pesto	800	35	83
Cordon Bleu	660	18	82
Cuban Pork Loin	745	30	82
Italian Vegetarian	640	16	93
Turkey Club	750	27	83
Salads: Caesar	190	10	11
Chicken Salad on Lettuce, no dr.	280	21	2
Chopstix Chicken	280	13	24
Fruit Salad, 10 oz	130	0	34
Greek Salad	200	13	13
House Salad, no dressing	50	0	11
Tuna Salad on Lettuce	360	32	4
Add Grilled Chicken, 2.5 oz	70	1.5	2
Extra Croutons, 0.5 oz	50	2	6

Atlanta Bread® cont...

Soups: Per Serving (10 oz)	C	F	Cb
Black Bean & Ham	250	9	40
Chicken Tortilla	190	9	20
Chunky Baked Potato	290	16	30
Classic Chicken Noodle	140	2.5	21
Cream of Broccoli	200	11	19
Creamy Tomato	130	9	10
French Onion w. Toppings	200	10	16
Garden Vegetable	100	1.5	19
Homestyle Chicken 'n Dumpling	290	18	25
New England Clam Chowder	280	16	24
Pasta Fagioli	170	6	24
Spicy Chicken Gumbo	120	2.5	16
Wisconsin Cheese	240	14	21
Breads: Per Thick Slice (2 oz)			
ABC Roll, 1 roll	260	1	54
Asiago	160	2	29
Challah	150	2.5	28
Cinnamon Raisin Loaf	150	2	28
Focaccia, round, ⅛ loaf	180	5	26
Pumpernickel	140	1.5	28
Rye; Nine Grain, avg.	155	2	28
Sourdough	140	0	29
Muffin Tops: Banana Nut	420	26	39
Blueberry	250	12	31
Chocolate Chip, 3 oz	400	19	52
Mocha	410	20	53
Pumpkin	350	13	54

For Complete Nutritional Data ~ see CalorieKing.com

Au Bon Pain®

	C	F	Cb
Bagels: *Per Bagel*			
Asiago Cheese	360	8	57
Cinnamon Raisin	290	1	62
Dutch Apple	450	3.5	93
French Toast	400	7	72
Plain	280	1	57
Spreads: Plain Cream Chse, 2 oz	120	11	4
Honey Walnut	140	9	12
Veggie, 2 oz	140	12	3
Breakfast Sandwiches: *Per Sandwich*			
Egg on a Bagel	400	4	63
w. Bacon	480	12	63
w. Bacon & Cheese	560	18	63
w. Cheese	480	11	63
Sandwiches			
Asian Chicken Salad	430	16	50
BBQ Pulled Pork	610	18	83
Chicken & Mozzarella Foccacia	740	24	73
Chicken Tarragon w. Field Onions	800	42	71
Fresh Mozzarella, Tomato w. Pesto	640	30	66
Grilled Chicken w. Blue Cheese	670	29	64
Spicy Tuna on Multigrain	690	33	72
Steak w. Swiss Cheese	690	28	68
Tuna w. Cheddar & Peppers	555	18	62
Turkey w. Guacamole & Swiss	760	28	77
Wraps: Chicken Caesar	590	24	63
Fields & Feta	550	16	90
Mediterranean Wrap	570	22	80
Southwest Tuna	540	25	68
Soups: *Per Serving (8 oz)*			
Broccoli Cheese	210	14	14
Chicken Noodle	100	2	14
Corn Chowder	230	13	28
Garden Vegetable	50	1	9
Split Pea w. Ham	140	1	28
Vegetarian Chili	120	1.5	29
Breads: Average, 1.75 oz slice	130	1	27
Artisan Multigrain Bread, 1 slice	170	2	31
Bread Bowl (1)	640	3	127
Foccacia (1)	310	3.5	58
Rosemary Garlic Breadstick	200	5	33
Bread Rolls, Soft (1)	400	11	65

Au Bon Pain® cont...

	C	F	Cb
Yogurt & Fruit Cups: *Per Serving*			
Yogurt & Fruit, average, 15 oz	380	4.5	75
Fruit Cup: Small, 6 oz	70	0	16
Large, 12 oz	140	0	32
Salads: *Per Container*			
Caesar Salad, 7 oz	240	11	23
Chef's Salad, 8⅓ oz	270	15	8
Garden Salad, Small, 4 oz	50	1	10
Gorgonzola & Walnut, 7 oz	340	28	10
Mediterranean Chicken, 11 oz	290	16	14
Thai Chicken, 11 oz	140	2.5	14
Tuna Garden, 11 oz	400	24	25
Turkey Medallion Cobb, 11 oz	370	18	27
Steak w. Cranb., Oranges, 11.5 oz	290	7	46
Cookies: *Per Cookie*			
Chocolate Chip	260	11	37
English Toffee	210	11	26
Oatmeal Raisin	230	8	37
Shortbread	310	18	34
Cakes & Bars: Apple Strudel	340	20	36
Blonde w. Nuts Brownie	570	36	57
Cheesecake Brownie	470	26	55
Cherry Strudel	330	20	34
Choc Chip Brownie	480	25	61
Pecan Roll	520	28	61
Croissants: Ham & Cheese	350	18	34
Spinach & Cheese	260	14	28
Filled: Plain	270	15	28
Almond	510	25	63
Apple	230	10	31
Chocolate	340	17	42
Raspberry	340	18	39
Sweet Cheese	350	20	36
Muffins: Blueberry	510	19	76
Cranberry Walnut	500	24	61
Chocolate Chunk	590	20	83
Corn	460	16	69
Raisin Bran	410	9	74
Low-Fat: Chocolate Cake	320	2	74
Triple Berry	290	2	61
Drinks			
Mocha Blast, 16 fl.oz	350	10	56
Frozen Mocha Blast, 16 fl.oz	320	13	57
Cappuccino, 16 fl.oz	105	4	11
Iced Tea, 22 fl.oz	120	0	30

For Complete Nutritional Data ~ see CalorieKing.com

Auntie Anne's®

Pretzels: With Butter	C	F	Cb
Almond	400	8	72
Cinnamon Sugar	450	9	83
Garlic	350	4.5	68
Glazin' Raisin®	510	4	107
Jalapeno	310	4.5	59
Original	370	4	72
Sesame	410	12	64
Sour Cream & Onion	340	5	66
Stix, 4 sticks	245	3	48
Whole Wheat	370	4.5	72

Pretzels: Without Butter			
Almond Pretzel; Whole Wheat	350	1.5	72
Cinnamon Sugar	350	2	74
Garlic Pretzel; Sour Crm & Onion	320	1	66
Glazin' Raisin®	470	0.5	104
Jalapeno	270	1	58
Original	340	1	72
Sesame	350	6	63
Stix, 4 sticks	225	1	48

Dipping Sauces			
Caramel Dip, 1.5 oz	135	3	27
Cheese Sce; Hot Salsa Chse, avg.	100	8	4
Chocolate Flavored Dip, 1¼ oz	130	4	24
Light Cream Cheese, 1¼ oz	70	6	1
Marinara Sauce, 1¼ oz	10	0	4
Strawberry Cream Cheese, 1¼ oz	110	10	4
Sweet Mustard, 1¼ oz	60	1.5	8

Beverages: Per Serving			
Auntie Anne's Lemonade, 22 fl.oz	180	0	43
Dutch Ice (20 fl.oz): Kiwi-Banana	270	0	63
Blue Raspberry	230	0	55
Lemonade	450	0	110
Mocha	570	15	105
Orange Crème	400	0	92
Pina Colada; Strawberry	535	0	125
Wild Cherry	300	0	69

Dutch Smoothie: Per 20 fl.oz			
Blue Raspberry	400	14	61
Kiwi-Banana	430	14	68
Lemonade	540	14	95
Mocha	590	23	90
Orange Crème	500	14	83
Pina Colada	470	14	79
Strawberry; Wild Cherry, avg.	450	14	74

Backyard Burgers®

Burgers	C	F	Cb
Back Yard Burger ⅓ lb.	470	29	38
Cheeseburger ⅓ lb	520	34	38
Bacon Cheddar	620	42	38
Barbecue Bacon	630	39	47
Black Jack	580	39	36
Chili Cheese	560	36	41
Garden Veggie Sandwich	240	6	47
Jr Burger	310	17	38
Hawaiian	550	33	44
Miz Grazi	530	34	39
Mushroom Swiss	540	36	37
Low-Carb Burger	350	27	3

Chicken Sandwiches			
Bacon Swiss	390	20	37
Barbecue	280	8	44
Blackened	290	11	39
Buffalo Ranch	540	30	51
Hawaiian Chicken	280	8	45
Honey Mustard	320	11	46
Lemon Butter Chicken	260	9	37
Savory Chicken	230	6	36
Specialities: BLT	270	16	36
Chicken Tenderloins, 3 piece	400	28	22
Chili Dog	340	20	29
Chili Cheese Dog	400	25	29
Hot Dog	310	18	27

Baked Potatoes			
Chili & Cheddar, 9 oz	330	11	48
Ranch, 7.7 oz	410	22	45
Salsa, 7.7 oz	250	5	47
Traditional/Plain, 6 oz	190	0	43

Fries			
Chili Cheese Fries, 6.7 oz	350	22	28
Seasoned Fries, regular, 3 oz	260	16	26
Waffle Fries, regular, 3 oz	240	16	23

Salads (No Dressing)			
Blackened Chicken	160	4	11
Charbroiled Chicken	140	3	11
Garden Fresh	25	0	5

Cobblers: Apple, 6 oz			
Apple, 6 oz	430	20	61
Blackberry; Peach, 6 oz	420	20	60
Cherry, 6 oz	460	20	68

Shakes: Per 12 fl.oz			
Chocolate; Strawberry	560	26	79
Vanilla	540	26	71

For Complete Nutritional Data ~ see CalorieKing.com

Baja Fresh®

Burritos: Includes Cheese	C	F	Cb
Baja Burrito: w. Charbroiled Chicken	930	45	83
w. Charbroiled Steak	1030	52	83
Bare Burrito: w. Charbroiled Chkn	640	7	97
Vegetarian	580	10	101
Bean & Cheese Burrito: w. Chkn	1120	42	114
w. Charbroiled Steak	1210	49	114
Vegetarian	980	42	114
Burrito Dos Manos: w. Chicken	835	29	103
w. Charbroiled Steak	885	33	103
Burrito Mexicano: w. Chicken	940	20	135
w. Charbroiled Steak	1030	27	135
Burrito Ultimo: w. Charbroiled Chkn	1030	43	102
w. Charbroiled Steak	1120	50	102
Grilled Vegetarian	950	40	112
Fajita Burrito w. Chicken	890	38	85
w. Steak	990	45	85
Fajitas			
Charbroiled Chkn w. Corn Tortillas	1010	31	123
Charbroiled Steak w. Corn Tortillas	1150	41	123
Nachos: w. Charbroiled Steak	2120	118	163
w. Cheese	1890	108	163
w. Chicken	2020	110	164
Quesadilla: w. Chicken & Chips	1330	80	84
w. Charbroiled Steak & Chips	1430	87	84
w. Cheese & Chips	1200	78	84
Vegetarian w. Chips	1260	78	96
Tacos			
Baja Fish Taco w. Breaded Fish	320	16	35
Grilled Mahi Mahi Taco	300	12	34
Baja Style Taco w. Charbroiled Chkn	250	8	30
w. Charbroiled Steak	280	10	30
w. Charbroiled Gulf Shrimp	250	8	31
Salads			
Baja Ensalada: *No Dressing*			
w. Charbroiled Chicken	310	7	18
w. Charbroiled Shrimp	230	6	18
w. Charbroiled Steak	450	18	18
Chipotle Glaze Charbroiled Chicken	590	22	54
Mahi Mahi Ensalada	310	12	22
Taquitos: w. Chicken & Beans	780	40	68
w. Charbroiled Chicken & Rice	740	40	66
w. Charbroiled Steak & Beans	800	42	68
w. Charbroiled Steak & Rice	770	42	66
Tostadas: Chicken	1140	55	98
Fish	1130	55	99
Pork Carnitas	1180	62	100
Steak Carnitas	1230	63	98

For Complete Nutritional Data ~ see CalorieKing.com

Baskin Robbins®

Hard Scooped Ice Cream	C	F	Cb
Classic: Per Regular Scoop			
Chocolate	260	14	33
Chocolate Chip	270	16	28
Chocolate Chip Cookie Dough	290	15	36
Chocolate Fudge	270	15	35
French Vanilla	280	18	26
German Choc Cake	300	16	36
Gold Medal Ribbon	260	13	34
Jamoca	240	13	26
Jamoca Almond Fudge	270	15	31
Mint Choc Chip	270	16	28
Old Fashion Butter Pecan	280	18	24
Oreo Cookies 'N Cream	280	15	32
Peanut Butter 'N Chocolate	320	20	31
Pistachio Almond	290	19	25
Pralines 'N Cream	270	14	34
Reeses Peanut Butter	300	18	31
Rocky Road	290	15	36
Vanilla	260	16	26
Very Berry Strawberry	220	11	28
World Class Chocolate	270	15	33
Chocolate Roll Cake: Per Slice (4.1 oz)			
Average all flavors	290	14	36
Low-Fat Ice Cream: Espresso 'N Crm	180	4	32
No Sugar Added Ice Cream, avg.	160	4	27
Ices, Sherbets, Sorbets: Regular Scoop			
Ices, Daiquiri; Margarita	135	0	34
Sherbets, average all flavors	160	2	34
Sorbets, average all flavors	115	0	29
Signature Sundaes			
Chocolate Bliss, 10 oz	880	42	121
Peanut Butter Pie, 8 oz	850	59	68
Tiramisu, 9.6 oz	790	39	101
Low-Fat Yogurt (Hard): Regular Scoop			
Average all flavors	200	4	38
Non-Fat Yogurt (Soft Serve): Per ½ Cup			
Vanilla, 4 oz	220	0	46
Other flavors, 3 oz	180	0	34
Shakes, Smoothies, Blasts: Regular (16 fl.oz)			
Shakes: Chocolate Ice Cream	675	26	98
Vanilla Ice Cream	690	33	85
Smoothies: Average all flavors	365	1	82
Blasts: Cappuccino w/whip cream	325	14	44
Cones: Sugar Cone	60	3	7
Cake Cone	25	0.5	4
Waffle Cone: Large	120	1.5	14
Fresh Baked	145	2	3

For Complete Nutritional Data ~ see CalorieKing.com

Fast - Foods & *Restaurants*

Ben & Jerry's® ⒸⒻⒸⓑ

Ice Cream & Frozen Yogurt ~ See Page 32
Novelty Bars ~ See Page 36

Big Apple Bagels®

	C	F	Cb
Bagels: All types, avg., 5 oz	340	2	68
½ bagel, 2.5 oz	170	1	34
My Favorite Muffin® : Per ⅓ Jumbo or 2 Minis			
Regular: Blueberry	170	8	22
Chocolate Chip	210	11	27
Pumpkin Spice	180	8	26
Cinnamon Swirl Cheesecake	215	11	28
Fat Free: Blueberry	110	0	26
Chocolate Eclair	120	0	27
Cinnamon Bun	170	0	42
Cream Cheese: Per 2 Tbsp (1 oz)			
Plain	100	10	2
Honey Cinnamon; Very Berry, avg.	130	12	3
Lite varieties, average	65	5	2
Soups: Per Cup (8 oz)			
Boston Clam/Potato Chowder	210	13	20
Chicken Noodle; Beef Pot Roast	110	4	12
Garden Vegetable	110	1	22
Minestrone	150	3	26
Split Pea w. Ham; Hearty Vege	95	2	16
For Complete Nutritional Data ~ see CalorieKing.com			

Big Boy® ⒸⒻⒸⓑ

	C	F	Cb
Breakfast: HealthSmart, Egg Beaters,			
Plain Omelette	310	8.5	38
Scrambled	310	8.5	38
Vegetarian Omelette	340	8.5	45
Health Smart Meals: Tossed Salad	45	1.5	6
Grilled Chicken Breast	325	10	22
Lemon Baked Cod	490	4.5	72
Spaghetti Marinara	420	6.5	76
Vegetable Stir-Fry	610	3.5	134
Sandwiches: Big Boy	600	26	35
Brawny Lad	420	21	30
Buddie Boy	760	34	80
Fish Sandwich	690	48	41
Small Hamburger	445	30	30
Super Big Boy	830	66	35
Swiss Miss	635	44	28
Sides: Chili	315	18	19
French Fries	360	19	45
Onion Rings	580	41	45
Tartare Sauce	370	40	1
Trio Salad	620	46	18
Soups: HealthSmart Cabbage Soup	50	0.5	9
Beverages: HealthSmart Shake	160	0	33

Blimpie® ⒸⒻⒸⓑ

	C	F	Cb
Cold Deli Subs: Per 6" Sub on White (w. Cheese)			
Blimpie Best	475	16	52
Club	440	12	50
Ham & Swiss Cheese	435	13	52
Roast Beef	450	13	49
Seafood, no Cheese	350	8	58
Tuna	495	23	51
Turkey	420	11	49
Paninis: Cuban	460	12	50
Grilled Chicken Caesar	560	26	50
Turkey Italiano	390	10	44
Wraps: Chicken Caesar	650	35	56
Zesty Italian	680	33	74
Hot Deli Subs: Per 6" Sub on White			
Grilled Chicken	375	9	50
Meatball w. Cheese	570	27	55
Mexi Max	430	9	65
Steak & Onion Melt w. Cheese	440	16	49
VegiMax	395	7	60
Salads: Chef Salad	210	9	9
Macaroni Salad, ⅓ container	360	25	25
Seafood Salad	120	4.5	16
Tuna Salad	260	19	8
Dressings & Sauces: Caesar	210	22	2
Blimpie, 1.5 oz	180	12	24
Soups: Per Serving			
Cream of Broccoli & Cheese	190	12	15
Garden Vegetable	80	0.5	14
Homestyle Chicken Noodle	120	2.5	18
Vegetable Beef	80	1.5	13
Desserts			
Cookies: Oatmeal Raisin	190	8	27
Sugar	330	17	24
Other varieties, average	200	10	26
For Complete Nutritional Data ~ see CalorieKing.com			

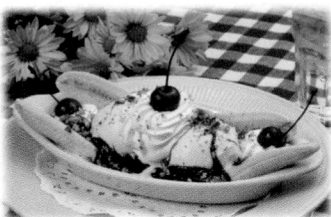

Restaurants & Fast - Foods

Bob Evans®

Breakfast

	C	F	Cb
Combinations: Country Biscuit	830	59	51
Fruit & Yogurt Plate	400	2	96
Home Fries	195	7	28
Lite Sausage Breakfast	470	21	48
Pot Roast Hash Breakfast	675	41	35
Sausage Benedict	950	67	40
Farm Fresh Eggs: Eggs Benedict	435	21	35
Hardboiled (1)	60	4	1
Over Easy (1)	100	8	1
Scrambled	255	17	2
Scrambled Egg Beaters	275	24	4
Hotcake: Blueberry (1)	370	10	62
Buttermilk (1)	355	10	58
Omelets: Three Cheese	770	67	4
Farmer's Market	910	74	15
Ham & Cheese	760	62	3
Western	780	63	8
Crepes: Raspberry (2)	780	44	82
Plain (2)	305	19	26

Dinners: *Per Serving*

	C	F	Cb
Beef & Pork: Meat Loaf	260	19	10
Country Fried Steak w. Gravy	635	45	43
no Gravy	480	33	26
Slow Roasted Pork Loin	520	30	30
Chicken & Turkey:			
Chicken Dinner, Fried, 1 piece	325	16	14
Chicken Dinner, Grilled, 1 piece	230	13	0
Chicken Pot Pie	900	61	62
Chicken-n-Noodles	295	16	23
Slow Roasted Turkey	115	4	1
Seafood: Salmon Dinner	290	13	0
Kid's Menu: Mac & Cheese	330	12	45
Mini Cheeseburgers (1)	255	14	20
Pasta	200	5	35
Plenty-O-Pancakes	500	17	79
Smiley Face Potatoes	340	40	48

Lunch Savors: *Per Serving*

	C	F	Cb
Chicken Parmesan Pasta	645	29	53
Salads: Cobb Grilled Chicken	470	30	10
Country Spinach	510	35	12
Wildfire Chkn: w. Fried Chicken	660	29	65
w. Grilled Chicken	540	26	49
Stir-Fry: Chicken	400	16	31

Bob Evans® cont...

Sandwiches & Burgers

	C	F	Cb
Burgers: Bacon Cheeseburger	710	49	32
Cheeseburger	640	42	32
Hamburger	540	32	31
Sandwiches: Bob's BLT	640	39	27
Fried Chicken Club	700	38	45
Grilled Chicken Club	605	35	31
Grilled Chicken	400	15	30
Pot Roast	605	28	58
Turkey Bacon Melt	615	29	53

Sides

	C	F	Cb
Baked Potato Seasoned, Loaded	375	13	56
Baked Potato Seasoned, Plain	210	0	54
Broccoli Florets, 4 oz	30	0	6
Coleslaw, 4 oz	210	14	19
French Fries, 3 oz	120	13	20
Garden Side Salad, 5.3 oz	140	4	22
Garden Vegetables, 6 oz	120	7	14
Glazed Carrots, 4 oz	85	3	14
Green Beans w. Ham, 6 oz	80	3	9
Mashed Potatoes, 5 oz	170	6	15
Vegetable Rice Pilaf, 6 oz	130	4	20
Specialty Breads: Banana Nut, 6 oz	430	16	68
Cinnamon Swirl Roll, Frosted	575	25	79
Dinner Roll (1)	200	5	34
English Muffin (1)	140	1	28
Garlic Bread, 2 oz	215	13	20
Sourdough, 1.7 oz	135	1	25
Texas Toast, 1.8 oz	120	1	12

Beverages

	C	F	Cb
Iced Tea: Regular	5	0	1
Raspberry/Strawberry	80	0	20

Desserts, Pies, Sundaes

	C	F	Cb
Pie: Apple Dumpling Pie, 1 slice	605	28	83
Apple Dumpling A La Mode, 1 sl.	790	38	108
Apple Pie, N.S.A., 1 slice	490	30	55
Coconut Cream Pie, 1 slice	555	29	67
French Silk Pie, 1 slice	695	47	62
Oreo Cookies & Cream, 1 slice	805	45	95
Pumpkin Pie, 1 slice	575	31	71
Kids Sundae: Fudge Blast, 5 oz	270	13	36
Reese's, 5.6 oz	355	18	44

For Complete Nutritional Data ~ see CalorieKing.com

Fast - Foods & *Restaurants*

Bojangles®

Cajun & Southern Style Chicken	C	F	Cb
Breast, average	280	17	12
Leg, average	265	16	11
Thigh, average	310	23	11
Wing, average	355	25	11
Sandwiches			
Cajun Filet: no Mayo	340	11	41
w. Mayonnaise	440	22	41
Grilled Filet: no Mayo	235	5	25
w. Mayonnaise	335	16	25
Snacks: Buffalo Bites	180	5	5
Chicken Supremes	335	16	26
Biscuit Sandwiches: Biscuit (plain)	245	12	29
Bacon	290	17	26
Bacon, Egg & Cheese	550	42	27
Cajun Filet	455	21	46
Country Ham	270	15	26
Egg	400	30	26
Sausage	350	23	26
Smoked Sausage	380	26	27
Steak	650	49	37
Fixins': Botato Rounds	235	11	31
Cajun Pintos	110	0	18
Corn on the Cob	140	2	34
Dirty Rice	165	6	24
Green Beans	25	0	5
Macaroni & Cheese	200	14	12
Marinated Cole Slaw	135	3	26
Potatoes, no Gravy	80	1	16
Seasoned Fries	345	19	39
Sweet Biscuits: Bo Berry	220	10	29
Cinnamon	320	18	37

For Complete Nutritional Data ~ see CalorieKing.com

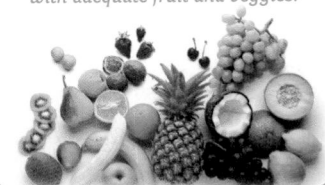

Be sure to balance 'eating out' with adequate fruit and veggies.

Boston Market®

Sandwiches & Burgers	C	F	Cb
Chicken Carver	690	32	57
Meatloaf Carver	940	45	96
Sirloin Dip Carver w. Beef Au Jus	940	43	74
Sirloin Dip Carver, no Beef Au Jus	920	43	70
Turkey Carver	830	36	70
Turkey Dip Carver: w. Poultry Au Jus	785	28	71
no Poultry Au Jus	770	27	67
Salads: Per Serving (w. Dressing)			
Caesar Entree: w. Roasted Sirloin	660	96	12
w. Roasted Turkey	640	52	13
w. Rotisserie Chicken	600	49	13
Market Chopped: w. Rsd Sirloin	580	48	31
w. Roasted Turkey	720	54	32
w. Rotisserie Chicken	680	50	32
Sides: Per Serving			
Caesar Side Salad: w. Dressing	400	40	7
no Dressing	40	2	3
Cinnamon Apples, 5 oz	210	3	47
Creamed Spinach, 6.7 oz	280	23	12
Fresh Steamed Vegetables, 4.8 oz	50	2	8
Fresh Vegetable Stuffing, 4.8 oz	190	8	25
Garden Fresh Coleslaw, 3.8 oz	190	16	9
Garlic Dill New Potatoes, 5½ oz	140	3	24
Green Beans, 4.7 oz	90	5	10
Macaroni & Cheese, 7.8 oz	330	12	39
Mashed Potatoes (7.8 oz): no Gravy	210	9	29
w. 2 oz Poultry Gravy	235	10	32
Seasonal Fresh Fruit Salad, 5 oz	60	0	15
Sweet Corn, 6.2 oz	170	4	37
Sweet Potato Casserole, 7 oz	460	17	77
Soups: Per Serving			
Chicken Noodle, 10 oz	180	7	16
Chicken Tortilla, 8 oz	340	22	24
Desserts: Per Serving			
Apple Pie, 1 slice, 6 oz	420	20	56
Chocolate Cake, 5.1 oz	600	32	75
Choc. Chip Fudge Brownie, 5 oz	580	23	81
Cornbread, 1.6 oz	130	3.5	21
Nestle Toll House Choc. Chip Cookie (1)	370	19	49

For Complete Nutritional Data ~ see CalorieKing.com

Boston Pizza® | C | F | Cb

	C	F	Cb
Starters: Cactus Cut Potatoes/Dip	780	41	91
Boston's BBQ Wings	690	42	24
Boston's Pizza Bread, no dip	510	13	83
Soup: Baked Onion	160	4	24
Salads: Caesar, reg., w. dressing	240	18	15
Greek, regular, w. dressing	600	57	18
Sirloin Steak w. dressing	640	48	17
Entrees: See CalorieKing.com			
Sandwiches: Boston Brute & Fries	1010	30	144
Boston Cheesesteak & Fries	1640	65	213
Chicken Santa Fe Stromboli & Caesar	720	22	106
New York Steak & Tossed Greens	510	33	12
Pizzas (Medium): Per 2 Slices			
BBQ Chicken	380	12	50
Boston Royal	440	12	54
Californian	320	4	62
Hawaiian	420	10	56
Meatlovers	520	20	58
Spicey	560	24	56
Ultimate Pepperoni	460	20	48
Vegetarian	360	8	54
Other Sizes: See CalorieKing.com			
Pastas (Full Order): Lasagna	670	22	83
Chicken & Mushroom Fettucini	1200	57	134
Spaghetti with Bolognese	780	13	138
Desserts: Chocolate Explosion	880	51	105
New York Cheesecake	620	33	80

For Complete Nutritional Data ~ see CalorieKing.com

Braum's®

Cinnamon Rolls, with Icing	340	11	56
Frozen Yogurt: Per Cup (8 fl.oz)			
Vanilla, Peach, Strawb./Banana	260	7	50
Other flavors, average	320	12	50
Ice Cream: Per Cup (8 fl.oz)			
Light: Average all varieties	300	10	52
Premium: Peanut Buttercup	440	28	46
Other flavors, average	380	20	45
Sherbet: Avg. all varieties, 1 cup	140	3	36
Pies (Baked): Average, 1 slice	400	20	50

For Complete Nutritional Data ~ see CalorieKing.com

Buck's Pizza®

Buck's Deluxe: Med. (12"), 1 sl, ⅙	265	13	28
Large (14"), 1 slice, ⅛	270	13	29
X-Large (16"), 1 slice, ¹/₁₂	240	11	38
Small (9"), Whole Pizza	900	44	96
Personal (6"), Whole Pizza	400	17	69

Bruegger's Bagels® | C | F | Cb

	C	F	Cb
Bagels			
Plain/Salt/Sesame/Garlic, avg.	350	2.5	68
Blueberry/Cranb. Or./Cinn. Raisin	340	2	68
Chocolate Chip	310	4.5	69
Everything/Onion/Sundried Tom.	320	2	65
Cream Cheese: Average, 2 oz	180	15	8
Light varieties, average, 2 oz	115	8	6
Hummus, 2 oz	120	7	8
Breakfast Sandwiches: Per Sandwich			
Egg, Cheese	420	18	71
Egg, Cheese & Bacon	460	23	65
Egg, Cheese & Ham	460	18	73
Egg, Cheese & Sausage	640	38	72
Sandwiches			
Bagel: Chicken Fajita	530	11	81
Smoked Salmon	490	10	74
Garden Veggie	400	2.5	82
Herby Turkey	560	14	78
Santa Fe Turkey	490	9	75
Deli: Chicken Breast w. Mustard	660	11	87
Chicken Salad w. Mayo	630	26	73
Ham w. Mustard	470	5	82
Turkey w. Mayonnaise	510	14	70

For Complete Nutritional Data ~ see CalorieKing.com

Burgerville® | C | F | Cb

	C	F	Cb
Hamburger	300	15	29
Cheeseburger	350	19	29
Double Beef Cheeseburger	430	25	29
Half Pound Colossal	730	45	31
Colossal	520	30	30
Tillamook Cheeseburger	630	40	32
Pepper Bacon Cheeseburger	680	45	28
Gardenburger	460	19	53
Spicy Black Bean Gardenburger	550	32	45
Turkey Burger	540	29	33
Turkey Club Sandwich	540	32	38
Deluxe Crispy Chicken	610	30	56
Crispy Chicken	450	18	55
Grilled Chicken	350	3	45
Halibut Fillet Sandwich	480	27	42
Halibut Fish, 3 pieces	330	16	25
Chicken Strips, 5 pieces	550	30	36
Protein Platter	530	40	6
French Fries: Regular, 5 oz	390	22	44
Large, 6½ oz	510	29	57

For Complete Nutritional Data ~ see CalorieKing.com

Burger King®

Burgers & Sandwiches	C	F	Cb
Bacon Cheeseburger	360	18	31
Bacon Double Cheeseburger	530	31	32
BK Veggie Burger (with mayo)	420	16	46
without mayonnaise	340	8	46
Cheeseburger	330	16	31
Double Cheeseburger	500	29	31
Hamburger	290	12	30
Double Hamburger	410	21	30
The Angus Steak Burger	560	22	59
Stackers: Double	610	39	32
Triple	800	54	33
Quadruple	1000	68	34
Whoppers®			
Whopper	670	39	51
without mayonnaise	510	22	51
Double Whopper	900	57	51
with Cheese, Mayo	990	64	52
without mayonnaise	740	39	51
Whopper JR	370	21	31
without mayonnaise	290	12	31
Triple Whopper	1130	74	51
Chicken & Fish			
BK Big Fish Sandwich w. tartar sce	620	29	67
Original Chicken Sandwich	660	40	52
without mayonnaise	450	17	52
Spicy TenderCrisp Chicken S'wich	720	36	74
without mayonnaise	570	21	73
TenderCrisp Chicken S'wich	780	43	73
TenderGrill Chkn S'wich w. mayo	510	19	49
without sauce	400	7	49
Chicken Fries: 6 pieces, no sauce	260	15	18
Chicken Tenders: 5 pieces, no sauce	210	12	13
Big Kid's Meal, 6 pces	250	15	16
Kid's Meal, 4 pieces	170	10	11
Dipping Sauces, (1 oz): Buffalo Sce	80	5	2
Honey Flavored	90	0	23
Honey Mustard	90	6	8
Ranch; Zesty Onion Ring, avg.	145	15	2
Sweet & Sour; Barbecue, avg.	40	0	11
French Fries: Small, 2.6 oz	230	13	26
Medium, 4 oz	360	20	41
Large, 5.6 oz	500	28	57
King Size, 6.8 oz	600	33	69
Ketchup, 1 packet	10	0	3
Onion Rings: Small, 1½ oz	150	7	19
Medium, 3.2 oz	320	16	40
Large, 4.8 oz	450	22	57
King Size, 5.3 oz	520	26	60
Cheesy Tots: Small, 6 pieces	210	12	20
Medium, 9 pieces	320	18	30

Burger King® cont..

Breakfast	C	F	Cb
Biscuits: Ham, Egg & Cheese	390	22	31
Sausage, Egg & Cheese	530	37	31
Croissan'wich: Egg & Cheese	300	17	26
Bacon/Ham, Egg & Cheese, avg.	340	20	26
Sausage & Cheese	370	25	23
Sausage, Egg & Cheese	470	32	26
Double Croissan'wich:			
Bacon, Egg & Cheese	430	27	27
Sausage, Bacon, Egg & Cheese	560	39	27
Sausage, Egg & Cheese	680	51	26
Omelet Sandwich: Enormous	730	45	44
Ham	330	14	35
French Toast: Sticks, 5 sticks	380	19	45
Kid's Meal (w. syrup)	660	22	102
Breakfast Syrup, 1 oz	80	0	21
Jam, Grape/Strawberry, 1 pkg	30	0	7
Hash Brown Rounds: Medium	430	28	42
Small, 3 oz	260	17	25
Cini-Minis (4), with Vanilla Icing	500	21	72
Salads: (No Dressing or Croutons)			
Garden Salad, no Chicken, 6½ oz	90	5	7
Side Garden Salad, 3½ oz	15	0	3
TenderGrill Chicken Garden Salad	240	9	8
TenderCrisp Chicken Garden Salad	400	21	32
Garlic Parmesan Croutons, ½ oz	60	2	9
Salad Dressings: Per 2 oz			
Ken's Fat-Free Ranch	60	0	15
Ken's Creamy Caesar	210	21	4
Ken's Honey Mustard	270	23	15
Ken's Light Italian	120	11	5
Ken's Ranch	190	20	2
Desserts: Dutch Apple Pie	300	13	45
Hershey's Sundae Pie	310	19	32
Drinks & Shakes: Coffee, Medium	5	0	1
Coca-Cola/Sprite/Dr Pepper (with ¼ Ice):			
Kids, 12 fl.oz	110	0	30
Small, 16 fl.oz	140	0	39
Medium, 22 fl.oz	200	0	53
Large, 32 fl.oz	290	0	79
King, 42 fl.oz	390	0	104
Icee (Coke/Minute Maid): Small	110	0	31
Medium, 11 fl.oz	140	0	40
Low-Fat Milk (1%), 8 fl.oz	100	2.5	12
Milk Shakes (Choc./Strawb.): Small	470	14	75
Medium	690	20	114
Large	950	29	151
Orange Juice, 8 fl.oz	140	0	33

For Complete Nutritional Data ~ see CalorieKing.com

California Pizza Kitchen
~ See CalorieKing.com

Captain D's Seafood®

	C	**F**	**Cb**
Platters: Per Platter			
Broiled Chicken/Fish, average	1015	8	194
Broiled Fish & Chicken	1005	7	194
Broiled Shrimp	1030	8	195
Lunches: Per Lunch Platter			
Broiled Chicken	490	9	63
Broiled Fish/Shrimp	425	7	63
Broiled Fish & Chicken	460	8	63
Stuffed Crab	155	6	16
Carb Counters: Fish Dinner	350	17	19
Chicken Dinner	320	15	19
Low-Cal Fare: w. Rice & Vegetables			
Baked Chicken Dinner, 1 piece	350	3.5	49
Baked Fish Dinner, 3 pieces	390	5	49
Baked Salmon Dinner, 1 piece	470	8	58
Shrimp Scampi Dinner, 10 pieces	370	5	50
Sandwiches: Broiled Chicken	445	18	29
Broiled Fish	520	18	51
Desserts: Carrot Cake	430	22	49
Cheesecake	425	31	30
Chocolate Cake	300	10	49
Pecan Pie	455	20	64

Caribou Coffee®

Beverages Based on 2% Milk Unless Indicated

Drinks: Per Cup (16 fl.oz)			
Alaskan Fruit Smoothies: Creampop	470	22	66
Passion Green Tea	200	0	48
Strawberry Banana	260	0	65
Wildberry	230	0	57
Coffee Coolers: Caramel	490	15	85
Chocolate	410	16	63
Espresso; Coffee, average	230	4	47
Mint Oreo	620	26	94
Vanilla	420	17	65
Espresso: Breve	440	38	16
Campfire Mocha	600	18	97
Cappuccino	180	7	18
Espresso	10	0	2
Latte	200	8	20
Macchiato	15	0.5	2
Mocha	480	19	63
White Chocolate Mocha	540	25	69
Skinny Bou Latte: Low Cal	120	0.5	17
Wild: Caramel Highrise	420	17	55
Hot Apple Blast	470	11	91
Lite White Berry	480	8	94
Mint Condition	580	19	89

& Fast - Foods

Carl's Jr.®

Burgers/Sandwiches	**C**	**F**	**Cb**
Bacon Swiss Crispy Chicken	770	38	74
Catch Fish Sandwich	560	27	58
Famous Star Hamburger	590	32	50
Charboiled: BBQ Chicken S'wich	370	4	47
Chicken Club Sandwich	545	23	43
Santa Fe Chicken Sandwich	610	32	43
Dble Sourdough Bacon Chseburger	920	59	45
Dble Western Bacon Chseburger	920	50	65
JR. Hamburger	280	9	36
Low Carb Chicken Club S'wich	380	21	10
Ranch Crispy Chicken Sandwich	660	31	72
Sourdough Bacon Cheeseburger	550	29	41
Spicy Chicken Sandwich	480	26	48
Super Star Hamburger	790	47	52
The Six Dollar Burger	960	62	52
Chili Cheese Burger	930	57	57
Jalapeno	1010	72	52
Low-Carb Burger	490	37	6
Western Bacon Burger	1080	62	84
Western Bacon Cheeseburger	660	30	64
Western Bacon Crispy Swiss Chkn	770	38	74
Potatoes: Plain, no marg.	280	0	63
Bacon & Cheese	620	29	71
Broccoli & Cheese	510	21	71
Sour Cream & Chives	410	14	65
Breakfast: Breakfast Burger	830	46	65
Breakfast Burrito	560	32	37
Loaded Breakfast Burrito	810	49	53
Breakfast Bowl, Low Carb	900	73	5
Breakfast Quesadilla	390	18	38
French Toast Dip (6), no Syrup	450	20	59
Sourdough Sandwich, no meat	410	19	39
Scrambled Eggs & Bacon	760	42	69
Bakery/Desserts: Chocolate Cake	300	12	48
Chocolate Chip Cookie (1)	350	18	46
Strawberry Swirl Chsecake, 3.5 oz	290	17	30
Side Orders: Chicken Stars, 9 pces	405	25	22
Chicken Breast Strips (5)	630	35	45
CrissCut Fries, 5 oz	410	24	43
French Fries, small, 3.2 oz	290	14	37
Hash Brown Nuggets, 4 oz	330	21	32
Onion Rings, 4.5 oz	440	22	53
Salads: No Dressing			
Charbroiled Chicken Salad-to-Go	330	7	17
Garden Salad-to-Go	120	3	5

Carvel®

Sundaes: Per Small	C	F	Cb
Thinny-Thin: Fudge No-Fat	380	0	84
Strawberry No-Fat	290	0	63
Classic Regular: Caramel	500	27	58
Bittersweet Fudge; Hot Fudge	500	29	54
Bordeaux Fudge	460	25	52
Strawberry	430	25	46
Metropolitan Coladas: Per Small			
Pina Colada	340	14	53
Other varieties	320	9	60
Novelties: Per Small			
Flying Sauces 98% Fat-Free	190	1.5	40
Parfait; Miniature Sundae No-Fat	190	0	42
Parfait; No Sugar Added	200	2.5	42
Old Fashioned Sundae No-Fat	300	0	66
No Sugar Added	360	4.5	76
Uptown Smoothies: Per Small			
Broadway Banana	280	0.5	69
Grand Central Cooler	280	0.5	70
Other varieties, average	280	0.5	70
Thinny-Thin: Berry Times Square	300	0	73
Grand Central Cooler	250	0	63
Other varieties, average	270	0	68
Creammaccino: Classic, 16 fl.oz	520	21	72
Caramel Cream, 16 fl.oz	670	14	108
Mocha Fudge, 16 fl.oz	690	30	94

Checkers®

~ Same Menu & Data as Rally's Hamburgers®
See Page 240 ~

Cheesecake Factory®

10" Cheesecake: Per Slice			
P. B. Cup Fudge Ripple	930	59	93
Banana Cream	860	63	70
Brownie Sundae	970	63	96
Choc Chip Cookie Dough	1910	72	102
Dulce de Leche	1010	74	83
Kahlua Cocoa Coffee	840	55	80
Keylime Cheesecake	710	49	64
Original Cheesecake	630	45	53
Vanilla Bean Cheesecake	870	64	69
White Choc. Raspberry Truffle	900	62	80

Charley's Grilled Subs®

Subs: Regular w. Dressing	C	F	Cb
BBQ Cheddar	730	28	83
Bacon 3 Cheese Steak	740	37	57
Chicken Buffalo, no cheese/dress.	680	31	62
Chicken Bacon Club	640	27	57
Chicken Cordon Bleu	650	24	61
Chicken Teriyaki, no chse./dress.	520	13	61
Italian Deli	620	29	56
Philly Cheese Steak	600	24	60
Philly Chicken, no cheese/dressing	570	20	59
Philly Ham & Swiss	600	25	58
Philly Steak Deluxe	600	24	60
Philly Veggie	600	28	65
Steak Siciliano	720	36	53
Turkey Melt, no cheese/dress.	590	22	59
Ultimate Club	660	32	54
Fresh Salads: Garden no dressing	155	9	13
Fries (Per Regular): Original	680	53	46
Cheddar & Bacon	1130	91	60
Cheddar Ranch & Bacon	1310	110	61
Ranch & Bacon	1210	102	56
Beverages: Natural Lemonade, reg.	130	0	32

Chevys Fresh Mex®

Burritos	C	F	Cb
Veggie w. Tortilla, Marinated Veges,			
San Antonio Veges,			
Pico de Gallo & Ranchero Sauce	430	19	49
Catch of the Day			
Fish/Veges/Salsa/Tomalito	430	16	16
Fajitas: With San Antonio Veges & Tomalito			
Chicken	285	6	13
Shrimp	285	7	13
Veggie w. Marinated Veges	345	28	16
Salad: With Salsa Vinaigrette Dressing			
Chicken, Grilled	535	18	53
Mixed Green	360	16	42
Sides: Black Beans	60	0	11
Guacamole, 2 oz	105	10	3
Mexican Rice	210	3	39
Salsa for Chips, 5 oz	40	0	8
Sour Cream	120	12	2
Tortilla: Corn	80	1	17
El Machino	165	4	27

Corner Bakery Cafe®

For Complete Nutritional Data ~ see CalorieKing.com

Chick-fil-A®

Chick-fil-A Sandwiches	C	F	Cb
Chicken Sandwich	410	16	38
Chargrilled Chicken Sandwich	270	3.5	33
Chicken Salad Sandwich	350	15	32
Cool Wraps: Chicken Caesar	460	10	52
Chargrilled/Spicy Chicken, avg.	395	7	54
Breakfast: Plain Biscuit, 2.8 oz	260	11	38
Biscuit and Gravy	330	15	43
Biscuit: w. Bacon, Egg & Cheese	470	26	39
w. Sausage	490	32	38
Hash Browns, 3 oz	260	17	25
Chick-n-Minis, 3 count	270	11	28
Chicken Biscuit	420	19	44
Platter: Chicken	630	32	51
Bacon	550	30	44
Breakfast Burrito: Chicken	410	16	42
Sausage	450	23	39
Chicken, Egg & Cheese Bagel	500	20	49
Salads: Chick-n-Strips® Salad	390	18	22
Chargrilled Chicken Garden	180	6	9
Southwest Chargrilled Chicken	240	8	17
Salad Dressing: Per Packet (1.25 oz)			
Caesar Dressing	160	17	1
Raspberry Vinaigrette	80	2	15
Bleu Cheese; Buttermilk, avg.	150	16	1
Fat Free Honey Mustard	60	0	14
Light Italian Dressing	15	0.5	2
Spicy Dressing	140	14	2
Thousand Island	150	14	5
Strips, Nuggets: Nuggets (8-pack)	260	12	12
Chick-n-Strips® (4-count)	290	13	14
Dipping Sauces: Polynesian, 1 oz	110	6	13
Barbecue; Honey Mustard, avg.,1 oz	45	0	10
Buffalo Sce, ¾ oz	15	1.5	1
Sides: Carrot & Raisin Salad, small	170	6	28
Fresh Fruit Cups, medium	70	0	17
Coleslaw, small	260	21	17
Garlic and Butter Croutons, ½ oz	70	2.5	9
Side Salad, 3.8 oz	60	3	4
Tortilla Strips, 1 pkt, ½ oz	70	3.5	9
Waffle Potato Fries, 4 oz	350	17	46
Desserts: Cheesecake, 3.3 oz slice	340	21	30
Icedream® Cup, small	240	6	41
Icedream® Cone, small	160	4	28
Lemon Pie, 4 oz slice	390	13	63
Fudge Nut Brownie (1), 2.6 oz	330	15	45

Chili's®

Starters: Per Serving	C	F	Cb
Awesome Blossom w. Sauce	2710	203	194
¼ Whole w. Blossom Sauce	680	51	48
Boneless Buffalo Wings + Sauce	1250	89	55
Boneless Shanghai Wings	1260	71	97
Bottomless Tostada Chips w. Sce	480	36	26
Fried Cheese w. Marinara Sauce	1210	89	62
Skillet Queso w. Tortilla Chips	1070	89	30
South Western Egg Rolls	810	51	59
Wings over Buffalo	1140	100	4
Guiltless Grill: Chicken Platter	580	9	85
Chicken Sandwich	490	8	63
Grilled Chicken Pita	550	9	70
Tomato Basil Pasta	650	14	107
Burgers (No Fries): BBQ Ranch	1110	71	60
Bunless Burgers	360	25	0
Chipotle Bleu Chse Bacon Burger	1090	71	57
Ground Peppercorn	1050	68	61
Meals: Chili's Sirloin, no sides	530	41	1
Cajun Chicken Pasta	1460	75	118
Cajun Chicken Sandwich, no Fries	820	43	66
Cheese Steak Sandwich, no Fries	1010	70	82
Chicken Caesar Pita, no Fries	650	41	31
Citrus Fire Chicken & Shrimp Fajita	720	42	34
Classic Nachos	1570	115	66
Country Fried Steak	1890	107	148
Flame Grilled Rib Eye, no Fries	960	87	1
Grilled Baby Back Ribs	1370	82	112
Grilled Salmon w. Garlic & Herbs	480	4	31
Grilled Shrimp Alfredo Pasta	1340	72	102
Margarita Grilled Chicken	690	14	85
Fajitas: Includes 3 Tortillas & Garnishes			
Mushroom Jack	1360	74	98
Chicken	940	30	90
Steak	1400	78	87
Salads: No Dressing Unless Indicated			
Chicken Caesar Salad w. Dressing	1010	76	39
Dinner Caesar Salad w. Dressing	430	34	20
Dinner House Salad	140	7	12
Quesadilla Explosion	850	45	60
Desserts: Choc Chip Paradise Pie	1600	78	215
Molten Choc Cake	1270	62	172

For Complete Nutritional Data ~ see CalorieKing.com

Chipotle®

	C	F	Cb
Bol Salad: Per Bowl (no Rice or Tortilla)			
Burrito w. Beans: Meat & Chse	475	22	24
Meat & Corn Salsa	475	14	45
Meat & Sour Cream or Cheese	470	23	25
Meat & Tomato Salsa	395	13	29
Fajita w. Vege: Meat & Corn Salsa	435	21	28
Meat & Sour Cream or Cheese	435	30	8.5
Meat & Tomato Salsa	355	20	12
Vegetarian: w. Guacamole			
w. Beans/Corn Salsa	420	17	52
w. Beans, Tomato Salsa	340	16	36
Burrito Bol: with Rice & Beans			
Meat & Cheese	710	29	63
Meat & Corn Salsa	710	21	85
Meat & Sour Cream or Cheese	705	30	65
Meat & Tomato Salsa	630	20	69
Vegetarian w. Guacamole:			
Rice & Beans	545	23	70
Tomato Salsa	575	23	76
Corn Salsa	655	24	92
Fajita Burrito Bol: with Rice & Beans			
Meat & Corn Salsa	1040	30	139
Meat & Sour Cream	1040	39	119
Meat & Tomato Salsa	960	29	123
Vegetables: Meat & Cheese	675	36	46
Meat & Corn Salsa	670	28	68
Meat & Sour Cream or Cheese	670	37	48
Vegetables & Meat: & Tom. Salsa	590	27	52
& Cheese or Sour Cream	1005	45	100
& Corn Salsa	1005	37	122
& Tomato Salsa	925	36	106
Taco w. 4 Crispy Shells: Per Serving			
Meat, Corn Salsa: & Cheese	705	31	57
& Sour Cream	675	32	58
Meat, Tomato Salsa: & Cheese	600	30	41
& Sour Cream	595	31	42
Vegetarian Burrito: w. Rice, Beans & Guacamole			
Black Beans	880	32	124
Corn Salsa	990	33	146
Sour Cream	985	42	126
Tomato Salsa	910	32	130

CinnaMonster®

	C	F	Cb
Cinnamon Roll: Per Roll			
Caramel Pecan	840	32	120
Original	880	24	100

Chuck E. Cheese®

	C	F	Cb
Appetizers: Per Serving			
Buffalo Wings (12)	660	45	3
French Fries (for s'wiches), 5 oz	240	9	37
French Fries ala Carte, 10 oz	480	17	74
Italian Bread Sticks (1)	195	8	27
Sargento Mozzarella Sticks (1)	105	6	7
Pizzas: Per Slice (Medium)			
BBQ Chicken	270	8	43
Cheese	235	7	33
Pepperoni	265	10	33
Vegetarian	235	7	36
Sandwiches: Ham & Chse, no Fries	620	28	70
Grilled Chicken Sub, no Fries	650	31	70
Italian Sub, no Fries	730	40	69
Hot Dog, no Fries	170	17	27
Hot Dog w. Cheese, no Fries	335	30	28
Desserts: Apple Pie Pizza 1 slice	195	2	40
Birthday Cake (8"), 1 slice (¹⁄₁₀)	310	13	45
Cinnamon Sticks, 1 stick	200	5	33

Church's Chicken®

	C	F	Cb
Fried Chicken: Per Piece			
Original: Breast	200	11	3
Leg	110	6	3
Thigh	330	23	8
Wing	300	19	7
Spicy: Breast	320	20	12
Leg	180	11	8
Thigh	480	35	20
Wing	430	27	17
Tender Strips: Original (1)	120	6	6
Spicy, 1 piece	135	7	7
Spicy Chicken Sandwich	360	18	35
Sides: Cajun Rice, regular, 3 oz	130	7	16
Cole Slaw, regular, 4.2 oz	150	10	15
Corn on the Cob, 1 ear	140	3	24
French Fries, regular, 5 oz	420	20	55
Fried Okra, 4 oz	300	23	27
Honey Butter Biscuits (1)	250	16	26
Jalapeno Cheese Bombers, 4 oz	240	10	29
Mashed Pot. & Gravy, reg., 3.6 oz	70	2	12
Apple Pie (Fried), 3 oz	260	11	39
Sauces: Per Pkg			
BBQ; Sweet & Sour	30	0	7
Creamy Jalapeno	100	11	1
Honey Mustard	110	11	4
Purple Pepper	45	0	12
Ranch	130	13	1

Cinnabon®

Sweet Rolls:	C	F	Cb
Cinnabon Bites (6)	510	19	77
Classic Cinnamon Roll (1)	815	32	117
Cinnabon Stix, 5 pieces, 85g	380	21	41
Minibon (1) 92g	340	13	49
Caramel Pecanbon (1)	1100	56	141
CinnaPretzel (1)	755	6	156
Sweet Roll Icing: Frosting Cup, 1.4 oz	180	11	20
Drinks: Mochalatta Chill, 480ml	360	13	55

For Complete Nutritional Data ~ see CalorieKing.com

Cici's Pizza®

Buffet Pizza (12"): *Per Slice (¹⁄₁₀)*

	C	F	Cb
Alfredo; Ham & Pineapple, avg.	140	5	18
Beef	170	6.5	18
Cheese	150	5	20
Pepperoni	175	7	21
Sausage	200	7	19
Zesty Ham & Cheddar	150	6	18

Cosi®

Pasta: Penne Marinara	930	9	180
Penne Pesto w. Chicken	1285	36	178
Penne a la Cosi	1300	37	189
Thai Chicken & Peanut Noodles	1600	28	276
Pizza: Four Cheese, 1 pizza	1280	38	185
Meatlovers, 1 pizza	1610	63	187
Spinach & Fresh Tomato, 1 pizza	1320	43	190
Sandwiches: Buffalo Blue	650	30	57
Cosi Club	680	34	59
Country Ham & Brie	790	39	69
Grilled Chicken TBM	790	43	60
Hummus & Fresh Veggies	430	8	77
Sesame Ginger Chicken	510	11	70
Tandoori Chicken	635	26	58
Tuna & Cheddar	955	55	55
Turkey Light	475	9	73
Melts: Bacon Turkey Cheddar	660	24	74
Grilled Chicken Parmesan	700	27	64
Salads *(No Dressing):* Bombay	175	3	13
Caesar	180	8	20
Chicken Caesar	340	16	21
Cobb	420	28	8
Greek	235	17	9
Mixed Greens	45	1	9
Shanghai Chicken	220	9	16
Signature	375	21	40

Regular Dressings: *Per Serving (2 oz)*

Regular: Cosi Vinaigrette	355	39	2
Other varieties, average	300	30	2

For Complete Nutritional Data ~ see CalorieKing.com

Cousins Subs®

Ciabatta Sandwiches	C	F	Cb
Classic Cubano Pork	590	34	38
Spicy Chicken Sedona	480	23	36
Tuscan Market Club	440	23	33
Salads: Chef Salad, no dressing	280	15	15
Garden Salad, no dressing	195	13	14
Garden Salad w. Chicken, no dr.	335	17	15
Italian Salad, no dressing	360	25	15
Oriental Sesame Chicken, no dr.	265	8	20
Seafood Salad, no dressing	440	35	19
Side Salad, no dressing	105	7	7
Tuna Salad, no dressing	370	28	14
French Fries: Medium	400	19	55
Large	525	24	72
Soups: *Per Regular Serving*			
Cheese	240	16	18
Chicken Dumpling	170	5	19
Chicken w. Rice	230	12	21
Chili	250	9	26
Cream of Broccoli w. Cheese	190	12	15
Cream of Potato	190	9	24
New England Clam Chowder	150	5	19
Subs 7½": *Per Sandwich (With Dressing)*			
BLT	615	42	45
Cappacola & Cheese	635	39	48
Cappacola & Genoa	630	40	48
Cheese Steak	540	24	46
Double Cheese Steak	850	46	46
Chicken Breast	620	34	46
Chicken Breast, Lower Fat	365	6	46
Club	705	40	48
Club Sub, Lower-Fat	705	40	48
Garden Veggie	365	11	49
Genoa & Provolone	730	49	48
Gyro	680	40	55
Hot Veggie	490	23	49
Italian Special	795	53	48
Meatball & Provolone	585	27	50
Pepperoni Melt	785	52	47
Philly Cheese Steak	600	29	49
Pizza Sub	770	49	50
Roast Beef	620	36	46
Seafood w. Crab	555	32	53
Tuna	830	60	46
Turkey Breast	560	32	48

For Complete Nutritional Data ~ see CalorieKing.com

Cold Stone Creamery®

	C	F	Cb
Sweet Cream Ice Cream			
Like It, average all flavors	400	24	40
Love It, average all flavors	660	40	67
Gotta Have It, average all flavors	920	56	93
Cake Batter, Like It	410	23	50
Low-Fat Frozen Yogurt (Choc)			
Like It	230	1.5	48
Love It	380	3	79
Non-Fat Frozen Yogurt: Like It	230	0	48
Love It, average all flavors	380	0.5	80
Gotta Have It, average all flavors	540	1	113
Sinless Sorbet: Like It, avg.	180	0	48
Love It, avg.	300	0	80
Gotta Have It, avg.	420	0	112
Ice Cream Cake: Per Slice (⅛ of 6" Cake)			
Butterfinger Bonanza	450	21	59
Celebration Sensation	350	17	46
Cheesecake Named Desire	420	19	56
Chocolate Chipper	450	26	50
Midnight Delight	510	28	60
Peanut Butter Playground	490	29	54
Strawberry Passion	390	19	50
Zebra Stripes Dark	480	29	53
Waffle Cone or Bowl	160	4	29

Culver's®

	C	F	Cb
Butterburgers: Cheese, Double	580	32	37
Bacon Deluxe	765	51	34
Deluxe Single	505	32	34
Deluxe, Double	685	44	34
Low-Carb	445	32	1
Favorite Sandwiches: Chkn Filet	620	28	68
Beef Pot Roast	305	10	33
Chicken Salad Sourdough	555	29	37
Grilled Chicken Breast	375	8	47
Grilled Ham & Swiss	520	26	35
Philly Ribeye Steak	515	21	46
Pork Tenderloin	705	29	87
Turkey Stacked	465	20	47
Turkey Sourdough BLT	565	31	39
Garden Fresh Salads: Chkn Caesar	400	19	14
Chicken Cashew	485	27	25
Garden Fresco Salad	250	12	29
Taco Salad	780	51	59
Side Salad	90	5	7
Fish & Chicken			
Breaded Shrimp Dinner, 8 pieces	1215	61	140
Chicken Dinner, 2 pieces	1740	94	137
Fish n' Chips Dinner, 6 pieces	1210	68	100
North Atlantic Cod, 2 pieces	1520	88	130

Culver's® cont...

	C	F	Cb
Sides			
Chili Cheddar Fries, 9.3 oz	705	41	73
French Fries, regular, 5 oz	420	22	53
Mashed Potatoes & Gravy, small	150	3	27
Onion Rings, breaded, 6.7 oz	580	30	73
Desserts: Lemon Ice, 7 oz	140	0	35
Lemon Ice Smoothie, 11 oz	405	16	61
Root Beer Float, 15 oz	470	18	70
Cookie Custard Sandwich	765	38	94
Custard Dishes: 1 Scoop	310	18	30
2 Scoops	590	35	58
3 Scoops	745	44	73
Custard Cake: Turtle, 3½ oz	270	16	30
Cookies & Cream, 3½ oz	245	14	26

For Complete Nutritional Data ~ see CalorieKing.com

D'Angelo's®

	C	F	Cb
Sandwiches			
Cheeseburger: Pokket	480	25	37
Sub	525	26	44
Wrap	570	25	52
Chicken Stir Fry: D'Lite Pokket	425	6	57
Sub	450	11	53
Wrap	490	10	61
Classic Veggie: D'Lite Pokket	360	7	63
Wrap	395	13	52
Grilled Chkn Breast D'Lite Pokket	390	7	52
Italian Sub	550	27	54
Number 9 Steak Sandwich: Pokket	435	18	36
Roast Beef: D'Lite Pokket	355	5	51
Sub	320	5	48
Turkey: D'Lite Pokket	365	4	51
Sub	315	4	45
Salads: No Dressing Unless Indicated			
Caesar Salad w. Dressing	480	39	25
Chicken Stir Fry	170	3	11
Greek Salad	300	23	17
Roast Beef	145	3	10
Lobster	385	27	10
Tossed Salad	50	1	11
Turkey	155	2	10

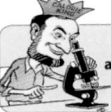

For Extra Menu Items
and Complete Nutritional Data
~ See Author's Website
www.CalorieKing.com

Dairy Queen®

Burgers/Sandwiches	C	F	Cb
GrillBurger: ½ lb Burger, no cheese	800	50	41
Classic, no cheese	540	30	41
Bacon Cheeseburger	710	45	40
Crispy Chicken Sandwich	590	34	50
DQ Homestyle: Hamburger	290	12	29
Bacon Double Cheeseburger	610	36	31
Cheeseburger	340	17	29
Double Cheeseburger	540	31	30
Ultimate Burger	670	43	29
Grilled Chicken Sandwich	340	16	26
Hot Dog, regular	240	14	19
Chili 'n' Cheese Dog, regular	330	21	22
Entrees/Sides: Chicken Strips (4)	400	24	21
Onion Rings, small, 4 oz	470	30	45
French Fries, small, 4 oz	300	12	45
Chicken Quesadilla, no dressing	550	31	35
Salads: No Dressing			
Crispy Chicken Salad	350	20	21
Grilled Chicken Salad	240	10	12
Ice Cream Cones/Soft Serve			
DQ Vanilla Soft Serve, ½ cup	140	4.5	22
DQ Choc. Soft Serve, ½ cup	150	5	22
Chocolate Cone, medium	335	11	51
Dipped Cone, medium	480	24	59
Vanilla Cone, medium	320	10	53
Novelties: Buster Bar	500	28	45
Chocolate Dilly Bar	220	13	25
DQ Fudge Bar, No Sugar Added	50	0	13
DQ Sandwich	200	6	31
DQ Vanilla Orange Bar, NAS	60	0	17
Lemon DQ Freez'r; Starkiss, avg.	80	0	20
Blizzards® & Sundaes			
Banana Split	590	18	94
Choc. Chip Cookie Dough, med.	1005	39	147
Oreo Cookie, medium	675	25	98
Chocolate Sundae, medium	400	10	70
DQ Treatzza Cake ⅛ cake	370	13	56
DQ Treatzza Pizza ⅛ pizza	180	7	28
Reese's Peanut Butter Cup	755	27	109
Strawberry CheeseQuake	705	28	101
Drinks: Chocolate Shake, medium	760	20	129
Malts, medium	870	22	153
Misty Slushes, medium	290	0	74
MooLatte: Cappuccino	490	18	68
Mocha	590	23	80

For Complete Nutritional Data ~ see CalorieKing.com

Daphne's®

Meals: Per Plate	C	F	Cb
Chicken: Combo	530	37	9
Kabob Plate	350	10	5.5
White Meat	370	16	6
Hummus & Pita	230	12	45
Kabob Lunch w. Chicken	210	9	2
Sandwich: Gyros Pita	650	46	38
w. Chicken Breast	565	22	34
Salads			
Greek Chicken	415	18	9
Spicy Greek Chicken w. 1 oz Fire Feta	510	24	12
Soups: Avgolemono, 1 cup	100	8	7
Extras			
Fire Feta, 2 Tbsp	100	7	2
Gyros, 4 oz	380	33	6
Pita Bread, whole	190	4	33
Rice Pilaf, 6 oz	275	7.5	47
Salad Dressing, 2 Tbsp	150	16	0
Tzatziki Sauce, 1.5 oz	60	6	3

Davanni's®

Hoagies: Per Half Hoagie (6") w. Mayonnaise			
Assorted	405	31	21
Cheese	400	29	21
Chicken Breast	495	33	23
Chicken Parmigiana	385	19	22
Club	400	27	22
Italian Sausage	520	37	28
Meatball	465	31	31
Mediterranean	510	38	22
Pastrami	460	27	22
Pizza	315	18	23
Roast Beef	385	25	21
Salami	485	38	21
Tuna	565	44	24
Turkey	370	24	22
Vegie	445	29	29
Without Cheese ~ Deduct	40	3	0
Without Mayo ~ Deduct	100	11	1
Calzones, average all varieties	700	35	65
Pizzas			
Pepperoni & Vegie Works:			
Thin, 1 slice	245	12	18
Traditional, 1 slice	295	12	28
Solo	775	35	70
The Works: Thin, 1 slice	250	13	18
Traditional, 1 slice	300	14	28
Solo	735	32	70
Vegie Works: Thin, 1 slice	210	9	18
Traditional, 1 slice	260	9	28
Solo	635	22	70

Deep Dish ~ Similar to Traditional slice

Del Taco®

Breakfast	C	F	Cb
Breakfast Burrito	250	11	24
Bacon & Egg Quesadilla	450	23	40
Egg & Cheese Burrito	450	24	39
Macho Bacon & Egg Burrito	1030	60	82
Steak & Egg Burrito	580	34	41
Hash Brown Sticks (5)	250	19	20
Tacos: Big Fat Chicken Taco	340	13	38
Big Fat Steak Taco	390	19	38
Big Fat Taco	320	11	39
Chicken Del Carbon	170	5	19
Steak Taco Del Carbon	220	11	19
Taco; Soft Taco, average	160	10	13
Burritos: Combo Burrito	530	22	61
Bean & Cheese Red/Green Burrito	270	8	38
Chicken Works Burrito	520	23	57
Del Beef Burrito	550	30	42
Del Classic Chicken Burrito	560	36	41
Deluxe Combo Burrito	570	25	64
Deluxe Del Beef Burrito	590	33	45
Half Pound Red/Green Burrito, avg.	430	12	63
Macho Beef Burrito	1170	62	89
Macho Combo Burrito	1050	44	113
Spicy Chicken/Veggie Works, avg.	480	17	68
Steak Works Burrito	590	31	58
Quesadillas: Cheddar	500	27	39
Chicken Cheddar	580	31	41
Spicy Jack Chicken	570	30	40
Spicy Jack	490	26	38
Salads: Deluxe Chicken Salad	740	34	77
Deluxe Taco Salad	780	40	76
Taco Salad	350	30	10
Burgers: Cheeseburger	330	13	37
Double Del Cheeseburger	560	35	35
Del Cheeseburger	430	25	35
Nachos: Regular, 4 oz	380	24	40
Macho Nachos, 16 oz	1100	63	113
Sides: Rice Cup, 4 oz	140	2	27
Beans 'n Cheese Cup, 7.8 oz	260	3	44
Fries: Chili Cheese, 10.5 oz	670	46	51
Deluxe Chili Cheese, 12 oz	710	49	53
Medium, 7 oz	490	32	47
Macho, 10 oz	690	46	68
Shakes: Chocolate, 15 fl.oz	680	16	117
Vanilla; Strawbrttu. 15 fl.oz	545	9	97

Denny's®

Breakfast	C	F	Cb
All American Slam, no toast	970	76	21
Country Sausage Bowl, no syrup	1680	108	127
French Slam, no syrup/marg.	1180	75	74
Grand Slam Slugger, no bread	1050	55	96
Heartland Scramble, no syrup	1210	61	118
Lumberjack Slam, no bread/syrup	1170	57	109
Meat Lovers Bowl, no syrup	1540	94	121
Moons Over My Hammy, no pot.	840	51	42
Original Grand Slam	770	44	56
w. Syrup & Margarine	1000	54	92
Two Egg Breakfast w. hash browns	680	55	20
Ultimate Omelette, no brd/pot.	600	49	7
Pancakes Platter (3), no syrup/marg.	420	5	82
Fruit Filled Pancakes, average	1075	55	105
Extra Breakfast Items ~ See CalorieKing.com			
Soup: Chicken Noodle, 8 oz	110	6	16
Vegetable Beef, 8 oz	80	1	11
Sandwiches (No Fries/Sauces)			
BBQ Chicken	1090	62	86
Bacon, Lettuce, Tomato	610	38	50
Boca Burger	450	11	64
Chicken Ranch Melt	840	47	57
Classic Burger, no cheese	695	35	56
Club Sandwich	600	38	45
Fish Sandwich	590	30	30
Grilled Chicken, no dressing	475	14	56
Italian Chicken Melt	1135	62	68
Mushroom Swiss Burger	880	49	63
Philly Melt	875	50	58
The Super Bird Sandwich	480	29	32
Appetizers/Entrees: No Sides/Condiments			
Buffalo Wings (9)	975	72	11
Buffalo Chicken Strips (5)	735	42	43
Chicken Strips (5)	720	33	56
Country Fried Steak	645	46	30
Fish & Chips	960	54	83
Fried Shrimp Dinner	260	11	19
Grilled Chicken Dinner	200	5	15
Grilled Tilapia Dinner	470	18	33
Hickory Grilled Chicken	765	48	18
Mini Burgers (6) w. Onion Rings	2045	122	179
Mozzarella Sticks (8)	710	41	49
Roast Turkey & Stuffing w. Gravy	435	10	62
Sampler, no condiments	1405	80	124
Smothered Cheese Fries	765	48	69
Steakhouse Strip Dinner	410	27	3
Steakhouse Strip & Shrimp	520	33	7
T-Bone Steak Dinner	860	65	0

Restaurants & Fast - Foods

Denny's® cont...

Sides	C	F	Cb
Garlic Bread, 2 pces	170	11	5
Corn, 4 oz	100	2	23
Onion Rings, 4 oz	380	23	38
Fries: Unsalted, 5 oz	425	20	57
Seasoned, 4 oz	260	12	35
Gravy, all types, average	15	0.5	2
Green Beans, 4 oz	40	1	8
Potato: Baked, plain with skin	220	0	51
Mashed, 5 oz	170	7	23

Salads (No Dressing/Bread Unless Indicated)	C	F	Cb
Fried Chicken Strips Salad	440	26	26
Grilled Chkn Caesar w. Dressing	600	41	20
Grilled Chicken Breast Salad	260	11	10
Side Caesar with Dressing	360	26	20
Side Garden Salad, no Dressing	115	7	6
Taco Salad	505	22	57

Dressings & Sauces	C	F	Cb
BBQ Sauce, 1.5 oz	50	1	11
Blue Cheese, 1 oz	165	18	1
Caesar; Ranch, avg., 1 oz	135	14	1
French, regular, 1 oz	105	10	3
Honey Mustard, 1 oz	160	15	20
Italian Dressing, Fat-Free; Salsa	15	0.5	3
Sour Cream, 1.5 oz	90	9	2
Thousand Island, 1 oz	120	11	5

Desserts: Carrot Cake, 8 oz	800	45	99
Hershey's Chocolate Cake	630	33	79
Hot Fudge Brownie, Kids	345	16	49
Pies (⅛ Whole): Apple, 7 oz	470	21	68
Cheesecake, no topping, 4 oz	580	38	51
Chocolate Peanut Butter, 6 oz	655	39	64
French Silk Pie	740	56	58
Sundaes: Banana Split	895	43	121
Single Scoop, no topping	190	14	14
Double Scoop, no topping	380	27	29
Dessert Toppings: Choc., 2 oz	135	0.5	34
Blueberry, 3 oz	70	0	17
Fudge, 2 oz	200	10	30
Strawberry, 3 oz	80	1	17

Drinks: Cappuccino, 8 fl.oz	100	3	28
Floats, Rootbeer/Cola, 12 fl.oz	280	10	47
Milkshake, Van/Choc., 12 fl.oz	560	26	76
Oreo Blender Blaster, 15 oz	895	46	112
Ruby Red Grapefruit Juice, 10 oz	160	0	41
Raspberry Iced Tea, 16 fl.oz	80	0	21

For Complete Nutritional Data ~ see CalorieKing.com

Dippin' Dots®

Flavored Ices	C	F	Cb
All flavors, ½ cup, 3 oz	90	0	23
Frozen Yogurt: All flavors, ½ cup	100	0	21
Ice Cream: Per Serving (½ Cup)			
Average all flavors	180	9	20
Fat-Free, Fudge, No Sugar Added	90	1	18
Low-Fat, Vanilla, No Sugar Added	125	6	13
Sherbet, ½ Cup	100	1	21

Donato's® Pizza

14" Traditional Pizza: Per Slice (⅛ Large)	C	F	Cb
Chicken Vegy Medley	310	10	37
Founders Fav.; The Works, avg.	460	20	40
Hawaiian; Serious Cheese, avg.	390	16	40
Mariachi Beef/Mariachi Chkn, avg.	405	18	41
Serious Meat	460	23	40
Vegy	365	14	42
Vegy (without Cheese)	250	5	40
Salads: Tuscan Chicken, no dress.	200	8	6
Tuscan Caesar, no dressing	90	6	3

Subs	C	F	Cb
Big Steak Hoagy w. Sauce	800	39	68
Grilled Chicken Club	900	44	71
Meatball	1135	64	78
Roasted Vegy	730	37	74
Steak & Cheese	780	34	69
Big Don: Italian	720	34	67
w. Pizza Sauce	655	26	69
Sausage Italian	1000	56	68

Individual No Dough Pizza: Per Whole Pizza	C	F	Cb
Chicken Vegy Medley	495	29	20
Classic Trio	530	37	18
Founder's Favorite	560	38	18
Hawaiian	435	26	22
Mariachi Beef	530	34	23
Mariachi Chicken	495	30	21
Pepperoni	500	35	17
Philly Cheese Steak	520	33	19
Serious Cheese	455	31	17
Serious Meat	655	46	19
Spinach	455	29	21
Vegy	420	25	23
White	390	26	15
Works	545	37	21

For Complete Nutritional Data ~ see CalorieKing.com

Domino's® Pizza

Feast Pizza Classic Hand-Tossed

14" Large: *Per Slice (⅛ Pizza)*	C	F	Cb
American Favorite	390	18	44
Bacon Cheeseburger	420	19	42
Barbecue Feast	390	15	49
Deluxe Feast	350	14	45
ExtravaganZZa	420	20	45
Hawaiian Feast	350	12	45
MeatZZa Feast	430	21	44
Pepperoni Feast	400	19	43
Philly Cheese Steak	350	13	40
Vegi Feast	340	12	44

Feast Pizza Crunchy Thin Crust

14" Large: *Per Slice (⅛ Pizza)*			
American Favorite	280	19	22
Bacon Cheeseburger	310	20	20
Barbecue Feast	280	16	27
Deluxe Feast	240	15	21
ExtravaganZZa	310	21	23
Hawaiian Feast	240	13	23
MeatZZa Feast	320	22	22
Pepperoni Feast	290	20	21
Philly Cheese Steak	240	14	18
Vegi Feast	230	13	22

Feast Pizza Ultimate Deep Dish

14" Large: *Per Slice (⅛ Pizza)*			
American Favorite	400	21	42
Bacon Cheeseburger	430	22	40
Barbecue Feast	400	18	47
Deluxe Feast	360	17	41
ExtravaganZZa	430	23	43
Hawaiian Feast	360	15	43
MeatZZa Feast	440	24	42
Pepperoni Feast	410	22	41
Philly Cheese Steak	360	16	38
Vegi Feast	350	15	42

Classic Hand-Tossed

14" Large: *Per Slice (⅛ Pizza)*			
Cheese only	290	9	42
Pepperoni	340	14	42
Ham	305	9.5	42
Sausage	350	15	44
Beef	340	15	42
Ham & Pineapple	320	9.5	45
Pepperoni & Sausage	400	19	44

Domino's® Pizza cont...

Crunchy Thin Crust

14" Large: *Per Slice (⅛ Pizza)*	C	F	Cb
Cheese only	180	9.5	20
Pepperoni	230	14	20
Ham	195	10	20
Sausage	240	15	22
Beef	230	14	20
Ham & Pineapple	210	10	23
Pepperoni & Sausage	290	20	22

Ultimate Deep Dish

14" Large: *Per Slice (⅛ Pizza)*			
Cheese only	320	14	40
Pepperoni	370	19	40
Ham	335	15	40
Sausage	380	20	42
Beef	370	19	40
Ham & Pineapple	350	15	43
Pepperoni & Sausage	430	24	42

Salads: *Per Serving*

Garden Fresh, ½ container	70	4	6
Grilled Chicken Caesar	105	4	6
Salad Dressing: Blue Cheese	230	24	2
Creamy Caesar	210	22	2
Italian	220	23	2
Lite	20	1	2
Ranch	220	24	2

Side Dishes: Breadsticks (1) | 130 | 7 | 14 |

Chicken Kickers (1), 0.8 oz	45	2	3
Buffalo Wings: Barbecue (1)	90	4.5	2
Hot (1)	85	4.5	2
Cheesy Bread (1), 1.3 oz	140	7	14
Cinna Stix (1), 1.2 oz	140	7	17
Sweet Icing	250	3	57
Dipping Sauce: Blue Cheese	230	24	2
Hot	120	12	3
Marinara	25	0	5
Ranch	200	21	2
Garlic Sauce	440	50	0

For Complete Nutritional Data ~ see CalorieKing.com

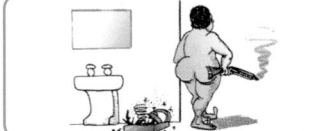

Restaurants & Fast-Foods

Don Pablos®

	C	F	Cb
Appetizers: Per Serving			
Beef Taquito (1), no garnish	65	3	5
Buffalo Chicken Wings (8)	1035	78	43
Chicken Flauta (1), no garnish	65	4	6
Nachos (1 order): Taco Beef	1625	113	85
Beef Fajita	1430	99	71
Chicken Fajita	1395	87	73
Quesadillas: Incl. Sour Cream & Guacamole			
Cheese Quesadilla, 8 slices	1595	99	105
Mesquite Grilled Chicken, 4 slices	665	32	55
Mesquite Grilled Steak, 8 slices	1560	91	122
Portabello Mushr. & Veges, 8 slices	1505	83	136
Primo Club, 8 slices	1745	100	114
Dips: Per 6 oz Cup (No Chips)			
Queso Blanco	340	27	13
Prairie Fire Bean w. Cheese	380	25	23
Spinach	315	28	8
Burritos (No Sides): Chicken	880	48	70
Beef & Bean	1390	73	123
Chimichangas: Includes Rice & Refritos			
Spicy Beef Chimi De Oro	1190	63	109
Chicken Chimi	815	44	71
Rellenos: Beef w. Sauce/Cheese	300	17	20
Cheese w. Sauce/Cheese	395	26	19
Chicken w. Sauce/Cheese	235	11	21
Salads (No Dress.): Steak Fajita	620	35	27
Chicken Fajita	565	30	28
Traditional Taco Salad, Beef	1290	80	94
Salad Dressing: Per 3 oz			
Blue Cheese	450	48	3
House Vinaigrette	355	31	10
Honey Mustard	315	27	17
Low Fat French	150	4	30
Ranch	320	34	3
Sides: Chips & Salsa, 1 order	340	17	43
Guacamole, 1.5 oz	50	5	2
Mexican Rice, 3 oz	105	1	21
Refritos, 5 oz	180	6	23
Salsa, 1 oz	5	0	1
Side Salad	110	7	8
Sour Cream, 1.25 oz	75	7	2
Sour Crema, 1 oz	55	5	1
Flour Tortilla , 7"	125	4	20

Extra Menu Items ~ see CalorieKing.com

Dunkin Donuts®

	C	F	Cb
Donuts			
Apple/Blueberry Crumb Donut	240	10	36
Apple N' Spice Donut	200	8	29
Black Raspberry/Strawberry Donut	210	8	32
Blueberry Cake Donut	290	16	35
Boston Kreme Donut	240	9	36
Chocolate Coconut Cake Donut	300	19	31
Chocolate Frosted Cake Donut	360	20	40
Chocolate Frosted Donut	200	9	29
Chocolate Glazed Cake Donut	290	16	33
Cinnamon Cake Donut	330	20	34
French Cruller	150	8	17
Glazed Cake Donut	350	19	41
Jelly Filled Donut	210	8	32
Kreme Filled (Choc./Vanilla)Donut	270	13	35
Lemon Glazed/Frosted Cake Donut	240	14	28
Maple/Marble Frosted Donut, avg.	210	9	29
Old Fashioned Cake Donut	300	19	28
Powdered Cake Donut	330	19	36
Strawberry Frosted; Bavarian	210	9	30
Sugar Raised Donut	170	8	22
Whole Wheat Glazed Cake Donut	310	19	32
Muffins: Banana Walnut	540	25	69
Blueberry: Regular	470	17	73
Reduced Fat	400	5	78
Chocolate Chip	630	26	89
Coffee Cake Muffin, 6.5 oz	580	19	78
Corn	510	18	77
Cranberry Orange	440	17	66
Honey Raisin Bran	480	15	79
Danishes: Apple	330	20	32
Cheese	340	22	30
Strawberry Cheese	320	20	31
Sandwiches: Per Sandwich			
Biscuit Sandwiches:			
Egg/Cheese Sandwich	410	25	32
Sausage/Egg/Cheese Sandwich	610	43	32
Croissant: Egg & Cheese	480	31	40
Sausage, Egg & Cheese	690	51	40
Eng. Muffin S'wich: Ham/Egg/Chse	310	10	34
Paninis: Meatball	480	19	56
Southwestern Chicken	420	10	57
Meatball	480	19	56

Continued Next Page ...

Dunkin Donuts® cont...

	C	F	Cb
Bagels: Per Bagel			
Reduced Carb w. Cheese	380	12	45
Everything	370	6	67
Onion	320	3.5	61
Sesame	380	8	64
Salt; Plain	320	2.5	62
Cream Cheese (Per Packet): Lite	110	9	6
Average of other flavors	180	17	4
Cake Munchkins: Plain (4)	270	16	27
Cinnamon; Powdered (4)	270	14	29
Glazed (5)	200	9	27
Lemon Filled (4)	170	8	23
Sugar Raised (7)	220	12	26
Cake Sticks: Per Stick			
Cinnamon	450	30	42
Glazed/Chocolate	470	29	50
Jelly	530	29	61
Plain	420	29	35
Powdered	450	29	42
Cookies: Chocolate varieties, avg. (1)	220	11	27
Oatmeal Raisin Pecan	220	10	29
Drinks: Dunkacino, 10 fl.oz	230	10	35
Hot Chocolate, 10 fl.oz	220	8	38
Iced Coffee: 16 fl.oz	15	0	3
w. Cream, 16 fl.oz	70	6	4
w. Milk, 16 fl.oz	35	1	4
Berry Bliss; Choc-Nilla, 16 fl.oz	90	6	8
Turbo Ice, 16 fl.ox	120	7	14
Vanilla Iced Latte Lite, 16 fl.oz	80	0	3
Vanilla Chai, 10 fl.oz	230	8	40
Smoothies, all flavors, 16 fl.oz	360	2.5	79
Coolatta: Per 16 fl.oz			
Coffee Coolatta®: w. Cream	350	22	40
w. Milk	210	4	42
w. 2% Milk	190	2	41
Orange Tropical Fruit Coolatta®	370	0	92
Strawberry Fruit Coolatta®	290	0	72
Vanilla Bean Coolatta®	440	17	70

Eat 'N Park®

	C	F	Cb
Breakfast			
Apple Waffles	960	44	125
Cornbeef Hash, 7.5 oz	340	23	16
Egg Beaters Breakfast	75	0	5.5
Fruit Cup	60	0.5	14
Hash Browns, 6 oz	235	12	28
Homefries, 6 oz	210	12	24
Omelette: Cheese	390	30	2.5
Ham & Cheese	465	33	3
Supreme	420	30	9
Pancake, Plain (1)	225	3	43
Burgers: American Grill	790	50	31
Bacon & Cheddar	1035	69	50
Cheeseburger	540	30	32
Classic Burger	815	50	40
Hamburger	495	26	32
Mushroom & Onion	885	56	44
Superburger	705	49	37
Swiss Burger	580	32	34
Swiss, Mushroom & Onion	880	55	45
Turkey Burger	500	22	37
Sandwiches: Tuna Melt	610	40	35
Bacon Turkey Swiss	525	37	16
Chicken Bacon Deluxe	565	23	50
Chicken (Breaded)	515	20	50
Chicken Chargrill/Spicy, 4 oz	320	6.5	32
Chicken Fiesta, 4 oz	325	11	21
Dutch Ham & Swiss	570	30	35
Grilled Cheese	505	35	26
Hot Roast Beef	310	6.5	32
Hot Turkey	260	5	27
Reuben	720	49	31
Steak'n Cheese	765	50	42
Tuna Melt	610	40	35
Turkey Club	775	46	50
Turkey Pastrami	715	46	40
Croissants, Chicken Salad; Tuna	595	39	36
Pita: Chicken Fajita	620	18	68
Tuna	640	25	72
Turkey	445	5	67
Appetizers: Cheese Fries	880	50	93
Cheese Sticks	410	24	17
Onion Rings	210	13	20
Wings	400	28	0.5

**For Extra Menu Items
+ Full Nutritional Data**
~ See Author's Website
www.CalorieKing.com

Eat 'N Park® cont...

	C	F	Cb
Dinners: Chicken Breast, stuffed	370	16	27
Chicken Fillets (5)	530	26	28
Chicken Naturelle, reg., 6 oz	210	5.5	0
Chicken Parmigiana Marinara	840	33	90
Chicken Stir-Fry	555	24	47
Country Fried Chicken Steak	790	40	43
Floridian Scrod, 4 oz	120	1.5	4
Rib-Eye	615	42	1
Spaghetti Marinara	620	8	120
Veal Parmigiana w. Meat Sauce	820	26	107
Ziti w. Meat Balls & Meat Sauce	960	42	102
Salads & Dressings			
Buffalo Chicken Salad	605	42	42
Chicken Caesar Salad	270	9	15
Chicken Portabella Salad	330	12	22
Garden Salad	100	3	16
Steak Salad	635	39	34
Taco Salad	805	40	70
Dressings: Bleu Cheese, 2 Tbsp	90	7	7
French Fat Free	70	0	17
Italian Fat Free	10	0	3
House, 2 Tbsp	115	11	2.5
Thousand Island , 2 Tbsp	95	9	3
Desserts: Cheesecake, Plain	505	36	40
Banana Fudge Sensation	975	44	147
Grilled Sticky A La Mode	730	38	80
Ice Cream, 2 scoops	285	16	33
Pies: Apple (NAS)	340	10	62
Peach (NAS)	300	10	50
Chocolate Pudding (Sugar Free)	90	2.5	13
Strawberry Shortcake	685	26	114

Edo Japan®

Meals: Per Regular Serving	C	F	Cb
Beef Yakisoba	575	26	54
Chicken & Beef	560	17	68
Chicken Yakisoba	430	6	52
Curry Chicken	395	5	87
Ginger Pork	520	10	71
Grilled Vegetables	325	1	71
Hawaiian Chicken	500	7.5	71
Seafood Grill	495	8	73
Sukiyaki Beef	635	26	68
Teriyaki Chicken	490	7.5	68
Teriyaki Shrimp	465	6	72

Einstein Bros®/Noahs®

	C	F	Cb
Bagels: Average, 4.2 oz	350	1	75
Chocolate Chip Bagel, 4 oz	370	3	76
Egg Bagel	340	3	69
Sesame Dip'd	380	5	75
Cream Cheese Shmear: Plain, 2 T.	70	7	1
Plain Reduced Fat, 2 Tbsp	60	5	2
Smoked Salmon, 2 Tbsp	65	6	2
Flavors, average, 2 Tbsp	70	5	2
Spreads: Fruit, 2 Tbsp	75	0	19
Honey Butter, 1 Tbsp	90	8	4
Peanut Butter, 2 Tbsp	190	15	8
Breakfast Sandwiches			
Lox & Bagel Sandwich	660	27	79
Spicy Elmo Egg Sandwich	650	35	50
Bagel Omelet Sandwiches:			
Black Forest Ham & Swiss	660	21	76
Cheddar	590	20	74
Santa Fe	720	28	78
Smoked Bacon & Cheddar	680	26	75
Turkey Sausage & Cheddar	660	23	74
Grilled Panini Omelet Sandwiches:			
Spinach & Bacon	930	49	72
Steak & Egg Ranchero	690	27	67
Sandwiches			
Grilled Panini: Cheese Steak	690	29	69
Country Cheese	540	20	49
Italian Chicken	690	27	68
Signature: Club Mex on Challah	730	38	60
Einstein Club on Grilled White	670	29	54
Tasty Turkey on Asiago Bagel	600	18	81
Veg Out on Sesame Bagel	500	13	82
Salads: Asiago Chicken Caesar	740	54	25
Bros Bistro	810	69	37
Chicken Chipotle	630	40	38
Soups: Per Bowl (14 oz)			
Broccoli Sharp Cheddar	380	23	43
Crab Chowder	370	25	25
Chicken & Wild Rice	440	9	67
Chicken Noodle	160	7	13
Cookies: Chocolate Chip	520	24	68
Trail Mix	480	19	70
Coffee: Cafe Latte, 12 fl.oz	135	5	13
Cappuccino, 12 fl.oz	90	3.5	9

Fast - Foods & 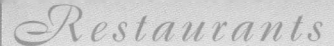Restaurants

El Pollo Loco®

Flame-Grilled Chicken	C	F	Cb
Chicken Breast w. Skin	185	7	0
Leg	85	3	0
Thigh	120	7	0
Wing	85	3	0
Burritos: Chicken Guacamole	535	17	59
Classic: BRC	530	15	79
Chicken Lovers	525	18	55
Classic Chicken	635	19	81
Grilled Signature: Grilled Fiesta	1070	54	91
Twice Grilled	855	41	62
Ultimate Chicken	700	24	84
Bowls: Chicken Caesar Salad	535	29	47
Pollo	545	10	84
Loco Favorites			
Cheese Quesadilla	545	26	51
Chicken Nachos	1300	77	90
Chicken Quesadilla	655	30	53
Chicken Soft Taco	235	11	18
Chicken Taquitos	370	17	43
Taco Al Carbon	135	3	18
Salads: Per Serving (With Dressing)			
Chicken Caesar	535	42	17
Chicken Fiesta	745	57	29
Chicken Tostada	745	37	84
Monterrey Pollo	260	13	17
Tostada Salad no Shell	415	16	42
Tamales (1)	180	8	21
Side Dishes: Per Individual Serving			
Cole Slaw, 5 oz	205	16	12
Corn Cobbette, 3 oz	40	0	10
French Fries, 5.5 oz	445	19	61
Fresh Vegetables, 4 oz	70	4	6
Garden Salad, 4.8 oz	120	11	9
Pinto Beans, 6 oz	155	4	24
Spanish Rice, 4 oz	160	1	33
Tortilla Chips, small, 2 oz	395	21	50
Tortillas: 6" Corn (3) 3 oz	210	3	42
6½" Flour (3), 3 oz	330	12	48
Condiments			
Dressings: Creamy Chipotle	270	28	3
Creamy Cilantro	275	29	3
Guacamole, 1.7 oz	50	3	5
Jalapeno Hot Sauce, 0.3 oz pkg	5	0	0
Sour Cream	105	10	2
Salsa: Avocado	20	1	1
Chipotle; House	5	0	1
Pico de Gallo	10	0	1
Desserts: Churro (1)	180	11	24
Flan, 5.5 oz	305	12	43
Soft Serve, Regular, 5 oz	180	5	30

For Complete Nutritional Data ~ see CalorieKing.com

Fatburger®

	C	F	Cb
Burgers: Baby Fat	295	13	25
Bacon & Egg Sandwich	440	27	31
Chicken Sandwich	400	15	32
Chili Dog	510	26	45
Fatburger	600	34	39
Fatburger w. Cheese	625	36	38
Kingburger	825	46	56
Kingburger w. Cheese	1020	58	65
Turkey Burger	590	33	41
Shakes (21 fl.oz): Vanilla	810	44	85
Chocolate, Strawberry, average	900	42	110
Fries & Sides: Chili Cup, 7.2 oz	345	23	14
Fat Fries, 7.6 oz	540	26	70
Skinny Fries, 5 oz	515	26	65
Onion Rings, 6.1 oz	235	23	56

For Complete Nutritional Data ~ see CalorieKing.com

Fazoli's® Italian Food

Classic Pasta: Per Serving	C	F	Cb
Classic Sampler Platter	810	20	123
Classic Ziti w. Meat Sauce, regular	700	26	76
Classic Ziti w. Meat Sauce, small	450	17	49
Ravioli w. Marinara Sauce	600	15	89
Ravioli w. Meat Sauce	630	17	89
Six Layer Lasagna	630	23	75
Six Layer Lasagna w. Broccoli	690	28	79
Spaghetti w. Marinara Sauce, reg.	670	3.5	132
Ultimate Sampler Platter	1020	27	145
Oven-Baked Pasta: Per Serving			
Baked Chicken Parmesan	1010	35	115
Baked Spaghetti	720	24	88
Baked Spaghetti w. Meatballs	990	42	98
Twice Baked Lasagna	800	36	78
Twice Baked Ziti	830	37	76
Paninis: Four Cheese & Tomato	820	52	51
Grilled Chicken	420	7	51
Smoked Turkey	710	40	51
Pizzas: Per Serving			
Double Slice, Cheese	500	20	57
Double Slice, Pepperoni	560	25	57
Mega Slice, Cheese	750	30	85
Mega Slice, Pepperoni	840	38	85

Fazoli's® cont...

Submarinos (7")

	C	F	Cb
Club	1040	44	117
Ham n' Swiss	980	38	117
Original	1390	78	116

Salads: Dressing Not Included

Garden Side Salad	25	0	4
Caesar Side Salad	110	5	12
Chicken Caesar Salad	200	7	14
Chicken and Pasta Caesar Salad	350	17	27
Grilled Chicken Salad	100	2	6
Italian Market Salad	620	41	32
Pasta Side Salad	230	13	22

Salad Dressing: Italian Dressing

Italian Dressing	160	14	7
Fat Free Honey Mustard	60	0	15
Caesar Dressing	230	25	1
Honey French	220	18	14
Thousand Island	210	20	6
Ranch Dressing	220	24	2
Lite Ranch Dressing	120	12	2

Breadsticks, Soup, Meatballs

Breadstick (1), dry	100	1.5	18
Minestrone Soup, small bowl	90	2	19

Desserts

Chocolate Chunk Cookie	590	28	77
Cheesecake: Plain	290	22	17
Turtle	450	28	43
Freezi's, average all flavors	380	3.5	92

Kids Meals: Lasagna

Lasagna	310	11	37
Fettuccine Alfredo	290	5	50
Cheese Ravioli w. Meat Sauce	300	8	42
Pizza: Cheese	500	20	57
Pepperoni	560	25	57
Spaghetti: w. Meatballs	340	7	53
w. Marinara or Meat Sauce, avg.	270	2	51

For Complete Nutritional Data ~ see CalorieKing.com

Fox's Pizza Den®

12" Pizzas: Per Slice (⅛ Pizza)

	C	F	Cb
Cheese	155	5	21
Pepperoni	180	7	21

16" Pizzas: Per Slice (⅒ pizza)

Cheese	220	7	30
Pepperoni	250	9	30

Firehouse Subs®

Subs: Per Medium

	C	F	Cb
Chicken Salad	765	46	63
Engine Co	385	7	56
Engineer	380	6	60
Ham Sub	425	7	70
Hero Sub	460	9	64
Hook & Ladder	400	6	64
Italian Sub	655	33	64
NY Steamer	470	16	53
Roast Beef	400	9	54
Tuna Salad	615	28	62
Turkey Sub	370	5	58
Veggie Sub	320	6	59

Frisch's Big Boy®

~ Same Menu & Data as Big Boy®
See Page 190 ~

Freshens®

Frozen Yogurt: Per Serving

	C	F	Cb
Soft Serve Yogurt, 1 oz	25	0.5	5

Ice Creams

Hand Dipped Ice Cream, ½ cup	150	12	21

Smoothies: Per Container (21 fl.oz)

All That Razz	360	0	79
Berry Breeze	305	0	77
Blueberry Bay	375	0	81
Caribbean Craze	290	0	73
Fitness Fuel	520	5	81
Jamaican Jammer	355	0	78
Mango Beach	90	0	48
Maui Mango	290	0	74
Mystic Mango	355	3	82
Orange: Shooter	335	3	77
Sunrise	355	3	64
Peach: Passion	150	0	32
Sunset	270	0	67
Peachy Pineapple	325	0	69
Pina Collider	430	4	88
Pineapple Paradise	330	4	77
Raspberry Royale	270	0	67
Strawberry: Oasis	80	0	49
Shooter	245	0	64
Squeeze	315	0	68
Sunrise	155	0	35

Snacks: Per Serving (3 oz)

Pretzel Logic: Gourmet Bites	115	9	4
Gourmet Pretzels, ½ pretzel	255	3	49

Gino's East®

	C	F	Cb
Deep Dish Pizza: Medium 11" ~ Per Slice (⅙ Pizza)			
Cheese	410	11	58
Crumbled Sausage	420	21	38
Pepperoni	445	15	57
Spinach	410	11	59
Deep Dish Pizza: Small 6" ~ Per Whole Pizza			
Cheese	720	16	116
Crumbled Sausage	800	22	116
Pepperoni	780	20	116

Gold Star Chili®

Meals

	C	F	Cb
Bowls: Low Carb Coney, 10.4 oz	570	47	7
Veggie Chili, 9 oz	160	2	29
Coney	285	14	30
Cheese Coney, 5.6 oz	345	18	18
Chili, 8 oz	215	12	8
Chili Cheese Nachos, 8½ oz	410	25	30
Chili Cheese Sandwich	285	12	30
Chili Sandwich	210	5	32
Regular 2-Way	420	11	58
Bean	490	12	71
Onion	435	11	62
Onion Bean	505	12	75
Regular 3-Way	650	30	59
Regular 4-Way	665	30	63
Regular 5-Way	735	30	76
Super 5-Way	1140	51	109
Tex Mex	210	9	17
Sides: Fries, 5 oz	365	19	44
Garlic Bread: Without Cheese, 2 oz	215	13	19
w. Cheese, 2½ oz	270	18	19
Side Salad	70	5	2

Golden Corral®

Meals

	C	F	Cb
Bourbon Street Chicken, 3.5 oz	210	11	5
Fish Fillet Cajun Style, 2 pces	210	10	18
Fresh Fried Chkn, Leg or Thigh (1)	250	19	2
Meatloaf, 3.5 oz	190	10	10
Sirloin Steak, Buffet, 3 oz	220	13	0
Steakburgers, Lunch, 6 oz	860	55	0
Turkey Breast w. Wing, 2 oz	70	3	1
Whitefish Cajun, 3 oz	110	7	0
Sides: Baked Potato, plain (1)	110	0	25
Carrot & Raisin Salad, ½ cup	115	5	17
Macaroni Salad, ½ cup	190	8	26

Godfather's™ Pizza

	C	F	Cb
Golden Pizza: Per Slice			
Cheese: Medium, ⅛ pizza	220	8	26
Large, ¹⁄₁₀ pizza	250	9	28
Combo: Medium, ⅛ pizza	275	13	27
Large, slice, ¹⁄₁₀ pizza	330	15	30
Original Pizza			
Cheese: Mini, ¼ pizza	150	4	20
Medium, ⅛ pizza	260	7	34
Jumbo, ¹⁄₁₀ pizza	430	13	53
Combo: Mini, ¼ pizza	210	8	22
Medium, ⅛ pizza	350	14	37
Jumbo, ¹⁄₁₀ pizza	580	24	57
Thin Pizza			
Cheese: Medium, ⅛ pizza	180	8	16
Large, ¹⁄₁₀ pizza	220	10	19
Combo: Medium, ⅛ pizza	250	13	18
Large, ¹⁄₁₀ pizza	290	16	21
Sides			
Breadstick (1)	80	2	14
Cheesestick, 1 piece, ⅙ whole	130	1	18
Choc. Chip Cookie, slice , ⅙ whole	200	8	30
Potato Wedges, 4 oz	190	9	24

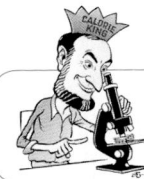

For full nutritional data and product updates
check the food database of the author's
website www.CalorieKing.com

(The) Great American Bagel Co®

	C	F	Cb
Bagels: Plain	390	1.5	85
4-Grain Honey; Cinn. Raisin	420	1.5	88
Apple/Blueberry Crumb, average	570	8	106
Banana Nut; Cheddar Herb, avg.	410	5	82
Blueberry; Onion; Strawberry	380	1	83
Cheddar Salsa	430	11	63
Cheese Twist	740	20	107
Chocolate Chip	390	4	75
Cinnamon Sugar; Egg	390	2	83
Cranb. Nut; P'nut Butter Choc Chip	400	6	72
Jalapeno Cheddar	330	4.5	58
Pumpernickel; Pumpkin, average	330	1.5	72
Pumpkin Chocolate Chip	350	3.5	67
Spinach Herb	300	1	60
Stuffed Pepperoni	500	12	74
Stuffed Spinach	720	22	98
Sun-Dried Tomato Basil	390	1.5	71
Other varieties, average	370	2	75

Green Burrito

	C	F	Cb
Burritos: Bean & Cheese	760	36	87
Grilled Chicken	1030	52	91
Meat Bean & Cheese: Chicken	660	28	67
Ground Beef	820	43	71
Steak	700	31	68
The Green Burrito w. Steak	920	34	117
Sides: Chips, 2 oz	300	15	75
Chips & Cheese, 5 oz	690	40	133
Guacamole, 1.4 oz	50	3	6
Green Sauce w. Jack & Cheese	400	27	43
Make Any Entree a Plate			
Beans Rice & Tortilla Chips	440	17	85
Pinto Beans & Cheese	330	16	43
Rice, 5 oz	220	3.5	43
Sour Cream, 1.4 oz	50	3.5	3
Specialties: Enchiladas w. Cheese	420	26	31
Super Nachos: Chicken; Steak	1020	56	165
Ground Beef	1170	70	167
Taco Salad: Chicken	790	45	68
Ground Beef	950	59	71
Steak	830	47	68
Taquitos: Chicken, 2 taquitos	160	8	18
Chicken, 5 taquitos	370	17	42
Tacos: Fish, 6 oz	290	14	34
Hard: Chicken; Steak	200	11	14
Ground Beef	300	19	16
Soft: Chicken	200	8	19
Ground Beef	270	14	20

(The) Great Steak & Potato Company®

	C	F	Cb
Sandwiches			
Cheeseburger, Kids	350	19	20
Chicken Philly	715	34	64
Chicken Teriyaki	760	34	74
Ham Delight	675	31	64
Ham Explosion	530	15	63
Phillyburger	615	41	23
Super Steak	710	34	60
Turkey Philly	640	28	60
Veggie Delight	700	38	62
Sides: Per Serving			
Bacon, 2 slices	85	4	1
Chicken Nuggets, Kids, 2.8 oz	185	10	11
Fries: Kids, 11.5 oz	850	44	128
Small, 13.9 oz	1065	55	142
Regular, 15.6 oz	1195	62	159
Large, 27.5 oz	2105	109	281
Potato Skins, 7 oz	755	57	54
Potato, Plain, 10.5 oz	215	0	45
Meat: Per Serving (Sides Not Included)			
Chicken, 5 oz	125	1	1
Gyro, 4 oz	280	29	14
Ham, 4 oz	165	6	2
Salami, 2 oz	145	11	1
Steak, 4 oz	140	6	0
Turkey, 4 oz	155	1	0
Salad: Chef Salad	300	12	9
Tossed Salad	40	0	8
Side Salad	20	0	4
Vegetables: Broccoli, 3 oz	25	0	4
Other vegetables, avg., 1 serving	10	0	2
Salad Dressings: Per Serving			
Low-Cal Mayo, ½ oz	40	4	1
Mayonnaise, ½ oz	100	11	0
Sauces: Cheese, 2 oz	80	5	0
Teriyaki Glaze, 1.2 oz	45	0	10
Tzatziki, 1 oz	90	9	1
Bun: Regular Bun, 3.5 oz	290	3	55
Large Bun, 5 oz	380	4	72
Pita, 3 oz	165	1	33
Drinks: Medium, 16 fl.oz			
Lemonade	210	0	56
Mountain Dew	240	0	59
Pepsi; Sierra Mist	210	0	54

Haagen-Dazs®

Ice Cream: Per ½ Cup	C	F	Cb
Almond Hazelnut Swirl	320	22	26
Baileys Irish Cream	270	17	23
Banana Split	280	16	31
Bananas Foster	260	15	28
Black Walnut	300	22	21
Butter Pecan	310	23	21
Caramel Cone	320	19	32
Cherry Vanilla	240	15	23
Chocolate	270	18	22
Chocolate Chip Cookie Dough	310	20	29
Chocolate Chocolate Chip	300	20	26
Chocolate Peanut Butter	360	24	27
Coffee	270	18	21
Cookies & Cream	270	17	23
Creme Brulee	280	19	23
Dulce De Leche	290	17	28
Eggnog	300	18	30
Macadamia Brittle	300	20	25
Mango	250	14	28
Mint Chip	300	19	26
Mocha Almond Fudge	340	23	28
Peaches & Cream	240	12	29
Pineapple Coconut	230	13	25
Pistachio	290	20	22
Rocky Road	300	18	29
Rum Raisin	270	17	22
Strawberry	250	16	23
Strawberry Cheesecake	270	16	28
Strawberry Shortcake	260	14	29
Triple Chocolate	330	21	31
Vanilla	270	18	21
Vanilla Bean	290	18	26
Vanilla Chocolate Chip	310	20	26
Vanilla Fudge	290	18	26
Vanilla Fudge Brownie	300	19	28
Vanilla Swiss Almond	300	20	24
White Chocolate Raspberry Truffle	310	18	32
Light Ice Cream: Dutch Chocolate	190	5	33
S'mores	240	6	42
Other varieties, average	220	7	33
Sorbet: Tropical	150	0	38
Other varieties, average	120	0	33
Frozen Yogurt: Per ½ Cup			
Choc. Fudge Brownie	200	2.5	35
Coffee; Vanilla; avg.	200	4.5	31
Dulce De Leche	190	2.5	35
Strawberry Fat Free	140	0	31
Strawberry Banana	160	2	32
Vanilla Raspberry Swirl	170	2.5	32
Ice Cream Bars: See Page 37			

Hardee's®

Sandwiches	C	F	Cb
Big Chicken Filet Sandwich	850	42	76
Hot Ham N Cheese	420	18	39
Big Hot Ham N Cheese	520	24	40
Regular Roast Beef Sandwich	330	16	29
Big Roast Beef Sandwich	470	23	38
Charbroiled BBQ Chicken S'wich	415	5	58
Charbroiled Chicken Club	560	30	33
Cheeseburger ⅓ lb	680	39	52
Double Cheeseburger ¼lb	510	26	38
Hamburger	310	12	36
Double Hamburger ¼lb	420	19	37
Fish Supreme Sandwich	500	27	38
Hot Dog	420	30	22
Six Dollar Burger ½ lb	1060	72	60
Spicy Chicken Sandwich	470	26	46
Thickburger ⅓ lb	850	57	54
Double Thickburger ⅔ lb	1240	90	55
Grilled Sourdough Thickburger ½ lb	1080	82	42
Bacon Cheese Thickburger ⅓ lb	910	63	50
Dble Bacon Chse Thickburger ⅔ lb	1300	96	51
Mushroom N Swiss Thickburger ⅓ lb	720	42	48
Monster Thickburger ⅔ lb	1410	107	47
Low Carb Thickburger ⅓ lb	420	32	5
Fried Chicken: Per Portion (edible portion, no bone)			
Breast portion	370	15	29
Leg portion	170	7	15
Thigh portion	330	15	30
Wing portion	200	8	23
Sides: Per Serving			
Crispy Curls, medium	410	20	52
Chicken Strips (3), 5 oz	380	21	27
Chicken Strips (5), 8.5 oz	630	34	45
Coleslaw, small, 4 oz	170	10	20
French Fries: Small, 4.4 oz	390	19	51
Medium, 5.2 oz	515	25	67
Large, 6 oz	595	29	78
Mashed Potato & Gravy, small	90	2	17
Breakfast: Bacon Platter	980	56	90
Low Carb Breakfast Bowl	620	50	6
Loaded Burrito	780	51	38
Chicken Platter	1140	61	105
Country Ham Platter	970	53	90
Country Steak Platter	1150	68	98
Dessert: Apple Turnover	290	15	36
Chocolate Chip Cookie	290	11	44
Peach Cobbler	280	7	56
For Complete Nutritional Data ~ see CalorieKing.com			

Harvey's®

Main Menu	C	F	Cb
Angus Burger	390	17	34
Angus Burger w. Cheese	440	21	35
Original Hamburger	380	16	35
Original Cheeseburger	430	22	36
Chicken Nuggets, 2.3 oz	170	9	11
Deluxe Burger	510	28	33
Fried Fish Sandwich	390	14	50
Harvey Jr. Burger	340	15	32
Hot Dog, 4.2 oz	320	14	34
Harvey's Grilled Chicken	340	6	32
Harvey's Crispy Chicken	460	15	56
Veggie Burger	315	9	39
Toasted Sandwiches: BLT w. Sauce	630	31	66
Grilled Chicken Club w. Sauce	670	29	62
Crispy Fries: Junior, 3.2 oz	240	10	35
Regular, 4.2 oz	320	13	47
Large, 5.3 oz	400	17	58
Onion Rings: Regular, 2.9 oz	280	14	34
Large, 4.3 oz	420	21	51
Side Orders: Per Serving			
Poutine, 10 oz	640	33	67
Gravy, 3 oz	35	1	5
Salads: Dressing Not Included			
Garden Salad	130	6	11
Caesar Salad	80	4	5
Chicken Caesar Salad	280	14	5
Grilled Chicken BLT	290	12	11
Soup: Harvest Vegetable, 1 cup	120	1	26
Cream of Mushroom, 1 cup	150	5	24
Chicken Noodle, 1 cup	90	1	14
Breakfast: Bagel, 4 oz	290	2	58
Breakfast Club Sandwich	400	20	35
Eggs (2): Fried	180	13	0
Scrambled Eggs	170	12	0
Hashbrowns, 2 oz	180	9	23
Home Fries, 4.6 oz	300	19	29
Pancakes (2), 4 oz	150	2	29
Pancake Syrup, 1.4 fl.oz	180	0	44
Sausage Patty, 1½ oz	130	9	3
Toasted Western Sandwich	370	20	37
Dressings: Light Caesar/Italian, 1 oz	60	4	5
Other varieties, average	140	14	2
Desserts & Shakes			
Apple Turnover, 3 oz	260	13	34
Shakes: Choc.; Vanilla, 14.5 fl.oz	540	13	88
Strawberry, 14.5 fl.oz	550	12	99

Hogi Yogi®

Frozen Yogurt: Per ½ Cup	C	F	Cb
Chocolate Base, 2.5 oz	80	0	17
Vanilla (No Sugar Added): Base, 2.6 oz	100	0	22
Regular Sandwiches: Club	340	5	47
BBQ Chicken	360	4.5	59
Roast Beef	300	4.5	46
Smokey Turkey	320	3	46
Turkey	290	3	57
Vegetarian	240	2.5	45
Smoothies: Per 24 oz			
Berry Blast	310	0	70
Fruit Safari	370	3.5	84
Jungle Mist	430	4	101
Peach Treat	430	0	105
Pina Collision	450	4.5	105
Pure Passion	430	4	99
Ragin Rasberry	370	3.5	84
Strawberry Kist	420	0.5	98

Hot Dog on a Stick®

Menu Items	C	F	Cb
Hot Dog on a Bun	470	26	41
Hot Dog on a Stick	255	14	23
Veggie Dog	175	3	24
American Cheese on a Stick	240	13	22
Pepper Jack Cheese on a Stick	235	13	21
French Fries, 7 oz	700	37	83
Lemonade (12 fl.oz): Original	135	0	34
Cherry/Lime, average	170	0	42
Sugar Free Lemonade	10	0	2

Hot Stuff Pizza®

	C	F	Cb
Pizza: Per Slice (⅛ Medium or ⅒ Large)			
Beef	320	12	34
Canadian Bacon	320	11	25
Cheese	350	12	25
Double Pepperoni	390	18	37
Garden Style	300	11	34
Italian Sausage	340	15	37
Masterpiece Supreme	330	14	34
Pepperoni	350	14	37
Pork Sausage	340	15	33
Western Omelet	320	15	30

Hungry Howie's Pizza®

Pizzas: Per Slice (Cheese Only)

	C	F	Cb
Small, ⅙ pizza	160	3.5	20
Medium, ⅛ pizza	190	5.5	23
Large, ⅒ pizza	210	5	25
X-Large, ⅛ pizza	395	9.5	42
Calzone Subs: Pizza, ½ sub	690	34	67
Deluxe Italian, ½ sub	505	19	61
Sides: Chicken Tenders, 2 pieces	140	4.5	11
Howie Wings, 5 wings	180	13	0

Toppings: Per Slice (For Medium or Large Pizza)

	C	F	Cb
Anchovies	55	3	0
Bacon	40	0.5	0.5
Banana Peppers	10	0	1.5
Beef; Pepperoni; Sausage	30	2	0.5
Black Olives; Green Olives	10	0.5	0.5
Green Peppers; Mushroom	0	0	0.5
Ham	5	0.5	0
Onions	5	1	0.5
Pineapple	5	0.5	1.5

I Can't Believe It's Yogurt®

Original Frozen Yogurt: Per Serving (4 oz)

	C	F	Cb
Chocolate; Vanilla	140	8	17
Strawberry	150	7	19

Low-Fat Frozen Yogurt: Per Bar (5.5 oz)

	C	F	Cb
Chocolate	120	2.5	23

Smoothies: Per Serving (8.5 oz)

	C	F	Cb
Ana-Bana-Berry	80	0	21
Might Berry	130	0.5	30
Raspberry Rush	110	0.5	26
Strawbapple; Strawberry Skinny	60	0	16
Strawberry Banana	130	0.5	30

In-N-Out Burger®

Burgers:

	C	F	Cb
Hamburger w. Onion	390	19	39
w. Mustard/Ketchup, no Spread	310	10	41
Protein Style, no Bun	240	17	11
Cheeseburger w. Onion	480	27	39
w. Mustard/Ketchup, no Spread	400	18	41
Protein Style, no Bun	330	25	11
Double Double® (2 patty/2 sl. chse)	670	41	39
w. Mustard/Ketchup, no Spread	590	32	41
Protein Style, no Bun	520	39	11
French Fries, 4.4 oz	400	18	54
Drinks: Milk, 10 fl.oz	180	6	18
Coca-Cola®; Dr. Pepper, 16 fl.oz	200	0	54
Lemonade, 16 fl.oz	180	0	40
Root Beer; Seven-Up® 16 fl.oz	220	0	54
Shakes, average all flavors, 15 fl.oz	690	36	83

For Complete Nutritional Data ~ see CalorieKing.com

IHOP®

Pancakes: (Syrup/Butter extra)

	C	F	Cb
Buttermilk (1), 1.7 oz	110	3	17
Short Stack, 3	330	9	51
Full Stack, 5	550	15	85
Country Griddle Cakes (1), 2 oz	120	3.5	19
Harvest Grain 'N Nut (1) 2¼ oz	180	9	20
Crepe-Style, 2 oz	120	6	14
Syrup: 1 Tbsp	50	0	12
Whipped Butter, 1 Tbsp	80	9	0
Waffles (Plain): Regular (1), 3 oz	310	15	37
Belgian, Regular (1), 4 oz	390	19	48

Breakfast: Per Serving

	C	F	Cb
Classic Combos: Cntry Fried Steak/Eggs	1530	105	73
Fruity Country Griddle Cakes Combo	960	56	83
Harvest Grain 'N Nut Combo	1035	65	80
T-Bone Steak & Eggs	1310	86	63
Signature, Rooty Tooty Fresh & Fruity, average all flavors	855	45	84

Omlette Feast

	C	F	Cb
Colorado Omelette: No pancakes	790	68	5
with 3 buttermilk pancakes	1205	83	66
The Big Steak Omelette: No pancakes	910	72	14
with 3 buttermilk pancakes	1325	87	75

Burgers

	C	F	Cb
Sourdough Bacon Burger Melt:			
Burger Only	690	41	37
with French Fries	1265	74	104
with Onion Rings	1230	88	64
with Salad & 2 ½ T. Reg. Dress.	870	56	47
Entrees: Old Fashioned Pot Roast	765	48	30
with Mashed Potatoes	965	53	65
Salad: Southwestern Chicken Fajita,			
with Tortilla Shell	1110	82	48
no Tortilla Shell	890	67	35

Jack's®

Sandwiches:

	C	F	Cb
Big Bacon Burger	700	42	45
Big Jack Burger	500	27	40
Cheeseburger	380	17	35
Chicken Fillet Sandwich	640	31	69
Double Big Jack Cheese Burger	930	60	43
Double Cheeseburger	595	33	37
Grilled Chicken	410	15	44
Hamburger	270	8	35
Sides: Brown Gravy, 1 oz	10	0	2
Coleslaw, 4 oz	210	16	14
Green Beans, 4 oz	25	0	5
Mashed Potatoes, 4 oz	70	0.5	15

For Complete Nutritional Data ~ see CalorieKing.com

Jack in the Box®

Breakfast	C	F	Cb
Biscuit: Bacon, Egg & Cheese	430	25	34
Sausage	440	29	32
Sausage, Egg & Cheese	740	55	35
Spicy Chicken	460	22	44
Breakfast Jack: Regular	290	12	28
w. Sausage	450	28	29
Sourdough	425	24	31
Ultimate	575	27	49
Croissant: Sausage	580	39	37
Supreme	455	26	36
Extreme Sausage Sandwich	675	48	31
Hash Browns (1), 2 oz	150	10	13
Meaty Breakfast Burrito: w. Salsa	490	29	30
No Salsa	480	29	29

Sandwiches & Burgers	C	F	Cb
Bacon Bacon Cheeseburger	840	56	51
Bacon Ultimate Cheeseburger	1095	77	53
Junior Bacon Cheeseburger	430	25	30
Ultimate Cheeseburger	1010	71	53
Hamburger	310	14	30
Hamburger w. Cheese	355	18	31
Deluxe Hamburger: No Cheese	370	21	31
w. Cheese	460	28	33
Jumbo Jack: Regular	595	34	51
w. Cheese	685	41	49
Sourdough Jack	715	51	36
Pannido: Deli Trio	665	35	56
Ham & Turkey	690	34	57
Zesty Turkey	835	48	55

Chicken & Fish	C	F	Cb
Bacon Chicken Sandwich	440	24	39
Chicken Breast Strips (4)	505	25	36
Chicken Fajita Pita, no salsa	300	10	31
Chicken Sandwich	400	21	39
Ciabatta: Bruschetta Chicken	660	26	69
Classic Chicken	510	13	69
Fish & Chips	680	41	60
Jack's Spicy Chicken Sandwich	615	31	61
w. Cheese	700	37	62
Sourdough Grilled Chicken Club	535	34	34
Southwest Chicken Pita, no salsa	230	3	34

Tacos & Snacks	C	F	Cb
Bacon Cheddar Potato Wedges	560	36	43
Beef Taco (1), regular	160	8	15
Egg Rolls (3)	400	19	44
Monster Beef Taco (1)	240	14	20
Stuffed Jalapenos (3)	230	13	22

Fries & Rings	C	F	Cb
Natural Cut Fries, medium, 4.7 oz	365	16	47
Seasoned Curly Fries, med., 4.4 oz	400	22	45
Onion Rings, 4.2 oz	500	30	51

Salads: No Dressing	C	F	Cb
Asian Chicken	140	1	20
Chicken Caesar	220	8.5	10
Chicken Club	300	16	13
Side Salad	60	3	5
Southwest Chicken	300	11	29

Sauces & Dressings	C	F	Cb
Dipping Sauce: Barbecue, 1 oz	45	0	11
Buttermilk House, 1 oz	130	13	3
Frank's Red Hot Buffalo, 1 oz	10	0	2
Sweet & Sour, 1 oz	45	0	11
Tartar, 1½ oz	210	22	2
Sauce: Mayo-Onion, ½ oz	90	10	1
Soy, 0.3 oz	5	0	1
Taco, 0.3 oz	0	0	0

Condiments	C	F	Cb
Cheese: American; Swiss	45	3.5	1
Provolone	70	6	0
Ketchup	10	0	2
Mustard	5	0	1
Salsa	5	0	1
Sour Cream	60	5	2

Desserts	C	F	Cb
Cheesecake	310	16	34
Double Fudge Cake	310	11	49

Ice Cream Shakes: Per Medium (14.5 oz)	C	F	Cb
Chocolate Ice Cream	865	38	117
Choc. Malted Crunch Ice Cream	940	42	122
Oreo Cookie Ice Cream	890	44	108
Strawberry Ice Cream	840	37	110
Vanilla Ice Cream	745	38	85

For Complete Nutritional Data ~ see CalorieKing.com

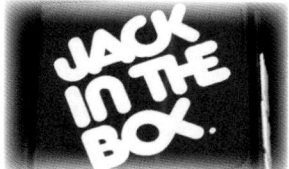

Jamba Juice®

	C	F	Cb
Juices: Per Original			
Carrot	150	1	34
Lemonade	450	0	112
Orange Banana	350	1.5	84
Orange Carrot	240	1.5	56
Orange	330	1.5	77
Vibrant C	380	1	92
Shots: Average all, 4 fl.oz	70	0	14
Wheatgrass, 1 fl.oz	10	0	1
Yogurt Blend:			
Bright Eyed & Blueberry	380	1	76
Sunrise Strawberry	400	1	83
Smoothies: Per Original			
Aloha Pineapple	500	1.5	117
Banana Berry	480	1	112
Berry Lime Sublime	460	2	106
Caribbean Passion	440	2	102
Chocolate Moo'd	680	8	138
Citrus Squeeze	470	2	110
Coldbuster	430	2.5	100
Cranberry Craze	460	0.5	104
Jamba Powerboost	440	1.5	103
Kiwi Berry Burner	470	0.5	112
Mango A Go-Go	440	1.5	104
Orange A Peel	440	1.5	102
Orange Berry Blitz	410	2.5	94
Orange Dream Machine	540	2.5	111
Peach Pleasure	460	2	108
Peanut Butter Moo'd	840	21	139
Peenya Kowlada	690	5	152
Protein Berry Pizzazz	440	1.5	92
Razzmatazz	480	2	112
Strawberries Wild	450	0.5	105
Energy: Acai Supercharger	420	5	86
Matcha Green Tea Blast	440	0.5	97
Turbo Tropic	470	1.5	112
Enlightened:			
Berry Fulfilling	290	1	62
Mango Mantra	310	1	71
Strawberry Nirvana	280	1	64
Tropical Awakening	320	1	73
Baked Goods			
Pretzels: Apple Cinnamon	410	5	78
Savory: Cheddar Jalapeno Twist	250	5	41
Grin n' Carrot	250	10	36
Pizza Protein Stick	230	6	33
Sweet: Blueberry Cinnamon Swirl	320	6	55
Honey Berry Bran	320	12	48
Lemon Poppyseed Bundt	300	12	44

Jimmy John's®

	C	F	Cb
Club Sandwiches			
Beach Club	775	36	78
Billy Club	840	39	77
Bootlegger's Club	710	28	74
Country Club	955	45	75
Gourmet Smoked Ham Club	825	38	76
Gourmet Veggie Club	1100	66	80
Hunter's Club	825	37	75
Italian Night Club	955	51	77
Lulu Club	755	33	74
Tuna Club	845	39	80
Plain Slims: Figures based on French Bread			
Bacon	490	8.5	71
John	415	1.5	71
Pepe	520	10	72
Tom	400	0.5	70
Tuna	580	19	74
Veggie	560	17	71
Vito	610	20	72
Subs: Figures based on 8" French Bread, Mayo, Cheese, Sce			
Big John	555	27	57
JJBLT	635	34	54
Sorry Charlie	505	20	59
The J.J. Gargantuan	980	53	61
The Pepe	660	36	55
Turkey Tom	555	26	54
Vegetarian	640	36	58
Vito	565	24	57
Unwich Wraps: Includes Mayo, Cheese & Sauce			
Beach Club	440	36	10
Big John	320	27	5.5
Billy Club	505	38	9
Bootlegger Club	375	27	6.5
Club Lulu	420	33	6.5
Country Club	480	36	7.5
Gourmet Smoked Ham Club	490	38	8
Gourmet Veggie Club	765	65	13
Hunter's Club	495	37	8
Italian Night Club	620	51	9.5
J.J.B.L.T.	395	34	5.5
The J.J. Gargantuan	745	53	13
The Pepe	425	36	6.5
Tuna Club	390	29	12
Turkey Tom	315	26	5.5
Vegetarian	400	36	9
Vito Wrap	325	24	8
Sides: Jimmy Chips, average 1 oz	160	8	18
Cookies, average	420	18	63

Restaurants & Fast - Foods

Johnny Rockets®

Original Hamburgers

	C	F	Cb
Hamburger #12	905	60	54
Chili Size	920	56	59
Original Burger	620	35	44
Patty Melt	940	60	51
Rocket Double	1240	84	57
Rocket Single	880	57	56
Route 66	890	61	45
Smoke House	990	59	70
St Louis	960	61	53
Streamliner	420	16	50
Sandwiches: Chicken Club	870	50	62
Bacon, Lettuce and Tomato	530	33	44
Egg Salad	700	49	40
Grilled Breast of Chicken	600	29	54
Grilled Cheese	520	31	42
Grilled Ham & Cheese	450	17	48
Tuna Melt	830	54	42
Tuna Salad	720	46	41

Other Favorites

	C	F	Cb
Chicken Club Salad:			
with Chicken Tenders	670	40	37
with Grilled Chicken Breast	440	25	8
Chicken Tenders	520	22	47
Chili Dog	570	33	46
Garden Salad	250	20	5
Hot Dog	430	23	39
Extras: Bacon, 0.7 oz	100	7	0
Extra Patty, 3 oz	270	20	1
Chili, 2½ oz	170	15	3
Grilled Onions or Mushrooms, 1 oz	20	2	2

Starters

	C	F	Cb
American Fries, 8 oz	530	23	77
½ Fries & ½ Rings, 9.3 oz	720	36	92
Cheese Fries, 10 oz	760	43	77
Chili Bowl, 10 oz	680	59	12
Chili Fries, 12 oz	710	40	76
Onion Rings, 6.8 oz	500	34	22
Desserts: Apple Pie	930	59	88
Hot Fudge Sundae	830	47	93
A la mode, 4 oz	260	16	26
Drinks (Medium): Rootbeer	170	0	49
Coke; Sprite	170	0	43
Lemonade	170	0	49
Float	420	26	42
Shakes: Chocolate, 20 oz	1100	60	120
Strawberry, 20 oz	810	48	82
Vanilla, 20 oz	1120	60	130
Extra for Malt, ½ oz	60	2	10

Kenny Rogers Roasters®

Chicken

	C	F	Cb
½ Chicken, No Skin or Wing	315	10	1
with Skin	515	28	2
¼ Dark Meat, No Skin	170	7	1
with Skin	270	17	1
¼ White Meat, No Skin or Wing	145	2	1
with Skin, serving	245	11	1
Grilled Breast Platter	990	52	100
Tenders (3)	510	37	24
Tenders Platter	1315	79	119
Pies: Chicken Pot Pie	710	33	78
Pitas: BBQ Chicken	400	7	51
Chicken Caesar	605	35	34
Roasted Chicken	685	35	42
Turkey: Sliced Breast	160	2	1
Salads (No Dressing): Side Salad	25	0	5
Chicken Caesar	285	9	18
Pasta	230	12	28
Roasted Chicken	290	10	19
Sour Cream & Dill Pasta	230	16	20
Tomato Cucumber	125	2	10

Sandwiches

	C	F	Cb
Chicken Tender	695	46	45
Chicken Tender Pita	610	38	45
Grilled Chicken	525	29	32
Turkey	385	12	30
Side Dishes: Cinnamon Apples	200	5	41
Cole Slaw	225	16	18
Cornbread Stuffing	325	19	34
Corn Cob	70	0.5	14
Corn Muffin	165	6	25
Sweet Corn Niblets	115	0.5	28
Creamy Parmesan Spinach	120	6	10
Honey Baked Beans	150	1	32
Italian Green Beans	115	8	10
Macaroni & Cheese	200	6	24
Potatoes: Baked Sweet	265	0	62
Garlic Parsley	260	12	37
Potato Salad	390	27	34
Real Mashed	295	14	39
Rice Pilaf	175	5	43
Steamed Vegetables	50	0	8
Zucchini & Squash Santa Fe	70	5	8
Soups: Chicken Noodle, 1 bowl	90	2	12
Chicken Noodle, 1 cup	55	1	7

KFC®

Extra Crispy™	C	F	Cb
Breast, 5.7 oz	460	28	19
Drumstick, 2.1 oz	160	10	5
Thigh, 4 oz	370	26	12
Whole Wing, 1.8 oz	190	12	10
Original Recipe®: Breast, 5.7 oz	380	19	11
Breast, no skin or breading	140	3	0
Drumstick, 2 oz	140	8	4
Thigh, 4.4 oz	360	25	12
Whole Wing, 1.6 oz	150	9	5
Crispy Strips, 3 pieces	400	24	17
Sandwiches: Honey BBQ	300	6	41
Double Crunch	530	28	42
Crispy Twister	670	38	55
Oven Roasted Twister	510	23	46
Tender Roast Chicken: w. Sauce	390	19	24
without Sauce	260	5	23
Triple Crunch	650	34	49
Snacker Sandwich: Regular	320	16	31
Buffalo	260	8	32
Fish	270	10	34
Honey BBQ	220	3.5	32
Entrees: Chicken Pot Pie, 13 oz	770	40	70
Boneless Wings (6), avg.	520	25	44
Honey BBQ Wings, 6 pces	540	33	36
Hot Wings, 6 pieces	450	29	23
Popcorn Chicken: Large, 6 oz	560	31	34
Individual, 4 oz	380	21	23
Salads: (No Dressing or Croutons)			
Crispy BLT/Caesar Salad, avg.	370	19	20
Rstd BLT/Caesar Salad, avg.	220	9	6
Parm. Garlic Croutons, ½ oz pouch	70	3	9
Side Dishes: Beans, 4.8 oz	230	1	46
Biscuit, 2 oz	190	10	23
Coleslaw, 4.6 oz	190	11	22
Corn on the Cob (3") 2.9 oz	70	1.5	13
Famous Bowls: Potato w. Gravy	690	31	77
Rice w. Gravy, 16.6 oz	770	25	107
Green Beans, 4 oz	50	1.5	7
Macaroni & Cheese, 4.8 oz	180	8	18
Mashed Potatoes: w. Gravy, 4.8 oz	130	4.5	19
without Gravy, 3.8 oz	110	4	16
Potato Salad, 4.5 oz	180	9	22
Potato Wedges, small, 3.6 oz	240	12	30
Desserts: Apple Pie Slice, 4 oz	290	11	44
Pecan Pie Slice, 4 oz	480	21	68
Sweet Potato Pie Slice, 4 oz	340	16	44
Double Choc. Chip Cake, 2.7 oz	400	29	31
Little Bucket™ Parfaits:			
Chocolate Cream, 4 oz	270	13	37
Fudge Brownie, 3.5 oz	270	9	44
Lemon Creme, 4.5 oz	400	14	65

Koo•Koo•Roo®

Rotisserie Chicken	C	F	Cb
Leg & Thigh, 4.8 oz	300	18	1
Breast & Wing, 6.5 oz	355	16	1
Half Rotisserie Chicken, 11.3 oz	655	34	2
Original Skinless Flame Broiled Chicken™			
3 Piece Original Dark, 5 oz	320	16	5
Original Breast, 4.1 oz	190	5.5	0
Roasted Turkey: Breast, sliced, 4 oz	180	8	0
Hand-Carved Turkey Sandwich	600	32	31
Traditional Turkey Dinner	690	29	67
Turkey Pot Pie	885	44	83
Salads: Per Regular (no Dressing)			
BBQ Chicken Salad	365	14	22
Chicken Caesar Salad	285	11	12
Chinese Chicken Salad	550	28	39
Koo Koo Roo House Salad	115	4	16
Chicken Bowls (No Sce): Chargrill	570	18	57
Southwest	570	18	66
Spicy Ginger Garlic	485	6	62
Tostada (no shell)	530	22	65
Soup: Ten Vegetable, 5 oz	95	2	16
Sandwiches: BBQ Chicken w. Sce	560	11	71
Original Chkn Breast w. Dressing	660	28	62
Chicken Caesar w. Dressing	780	35	62
Wraps: Caesar Chicken w. Dressing	755	39	60
Chipotle Chicken w. Dressing	925	43	88
Sides: Baked French Fries, 5 oz	250	7.5	42
Baked Yams, 6 oz	200	0	47
Black Beans, 6 oz	125	2.5	22
Buffalo Wings (no sauce), 6 wings	605	27	42
Creamed Spinach, 5 oz	100	6.5	10
Mashed Potatoes, 6.5 oz	185	5	32
Macaroni & Cheese, 6 oz	340	16	32
Roasted Garlic Potatoes, 5 oz	135	4.5	21
Extras/Dressings			
Lahvash (flatbread), each	60	0	12
BBQ Vinaigrette, 2 oz	100	4	14
Caesar Dressing, 1½ oz	235	26	1.5
Chinese Salad Dressing, 3 oz	325	26	26
Chipotle Sauce, 1 oz	130	14	0.5
Cranberry Sauce, 1 oz	45	0	11

For Complete Nutritional Data ~ see CalorieKing.com

Kilwin's® ~ *see CalorieKing.com*

Kohr Bros® ~ *see CalorieKing.com*

Kolache® ~ *see CalorieKing.com*

Restaurants & Fast - Foods

Krispy Kreme®

Doughnuts

	C	F	Cb
Caramel Kreme Crunch	350	19	43
Chocolate Glazed Cruller	290	15	37
Chocolate Iced Cake	270	14	36
Chocolate Iced Custard Filled	300	17	35
Chocolate Iced Glazed	250	12	33
Chocolate Iced Kreme Filled	350	20	38
Chocolate Iced w. Sprinkles	260	12	38
Cinnamon Apple Filled	290	16	32
Cinnamon Bun	260	16	28
Cinnamon Twist	230	9	33
Dulce de Leche	290	18	30
Glazed Blueberry	330	17	43
Glazed Chocolate Cake	300	15	41
Glazed Cinnamon	210	12	24
Glazed Cruller	240	14	26
Glazed Kreme Filled	340	20	38
Glazed Lemon Filled	290	16	35
Glazed Raspberry Filled	300	16	39
Glazed Sour Cream	340	18	42
Key Lime Pie	320	17	40
Maple Iced Cake	270	13	35
Maple Iced Glazed	240	12	32
New York Cheesecake	320	19	35
Original Glazed	200	12	22
Powdered Blueberry Filled	290	16	33
Powdered Cake	280	14	37
Powdered Strawberry Filled	290	16	33
Sugar Doughnut	200	12	21
Traditional Cake Doughnut	230	13	25
Doughnut Holes: Orig. Glazed (5)	200	11	24
Glazed Cake (4)	210	11	28

Beverages: Per Container (w. Whipped Cream)

	C	F	Cb
Frozen Double Chocolate Blend/w. Coffee:			
large, 20 fl.oz	750	28	116
medium, 16 fl.oz	600	22	93
Frozen Latte Blend: large, 20 fl.oz	765	28	115
medium, 16 fl.oz	610	22	92
Frozen Original Kreme Blend:			
large, 20 fl.oz	750	26	119
medium, 16 fl.oz	600	21	95
Frozen Original Kreme w. Coffee Blend:			
large, 20 fl.oz	750	26	117
medium, 16 fl.oz	600	21	95
Frozen Raspberry Blend:			
large, 20 fl.oz	740	24	124
medium, 16 fl.oz	590	19	99

For Complete Nutritional Data ~ see CalorieKing.com

Krystal®

Burgers/Sandwiches

	C	F	Cb
B.A. Burger	470	27	39
w. Cheese	530	32	40
Double B.A. Burger	800	53	41
Krystal Burger	160	7	17
Krystal Chik	240	11	24
Bacon Cheese Krystal	190	10	16
Cheese Krystal	180	9	17
Double Krystal	260	13	24
Double Cheese Krystal	310	16	26
Chili Cheese Pup	210	12	17
Corn Pup	260	19	19
Plain Pup	170	9	15
Sampler Combo (Krystal, Chik, Chili Cheese Pup, Fries, 24 oz drink)	1320	50	171

French Fries

	C	F	Cb
Regular, 4.2 oz	470	20	53
Chili Cheese Fries, 7.3 oz	540	28	59

Sides

	C	F	Cb
Krystal Chili	200	7	22
Chik'n Bites, Small, 4 oz	310	19	16
Chik'n Bites & Salad	290	20	12
Kryspers	190	13	17

Breakfast Items

	C	F	Cb
Krystal Sunriser Sandwich	240	14	14
Biscuit: Bacon, Egg & Cheese	390	23	33
Chik Biscuit	360	15	40
Plain Biscuit	270	13	33
Sausage Biscuit	480	33	33
Biscuit & Gravy	280	14	34
Country Breakfast	660	42	46
Scrambler, 11 oz	440	26	33
4-Carb Scrambler: Bacon	370	29	4
Sausage	600	51	3

Desserts: Apple Turnover, fried

	C	F	Cb
Apple Turnover, fried	220	10	31
Lemon Icebox Pie	260	9	41

Drinks: Per Small Serving (16 fl.oz w. ¼ ice)

	C	F	Cb
Coca-Cola Classic	160	0	40
Coca-Cola Classic, frozen	145	0	36
Diet Coke	0	0	0
Sprite	155	0	39

For Complete Nutritional Data ~ see CalorieKing.com

More extensive menu listings in website database www.calorieking.com

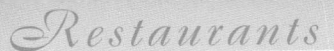

La Rosa's Pizzeria®

	C	F	Cb
***Pan Crust Medium Pizza:** Per Slice*			
Blanca, 1/10 pizza	350	22	28
Cheese	300	16	30
Deluxe/Pepperoni Topper	370	21	31
Meat Topper	400	23	30
Veggie Topper	320	16	32
***Traditional Crust Medium Pizza:** Per Slice*			
Blanca, 1/10 pizza	260	16	17
Cheese	200	10	19
Deluxe/Pepperoni Topper	280	16	20
Meat Topper	300	18	20
Veggie Topper	220	11	21
***Calzones:** Per Calzone (No Dipping Sauce)*			
3 Meat & 3 Cheese	1080	55	102
3 Veggie & 3 Cheese	860	34	105
Cheese	840	34	101
Cheese & Pepperoni	960	45	101
Philly Cheese Steak	865	39	90
***Hoagy:** No Cheese/Dressing/Sauce*			
Baked Buddy, 8.7 oz	665	28	62
Baked Royal, 9 oz	600	22	62
Meatball, 11.7 oz	690	26	77
Original Steak, 11.3 oz	730	35	65
Philly Steak, 9.3 oz	620	25	64
Hoagy Dressing: Chse on Hoagy	220	18	0
Italian Dressing, 1½ oz	230	26	2
Mayonnaise, 2 oz	400	11	0
Pizza Sauce, 2 oz	50	2	7
Tartar Sauce, 2 oz	260	24	11
Lite & Low Fat Menu			
Grilled Chicken Hoagy, low fat	520	9	56
Grilled Chicken Salad, low fat	380	10	40
Lite Deluxe Pizza, Medium, 1 slice	190	6	27
Minestrone Soup, 12 oz bowl	130	2	22
***Pasta Dinner:** No Sides*			
Cheese Ravioli	660	26	80
Lasagna w. Meat Sauce	735	38	61
Meat Ravioli	620	22	102
Spaghetti: w. Meat Sauce	700	18	104
w. Meatballs	870	28	119
w. Traditional Sauce	640	12	113
***Chicken Wings:** BBQ Wings (12)*	1255	77	48
Special Recipe Wings (12)	1260	87	21
Spicy Hot Wings (12)	1250	85	26

For Complete Nutritional Data ~ see CalorieKing.com

La Salsa Fresh Mexican Grill®

	C	F	Cb
***Appetizers:** Tortilla Chips, serving*	900	42	108
Chips, Guacamole & Salsa	1180	68	125
Nachos w. Chicken, no Beans	1515	86	128
Nachos w. Steak, no Beans	1530	90	127
***Burritos:** Chips and Salsa Not Included*			
Baja Fish	920	56	67
Bean & Cheese: w. Black Beans	635	20	87
w. Chicken/Carnitas, avg.	590	23	57
w. Pinto Beans	610	20	83
w. Steak, no beans	605	27	56
California Veggie: w. Beans, avg.	750	32	96
no Beans	660	31	80
California: w. Beans, avg.	750	32	96
w. Carnitas, no Beans	765	35	81
w. Chicken, no Beans	795	35	82
w. Steak, no Beans	810	39	81
Fire-Rstd Bowl: w. Steak, no Beans	665	38	65
w. Carnitas/Chkn, avg., no Beans	650	34	66
Grande: w. Steak, no Beans	810	41	81
w. Carnitas/Chkn, avg., no Beans	795	37	82
Los Cabos Shrimp, no Chips & Salsa	785	40	88
Original Gourmet: w. Steak	665	32	62
w. Carnitas, avg.	650	28	63
Sonora Fish, no Chips & Salsa	630	25	63
The No Rice No Beans: w. Carnitas	780	40	69
w. Chicken	810	40	70
w. Steak	825	44	69
Three Pepper Fajita: w. Carnitas	820	39	86
w. Chicken	850	39	87
w. Shrimp	785	37	86
w. Steak	865	43	86
***Meal Platters:** Beans, Chips and Salsa Not Included*			
Carnitas Guadalajara Taco	445	20	56
Cheese Enchilada	665	38	62
Enchilada: w. Carnitas	645	29	63
w. Chicken	685	29	65
w. Steak	705	34	67
Taquitos & Quesadilla: w. Carnitas	2125	120	173
w. Chicken	2160	120	174
w. Steak	2170	124	173
Three Pepper Fajita: w. Carnitas	1220	38	208
w. Chicken	1485	46	212
w. Steak	1515	53	210
Two Soft Tacos: w. Carnitas	550	22	77
w. Chicken	570	22	78
w. Steak	580	24	77

La Salsa Fresh® cont...

Quesadillas: No Chips/Salsa	C	F	Cb
Classic Quesadilla: w. Carnitas	995	61	61
w. Chicken	1025	61	62
w. Steak	1040	65	61
Grande: w. Carnitas, no Beans	1085	63	79
w. Chicken, no Beans	1115	63	80
w. Steak, no Beans	1130	67	79
Stuffed Fajita: w. Steak	955	60	55
w. Carnitas/Chicken, avg.	940	57	56
***Salads:** Chips and Salsa Not Included*			
Chile Lime Salad: w. Carnitas	645	46	49
w. Chicken	775	50	51
w. Steak	790	54	50
Chipotle Shrimp Salad	800	56	52
Taco Salad: w. Steak, no Beans	885	47	88
w. Carnitas/Chkn, avg., no Beans	870	43	89
Sides: Chips & Salsa	200	10	25
Black Beans: with Cheese	200	3	33
no Cheese	180	1	33
Pinto Beans: with Cheese	175	3	28
no Cheese	155	1	28
Rice: with Cotija Cheese	120	5	22
no Cotija Cheese	100	3	22
***Tacos:** Chips and Salsa Not Included*			
Baja Fish Taco	450	26	42
Baja Style Shrimp Taco	370	26	29
Carnitas Guadalajara Taco	320	17	30
La Salsa: w. Steak Taco	275	12	28
w. Carnitas/Chicken, avg.	265	10	29
Sonora Fish Taco	235	11	19
Taquitos (3)	1910	109	162

LaMar's®

Bars: Caramel Iced, Unfilled	430	18	59
Chocolate Iced: Unfilled	540	22	81
Bavarian Cream Filled	600	22	96
Chocolate/White Fluff Filled	810	35	120
Bizmarks: Bavarian Cream	620	22	101
Blueberry/Lemon Filled, avg.	530	21	80
Cherry Filled	550	19	88
Donuts: Apple Spice Cake	340	17	44
Bluberry Cake	350	17	44
Chocolate Iced Cake	330	18	37
Old Fashioned Sour Cream	420	18	60
Ray's Chocolate Glazed	290	11	44
Ray's Original Glazed	220	10	31
White Iced Cake	320	17	38
Other Items: Apple Fritter	650	26	91
German Chocolate Knot	480	27	54
Cinnamon Roll	690	25	106
Cinnamon Twist	770	26	120
Raisin Nut Cinnamon Roll	850	27	137

Little Caesar®

Pizza: Per Slice	C	F	Cb
12" Round: Cheese, 1/8 pizza	180	6	23
Pepperoni, 1/8 pizza	210	7.5	23
12" Thin Crust: Cheese, 1/8 pizza	140	7	13
Pepperoni, 1/8 pizza	150	8.5	13
14" Round: Cheese, 1/10 pizza	200	6.5	25
Meatsa, 1/10 pizza	280	13	26
Pepperoni, 1/10 pizza	230	8	25
Supreme, 1/10 pizza	270	10	31
Veggie, 1/10 pizza	240	7.5	32
14" Thin Crust: Cheese, 1/10 pizza	160	7.5	14
Pepperoni, 1/10 pizza	180	9	14
16" Round: Cheese, 1/12 pizza	220	7	27
Pepperoni, 1/12 pizza	240	8.5	27
18" Round: Cheese, 1/14 pizza	230	7	30
Pepperoni, 1/14 pizza	260	9	30
Large Deep Dish: Cheese, 1/8 pizza	320	12	37
Pepperoni, 1/8 pizza	350	14	38
Medium Deep Dish: Cheese, 1/8 pizza	320	12	37
Extras			
Baby Pan! Pan!, 1 piece, 5.1 oz	360	16	34
Chicken Wings (1)	70	5	0
Crazy Bread: 1 stick	90	2.5	15
Cinnamon, 2 sticks	100	2	19
Crazy Sauce, 4 oz	45	0	9
Italian Cheese Bread, 1 piece	130	6	13
Sandwiches			
Deli: Ham & Cheese	640	29	66
Italian	800	44	66
Veggie	600	27	67
Side Salads			
Antipasto	140	7.5	6
Caesar	90	3	12
Greek	120	6.5	11
Tossed	100	3	15
***Salad Dressings:** Per Serving*			
Caesar	230	25	1
Greek	270	29	0
Italian	220	23	2
Ranch	230	24	2
Fat-Free: Italian	25	0	5

For Complete Nutritional Data ~ see CalorieKing.com

Lone Star Steakhouse®

Meals	C	F	Cb
Grilled Chicken, 6 oz	185	2.5	0
Grilled Pork Chops (2) 16 oz	1430	100	0
Mesquite Grilled Steaks:			
Cajun Ribeye, 16 oz	1250	101	0
Chopped Steak, 12 oz	900	71	0
Delmonico, 11 oz	860	69	0
Five Star Filet, 9 oz	740	60	0
New York Strip, 14 oz	1035	80	0
San Antonio Sirloin, 12 oz	770	55	0
T-Bone, 20 oz	1540	124	0
Texas Ribeye, 14 oz	1090	88	0
Baby Back Ribs, 12 oz	970	80	0
Shrimp Dinner, 3.5 oz	105	1.5	1
Slow Roasted Prime Rib, 16 oz	1250	101	0
Sweet Bourbon Salmon, 6 oz	240	11	0
Texas Teasers Ribs, 6 oz	485	40	0
Sides: Per Serving			
Baked Potato	665	18	114
Baked Sweet Potato	635	8	137
Lone Star Chili, 6 fl.oz	230	15	8
Sauteed Mushrooms	115	9	6
Sauteed Onions	100	7	8
Steamed Vegetables	70	1	14
Texas Rice	80	2	11
Soups			
Black Bean, 6 fl.oz	190	4	31
Desserts			
Homemade Cobbler	240	8	43

Long John Silver's®

Sandwiches: Ultimate Fish	530	28	49
Fish Sandwich	470	23	48
Chicken Sandwich	410	22	39
Sides: Cheese Sticks (3)	140	8	12
Fries: Small, 3 oz	230	10	33
Large, 5 oz	385	17	55
Cheese Sticks (3)	140	8	12
Coleslaw, 4 oz	190	14	15
Corn Cobbette, no butter	90	3	14
Crumblies, 1 oz	170	13	14
Hushpuppy (1)	60	3	9
Rice, 4 oz	180	3.5	34
Soup: Clam Chowder, 1 bowl	220	10	23
Chicken: Battered Plank, 1 piece	140	8	9
Seafood: Battered Fish, 1 piece	260	16	17
Battered Shrimp, 1 piece	45	3	3
Clam Strips, 3 oz	240	13	22
Desserts: Per Serving			
Chocolate Cream Pie	310	22	34
Pecan Pie	370	15	23
Pineapple Cream Pie	290	13	39

For Complete Nutritional Data ~ see CalorieKing.com

Luby's®

Entrees: (Without Sides)	C	F	Cb
Blackened Chicken Breast	350	15	5
Blackened Tilapia	270	11	5
Carved Ham	300	11	6
Chicken Piccata	420	25	13
Grilled Chicken Breast w. skin	415	23	1
Lemon Basil Salmon	355	20	1
Pan Grilled Fillet	330	12	19
Roasted Chicken, ½, no skin	460	23	0
Roasted Turkey, no skin, no Gravy	280	3	0
Tuscan Chicken	525	25	15
Sides			
Bread Rolls: White	130	3	23
Whole Wheat	170	5	23
Black-eyed Peas	220	5	33
Blue Lake Green Beans	85	5	9
Broccoli	80	4	9
Cabbage	70	5	6
Carrots	95	4	15
Cauliflower Peas & Carrots	65	4	7
Corn	190	5	38
Fresh Green Beans	90	5	10
Grapefruit	45	0	12
Holiday Rice	165	3	30
Jello	100	0	24
Pineapple	50	0	12
Pinto Beans	190	5	28
Roasted Mixed Vegetables	135	8	16
Spinach	65	4	5
Salads: Marinated Cucumbers	115	8	13
Grilled Chicken Caesar w. Dressing	790	50	23
Grilled Chicken Caesar, no Dressing	550	26	23
Mediterranean Vegetables	140	10	9
Mixed Field Greens, no Dressing	35	0	7
Spinach Salad, no Dressing	50	2	5
Dressings: Per Tablespoon (½ fl.oz)			
Blue Cheese	90	9	0
Caesar	75	8	0
French	80	7	5
Greek	30	3	0
Honey Mustard; Italian	75	7	4
Ranch	55	6	1
Thousand Island	50	5	2
Soups: Chicken Noodle, 1 bowl	235	9	21

For Complete Nutritional Data ~ see CalorieKing.com

McDonald's®

Burgers/Sandwiches

	C	F	Cb
Big Mac	540	29	45
Big N'Tasty	460	24	37
Big N'Tasty w. Cheese	510	28	38
Cheeseburger	300	12	33
Cheeseburger Double	440	23	34
Filet-O-Fish Sandwich	380	18	38
Hamburger	250	9	31
McChicken	360	16	40
McRib Burger	490	25	44
McVeggie Burger	350	8	47
McVeggie Burger w. Cheese	400	12	49
Quarter Pounder	410	19	37
Quarter Pounder w. Cheese	510	26	40
Quarter Pounder Double w. Cheese	740	42	40
Chicken Fajita	220	8	26
Deli Sandwiches: Trio	410	7	61
Turkey BLT Toasted	500	15	61
Grilled Chicken Flatbread Sandwich	520	23	55
New York Reuben w. Corned Beef	560	23	58
New York Reuben w. Turkey	540	19	60
Premium Chicken Sandwiches:			
Crispy Chicken Classic	500	17	61
Crispy Chicken Club	660	28	63
Crispy Chicken Ranch BLT	600	23	64
Grilled Chicken Classic	420	10	51
Grilled Chicken Club	570	21	52
Grilled Chicken Ranch BLT	520	16	54
Spicy Chicken	510	18	63
Snack Wrap: w. Honey Mustard	320	15	34
w. Honey Mustard, Grilled	260	9	27
w. Ranch	330	16	33
w. Ranch, Grilled	270	10	26

Extra Value Meals

	C	F	Cb
Large Fries & Large Soda, add	880	30	156

French Fries

	C	F	Cb
Small, 2.6 oz	250	13	30
Medium, 4 oz	380	20	47
Large, 6 oz	570	30	70

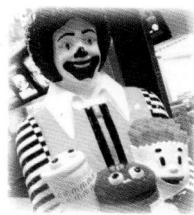

McDonald's® cont...

Chicken McNuggets®/Sauces

	C	F	Cb
Chicken McNuggets: 4 pieces	170	10	10
6 pieces	250	15	15
10 pieces	420	25	26
Sauce: Barbecue, 1 oz	50	0	12
Honey, ½ oz	50	0	12
Hot Mustard, 1 oz	60	2.5	9
Sweet 'N Sour, 1 oz	50	0	12
Chicken Selects® Breast Strips			
Strips: 3 pieces	380	20	28
5 pieces	635	33	46
10 pieces	1270	66	92
Sauces (1.5 oz pkg): Creamy Ranch	200	22	2
Spicy Buffalo	70	7	1
Tangy Honey Mustard	70	2.5	13
Chipotle Barbecue	70	0	18
Mozzarella Sticks w. Marinara Sce, 4 oz	290	18	21

Breakfast Menu

	C	F	Cb
Bagel: Plain	260	1	54
Ham, Egg & Cheese	550	24	57
Spanish Omelete	765	44	61
Steak, Egg & Cheese	640	32	55
Biscuit: Regular, 2.4 oz	230	10	32
Large, 2.9 oz	300	14	37
Bacon Egg & Cheese, large	500	29	42
Bacon Egg & Cheese, regular	450	25	36
Sausage w. Egg, large	550	36	40
Sausage w. Egg, regular	490	32	34
Breakfast Steak	120	8	0
Big Breakfast, regular	720	46	48
Deluxe Breakfast, regular	1220	61	133
English Muffin, 2 oz	140	1.5	27
Grape/Strawberry Jam	35	0	9
Hash Browns (1), 2 oz	140	8	15
Hotcakes: Plain (3)	350	9	60
w. Margarine (2 pats), no Syrup	430	18	60
w. Margarine (2 pats) & Syrup (1)	780	33	106
McGriddles: Bacon, Egg & Chse	460	21	48
Sausage	420	22	44
Sausage, Egg & Cheese	560	32	48
McMuffin: Egg	300	12	30
Sausage	370	22	29
Sausage w. Egg	450	27	30
Sausage, 1.5 oz patty	170	15	1
Sausage Breakfast Burrito	300	16	26
Scrambled Eggs (2)	170	11	1
Warm Cinnamon Roll: Regular	440	19	60
Deluxe	580	20	88

Breakfast Value Meal (Extras)

	C	F	Cb
If Hash Browns & Coffee (black/no sugar,) add	140	8	15
If Hash Browns & Orange Juice, add	280	8	48

Salads/Desserts/Drinks ~ Next Page ...

McDonald's® cont...

Salads: (No Dressing)	C	F	Cb
Asian Salad: No Chicken	150	7	15
w. Crispy Chicken	380	17	33
w. Grilled Chicken	300	10	23
Bacon Ranch Salad: No Chicken	140	7	10
w. Crispy Chicken	340	16	23
w. Grilled Chicken	260	9	12
Caesar Salad: No Chicken	90	4	9
w. Crispy Chicken	300	13	22
w. Grilled Chicken	220	6	12
Fruit & Walnut, Snack Size	210	8	31
Side Salad, 3.1 oz	20	0	4
Butter Garlic Croutons, ½ oz	60	1.5	10
Salad Dressings: Per Package			
Newman's Own: Cobb Dressing	120	9	9
Creamy Caesar Dressing	190	18	4
Ranch Dressing	170	15	9
Low-Fat: Balsamic Vinaigrette	40	3	4
Sesame Ginger Dressing	90	2.5	15
Soups: Broccoli Cheese	180	9	19
Chicken Noodle	100	0	16
Cream of Potato	190	7	27
Italian Wedding	150	3.5	18
Vegetable Beef	120	1	20
Desserts/Cookies/Shakes			
Apple Dippers w. Caramel Dip	100	0.5	23
Apple Dippers, 1 pkg	35	0	8
Caramel Dip, 0.7 oz	70	0.5	15
Baked Apple Pie, 2.7oz	270	12	36
Cookies: Oatmeal Raisin (1)	150	6	22
Chocolate Chip Cookie (1)	160	7	22
Sugar Cookie	150	6	21
McDonaldland® Cookies: 2 oz	250	8	42
Chocolate Chip Cookies, 2 oz	270	11	39
Fruit 'n Yogurt Parfait: Regular	160	2	31
without Granola	130	2	25
Ice Cream: Kiddie Cone	45	1	8
Vanilla Reduced Fat Cone	150	3.5	24
Vanilla Red.-Fat Ice Cream only, 3 oz	130	3.5	20
McFlurry™: M&M®, 12 fl.oz cup	620	20	96
Oreo®, 12 fl.oz cup	560	16	88
Sundaes: Nuts (Topping)	45	3.5	2
Hot Caramel Sundae	340	8	60
Hot Fudge Sundae	330	10	54
Strawberry Sundae	280	6	49
Triple Thick Shakes, average all flavors:			
12 fl.oz cup	430	10	76
16 fl.oz cup	580	14	102
21 fl.oz cup	750	18	180
32 fl.oz cup	1150	27	200

McDonald's® cont...

	C	F	Cb
Drinks: 1% Low Fat Milk, 8 fl.oz	100	2.5	12
Coffee (black), 16 fl.oz	0	0	0
Half & Half Creamer, 1 pkg	20	2	0
Cappuccino: Per 12 fl.oz			
French Vanilla	215	6	38
Original; Swiss Mocha	205	4	39
White Choc. Raspberry	225	9	34
Coca-Cola or Sprite (with ⅓ Ice):			
Childs, 12 fl.oz cup	115	0	33
Small, 16 fl.oz cup	155	0	43
Medium, 21 fl.oz cup	205	0	56
Large, 32 fl.oz cup	310	0	86
Diet Coke	0	0	0
Hi-C Orange Drink (with ⅓ Ice):			
Childs, 12 fl.oz cup	120	0	32
Small, 16 fl.oz cup	160	0	44
Medium, 21 fl.oz cup	240	0	64
Large, 32 fl.oz cup	350	0	94
Iced Tea	0	0	0
Orange Juice: 12 fl.oz cup	190	0	44
16 fl.oz cup	250	0	57
Powerade Mountain Blast (with ⅓ Ice):			
Childs, 12 fl.oz	85	0	22
Small, 16 fl.oz	110	0	29
Medium, 21 fl.oz	145	0	38
Large, 32 fl.oz	220	0	58
Whipped Hot Chocolate, 12 fl.oz	195	1	43

For Complete Nutritional Data ~ see CalorieKing.com

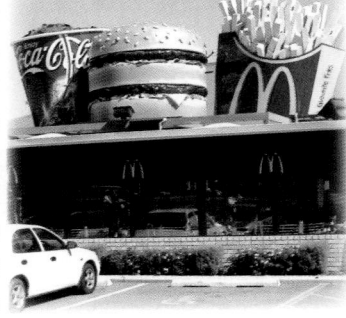

Manhattan Bagel®

Bagel: Per Bagel (4 oz)

	C	F	Cb
Blueberry	370	1	81
Cheddar Cheese	330	1	72
Chocolate Chip	370	3	76
Cinnamon Raisin	340	1	74
Cranberry Orange	350	1	76
Egg, 4 oz	330	1.5	71
Jalapeno Cheddar; Marble Rye	330	1	72
Lower Carb 9-Grain	210	3.5	28
Oat Goodness	350	3	71
Plain, 4 oz	330	1	72
Pumpernickel; Rye	340	1	73
Spinach	330	1	71
Sundried Tomato	330	1	73
Whole Wheat	320	1	69
Cream Cheese: Reduced Fat, 2 Tbsp	60	5	1

For Complete Nutritional Data ~ see CalorieKing.com

Max & Erma's®

Appetizers

	C	F	Cb
Black Bean Roll-Ups	575	10	95
Entrees: Blue Cheese NY Strip	1340	107	9
Caribbean Chicken (lunch)	535	20	60
Salads: No Breadstick			
Hula Bowl w. Dressing	575	7	79
Half Hula Bowl w. Dressing	365	4	57
Baby Greens Salad, no dressing	120	11	6
Shrimp Stack Salad	320	12	33
Sandwiches & Hamburgers			
Burger Stack w. Broccoli	1105	81	6.5
Chicken Stack w. Broccoli	825	51	6.5
Sides			
Buttered Broccoli, 3.5 oz	105	9	4.5
Fruit Salad, 4.5 oz	55	0	16
Garlic Breadstick (1)	155	6	21
Hearty Beef Chili Soup	390	15	39
Beverages: Fruit Smoothie	125	0.5	28
Dressings: Per 2 Tablespoons (1 fl.oz)			
Bleu Cheese	200	21	0.5
Italian	110	12	1
Ranch	120	12	0.5
Fat Free: French	125	0	31
Honey Mustard	60	0	14
Low-Fat Tex Mex Dressing	25	0	2.5

For Complete Nutritional Data ~ see CalorieKing.com

Mazzio's® Pizza

Appetizers: Per Serving

	C	F	Cb
Breadsticks, no sauce, ¼ order	150	3	26
Cheese Dippers, no sce, ⅓ order	410	18	47
Cinnamon Sticks, no sce, ¼ order	625	36	70
BBQ Chicken Wings, no sce, ⅓ order	190	12	7
Nachos: Beef w. Jalapenos, ½ order	485	34	20
Cheddar w. Jalapenos, ½ order	425	35	19
Calzones: Per Slice (⅓ Whole)			
Ham Bacon & Cheddar, no Sauce	245	7.5	32
Pepperoni	260	10	32
Pastas: Without Garlic Toast			
Fettuccine Alfredo	1060	56	106
Spaghetti w. Marinara Sce	640	8	120
Lasagna: w. Meat Sauce	950	52	64
w. Marinara Sauce	705	30	73
w. Alfredo Sauce	1265	94	55
Sandwiches			
Focaccia: Chicken, Bacon & Swiss	1020	70	49
Ham & Cheddar	745	47	47
Mazzio's Sub	770	50	45
Turkey & Swiss	720	38	46
Tuscan Smash	645	34	45
Hoagie: Chicken, Bacon & Swiss	1360	73	120
Ham & Cheddar	1090	50	119
Mazzio's Sub	1110	52	117
Turkey & Swiss	1060	41	118
Tuscan Smash	985	36	117
Pizzas: Per Slice (⅛ Medium Pizza)			
Cheese: Original Crust	235	9	30
Thin Crust	180	9	18
Chicken Club: Original Crust	260	9	31
Thin Crust	205	9	19
Mazzio's Works: Original Crust	310	14	31
Thin Crust	255	14	20
Meatbuster: Original Crust	285	13	30
Thin Crust	235	13	19
Mexican: Original Crust	315	14	35
Thin Crust	260	14	23
Pepperoni: Original Crust	255	11	30
Thin Crust	200	11	18
Sausage: Original Crust	275	12	30
Thin Crust	225	13	19
Supremebuster: Original Crust	260	10	31
Thin Crust	205	11	18
Veggie: Original Crust	230	8	31
Thin Crust	180	8	20
Sides: Garlic Toast, 1 pce, 1.4 oz	160	10	15
Kosher Pickle Spear, 1 oz	5	0	1
Potato Chips, 1 oz	150	10	15

For Complete Nutritional Data ~ see CalorieKing.com

Mimi's Cafe®

Breakfast	C	F	Cb
Hot off the Griddle, French Toast	305	13	40
Hot off the Griddle, Pancakes	955	35	139
Three Egg Omelette w. Sides, Low-Fat	480	5	69
Two Egg Breakfasts w. Sides	385	25	26
Carb Conscious Specialties			
Breakfast	680	22	21
Chicken & Vegetable Platter	765	42	18
Fresh Salmon w. Steamed Veges	460	28	8
Half Pound Cheeseburger in Lettuce	730	41	13
Mediterranean Omelette w. Tomato	545	35	25
Petite Chopped Cobb Salad, no Dr.	605	51	13
Top Sirloin Steak w. Steamed Veges	580	27	7
Two "AA" Large Eggs w. Tom./Saus.	415	32	5
Sandwiches			
Classic Beef Dip	520	15	43
Fresh Roasted Turkey Breast: Reg.	530	27	28
Low-Fat, ½ sandwich	335	9	42
Ham & Cheddar Grill	1210	77	7

For Complete Nutritional Data ~ see CalorieKing.com

Miami Subs®

Burgers	C	F	Cb
Deluxe Burger	785	59	31
Deluxe Cheeseburger	860	65	32
Deluxe Bacon Cheeseburger	920	69	32
Platters: Chicken Breast	745	41	57
Gyros	1420	93	81
10 Wings w. Fries & Blue Cheese	1020	67	50
Salads: Caesar w. Dressing	460	34	26
Chicken Caesar w. Dressing	610	39	28
Chicken Club	490	25	23
Garden	310	18	21
Greek	285	15	24
Side Greek w. Dressing	80	5	4
Cheesesteaks (6"): Original	410	11	45
Classic	420	11	47
Chicken Philly Classic	550	27	46
Works	530	22	51
Pitas: Gyros	660	39	46
Chicken	390	13	33
Subs(6"): Ham & Cheese	450	18	79
Italian Deli	515	24	49
Meatball	490	22	49
Tuna	470	18	44
Turkey	485	18	51
Sides: Mozzarella Sticks	755	56	34
Onion Rings	870	68	55
Spicy Fries: Regular	530	39	39
Large	1040	72	85

Mr. Goodcents®

	C	F	Cb
Cold Sub: Per Half Sandwich on Wheat Bread			
Centsable Sub	495	20	57
Cheese Mix	570	26	57
Ham & Cheese	420	10	62
Italian Sub	620	34	57
Mr. Goodcents Original	480	28	29
Oven Roasted Chicken Breast	355	6	54
Penny Club	365	7	56
Pepperoni & Cheese	750	54	32
Roast Beef	370	7	54
Hot Sub: Per Half Sandwich on Wheat Bread (w. Cheese)			
Chicken Bacon Ranch	580	31	28
Chicken Parmesan	525	15	61
Meatball	715	33	65
Pasta: Chicken Parmesan	695	12	100
Red Sauce on Mostaccioli	520	4	100

Mr. Hero®

Sandwiches: Per 7" Sub	C	F	Cb
Hot Subs: Grilled Chkn Philly	440	14	48
Cheesesteak: Grilled Steak Philly	450	14	48
Hot Buttered Deluxe	565	33	48
Cold Subs: Classic Italian	585	36	49
Tuna & Cheese	665	47	47
Turkey & Cheese	455	20	46
Ultimate Italian	610	33	51
Meatball	620	32	53
Romanburger	715	47	49
Round: Bacon Cheeseburger	350	23	23
Chicken	420	22	23
Fish	410	23	31
Tuna	430	33	22
Pasta: Breadsticks w. Sauce, 5 oz	290	9	47
Spaghetti Dinner, 16.8 oz	610	8	110
Spaghetti w. Meatballs, 19.8 oz	845	26	116
Salads: Garden Salad	35	0.5	7
Grilled Chicken	225	10	7
Seafood Crab	450	37	17
Side Salad	30	0.5	6
Tuna Salad	740	69	8
Dressings: Buttermilk, 2 oz	290	29	6
Creamy Italian, 2 oz	190	17	11
Croutons, ½ oz	60	2	8
Fat-Free: French ; Ranch	70	0	18
Side Orders: Onion Rings, 6 oz	565	32	64
Cheddar Cheese Sauce, 1.5 oz	60	4.5	5
Potato Waffers, 3.7 oz	335	17	42
Desserts: Cheesecake, plain, 3.5 oz	350	26	26
Cheesecake w. Cherries, 4.7 oz	385	26	35

Mrs Fields Cookies®

Brownies: Per Brownie (3 oz)

	C	F	Cb
Butterscotch Blondie	260	11	29
Double Fudge	260	14	35
Mint Fudge	260	14	35
Pecan Fudge	280	17	31
Pecan Pie	230	14	8
Pecan Pie Chocolate Chip	230	14	24
Special Walnut Fudge & Blondie	260	13	35
Toffee Fudge	260	14	35
Walnut Fudge	270	16	31
Cakes			
Blueberry, 3 oz slice	270	12	36
Carrot Cake, 3 oz slice	280	13	37
Chocolate, 3 oz slice	350	21	35
Chocolate Chip, 3 oz piece	350	17	45
Cinnamon Sugar Pecan, 2.1 oz slice	270	14	32
Lemon Bundt, 2.1 oz slice	300	14	40
Raspberry, 3 oz slice	270	12	36
Raspberry Chocolate Chip, 2.1 oz	260	12	36
Cookies			
Bite Size Nibblers: Cinn. Sugar (2)	120	4.5	17
Debra's Special (2)	100	4.5	15
Peanut Butter (2)	110	6	13
Semi-Sweet Chocolate (2)	110	5	15
Triple Chocolate (2)	110	6	15
White Chunk Macadamia (2)	120	7	13
Cinnamon Sugar (1)	300	12	41
Coconut & Macadamia (1)	280	13	39
Debra's Special (1)	280	12	39
Milk Chocolate & Walnuts (1)	320	17	37
Milk Chocolate Macadamia (1)	320	18	36
Milk Chocolate, no nuts (1)	280	13	38
Oatmeal Chocolate Chip (1)	280	13	40
Oatmeal Raisin (1)	180	7	29
Peanut Butter (1)	310	16	34
Semi-Sweet Chocolate (1)	280	14	40
w. Walnuts (1)	310	16	38
Triple Chocolate (1)	220	10	31
White Chunk Macadamia (1)	310	17	37

For Complete Nutritional Data ~ see CalorieKing.com

My Favorite Muffin®

*~ Same Menu & Data as
Big Apple Bagel (See Page 189) ~*

Nathan's Famous®

Burgers

	C	F	Cb
¼ lb Burger	535	30	42
¼ lb Burger w. Cheese	850	61	45
Bacon Cheeseburger	705	44	43
Super Burger	865	61	42
Cheesesteaks: Chicken	565	19	62
Original	740	43	50
Supreme	785	43	61
Fish Sandwich	465	20	41
Hot Dogs: Nathan's Famous (1)	310	20	22
Sides			
French Fries: Regular, 9.6 oz	545	37	46
Large, 13.4 oz	760	52	65
Super, 21 oz	1190	82	101
Nuggets (6), 3.5 oz	350	27	20
Onion Rings, 5.6 oz	560	44	36

For Complete Nutritional Data ~ see CalorieKing.com

Noodles & Company®

Classics

	C	F	Cb
Buttered Noodles & Parm.	1010	36	134
Chicken Noodle Soup	290	9	37
Mushroom Stroganoff	1000	45	116
Pad Thai	720	9	147
Pesto Cavatappi	760	30	89
Tomato Marinara	560	13	87
Wisconsin Mac & Cheese	970	44	99
Noodle-Less: Chicken Rustica	530	26	11
Mediterranean Mixed Grill	190	2	43
Shrimp Curry Saute	190	6	20
Sweet Chili Chicken	470	14	29
Specialties: Bangkok Curry	400	10	71
Indonesian Peanut Saute	820	21	128
Japanese Pan Noodle, no oil	620	1.5	128
Pasta Fresca	660	19	93
Penne Rosa	670	32	70
Thai Curry Soup	360	15	49
Whole Grain Tuscan Fettuccine	500	17	70
Salads			
Caesar Salad w. Dressing	440	35	28
Chinese Chop Salad	340	21	37
Market Salad w. Fat Free Dressing	190	2	43
The Med Salad	360	16	40
Spicy Peanut Noodle Salad	480	9	83
Spicy Thai Caesar Salad	220	19	11
Sides: Potstickers (3)	330	17	34
Cucumber Tomato Salad	100	0	21

Ninety Nine

	C	F	Cb
Appetizers			
All Star Sampler, ¼ platter	450	29	23
Boneless Wings & Skins Sampler, ¼	360	22	19
Outrageous Potato Skins, ¼ platter	300	23	13
Toasted Ravioli w. Marinara	410	24	32
Desserts			
Apple Fortune	870	39	123
Low Carb Cheesecake	380	29	35
Milky Way Madness, 1 pce	900	45	119
Strawberry Shortcake	590	25	88
Towering Midnight Oreo Fudge Cake	830	40	116
Sandwiches: No Sides			
BBQ Pulled Pork Sandwich	830	37	77
Cajun Mushroom Steakburger	1260	85	64
Louisiana Fish Sandwich	760	37	71
Philly Steakburger	990	53	68
Tuscan Steakburger	1170	79	55
Veggie Burger	910	41	95
Salads			
Boneless Buffalo Wing Salad	980	60	71
w/o dressing or bread	540	25	42
Calypso Coconut Shrimp Salad	1000	65	90
Tropical Chicken Salad	850	41	71
Wild Bleu Chicken & Spinach Salad	1270	82	67
Meals			
Cape Cod Seafood Trio, no pot./vege	670	40	20
Captain's Combo Platter	2310	143	165
Grilled Chicken Fajitas	1400	57	120
Grilled Double BBQ Turkey Tips	1620	65	138
no sides	610	3	42
Shrimp Parma Rosa Pasta	1320	57	151
Smothered Sirloin Tips, no vege	1200	49	78
Wild Bleu Cajun Sirloin Skillet, no pot.	870	55	18
Sides			
Double Bleu Iceberg Wedge	450	41	9
Garlic Redskin Mashed Potatoes	300	14	42
Honey Butter Biscuit w. honey butter	300	14	38
Honey Butter, ¼ oz	35	3	1
Onion Rings	360	24	32
Rice Side Dish, 8.5 oz	340	8	60
Cole Slaw, 7 oz	320	26	20
French Fries, 8 oz. raw weight	550	35	48
Rustic Bread w. Garlic Sauce	140	3	27
Soup			
Seafood Chowder, no topp., 8 oz. c.	220	6	19

O'Charley's®

	C	F	Cb
Appetizers: Per Serving			
Chicken Quesadilla, ½ order	490	30	26
Chicken O'Tenders, ½ order	580	15	74
Chips & Salsa, ½ order	470	23	62
Fried Cheese Wedges, ½ order	265	15	21
Over-Loaded Potato Skins, ½ order	570	40	19
Spinach & Artichoke Dip, ½ order	700	44	69
Brunch: Per Order (w. Brunch Potatoes & Bread)			
Cajun Chicken Omelette	1140	80	48
Spanish Omelette	960	70	47
Ultimate Omelette	970	66	50
Strawberry Waffle	975	33	158
Chicken: Per Order			
Chicken Parmesan w. Vegetables	835	27	90
Chkn Tenders Dinner, w. Sauce	1360	34	178
Chicken Teriyaki on Rice	690	17	69
Grilled Chicken Dinner	560	17	36
Salad: Black & Bleu Caesar	1010	66	15
O'Charley's Caesar Salad	465	38	11
Cajun Chicken w. Ranch Dressing	975	78	21
Island Chicken Salad w. dressing	1465	30	225
Southern Fried Chkn w. Dressing	1805	85	173
Sandwiches: No Sides			
Bacon & Cheese Trio Chicken	760	45	36
Buffalo Chicken	720	32	65
Cajun Chicken	480	21	38
French Dip	945	41	77
Grilled Chicken Sandwich	470	21	35
Half Pound Cheeseburger	1130	73	35
Three Cheese Bacon Burger	1305	88	36
Seafood: Per Order			
Fisherman's Platter w. Sides	1890	95	180
Fried Shrimp Platter (8) w. Sauce	550	28	26
Sides: Baked Potato, plain	205	0.5	46
Cole Slaw	220	14	21
French Fries	410	21	50
Rice Pilaf	220	6	38
Smashed Potatoes	365	12	44
Vegetable Medley	130	8	13
Steak & Ribs: Per Serving (No Sides or Fries)			
Steak Tips Monterey, 1 order	1140	82	46
Choice Sirloin, 10 oz	450	18	1
Filet Mignon, 9 oz	755	53	1
Flame Grilled Sirloin: 7 oz	320	13	1
10 oz	450	18	1
Prime Rib: 8 oz	930	80	0
10 oz	1165	100	0
16 oz	1865	159	0
Full Rack of Ribs w. Fries/Slaw	2915	193	164
Ribeye Steak, 12 oz	905	71	1

Old Country Buffet®

	C	F	Cb
Entrees: BBQ Beef Ribs, 5 oz	300	23	7
BBQ Smoked Sausage, 2.8 oz	140	10	9
Breakfast Quiche, 3.7 oz	220	15	12
Carved: Beef Brisket, 3 oz	200	11	1
Ham, 3 oz	140	9	0
Peppered Pork Loin, 3 oz	160	8	0
Roast Beef, 3 oz	230	15	0
Roast Turkey, 3 oz	170	8	0
Salmon Filet, 3 oz	190	12	0
Chicken Wings: Hot, Drummies (1)	35	2	0
Hot, Wing (1)	25	1.5	0
Teriyaki, Drummie (1)	50	2.5	2
Teriyaki, Wing (1)	50	2.5	2
Chicken Hand Breaded Fried:			
Breast, 5 oz	310	16	3
Drumstick (1), 1.4 oz	90	6	2
Thigh (1), 3.1 oz	210	14	4
Chicken, Traditional Baked: Breast	280	12	0
Drumstick (1), 1.4 oz	90	6	0
Thigh (1), 3.2 oz	160	11	0
Fish: Patties, 1 piece, 2.5 oz	160	9	13
Baked, 1 piece, 3 oz	120	4	0
Fried, 1 piece, 1.3 oz	80	3.5	9
Shrimp, fried, 6 shrimp, 1.9 oz	110	5	11
Smoked Sausage & Sauerkraut	195	17	3
Spanish Rice, 3 oz	140	9	9
Salads			
California Coleslaw, 3.5 oz	90	0.5	22
Macaroni Vegetable Salad, 3.5 oz	230	15	20
Marinated Vegetables, 3.5 oz	60	3.5	6
Seven Layer Salad, 2.6 oz	180	17	4
Tossed Green Salad, 1 cup, 1.6 oz	5	0	1
Sides: Baked Potato (1), 6.3 oz	160	0	39
Mashed Potato, 5 oz	150	2.5	30
Soups: Chili Bean, 4 fl.oz	100	3.5	11
Corn Chowder, 4 fl.oz	140	8	15
Navy Bean Soup w. Ham, 4 fl.oz	50	0	10
Desserts			
Cheesecake, plain, 1 piece, 2.8 oz	220	10	29
Chocolate Decadence Cake, 1 piece	200	9	27
Cookie, Sugar Free Ranger (1)	100	5	11
Hot Fudge Sundae Cake, 3 oz	160	3.5	32
Pumpkin Pie, reduced sugar, 4.2 oz	270	9	31
Pudding: Chocolate, 1 spoon, 3 oz	150	7	19
Reduced Sugar/Calorie, 3 oz	70	1	14
Vanilla, 1 spoon (3 oz), 86g	140	6	19
Soft Serve Ice Cream, avg., 4 oz	140	4.5	24

Olive Garden®

Appetizers	C	F	Cb
Bruschetta	440	21	57
Sicilian Scampi (4)	460	31	16
Stuffed Mushrooms (2)	385	31	12
Entrees (Includes Vegetables):			
Lunch: Lasagna Classico (4"x4½")	860	47	54
Eggplant Parmigiana	900	39	78
Fettuccine Alfredo	850	58	70
Sausage & Peppers Rustica	885	51	71
Dinner: Pork Fillettino	1010	58	116
Chicken Castellina	895	46	78
Manicotti Formaggio	800	38	57
Mixed Grill, 21.4 oz	840	43	65
Stuffed Chicken Marsala	1315	87	72
Garden Fare Selections (Lower Fat)			
Lunch: Capellini Pomodora, 13 oz	410	9	52
Chicken Giardino, 15.5 oz	410	12	40
Linguine alla Marinara, 10.6 oz	340	6	48
Shrimp Primavera, 19 oz	485	12	65
Dinner: Chicken Giardino, 21.5 oz	560	15	59
Capellini Pomodora, 21 oz	645	14	84
Linguine alla Marinara, 17 oz	550	8	79
Shrimp Primavera, 26 oz	705	24	84
Extras: Minestrone Soup, 6 fl.oz	160	1	30
Breadstick, plain, 1 stick	140	1.5	26
Dressing (Low Fat): Italian	37	2	4
Parmesan Peppercorn, 2 fl.oz	45	2	5

(The) Old Spaghetti Factory®

	C	F	Cb
Lunch Entrees: Fettuccine Alfredo	1130	83	71
Chicken Parmigiana, 19 oz	840	34	84
Garlic Cheese Bread Starter, 13½ oz	1220	85	105
Lasagna, 13 oz	520	27	29
Manicotti, 11½ oz	510	21	55
Pot Pourri, 10 oz	480	22	54
Spinach & Cheese Ravioli, 11 oz	480	15	59
Spinach Tortellini w. Alfredo, 12 oz	930	56	82
Spaghetti: w. Clam Sauce, 10 oz	460	19	56
w. Meatballs, 13.5 oz	610	24	62
w. Meat Sauce & Mizithra, 9.2 oz	450	19	53
w. Mizithra/Mushr./Tom. Sauce	450	19	52
w. Rich Meat Sauce, 10 oz	310	3.5	55
w. Sausage & Meat Sce, 13.7 oz	620	29	57
w. Tomato & Meat Sauce, 10 oz	300	3.5	56

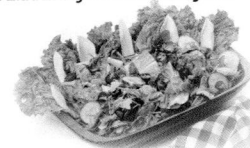

Fast - Foods & *Restaurants*

On the Border®

	C	**F**	**Cb**
Salads: *With Dressing Unless Indicated*			
Chicken Chopped Salad, w. dressing	1330	89	54
Chicken Fiesta, Blackened	1150	75	54
Chicken Fiesta, Grilled	1140	74	52
Grande Taco Salad, Beef, no dress.	1450	102	78
House Salad, no dressing	170	10	15
Sizzling Beef Fajita, no dressing	910	65	24
Sizzling Chicken Fajita, no dressing	760	48	23
Dressings: *Per Serving (2 fl.oz)*			
Chipotle Honey Mustard	310	29	11
Jalapeno Caesar	300	31	3
Ranch Dressing	220	23	2
Smoked Jalapeno Vinaigrette	230	22	8
Sweet Pepper Vinaigrette	270	25	10
Fat-Free, Balsamic Vinaigrette	50	0	10
Low-Fat, Ranch	110	6	11
Soups: Chicken Tortilla, 1 bowl	350	22	24
For Complete Nutritional Data ~ see CalorieKing.com			

Orange Julius®

	C	**F**	**Cb**
Original *(Orange, Strawberry):*			
Small, average, 16 fl.oz	220	0	55
Medium, average, 20 fl.oz	275	0	68
Large, average, 32 fl.oz	450	1	109
Classic Smoothy® Drinks: *Per 16 fl.oz*			
Bananarilla; Tropical, average	300	7	56
Cool Cappuccino	390	10	69
Pina Colada; Tripleberry, average	360	7	70
Strawberry Banana	400	7	77
20 fl.oz Size ~ Add 25% to above figures			
32 fl.oz Size ~ Double the above figures			
Premium Smoothy: *Per 20 fl.oz*			
Banana Chill	550	10	134
Berry Lively; Blackberry Toner	450	1	100
Blackberry Storm	630	8	130
Blueberrathon	350	1.5	90
Cocoa Latte Swirl	640	9	122
Orange Swirl	490	10	96
Raspberry Crush	330	2	83
Strawb. Treasure; Raspb. Creme	540	8	103
Strawberry Xtreme	410	0.5	87
Tart 'N' Berry	450	1	102
Tropi-Colada	560	8	110
Wild Blue Twist	490	0.5	115
Add Banana, 1 medium	110	0.5	27
Nutrifiers: Avg. all types, ¼ oz	15	0	4

Outback Steakhouse®

	C	**F**	**Cb**
Aussie-Tizers			
Aussie Chse Fries (28 oz), w. dress.	2900	182	240
Bloomin Onion (23 oz), w. dressing	2210	134	241
Gold Coast Coconut Shrimp, w. Sce	690	30	97
Grilled Shrimp on the Barbie w. Sce	660	42	32
Kookaburra Wings w. Sauce (10)	1160	75	65
Lobster-Crab Cakes w. Sauce (2)	840	72	33
Steaks: *Meat Only ~ Add Extra for Sides*			
Ayers Rock Strip (New York Strip) 12 oz	850	66	0
Outback Special, 12 oz Sirloin	780	55	0
Prime Minister's Prime Ribs:			
8 oz cut	450	38	0
12 oz cut	675	57	0
16 oz cut	905	77	0
Rockhampton Rib-Eye, 14 oz	730	40	0
The Melbourne, P/house, 20 oz	1365	110	0
Lean meat only	700	37	0
Victoria's "Center Cut Filet": *With ¼" Fat*			
Tenderloin, 7 oz	490	37	0
Tenderloin, 9 oz	630	48	0
Victoria's "Crowned Filet": *No Sides*			
Tenderloin (7 oz) w. Horseradish	840	64	21
Tenderloin (7 oz) w. Bleu Chse	1110	86	22
Tenderloin (9 oz) w. Horseradish	1005	79	22
Tenderloin (9 oz) w. Bleu Chse	1270	101	22
Meals: Hearts of Gold Chicken	870	55	22
Hearts of Gold Tilapia	640	31	23
Alice Springs Chicken	1080	60	23
Salad: Queensland w. Dressing	1100	88	45
Queensland Salad, no Dressing	705	47	37
Sides: Aussie Chips, 7½ oz, w. Ketchup	725	32	100
Fresh Veggies	80	1	14
Grilled Onions, 7.5 oz	180	11	19
Jacket Potato, Plain, 9 oz	270	0	63
Jacket Potato, w. Butter/Cheese	400	14	63
Mushrooms, Sauteed, 8 oz	150	11	12
Desserts: Cheesecake Olivia	700	38	79
Choc. Thunder from Down Under	1220	78	134
Most figures above are author calculations and not intended for clinical use.			
For Extra Listings ~ see CalorieKing.com			

Restaurants & Fast - Foods

Panda Express®

Meals	C	F	Cb
Chicken: Black Pepper, 5½ oz	200	12	11
Orange Chicken, 5½ oz	500	27	42
w. Mushrooms, 5½ oz	130	6	8
Chicken Kung Pao Cashew, 5½ oz	200	9	12
BBQ Pork, 5½ oz	440	23	15
Beef & Broccoli, 5½ oz	150	7	11
Sweet & Sour Pork, 5½ oz	400	23	35
Mixed Veges, 5½ oz	50	1.5	7
Fried Tofu w. Veges, 5½ oz	120	8	10
Rice & Noodles: Serving (8 oz)			
Chow Mein	390	12	59
Fried Rice	450	14	67
Steamed Rice	380	2.5	81
Appetizers: Chkn Egg Roll (1), 3 oz	170	8	17
Fried Shrimp, 6 pieces , 3½ oz	260	13	26
Spring Roll (1)	80	3.5	14

Panera Bread®

	C	F	Cb
Bagels: Blueberry	330	1	69
Dutch Apple & Raisin	370	3	78
Plain	290	1	61
Spreads: Plain Cream Cheese, 2 oz	200	19	2
Reduced Fat, average, 2 oz	140	13	2
Salad: Asian Sesame Chkn w. Dr.	430	19	33
Caesar w. Dressing	440	32	25
Classic Cafe w. Dressing	400	37	18
Greek w. Dressing	520	48	17
Grilled Chicken Caesar w. Dressing	560	34	26
Sandwiches: Asiago Roast Beef	670	27	55
Bacon Turkey Bravo	740	25	82
Chicken Salad on Whole Grain	580	25	71
Garden Veggie	590	13	100
Italian Combo	1110	56	91
Sierra Turkey	960	53	80
Smoked Ham & Swiss on Rye	680	34	52
Smoked Turkey Brst on Sourdough	430	14	44
Smokehouse Turkey on Artisan	690	15	77
Tuna Salad on Honey Wheat	720	44	51
Turkey Artichoke Panini	840	38	85
Tuscan Chicken	740	30	79
Soup (8 oz): Boston Clam Chowder	300	11	19
Broccoli Cheddar	230	16	13
Chicken Noodle, Low Fat	100	2	15
Cream of Chicken & Wild Rice	200	12	19
French Onion, no Cheese/Croutons	80	3	12
Vegetarian: Black Bean	160	1	31
Garden Vegetable	90	0.5	17
Muffins: Banana Nut Muffie	230	11	31
Chocolate Chip Muffie	240	10	36
Pumpkin Muffie	310	7	49
Low Fat Tripleberry Muffin	270	2.5	57

For Extra Listings ~ see CalorieKing.com

Papa Gino's®

Appetizers: Per Serving	C	F	Cb
Buffalo Chkn Tenders, small, 4.2 oz	200	7	20
Cheese Breadsticks, small, 5.8 oz	450	19	52
Cheese Garlic Bread, large, 3.8 oz	220	5	36
Chicken Tender, small, 3.9 oz	220	7	24
Cinnamon Sticks, small, 7.2 oz	620	18	105
French Fries, small, 12.7 oz	665	37	76
Mozzarella Sticks, small, 3.3 oz	230	10	23
Pastas: Entree Size			
Papa Platter, Penne/Spagh., plain	995	23	136
Ravioli	445	20	49
Spaghetti & Meatballs	885	19	123
Spaghetti Chicken Parmigiana	1035	34	129
Pizzas: Per Slice			
Large Thin Crust: BBQ Chicken	285	6	41
Buffalo Chicken	255	6	35
Cheese	240	6	36
Cheeseburger	330	13	38
Chicken Pepper	295	9	36
Fenway	325	12	40
Garlic Chicken	300	9	38
Hawaiian	295	8	38
Meat Combo; PapaRoni, avg.	335	15	36
Pepperoni	285	10	36
Super Veggie	260	7	39
Works	315	12	38
Subs: Per Small Sub			
BLT, 11 oz	670	30	72
Italian, 11 oz	890	48	70
Meatball, 11 oz	740	17	78
Meatball Parmesan, 11.5 oz	815	36	77
Seafood Salad, 10 oz	675	34	69
Steak & Cheese, 7.5 oz	615	35	45
Steak, 6.7 oz	555	31	43
Super Steak, 11.2 oz	560	25	51
Tuna, 9.9 oz	730	38	67
Turkey, 7.5 oz	425	1	73
Salads			
Buffalo Chicken Tender	320	15	32
Caesar	190	8	20
Chicken Bacon Cheddar	480	21	26
Chicken Tender	280	10	30
Garden	175	6	27
Italian Chopped	575	50	12
Side: Caesar	70	3	7
Garden	65	2	10
Dressings: Bleu Cheese, 1.1 oz	150	15	3
Caesar, 3 oz	395	43	0
Ranch, 3 oz	285	31	3
Honey Dijon, Fat-Free	60	0	13

Papa John's®

	C	F	Cb
Original Crust (14"): *Per Slice (1/8 Whole)*			
All the Meats w. Beef	370	17	38
BBQ Chicken & Bacon	340	11	44
Cheese	300	11	39
Garden Fresh	280	9	40
Hawaiian BBQ Chicken	340	11	46
Pepperoni	310	13	38
Sausage	330	15	37
Spinach Alfredo/Chicken	280	11	36
The Works	330	11	39
Thin Crust (14"): *Per Slice (1/8 Pizza)*			
All the Meat: w. Beef	320	20	23
BBQ Chicken & Bacon	290	14	29
Cheese	240	13	22
Garden Fresh	210	11	23
Grilled Chicken Alfredo	240	13	20
Grilled Chicken Club	270	14	25
Hawaiian BBQ Chicken	290	14	31
Pepperoni	260	15	23
Sausage	280	17	23
Spicy Italian	320	14	24
Spinach Alfredo/Chicken, avg.	240	14	21
The Works	280	14	24
Side Orders: Bread Sticks, 1 stick	140	2	26
Cheese Sticks, 2 sticks	370	16	42
Papa's Chickenstrips, 2 strips	160	8	10
Papa's Cinnapie, 2 slices, 2 oz	200	8	29
Sauce: Garlic, 1 oz	150	17	0
Honey Mustard, 1 oz	150	15	5
Pizza, 1 oz	20	0	3

Papa Murphy's®

	C	F	Cb
Pizzas: *Per Slice (Family Size)*			
Deeper Dish, Traditional, 1/8 pizza	440	24	34
Gourmet: Chicken Garlic, 1/12 pizza	320	14	30
Classic Italian, 1/12 pizza	350	18	30
Veggie, 1/12 pizza	300	13	31
Papa's: BBQ Chicken, 1/12 pizza	335	13	37
Cheese, 1/12 pizza	260	10	29
All Meat; Cowboy, 1/12 pizza, avg.	350	17	30
Hawaiian, 1/12 pizza	285	11	33
Murphy's Combo, 1/12 pizza	355	18	31
Pepperoni, 1/12 pizza	310	15	29
Specialty; Perfect, 1/12 pizza, avg.	310	14	31
Rancher, 1/12 pizza	325	15	30
Veggie Combo, 1/12 pizza	285	12	32

Continued Next Page . . .

Papa Murphy's® cont...

	C	F	Cb
Pizzas: *Per Slice (Family Size)*			
Stuffed: Big Murphy, 1/16 pizza	360	16	40
Other varieties, 1/16 pizza	370	16	39
Thin Crust deLITEs: Cheese, 1/10	140	6.5	13
Hawaiian, 1/10 pizza	150	6.5	15
Meat, 1/10 pizza	190	10	13
Pepperoni, 1/10 pizza	165	9	13
Veggie, 1/10 pizza	150	8	13
Salads: Club, no Dressing	315	19	18
Garden, no Dressing	160	11	10
Italian, no dressing	220	16	9

Pei Wei Asian Diner

	C	F	Cb
Appetizers: *Per Serving*			
Crab Wontons (4)	190	13	9
Crispy Potstickers (4)	130	7	10
Edamame, ½ dish	155	8	12
Minced Chicken w. Lettuce Wraps	250	4	31
Spring Rolls (2)	90	5	11
Meals: *Per ½ Dish/Bowl*			
Dan Dan Noodle, Chicken	390	7	54
Fried Rice: Beef	580	21	56
Chicken	470	11	56
Japanese Udon Noodles: Beef	600	26	57
Chicken	490	16	57
Lo Mein Noodles: Chicken	460	11	61
Beef	570	21	61
Pad Thai: Beef	670	30	63
Chicken	560	20	61
Soba Miso Bowls: Shrimp	360	6	51
Beef	530	18	53
Chicken	420	8	53
Teriyaki Bowl w. Brown Rice: Beef	580	17	66
Chicken	460	7	64
Teriyaki Bowl w. White Rice: Beef	560	16	62
Chicken	440	6	60
Salads: *Per ½ Dish (no Dressing)*			
Asian Chopped Chicken	200	8	10
Spicy Chicken	210	2.5	23
Salad Dressings: *Per Serving*			
Lime Vinaigrette, 2 oz	230	20	13
Sesame Ginger, 2 oz	70	16	5
Sauces: Lettuce Wrap, 2 oz	70	4.5	2
Sweet Chile, 2 oz	140	0	34
Thai Peanut, 2 oz	170	11	15
Sides: *Per ½ Dish*			
Noodles: Egg	210	2.5	39
Rice	130	0	32
Udon	100	0	20
Rice: Brown	170	1.5	37
White	200	0	44
Soups: Hot & Sour, 1 bowl	500	28	37
Wonton, 1 bowl	260	4.5	49

Penn Station®

Subs (6")	C	F	Cb
Artichoke: w. mayo	360	18	37
No mayo	260	7	37
Cheese Bread	250	5.5	42
Chicken Salad	360	15	41
Chicken Teriyaki	435	13	48
Grilled Vegetarian	245	4	46
Ham Dagwood, no cheese	260	6.5	35
Philadelphia Cheesesteak	500	25	45
Philadelphia Cheesesteak, no mayo	395	14	45
Reuben	500	21	40
Reuben, no 1000 Island Dressing	390	12	37
Tuna Salad	365	15	41
Turkey Dagwood	420	18	36
Turkey Dagwood, no Cheese/Mayo	240	4	34

Pepe's Mexican®

	C	F	Cb
Burritos: Beef & Bean	510	24	52
Beef & Bean Suizo	640	34	55
Chicken & Bean	480	21	51
Chicken & Bean Suizo	610	31	54
Pork & Bean	470	19	51
Pork & Bean Suizo	600	29	54
Flauta: Beef, plain	160	9	10
Beef w. cheese & sauce	190	12	11
Chicken, plain	190	10	16
Chicken w. cheese & sauce	230	13	17
Taco Salad: (Includes Taco Shell)			
Beef w. 4 oz salsa	550	26	52
Chicken w. 4 oz salsa	520	23	51
Pork w. 4 oz salsa	500	20	52
Without Taco Shell, deduct	210	7	32
Tacos: Beef Crisp	210	11	16
Beef Soft Corn	250	10	28
Beef Soft Flour	250	11	24
Chicken Crisp	190	9	15
Chicken Soft Corn	230	8	27
Chicken Soft Flour	230	9	23
Pork Crisp	170	6	16
Pork Soft Corn	220	6	27
Pork Soft Flour	220	7	24
Tostada			
Beef & Bean	380	23	26
Beef & Bean Suiza	440	29	26
Chicken & Bean	360	21	21
Chicken & Bean Suiza	410	26	25
Pork & Bean	350	20	26
Pork & Bean Suiza	410	25	26

Perkin's® Family Restaurant

Entrees	C	F	Cb
Chicken Dinner	620	13	60
Fish Dinner	470	7	60
Fruit Cup	50	0.5	12
'Lite & Healthy'	105	2	15
Omelettes: Country Club	930	79	6
Deli Ham & Cheese	960	79	8
'Everything' Omelette	695	54	9
Granny's Country Omelette	940	82	7
w. 9 oz Hash Browns	1245	90	57
Salads: Chef's, Mini	215	11	7
Muffins: Banana	650	33	78
Blueberry; Pumpkin	550	26	78
Bran Muffin	550	16	94
Carrot	455	26	55
Chocolate Chips	620	26	81
Cranberry Nut	585	29	75
Lemon Poppyseed	685	33	88
Oat Bran	455	15	68
Peaches & Cream; Apple, avg.	520	23	72
Raspberry & Cream	585	26	81
Pancakes: Buttermilk (1), no syrup	140	4.5	20
Short Stack (3), no syrup	425	14	60
Regular Stack (5), no syrup	705	24	100
Pies (Per Slice): Apple Pie, 1/6 pie	375	15	56
Wildberry, 1/6 pie	390	16	66
Bundt Cake, w. Icing (sugar free)	385	17	70
For Complete Nutritional Data ~ See CalorieKing.com			

Petro's®

Petro: Per Serving	C	F	Cb
Chicken: small	465	24	43
medium	665	36	59
large	970	52	88
Lite: small	380	12	48
medium	530	16	66
large	785	24	99
Original: small	515	30	43
medium	735	43	58
large	1075	63	87
Pasta Lite: small	335	2.5	52
medium	495	3.5	79
large	680	4.5	107
Pasta: small	405	16	45
medium	625	26	67
large	850	36	91
Veggie: small	525	28	52
medium	745	41	70
large	1090	60	105

Petro's® cont...

Chili: *Per Serving (Medium Container)*

	C	**F**	**Cb**
Chicken	275	4	43
Original	370	14	42
Veggie	385	11	58
Baked Potato: #1 Lite (1)	365	0.5	74
#2 Butter Sour Cream (1)	480	18	74
#3 Loaded (1)	680	33	78
#4 Loaded w. Chili (1)	780	37	90
#5 Broccoli 3 Cheese (1)	655	30	77
Hot Dogs			
Chili	315	17	28
Chili & Cheese	345	19	29
Loaded	350	19	30
Plain	265	14	22
Slaw	350	16	23
Tostitos Chips: *Per Serving*			
Loaded Ultimate Nachos	880	51	79
Tostitos Chips: Queso	500	27	60
Ransalsa	560	35	61
Salsa	415	18	62
Salads			
Garden, small	45	0.5	8
Petro, Original	570	36	42
Petrol, Grilled Chicken	740	41	42

For Complete Nutritional Data ~ see CalorieKing.com

Peter Piper® Pizza

Cheese Pizza: *Per Slice*

	C	**F**	**Cb**
Hand-Tossed Crust (14"), ⅛ pizza	290	9	38
Hand-Tossed Crust (16"), ¹⁄₁₂ pizza	260	8	33
Healthy Dining: Orig. Crust, 1 slice	300	6	38
Ultra Thin Crust, slice	130	4	15
Original Crust (14"), ⅛ pizza	300	9	37
Original Crust (16"), ¹⁄₁₂ pizza	260	8	32
Pan Crust (14"), ⅛ pizza	290	9	38
Pan Crust (16"), ¹⁄₁₂ pizza	290	8	38
Thin Crust (14"), ¹⁄₁₂ pizza	150	5	13
Thin Crust (16"), ¹⁄₁₆ pizza	140	5	13
Pepperoni Pizza: *Per Slice*			
Hand-Tossed Crust (14"), ⅛ pizza	290	10	37
Hand-Tossed Crust (16"), ¹⁄₁₂ pizza	260	8	33
Original Crust (14"), ⅛ pizza	300	10	36
Original Crust (16"), ¹⁄₁₂ pizza	260	8	32
Pan Crust (14"), ⅛ pizza	330	10	44
Pan Crust (16"), ¹⁄₁₂ pizza	280	9	37
Thin Crust (14"), ¹⁄₁₂ pizza, 48g	150	6	13
Thin Crust (16"), ¹⁄₁₆ pizza, 47g	140	6	13
Appetizers: Breadsticks (2)	250	10	36
Chicken Strips, 2 pieces	300	9	26
Garlic Cheese Bread, 2 slices	310	14	37
Wings, 2 pieces	110	8	0

For Complete Nutritional Data ~ see CalorieKing.com

P F Chang's®

Appetizers: *Per Whole Dish*

	C	**F**	**Cb**
Crab Wontons w. Plum Sauce	530	26	52
Harvest Spring Rolls (4)	350	15	46
Lettuce Wraps: Chicken	510	12	68
Vegetarian	420	4.5	70
Peking Dumplings: Pan-Fried	430	24	31
Steamed	390	19	31
Seared Ahi Tuna w. Mustard	260	6	21
Shrimp Dumplings: Pan-Fried	330	13	26
Steamed w. Ginger Sauce	290	9	26
Spare Ribs: w. Barbecue Sauce	1280	79	47
Northern Style	730	55	6
Vegetable Dumplings: Pan-Fried	370	12	53
Steamed	330	8	53
Desserts: Banana Spring Rolls	950	52	130
Great Wall of Chocolate	2240	89	376
New York Style Cheesecake	950	55	88
Meals: *Per Whole Dish*			
Beef: A La Sichuan	1180	64	56
Mongolian	1180	73	29
Orange Peel	1580	85	115
Chicken: w. Black Bean Sauce	700	25	33
Chang's Spicy	930	37	88
Ginger & Broccoli	660	26	45
Kung Pao, regular	1240	80	58
Mu Shu	720	38	50
Orange Peel	1280	60	127
Philip's Better Lemon	1060	42	113
Spicy Ground w. Eggplant	810	40	73
Sweet & Sour	770	20	107
Duck, Cantonese Roasted	900	54	63
Lamb, Wok Seared	1080	80	29
Seafood: Cantonese Scallops	400	16	26
Cantonese Shrimp	330	12	21
Chang's Lemon Scallops	950	27	100
Crispy Honey Shrimp	1380	64	147
Hot Fish	1340	71	111
Kung Pao Scallops	1130	56	66
Kung Pao Shrimp	980	58	58
Lemon Pepper Shrimp	710	36	59
Oolong Marinated Sea Bass	520	12	40
Orange Peel Shrimp	1020	41	118
Salt & Pepper Prawns w. Sauce	850	50	53
Sichuan From The Sea: Calamari	1000	39	110
Scallops	1030	35	98
Shrimp	730	37	55
Wild Alaskan Salmon Lemon Pepper	700	36	36
Traditions Lunch: Beef w. Broc.	900	54	28
Almond Cashew Chicken	670	28	47
Crispy Honey Chicken	1000	38	111
Lo Mein Beef	1530	112	74

P F Chang's® cont...

Meals (Cont): Per Whole Dish	C	F	Cb
Traditions Lunch: Lo Mein Chkn	1510	104	95
Moo Goo Gai Pan	660	34	32
Shrimp w. Lobster Sauce	410	21	18
Vegetarian Plate: Buddha's Feast	430	6	80
Coconut Curry Vegetables	690	46	48
Garlic Snap Peas	210	10	23
Ma Po Tofu	540	19	51
Shanghai Cucumbers	120	6	8
Sichuan Asparagus	200	6	34
Sichuan Green Beans	610	40	48
Spinach Stir-Fried w. Garlic	140	6	16
Stir-Fried Eggplant	600	34	64
Soups: Hot & Sour, 1 bowl	650	15	86
Pin Rice Noodle, 1 bowl	740	30	91
Wonton, 1 bowl	350	10	44

For Complete Nutritional Data ~ see CalorieKing.com

Philly Connection®

Sandwiches: Regular Serving	C	F	Cb
Cheesesteak: Hoagie	490	23	42
Mushroom	460	19	43
Pizza Steak	470	19	44
Steak	350	11	40
The Original	460	20	41
The Works	490	19	52
Hoagie: Chicken	430	19	42
Chicken Parmesan	440	14	45
Chicken Works	440	14	54
Italian	500	26	40
Tuna	580	35	39
Turkey	420	20	41
Veggie Delite	410	16	55
Philly Lite: Chicken Hoagie	290	3.5	42
Chicken Parmesan	330	6	44
Chicken Works	330	5	54
Grilled Chicken	290	3.5	42
Turkey Hoagie	280	4	41
Veggie Hoagie	260	2.5	54
Specialty: Cheese Chicken	400	12	43
Meatball Parmesan	590	33	46
Sides			
Chicken Tenders, 9.5 oz	600	28	44
Salads			
Cheesesteak	330	18	15
Chicken Tenders	360	15	33
Grilled Chicken Salad	150	2	15
Grilled Chicken Caesar	190	5	13
Philly Lite: Garden	40	0.5	8
Grilled Chicken	150	2	15
Turkey	130	2.5	11
Tuna	290	18	9
Turkey	130	2.5	11
Veggie Delite	230	10	27

Piccadilly Cafeteria®

Meals: No Sides Included	C	F	Cb
Beef: Chopped Steak Fried, 4.5 oz	415	33	6
Roast Leg, small, 4 oz	350	22	2
Steak: Filet Mignon, 6 oz	340	20	1
New York Strip, 10 oz	875	71	1
Ribeye, 10 oz	1040	91	2
Chicken: Breast, Mesquite Smoked	210	8	1
Baked Cajun, Boneless Breast	430	27	9
Fish: Catfish Cajun Baked	405	28	6
Catfish Filet Stuffed	550	40	9
Tilapia Baked	210	11	10
Trout Almondine Baked, large	490	22	11
Trout Cajun Baked	520	27	7
Trout Filets Baked	465	19	10
Pork Loin: Bone in Roast, 5 oz	375	13	10
Shrimp, Fried	460	19	34
Turkey Breast, Carved, 5.5 oz	265	10	5
Salads			
Caesar Salad, 3 oz	145	11	7
Chef's Salad, Small, 6 oz	145	9	4
Italian Coleslaw, 3.7 oz	165	16	5
Louisianne Bowl	45	3	2
Mexican	60	3	8
Piccadilly Bowl	25	0	6
Shrimp Remoulade	515	28	33
Dressings			
Au Jus, 3 fl.oz	5	0	1
Blue Cheese, 2 Tbsp	160	18	1
Cheese Sauce, 2 fl.oz	35	1	5
French, 2 Tbsp	130	13	5
Italian, 2 Tbsp	160	17	1
Ranch, 2 Tbsp	150	17	1
Ranch Fat-Free, 2 Tbsp	35	0	7
Thousand Island, 2 Tbsp	170	18	2
Soups: Per 9.5 oz (No Rice)			
Gumbo: Chicken	100	2	11
& Sausage	225	15	10
Extras			
Broccoli w. Cheese Sauce	105	7	9
Cabbage: Buttered, Steamed	70	5	6
Bacon Seasoned	105	8	6
Cauliflower, Buttered	90	6	8
Fried Okra	240	13	26
Greens: Collard Mustard & Turnip	135	10	3
Turnip w. Diced Turnips, 3.2 oz	150	12	4

Pizza Hut®

	C	F	Cb
Fit 'N Delicious Pizzas: *Per Slice (⅛ Medium Pizza)*			
Diced Chkn, Red Onion, Peppers	170	5	23
Diced Chkn, Mushroom, Jalapeno	170	5	22
Ham, Red Onion, Mushroom	160	4.5	23
Ham, Pineapple, Diced Red Tomato	160	5	24
Peppers, Red Onion, Diced Tom.	150	4	24
Tomato, Mushroom, Jalapeno	150	4	22
Carb Tracker: *Per 6" Pizza*			
Pepperoni	520	29	37
Pepperoni & Mushroom	490	25	39
Meat Lovers	740	46	41
Pan Pizza: *Per Slice (⅛ Medium Pizza)*			
Cheese	270	13	27
Chicken Supreme	270	12	28
Ham	250	11	27
Meat Lover's	370	22	27
Pepperoni	280	14	27
Pepperoni Lover's	330	18	28
Sausage Lover's	360	20	28
Super Supreme	330	17	29
Supreme	310	16	28
Veggie Lover's	250	11	28
Personal Pan Pizza: *Per Pizza*			
Cheese	620	26	69
Ham	570	22	67
Pepperoni	640	29	67
Sausage Lover's	850	47	71
Supreme	710	34	70
Veggie Lover's	560	22	70
Thin 'n Crispy: *Per Slice (⅛ Medium Pizza)*			
Cheese; Chicken Supreme, avg.	200	8	21
Ham	180	7	21
Meat Lover's	310	18	22
Pepperoni	210	10	21
Pepperoni Lover's	260	14	22
Sausage Lover's	280	16	22
Supreme	230	11	22
Super Supreme	250	13	23
Veggie Lover's	180	7	23
Hand Tossed: *Per Slice (⅛ Medium Pizza)*			
Cheese; Chicken Supreme, avg.	230	8	28
Ham	210	6	27
Meat Lover's	330	17	28
Pepperoni	240	9	27
Pepperoni Lover's	290	13	28
Sausage Lover's	310	16	28
Super Supreme	280	13	29
Supreme	260	11	29
Veggie Lover's	210	6	29

Pizza Hut® cont...

	C	F	Cb
Stuffed Crust: *Per Slice (⅛ Large Pizza)*			
Cheese	350	13	40
Chicken Supreme	350	12	41
Ham	340	12	40
Meat Lover's	500	27	41
Pepperoni	380	16	40
Pepperoni Lover's	440	21	41
Super Supreme	430	20	42
Supreme	410	18	42
Veggie Lover's	330	11	41
The Full House XL: *Per Slice*			
Cheese Only	280	12	30
Chicken Supreme	270	10	31
Meat Lover's	380	21	30
Pepperoni	290	13	30
Pepperoni Lover's	310	15	30
Quartered Ham	260	10	30
Sausage Lover's	350	19	31
Super Supreme	330	16	32
Supreme	310	15	31
Veggie Lover's	260	11	32
P'zone Pizza: *Per ½ Pizza*			
Classic	610	21	71
Meat Lover's	680	28	70
Pepperoni	610	22	69
Dessert Pizza: Apple Dessert	260	3.5	53
Cherry Dessert Pizza	240	3.5	47
Pasta: *Per Serving*			
Cavatini Pasta	420	15	55
Cavatini Supreme Pasta	460	18	56
Spaghetti: w. Marinara	490	8	90
w. Meat Sauce	640	20	92
Meatballs	630	19	92
Sides: Breadsticks, 1.3 oz	150	6	20
Buffalo Wings, Hot (1)	55	3	1
Buffalo Wings, Mild (1)	55	3.5	0
Ranch Dipping Cup, 1½ oz	210	24	2
Garlic Bread, 1 piece	170	12	13

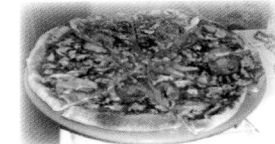

Pizza Pizza® (Canada)

Pizza: Per Slice (⅛ Classic Medium)	C	F	Cb
Bacon Dble Cheeseburger	220	7	29
Big Bacon Bonanza	220	7	29
Canadian Eh!	230	7	30
Cheese	200	5	29
Garden Veggie	190	4.5	30
Harvest Medley	200	4.5	31
New York Style Pepperoni	230	8	29
Pepperoni & Mushroom	210	6	30
Pepperoni	210	6	29
Sicilian	240	9	30
Spicy BBQ Chicken	200	4.5	30
Super	210	6	30
Tropical Hawaiian	220	7	30

Small Pizza: Per Slice
Deduct 10% fewer calories/fat/carbs from figures for medium pizza

Large Pizza: Per Slice
Add 10% more calories/fat/carbs from figures for medium pizza

Classic Slice: Big Bacon, 1 slice	710	26	88
Other varieties, average, 1 sl.	640	19	88
Signature Slice: Bacon Chkn, 1 sl.	830	39	88
Other varieties, average, 1 slice	620	22	85

Oven Toasted Sandwiches

BBQ Chicken	530	8	78
BBQ Chicken, no cheese	475	3	78
Italian Deli Classic	680	32	48
Meatball	520	23	52
Mediterranean Vegetable	560	27	57
Mesquite BBQ Chicken	500	11	62
Philly Cheese Steak	530	14	61
Stuffed S'wich: Classic Super	340	11	45
Mediterranean Vegetarian	390	15	49

Chicken

Bites, 3 pieces	230	11	14
Crispy Wings, 6 wings	720	46	22
Crunchers, 6 pieces	315	22	29
Lightly Breaded Wings, 6 wings	660	40	36
Strips, 3 pieces	310	16	22
Fries: Regular, 5 oz	410	20	55
Big Box, 16 oz	1320	64	176
Garlic Stix: Regular (3)	665	39	68
Four Cheese (3) w. 1 oz cheese	760	47	68
Garlic Bread: Regular, 5 pieces	760	42	79
with Cheese, 4 pieces	800	49	63

Drinks

Lipton's Brisk, 12 fl.oz	120	0	31
Mug Root Beer, 12 fl.oz	160	0	41
Orange Crush, 12 fl.oz	180	0	48
7-UP, 12 fl.oz	160	0	43

Pizza Ranch®

Pizzas, 12 ": Per Slice (⅛ Pizza)	C	F	Cb
Original: BBQ Beef	220	8	28
BBQ Chicken	210	6	27
Bacon Cheeseburger	220	9	26
Beef; Canadian Bacon, avg.	210	7	25
California Chicken	250	12	26
Cheese; Chicken Broccoli, avg.	220	8	26
Garlic Cheese	230	11	25
Italian Sausage; Pepperoni	220	9	25
Prairie; Sweet Swine, avg.	210	7	26
Roundup; Tabasco Pepperoni	230	10	26
Stampede	250	10	27
Texan	240	9	31
Skillet: BBQ Beef	230	8	30
BBQ Chicken	220	6	29
Bacon Cheeseburger	230	9	28
Beef; Canadian Bacon, avg.	220	7	27
Bronco; California Chicken, avg.	270	12	27
Cheese; Chicken Broccoli, avg.	230	8	28
Garlic Cheese	240	11	27
Italian Sausage; Pepperoni, avg.	230	9	27
Prairie; Sweet Swine	220	7	28
Roundup; Tabasco Pepperoni	240	10	28
Stampede	260	11	29
Texan	250	9	33
Thin: BBQ Beef	170	7	17
BBQ Chicken	150	6	16
Bacon Cheeseburger	170	8	15
Beef; Canadian Bacon, avg.	150	7	14
California Chicken; Bronco, avg.	200	11	15
Cheese; Chicken Broccoli, avg.	160	8	14
Garlic Cheese	170	10	14
Italian Sausage; Pepperoni, avg.	160	8	14
Prairie; Sweet Swine, avg.	150	7	15
Roundup; Tabasco Pepperoni	180	9	15
Stampede	190	10	16
Texan	190	9	20
Broasted Chicken: Breast, 1 pce	440	23	4
Leg, 1 piece	190	12	2
Thigh, 1 piece	370	26	4
Wing, 1 piece	190	13	2
Sides: Potato Wedges (1)	60	0	13

For Complete Nutritional Data ~ see CalorieKing.com

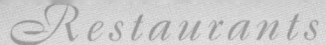

Planet Smoothie®

Cool Blended Smoothies	C	F	Cb
Per 22 fl.oz Unless Otherwise Stated			
Captain Kid, 12 fl oz	195	1.5	47
PBJ	560	17	97
Shag-a-delic	430	1	104
The Last Mango	355	3.5	83
Twig & Berries	300	0.5	74
Vinnie del Rocco	385	3.5	92
Energy Smoothies: Per 22 fl.oz			
Berry Bada-Bing	360	0.5	88
Chocolate Elvis	520	9	109
Frozen Goat	360	0.5	85
Grape Ape	305	0.5	78
Road Runner	280	0.5	72
Spazz	265	0.5	68
Workout Smoothies: Per 22 fl.oz			
Big Bang	350	0.5	80
Chocolate Chimp	400	1	94
Merlin's Planet Living Pineapple	340	1	35
Strawberry	415	1.5	55

Pollo Tropical®

Chicken			
Boneless Chicken Breast, 2 pieces	240	3	0
Quarter Chicken: Dark Meat w. skin	290	18	0
no skin	190	10	0
White Meat w. skin	325	16	0
no skin	205	6	0
TropiChop: Shrimp Creole	505	10	75
Chicken w. Rice & Black Bean	565	10	95
Chicken w. Yellow Rice & Veges	340	5	50
Grilled Chicken Deluxe	410	6	51
Pork w. Rice & Black Beans	715	23	97
Pork w. Yellow Rice & Vegetables	480	21	90
Ropa Vieja (shredded beef)	620	17	98
Vegetarian	580	13	109
Salads: With Dressing			
Balsamic Tomato & Chicken Salad	325	6.5	19
Chicken Caesar Salad w. dressing	670	41	13
Sandwiches			
Chicken Caesar	880	34	71
Grilled Chicken	825	25	84
Sides: Corn Combo, 4 oz	120	4	19
Black Beans: Combo, 4 oz	90	2.5	18
Small, 9 oz	205	5.5	40
Boiled Yucca, Combo, 7.5 oz	190	0	51
Tropical Favorites: Bananas	435	11	89
Yucatan Fries	495	24	69
White Rice, Combo, 4.5 oz	205	3.5	40

For Complete Nutritional Data ~ see CalorieKing.com

Popeye's®

	C	F	Cb
Chicken: Chkn Breast, Mild/Spicy	530	31	18
Chicken Leg, Mild/Spicy	200	12	7
Chicken Thigh, Mild/Spicy	390	29	12
Chicken Wing, Mild/Spicy	220	15	10
Sides: Biscuit, 2.1 oz	240	14	25
Cajun Rice, regular, 4.1 oz	180	7	23
Cinnamon Apple Turnover, 3 oz	250	10	37
Coleslaw, regular, 5 oz	230	17	20
Corn on the Cob (1), 7.8 oz	260	4	48
French Fries, 3 oz	260	12	34
Mashed Potatoes: no Gravy, reg.	100	3	17
w. Gravy, regular, 5 oz	120	4	18
Red Beans & Rice, regular, 6 oz	340	19	33

Port of Subs®

	C	F	Cb
Salads: Includes Dressing			
Caesa Salad	335	30	7
Chef Salad	390	25	13
Garden Salad	95	5	10
Grilled Chicken Caesar Salad	540	34	15
Grilled Chicken Salad	300	10	16
Macaroni Salad	440	30	36
Potato Salad	360	26	54
Tuna Salad	310	23	12
Sandwiches: Per 5" Sub (No Mayonnaise)			
#1 Ham Salami Capicolla			
& Pepperoni w. Provolone	530	26	45
#2 Ham & Turkey w. Provolone	435	15	46
#3 Salami & Turkey w. Provolone	465	20	46
#4 Ham & Salami w. Provolone	470	21	45
#5 Smkd Ham & Turkey w. Cheddar	430	15	47
#6 Vegetarian w. Avocado & Olives	355	15	48
#7 Roast Beef w. Provolone,	420	14	43
#8 Turkey w. Provolone	420	14	47
#9 Peppered Pastrami w. Swiss	440	17	44
#10 Rstd Chicken Brst w. Provolone	410	13	45
#11 Ham w. American	380	20	45
#12 Salami w. Provolone	480	25	45
#13 Combination of Cheeses	510	26	44
#14 Smoked Ham w. Swiss	445	17	45
#15 Salami & Pepperoni w. Prov.	510	27	45
#16 BLT no Cheese	400	19	43
#17 Tuna no Cheese	420	18	45
#18 Rst Beef & Turkey w. Provolone	420	14	45

Port of Subs® cont...

Hot Subs: Per 8" Sub	C	F	Cb
Grilled Chicken	565	11	68
Hot Pastrami	760	17	62
Meatball	655	25	76
Tortilla (1)	200	7	27

Tortilla Wrap: Per Wrap (12" Tortilla)			
Chicken Caesar	630	34	35
Hot Grilled Chkn & Smokey Cheddar	485	18	35
Turkey & Bacon Ranch	590	38	34

Sauces & Dressings: Per 2 Tablespoons			
Mayo & Mustard Mix	110	12	0
Mayonnaise	130	14	0
Mustard	0	0	0

Soups: Medium Bowl (6 oz)			
Campbell's: Boston Clam Chowder	105	4	13
Broccoli Cheese	120	6	13
Minestrone	55	1	8
Roasted Chicken Noodle	85	2	9

Pret A Manger®

Bakery: Almond Croissant	265	15	27
Banana Nut Muffin	600	36	77
Brownie	310	17	34
Carrot Card Box Cake, 4 oz	400	22	46
Oatmeal Muffin	530	10	99
Pecan Pie	240	14	27
Raspberry Bar	270	17	32

Salads: Per Pack			
Chef Salad & Greens	400	24	12
Cobb & Greens	460	25	47
Fresh Mozzarella, Tomato & Greens	380	31	17
Grilled Chicken & Citrus	300	13	20
Chicken Avocado	410	27	41
Tuna, Greens & Organic Egg	230	6	11

Sushi: Deluxe Sushi, 4 rolls, 9 oz	365	3.5	65
Salmon Nigiri, 7 pce, 6 oz	245	3.5	43

Sandwiches			
Bacon Lettuce & Tomato S'wich	550	21	51
Chicken & Avocado Sandwich	580	23	62
Chicken & Bacon Sandwich	520	15	59
Chicken & Mozzarella Baguette	580	19	72
Free-Range Egg Salad Sandwich	250	21	6
Ham & Swiss Baguette	620	16	66
New York Brunch Sandwich	590	18	53
Rst Beef Arugula & Parm. Baguette	670	13	65
Turkey Club Sandwich	530	21	59

Wraps: Avocado Salad	460	30	35
Just Made Mozzarella	630	32	43
Murray's Turkey Club	480	13	39

For Complete Menu ~ See CalorieKing.com

Pretzelmaker®

Pretzels	C	F	Cb
Bites: Small, 3½ oz	280	4.5	53
Medium, 4.6 oz	370	5	70
Large, ½ order, 4.1 oz	320	4.5	62
Cinnamon Sugar, 4.7 oz	410	12	70
Original: Pretzel (1) 4.4 oz	340	2	70
Butter Flavor & Salt (1) 4.6 oz	370	5	71
Caramel Crunch (1) 4.7 oz	390	6	74
Cinnamon (1) 4.6 oz	380	5	74
Garlic (1) 4.7 oz	380	6	72
Iced Cinnamon Swirl (1) 5.3 oz	470	9	87
Parmesan (1) 4.7 oz	390	6	72
Poppy Seed (1) 4.6 oz	380	6	71
Pretzel Dog (1) 5.6 oz	490	30	38
Sesame (1) 4.6 oz	380	6	71

Sauces: Per Container			
Caramel, 2 oz	140	0	35
Cheddar Cheese, 1½ oz	130	10	6
Chili Spice, 1½ oz	360	5	72
Cream Cheese/Icing, 2 oz	200	20	2
Honey Mustard, 1½ oz	80	0	20
Ketchup, 2 packets, 0.6 oz	20	0	4
Mustard, 2 packets, 0.3 oz	10	0	1
Nachos Cheese, 1½ oz	105	7.5	4
Pizza Sauce, 1½ oz	20	0.5	6

Beverages			
Smoothies (20 fl.oz): Coffee	640	21	107
Mocha	620	20	106
Peach; Raspberry	650	20	117
Strawberry Banana	650	20	115
Fat Free: Peach; Raspberry	480	0	130
Mrs Fields Lemonade: Small, 20 fl.oz	160	0	39
Medium, 32 fl.oz	255	0	63
Large, 44 fl.oz	350	0	86

Pretzel Time®

Pretzels			
Bites: Plain, small, 3 oz	210	0.5	45
medium, 4 oz	280	1	59
large, 3.5 oz	250	1	52
Whirl & Salt, small, 3.2 oz	240	3.5	45
medium, 4.2 oz	310	4	59
large, 4 oz	270	3.5	52
Caramel Crunch (1), 4.7 oz	335	4	66
Cinnamon Sugar (1), 4.1 oz	330	4	65
Italian Parmesan (1), 4.2 oz	310	3.5	60
Plain, 3.8 oz	280	1	59
Sour Cream & Onion (1), 4.2 oz	310	3.5	60

Pretzel Time® cont...

Pretzels	C	F	Cb
Stuffers: Cheese, regular, 13 oz	1200	69	95
small, 7.6 oz	700	36	82
Jalapeno, regular, 13.6 oz	1210	69	97
small, 8 oz	700	38	64
Whirl & Salt (1), 4 oz	310	4	59
Pretzel Dog, 5.5 oz	480	29	38
Sauces & Dressings: Per Container			
Caramel, 2 oz	190	0	47
Cream Cheese Icing, 2 oz	200	20	2
Cheddar/ Nacho Cheese, 2 oz	80	5	6
Cream Cheese, 2 oz	200	20	4
Ketchup, ½ oz	20	0	4
Mustard, ½ oz	10	0	1
Pizza Sauce	20	0.5	6
Mrs Fields Lemonade: 20 fl.oz	160	0	39
32 fl.oz	280	0	65

Quizno's Subs®

Signature Subs: No Dressing	C	F	Cb
Classic Italian Sub: Small, 9 oz	645	30	60
Regular, 11½ oz	730	33	69
Large, 19½ oz	1200	58	102
Honey Mustard Chkn w. bacon, large	1355	40	137
Philly Cheese Steak, large, 10½ oz	720	16	92
Steakhouse Sub (6"), 6½ oz	510	21	52
The Traditional (8") 16 oz	800	24	94
Turkey Ranch Swiss (8")	690	18	89
Low-Fat Subs (Small): Turkey Lite	335	6	52
Honey Bourbon Chicken	360	6	45
Sierra Smoked Turkey w. Sauce	350	6	53
Flatbread Sandwiches: No Dressing			
Antipasto	760	40	62
Classic Cobb	515	13	62
Chicken Caesar	560	12	62
Roasted Chicken	660	23	62
Flatbread Chopped Salads: No Dressing			
Classic Cobb	530	16	57
Chicken	745	33	57
Chicken Caesar	640	22	57
Antipasto	905	54	61
Dressings: Beef Au Jus, 4½ oz	25	0.5	3
Caesar Dressing	295	32	2
Honey Mustard, 2 oz	140	6	22
Italian Vinaigrette, 1 oz	130	14	3
Ranch Dressing, 2 oz	285	30	3
Toasted Gourmet Bread Bowls			
Country French Chicken	830	31	96
Southwest Chicken	850	33	96
Signature Steak 'N Chili	885	34	101

Rally's Hamburgers®

Burgers/Sandwiches	C	F	Cb
Rallyburger	435	22	35
with Cheese	490	27	35
Big Buford	745	48	35
Chicken Fillet Sandwich	400	15	43
Chili w. Cheese & Onion: 7 oz	360	22	20
13 oz size	670	41	37
Super Barbecue Bacon	595	31	49
Super Double Cheeseburger	760	48	37
French Fries: Regular	210	11	26
Large	320	16	39
X-Large	425	21	52
Shakes: Vanilla, small	320	11	49
Other flavors, small	410	12	73

Ranch 1®

	C	F	Cb
Salads: Gourmet Greens	220	7	31
Chicken on Gourmet Greens	350	11	31
Zesty Caesar Salad	180	3	31
Zesty Chicken Caesar Salad	280	6	31
Sandwiches: American Rancher	390	10	51
Club Sandwich	470	16	53
Grilled Chicken Philly	450	14	53
Ranch Classic	370	5	53
Spicy Grilled Chicken	420	11	58
Side Kicks: Fruit Cup, 8.3 oz	90	0.5	18
Ranch Fries, regular, 4.5 oz	350	14	51
Specialties: Chicken Tenders	370	15	7
Baked Potato: w. Broccoli	510	0.5	117
w. Cheese	790	25	118
w. Chicken	610	4	114
Grilled Chkn & Vegetable Platter	790	7	129
Grilled Chicken Fajita	330	16	25
Grilled Chicken Hot Pasta	580	10	86

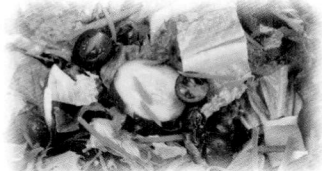

Note: Figures are only estimates
For extra listings and data ~ See CalorieKing.com

Rax®

Sandwiches	C	F	Cb
Regular Rax	390	22	32
Deluxe	520	35	35
BBC	715	51	37
Grilled Chicken: Philly Melt	535	32	35
Jr. Deluxe	365	25	25
BBQ Beef	400	20	43
Mushroom Melt	600	38	35
Turkey/Bacon Club	680	47	37
Turkey	485	32	33
Cheddar Melt	345	23	26
Potatoes: Cheese/Broccoli	285	0	72
Plain: No Topping	205	0	60
w. Butter	305	12	60
w. Sour Topping	255	4	62
Soups: Cream of Broccoli	95	4	14
Chicken Noodle	115	1	21
Chili	160	9	12
Salads: Grilled Chicken	160	5	6
Side Salad	40	4	2
Garden	220	9	12
Salad Dressings: Fat Free Italian	10	0	2
Fat Free Catalina; Ranch	30	0	6
1000 Island	130	13	5
Buttermilk Ranch	175	20	1
Blue Cheese; Creamy Caesar	145	16	1
Honey French	140	5	9
Vinaigrette	30	2	4

Red Lobster®

Lighthouse Menu	C	F	Cb
Fresh Fish: Per Serving			
Broiled Flounder, lunch portion	240	5	0
Atlantic Salmon, full portion	580	33	0
Atlantic Salmon, half portion	260	12	0
Broiled Flounder, dinner portion	240	5	0
Rainbow Trout, full portion	510	25	6
Rainbow Trout, half portion	275	14	0
Tilapia, full portion	345	10	0
Tilapia, half portion	185	6	0
Meals: Per Serving			
Grilled Chicken Breast	315	8	0
Signature Shellfish: Per Serving			
Garlic Chili Jumbo Shrimp	140	3	1
Grilled Jumbo Shrimp Dinner	140	3	1
Jumbo Shrimp Cocktail Dinner	230	4	2
Live Maine Lobster, 1¼lb	145	1	2
Lobster Chops	320	8.5	0
North Pacific King Crab Legs	490	9	0
Rock Lobster Tail	260	3	0
Snow Crab Legs	260	4.5	0

Red Lobster® cont...

Sides: Per Serving	C	F	Cb
100% Pure Melted Butter, 1 oz	190	21	0
Baked Potato w. Pico de Gallo	185	2	37
Baked Potato, no topping	180	2	36
Cheddar Bay Biscuit (1)	160	9	17
Cocktail Sauce, large	85	2	17
Garden Salad	50	2	9
Jumbo Shrimp Cocktail	140	2	1
King Crab Legs	165	3	0
Lemon Wedge (1)	10	0	2
Petite Shrimp Topping	30	1	1
Red Wine Vinaigrette Dressing	50	3	5
Seasonal Vegetables w. butter	145	11	9
Seasoned Broccoli	55	0	10
Snow Crab Legs	130	2	0
Wild Rice Pilaf	205	5	36

For Complete Nutritional Data ~ see CalorieKing.com

Rita's®

	C	F	Cb
Italian Ice: Kids, 7.5 oz	165	0	43
Regular, 12 oz	265	0	69
Large, 19 oz	415	0	109
Quart, 32 oz	705	0	185
Cream Ice: Kids, 7.5 oz	195	2	44
Regular, 12 oz	310	4	70
Large, 19 oz	495	6	109
Quart, 32 oz	830	11	187
Custard: Kids, 5 oz	285	15	32
Regular, 6.75 oz	555	30	62
Large, 9.75 oz	555	30	62
Gelati w. Custard: Vanilla, Reg., 10 oz	365	13	59
Vanilla, large, 17 oz	560	17	102
Chocolate, regular, 10 oz	350	11	60
Chocolate, large, 17 oz	535	14	101
Misto w. Custard: Van., reg., 15 oz	420	7	90
Vanilla, large, 23 oz	620	10	135
Chocolate, regular, 15 oz	410	7	90
Chocolate, large, 23 oz	605	9	135
Sugar Free: (w. Sorbitol)			
Ice: Kids, 7.5 oz	60	0	24
Regular, 12 oz	100	0	39
Gelati w. Van. Custard, reg., 10 oz	285	13	45
Misto w. Van. Custard, reg., 15 oz	245	8	57

For Complete Nutritional Data ~ see CalorieKing.com

Rocky Rococo®

C **F** **Cb**

Pastas: Per Serving	C	F	Cb
Can't Decide, 14 oz	465	9	77
Fettuccine w. Alfredo Sauce:			
Regular, 14 oz	460	14	66
Light, 7 oz	230	7	33
Spaghetti with Meat Sauce: Reg.	485	7	87
Light, 7 oz	250	3	44
Spaghetti w. Meatballs: Reg., 15 oz	630	16	89
Light, 7.5 oz	315	8	45
Spaghetti w. Tomato Sauce: Reg.	470	4	87
Light, 7 oz	235	2	44

Pizzas: Per Regular Slice			
Cheese	380	9	54
Garden	390	10	56
Pepperoni	425	13	54
Sausage	495	19	54
Sausage Mushroom	500	19	55

Sides			
Breadsticks: w. Marinara Sce (6)	420	7	72
w. Jalapeno Cheese Sauce (6)	530	18	72
Wheat Muffin (1)	200	4	38

Roly Poly®

C **F** **Cb**

Sandwiches: Per ½ Sandwich (Wheat Bread)	C	F	Cb
Baked Ham & Roast Pork:			
BarBQ Pork Melt	300	10	26
Italian Classic	330	12	28
Key West Cuban Mix	300	9	27
Peachtree Melt	330	11	28
Porky's Nightmare	310	12	26
Chicken: Basil Cashew Chicken	290	11	27
Catalina Chicken Salad	305	12	26
Chicken Caesar	310	12	28
Chicken Cordon Bleu	305	11	27
Chicken Fajita	280	8	27
Chicken Popper	245	7	29
Cobb Salad	320	14	28
Delhi Chicken	320	12	32
Hickory Chicken	335	11	27
Oriental Chicken	260	6	30
Santa Fe Chicken	285	8	29
Seafood: Salmon Club	295	13	28
Salmon Roll	280	11	28
Texas Tuna Melt	310	13	26
Thai Hot Tuna	330	13	27
Tuna Luau	325	15	28

Round Table® Pizza

C **F** **Cb**

Large Pizza (14"): Per Slice (½ Whole)	C	F	Cb
Cheese: Pan Crust	300	9	38
Skinny Crust	190	8	18
Chkn & Garlic Gourmet: Pan Crust	330	11	39
Skinny Crust	210	9	19
Chicken Smokehouse: Pan Crust	350	12	39
Skinny Crust	230	10	20
Gourmet Veggie: Pan Crust	320	11	40
Skinny Crust	200	9	19
Guinevere's Garden Delight: Pan Cr.	300	8	39
Skinny Crust	180	7	20
Hawaiian: Pan Crust	310	8	40
Skinny Crust	190	7	20
Italian Garlic Supreme: Pan Crust	360	15	39
Skinny Crust	240	13	18
King Arthur Supreme: Pan Crust	340	12	39
Skinny Crust	240	12	19
Maui Zaui w. Polynesian Sce: Pan	340	11	43
Skinny Crust	220	9	22
Maui Zaui w. Zesty Red Sce: Pan Cr.	330	11	40
Skinny Crust	220	9	20
Montague's All Meat Marvel: Pan	360	14	38
Skinny Crust	260	14	18
Pepperoni: Pan Crust	320	11	38
Skinny Crust	210	10	18
Smokehouse Combo: Pan Crust	370	14	40
Skinny Crust	250	13	20
Ulti-Meat Premium All-Meat: Pan	390	16	38
Skinny Crust	270	15	18
Wombo Combo: Pan Crust	360	14	39
Skinny Crust	240	12	19

Sandwiches			
Chicken Club	760	34	67
Ham Club	810	37	76
RT Pizza Sandwich	690	34	65
RT Veggie Sandwich	680	29	79
Turkey Club	800	37	75

Sides			
Buffalo Wings, 6 pieces	420	28	2
Garlic Bread, 4.7 oz	470	21	59
Garlic Bread with Cheese, 6.7 oz	630	33	59
Honey BBQ Wings, 6 pieces	390	25	8

For Complete Nutritional Data ~ see CalorieKing.com

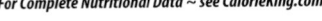

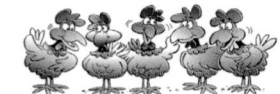

Roy Rogers®

Breakfast Itrems	C	F	Cb
Big Country Breakfast: w. Bacon	740	43	61
w. Sausage	920	60	61
w. Ham	710	39	67
Burgers			
Hamburger	260	9	33
Cheeseburger	300	13	34
¼ lb Hamburger	430	18	41
¼ lb Cheeseburger	470	22	42
Sourdough Grilled Chicken	500	21	46
Sandwiches: Roast Beef	260	4	30
Chicken Fillet	500	24	49
Grilled Chicken	340	11	32
Fries: Regular	350	15	49
Large	430	18	59
Desserts: Hot Fudge Sundae	320	10	50

Rubio's Fresh Mexican Grill®

Burritos	C	F	Cb
Baja Gourmet Seafood: Fish	740	40	70
Langostino Lobster	670	32	79
Baja Grill: Carne Asada	680	32	58
Carnitas	630	29	59
Chicken	630	24	59
Bean & Cheese Burrito	820	36	88
Especial: Carne Asada	940	37	117
Carnitas	890	33	118
Chicken	890	29	117
Fish Burrito	740	40	70
Grilled Mesquite Shrimp Burrito	710	31	77
HealthMex: Chicken	530	10	77
Veggie	520	8	98
Mahi Mahi Burrito	720	36	56
Street Burrito: Carne Asada	330	13	34
Carnitas	300	11	35
Chicken	300	7	34
Tacos			
Carne Asada w. Corn Tortilla	250	10	23
Carnitas w. Corn Tortilla	230	9	34
Chicken w. Corn Tortilla	300	15	24
Fish, Especial w. Corn Tortilla	370	22	29
Fish, Original w. Corn Tortilla	300	16	27
HealthMex: Chicken	170	3	22
Mahi Mahi	180	3	22
Mahi Mahi w. Corn Tortilla	310	16	23
Street Taco: Carne Asada	130	6	10
Carnitas	110	5	11
Chicken	110	3.5	10
Taquitos, Chicken (3)	290	11	34

Rubio's cont...

Quesadillas	C	F	Cb
Carne Asada Quesadilla	990	61	58
Cheese Quesadilla	830	52	56
Chicken Quesadilla	950	54	58
Shrimp Quesadilla	920	56	58
Torta Sandwiches: Carne Asada	390	26	23
Carnitas	370	24	23
Chicken	370	23	23
Salads			
Baja Caesar Salad	500	37	16
Chicken Chopped Salad	570	33	35
Chicken Fiesta Salad	480	33	12
Chipotle Ranch Salad	750	51	42
HealthMex Chicken Salad	260	2	34
Dressings: Serrano Grape, 1.3 oz	40	0	9
Meals			
Grilled Grande Bowl: Carne Asada	730	40	60
Chicken	690	33	60
Mahi Mahi	710	35	58
Shrimp	670	35	61
Nachos: Grande	1270	78	111
Carne Asada	1420	87	113
Chicken	1380	80	113
Three Taco Combos: w. Chips & Beans			
Carne Asada	1060	44	116
Carnitas	1010	41	118
Chicken	1220	59	117
Fish Especial	1420	78	134
Fish	1220	62	128
Burrito Combos: w. Chips & Beans			
Baja Grill Carne Asada	990	44	104
Baja Grill Carnitas	940	42	106
Baja Grill Chicken	940	36	105
Fish	1050	52	116
Sides			
Cheese, 1 oz	100	8	1
Sour Cream, 1 oz	60	6	1
Black Beans, 7 oz	170	2	28
Carne Asada, 3 oz	160	8	2
Carnitas, 3 oz	120	6	3
Chicken, 3 oz	120	2	2
Chips, 1½ oz	220	11	28
Chips, side order, 3 oz	430	22	56
Churro, 1½ oz	170	8	22
Guacamole: Small, 3.7 oz	170	16	8
Large, 7.7 oz	340	32	16
Original & Pinto Beans, 9.3 oz	420	18	50
Pinto Beans, 7 oz	190	3	37
Rice: 2 oz	80	1	16
Side order, 4 oz	160	1.5	33

For Complete Nutritional Data ~ see CalorieKing.com

243

Ruby Tuesday®

	C	F	Cb
Appetizers: Per ¼ Order (Sauces Not Included)			
Asian Spiced Dumplings	130	6	14
Bacon Cheese Fries	300	17	27
Chicken Quesadilla	225	14	12
Jumbo Lump Crabcake	70	4	4
Southwestern Spring Rolls	175	10	16
Spicy Buffalo Wings	220	16	3
Thai Phoon Shrimp	195	13	12
The Sampler	325	19	19
Tuesday Tenders, Classic	120	6	8
Tuesday Tenders, Spicy Buffalo	180	12	10
Beef: Sides and Sauces Not Included			
Peppercorn Mushroom Sirloin	495	28	10
Petitie Sirloin	205	5	2
Premium Aged Prime Sirloin	545	30	0
Ribeye	590	35	6
Petite Sirloin	205	5	2
Top Sirloin	255	6	2
Premium Baby Back Ribs:			
Classic BBQ, full rack	1600	96	92
Classic BBQ, half rack	1105	64	77
Memphis Dry Rub	1685	111	70
Memphis Dry Rub, half rack	1150	71	66
Triple Play	1670	91	120
Chicken & Seafood: No Sides, Bread, Sauces			
Baked Chicken & Broccoli Pasta	2060	128	122
Baked Chicken Parmesan Pasta	1655	96	126
Chicken Portobello	920	52	41
Gourmet Chicken Pot Pie	1325	105	34
Smoky Mountain Chicken	1065	58	48
Smart Eating: Chicken Portobello	520	27	9
Grilled Chicken	295	8	0
Creole Catch	660	31	43
Louisiana Fried Shrimp	825	42	73
New Orleans Seafood	845	46	45
Shrimp Pasta Parmesan	1220	64	108
Smart Eating, Creole Catch	310	16	0
Smart Eating, New Orleans Seafood	495	31	2
Salad Dressings & Sauces			
Avocado Ranch Dressing, 1 oz	60	5	3
Bleu Cheese Dressing, 1 oz	175	19	1
Caesar Dressing, 1 oz	95	10	2
Honey Mustard Dressing, 1 oz	90	8	5
Ranch Dressing, 1 oz	100	11	1
Light Ranch Dressing, 1 oz	55	5	1
Smoky Honey Dijon Dressing, 1 oz	100	8	7
Marinara Sauce, 1 oz	15	1	2
Sour Cream, 1 oz	30	2	2

	C	F	Cb
Salads: Dressing Not Included			
Carolina Chicken	1025	72	45
Club House	900	60	38
Fresh Tomato & Mozarella	110	7	7
Skinny Chicken	380	15	10
Tossed Caesar	175	15	7
Sandwiches & Burgers: No Sides			
Alpine Swiss Burger	1265	89	61
Bacon Avocado Turkey	1025	63	56
Bacon Cheeseburger	1195	85	52
Bison Bacon Cheeseburger	1070	71	53
Bison Burger	890	57	53
Buffalo Bleu Chicken	1030	71	67
Chicken BLT Burger	980	63	64
Classic Cheeseburger	1105	78	52
Colossal Burger	1945	141	81
Hickory Chicken Burger	910	51	64
Portobello Swiss Turkey	1040	62	56
Ruby's Classic	1015	71	52
Ruby's Minis, 4 burgers	1275	86	74
Smokehouse Burger	1390	96	78
Veggie Burger	945	52	75
Turkey Burger	810	45	53
Jumbo Lump Crab Burger	755	45	63
Ruby's Triple Prime Burger	885	56	53
Turkey Sandwich	655	34	53
Smart Eating Wraps: Chicken	450	26	21
Turkey Burger	420	17	21
Desserts			
Blondie	675	31	93
Chocolate Tallcake	590	23	85
Double Chocolate Cake	980	48	124
Fresh Strawberries & Cream	220	8	30
Sides			
Fresh Hot Fries	360	13	57
Baked Potato: Plain, no dressing	295	2	60
w. Butter & Sour Cream	460	19	62
w. Cheese & Bacon	615	32	63
Brown Rice Pilaf w. Cheese & Tom.	220	6	35
Creamy Mashed Cauliflower	165	11	15
Sauteed Portobello Mushroom Slices	130	11	6
White Cheddar Mashed Potatoes	275	16	24
Soups: No Bread or Crackers			
Broccoli & Cheese	335	27	15
Garden Vegetable	185	7	21
White Bean Chicken Chili	220	8	28
For Complete Menu ~ see CalorieKing.com			

Runza®

Sandwiches

	C	F	Cb
Original Overstuffed Sandwich	495	17	65
Cheese Overstuffed Sandwich	555	21	66
BBQ Chicken Sandwich, grilled	390	9	46
Fish Sandwich	485	23	49
Polish Dog	425	26	30
Smothered Chicken, grilled	380	10	41
Special Deluxe Chicken, grilled	380	12	40

Burgers

	C	F	Cb
Junior: Cheeseburger	325	17	28
Cheeseburger Runza	305	14	30
Swiss Mushroom	380	21	26
Legendary: ¼ lb Cheeseburger	430	21	32
½ lb Double Cheeseburger	640	32	37
¼ lb Bacon Cheeseburger	515	29	36
¼ lb Legend Supreme	765	37	62
¼ lb Swiss Cheese Mushroom	450	25	36

Sides

	C	F	Cb
French Fries: Small, 3.1 oz	280	15	31
Medium	410	23	46
Large	625	35	70
Frings, 6.3 oz	540	28	64
Onion Rings: Medium, 4 oz	370	20	41
Large, 6.5 oz	590	32	66
Onion Ring Dip, 2.1 oz	90	6	4

Salads: No Dressing

	C	F	Cb
Tossed Salad w. Crispy Chicken	435	27	29
Tossed Salad w. Grilled Chicken	275	13	13
Dressing: Ranch, 2.4 oz	300	32	5
Reduced Calorie Ranch, 2.5 oz	170	11	17
Lite Italian, 2.6 oz	85	5	10
Raspberry Vinaigrette	25	0	6

Soups: Per Bowl

	C	F	Cb
Boston Clam Chowder	320	23	33
Broccoli Cheese	360	27	35
Cauliflower Cheese	335	26	32
Chicken Noodle	170	5	21
Homemade Chili	310	10	26
Potato w. Bacon	305	20	40
Vegetable Cheese	330	22	28
Wisconsin Cheese	425	35	36
Kids-Size: Mini Corn Dogs (5)	275	17	25
Chicken Strips (2)	185	10	11

Desserts & Drinks

	C	F	Cb
Chocolate Chip Cookie (1)	310	16	34
Vanilla Shake, regular, 12 fl.oz	465	16	69
Oreo Shake, regular, 12 fl.oz	605	24	84
Pepsi Slushie, medium, 18 fl.oz	225	0	60

Ryan's® Family Steakhouse

Main Courses: Sides Not Included

	C	F	Cb
BBQ Beef, 6 oz	225	12	9
BBQ Chicken, ¼, 5 oz	230	15	5
Carved Turkey Breast, 6 oz	280	12	0
Chkn Fried Beef Steak (1), no gravy	180	9	16
Chkn Fried Beef Steak (1), w. gravy	220	11	24
Chicken Pot Pie, 8 oz	350	16	48
Grilled Chicken Breast, plain, 6 oz	280	18	0
Grilled Pork Chop: Plain, 1 chop	240	14	1
BBQ; Teriyaki, avg., 1 chop	160	8	8
Grilled Salmon, 7 oz entree	240	9	0
Grilled Sliced Sausage: BBQ Sce, 6 oz	555	48	0
in Peppers and Onions, 6 oz	450	42	6.5
Grilled Teriyaki Chicken Thighs, 6 oz	215	6	5
Macaroni and Cheese, 8 oz	350	16	40
Meat Lasagne, 8 oz	370	16	30
Meat Loaf, 4 oz	220	12	9
Mexican Casserole, 8 oz	415	16	46
Pizza: Cheese, 1 slice, 3½ oz	200	10	11
Pepperoni, 1 slice, 3½ oz	230	13	10
Rotisserie Chicken, ¼, 5 oz	250	15	0
Salisbury Steak w. gravy, 1 patty	200	11	11
Sirloin Steak: 8 oz	485	33	0
10½ oz	640	44	0
16 oz	970	67	0
Sirloin Tips, 5.5 oz	330	23	0
Stuffed Alaskan Pollock Fillet, 6 oz	360	30	18
Taco Beef, 4 oz	180	10	8
Vegetable Lasagne, 8 oz	355	16	30
White Turkey w. gravy, 6 oz	140	3	6.5

Sides: Baked Potato, plain, 8 oz

	C	F	Cb
Sides: Baked Potato, plain, 8 oz	250	0	57
Bowtie Pasta and Veges, 8 oz	210	0	38
Chicken Salad, Low-Fat, 8 oz	245	4	24
Coleslaw, 4 oz	180	12	12
Corn Cobbet (1) 4 oz	90	6	11
Garlic Mashed Potatoes, 4 oz	120	4	16
Glazed Baby Carrots w. Sauce, 4 oz	125	8	12
Low Carb Grilled Veges, 4 oz	40	0	8
Marinated 7-Bean Salad, 6 oz	300	0	66
Pinto Beans, 4 oz	105	2	16
Potato Salad, 6 oz	280	12	33
Sweet Pot. w. M'mallows, 4 oz	240	18	16
Yellow Squash w. Onions, 4 oz	50	2	7

Desserts: Cheesecake, plain, 1 sl.

	C	F	Cb
Desserts: Cheesecake, plain, 1 sl.	190	15	11
Ice Cream Cone (flat bottom)	20	0	4
Key Lime Pie, 1 slice	410	17	58
Lemon Creme Cake, 1 slice	170	15	9
Cookies: Oatmeal Raisin (1)	110	3.5	18
Sugar Cookie (1)	120	5	18

245

7-Eleven®

Breakfast Sandwiches	C	F	Cb
Big Bite Breakfast Sandwich	430	27	29
Croissant: w. Bacon, Egg & Chse	400	33	34
w. Ham, Egg & Chse	390	22	34
Engl. Muffin w. Saus., Egg, Chse	450	24	37
Sausage, Egg & Cheese Biscuit	500	31	34
Sausage, Egg & Twister Roll	430	27	29

Hot Dogs (Big Bite)			
¼ Pound Hot Dog, no bun	360	34	6
⅓ Pound Hot Dog, no bun	480	45	3
Spicy Bite, 1 link, 4 oz	425	38	2
Bacon Cheeseburger Bite, no bun	270	12	1

Reynoldos Jumbo Burritos (10 oz)			
Beef & Bean; Beef & Potato	590	20	82
Red Hot Burrito	640	20	88
Green Burrito	710	26	93

Sandwiches (7-Eleven)			
Black Forest Ham	380	6	59
Chicken Salad, 7.3 oz	500	28	44
Chicken w. Ancho Lime Spread	500	26	47
Classic Chicken Caesar, 8.3 oz	590	27	45
Classic Sub on Roll, 7.6 oz	380	6	49
Combo Sub w. Turkey, 5.5 oz	270	7	33
Ham & Swiss, 4.9 oz	330	11	39
Hearty Ham, 8.3 oz	570	30	48
Pastrami & Swiss on Wheat	480	21	48
Smoked Turkey w. Chse/Mayo	550	27	46
Turkey & Ham on Tom. Basil Brd	490	23	42
Turkey & Ham on White Bread	350	6	53
Tuna Salad, 7.5 oz	540	27	45

Bakery Stix™ Treats: Per Stick (3.5 oz)			
Grilled Cheese	270	11	30
Ham & Cheese	280	12	32
Pepperoni & Cheese	340	18	30

Sushi: California Rolls, 3 pieces	155	2	39
Imperial Rolls, 3 pieces	210	11	22

Salads			
Tuna Macaroni Salad, 8 oz	270	8	29
Reser's Coleslaw, 3 ½ oz	130	7	17
Reser's Macaroni Salad, 3 ½ oz	220	15	20
Reser's Potato Salad, 3 ½ oz	200	10	19

Go-Go Taquitos			
Beef Taco & Cheese, 3 oz (1)	250	11	30
Fiesta Chicken, 3 oz (1)	220	12	23
Jalapeno & Cream cheese, 3 oz	240	13	27
Monterey Jack Chkn, 3 oz (1)	280	14	30
Go-Go French Toast Sticks, 3 oz	270	16	23

7-Eleven® cont...

Donuts & Muffins (World Ovens)	C	F	Cb
Donuts: Blueberry Cake (1)	330	22	31
Chocolate Iced (1)	250	11	35
Glazed (1)	250	16	24
Jelly (1)	420	16	66
Sour Cream Donut (1)	450	19	65
Muffins: Banana Nut, 7 oz	660	26	97
Blueberry, 5.6 oz	310	8	54
Brownies: Original, 5 oz	570	28	83
Peanut Butter Cup Brownie, 4.4 oz	560	20	55
Walnut Brownie, 5 oz	600	31	78

Fountain Drinks (Figures Assume ⅓ Ice)			
Coca-Cola/Pepsi/Dr.Pepper/7Up:			
Gulp, 20 oz	195	0	51
Big Gulp, 32 oz	310	0	82
Super Gulp, 44 oz	430	0	112
Double Gulp, 64 oz	625	0	163
Diet Coke/Diet Pepsi, 16 oz	1	0	0
Slurpees: Average All Flavors,			
12 oz size	95	0	24
22 oz size	175	0	44
28 oz size	220	0	56
40 oz size	315	0	80
Crystal Light, 12 fl.oz	45	0	9
Hawaiian Punch; Dr Pepper, avg.,			
12 oz size	180	0	48
22 oz size	330	0	88
28 oz size	420	0	112
40 oz size	600	0	160
Cafe Select Coffee: 12 fl.oz	8	0	2
16 fl.oz size	10	0	2
20 fl.oz size	14	0	3
24 fl.oz size	16	0	4
Hot Drinks: Hot Chocolate, 8 fl.oz	180	3	36
French Vanilla Cappuccino, 8 fl.oz	160	6	26

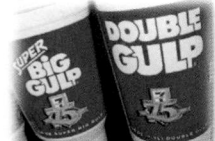

Sammy's®
Woodfired Pizza

Healthy Dining Meals	C	F	Cb
Pasta: Grilled Vegetable Penne	620	21	84
Tomato Angel Hair Pasta	700	18	115
Individual Salad: Chinese Chicken	450	12	47
Chopped Chicken	425	11	30
Oak Roasted Salmon on Ponzu	470	19	21
Fresh Tomato Basil Soup	110	5	10
Roast Chicken Pesto Wrap	480	20	22
Vegetarian Pizza, ½ pizza	885	21	130

Samurai Sam's®

Bowls: Per Regular Bowl (w with White Rice)			
Low-Carb Bowl	230	4	16
Spicy Beef'n Broccoli	620	13	97
Sweet & Sour Dark Chicken	610	10	96
Sweet & Sour White Chicken	580	4.5	96
Teriyaki Dark Chicken & Steak	540	9	83
Teriyaki Dark Chicken	540	10	79
Teriyaki Steak	530	8	86
Teriyaki Veggie	370	5	80
Teriyaki White Chicken & Steak	520	6	83
Teriyaki White Chicken	520	4	79
Salads: Oriental Chicken	220	4	9
Sesame Garden Toss	490	13	57
Sides: Grilled Chicken Egg Roll, 3 oz	150	7	17
Oriental Salad Dressing, 1 oz	70	2	12
Teriyaki Sauce, 1 oz	40	0	9
Wraps: with White Rice			
Teriyaki Dark Chicken	670	16	95
Teriyaki Steak	650	14	101
Teriyaki Veggie	510	8	94
Teriyaki White Chicken & Steak	650	13	98
Teriyaki White Chicken	640	11	96

Sbarro's®

Entrees	C	F	Cb
Baked Ziti w. Sauce	700	41	43
Chicken Parmigiana	520	22	16
Meat Lasagna	650	37	36
Spaghetti w. Sauce	820	28	120
Pizza: Per Slice			
Cheese	460	13	60
Pepperoni	730	37	61
Sausage	670	31	60
Supreme	630	27	63
Stuffed Pizza: Per Slice			
Spinach & Broccoli	790	34	89
Pepperoni	960	42	89

Schlotzsky's®

Oven-Toasted Sandwiches: Per Medium Sandwich	C	F	Cb
Angus, Beef & Provolone	750	28	78
Angus, Corned Beef Reuben	890	41	74
Angus, Corned Beef	570	13	76
Angus, Pastrami Reuben	890	40	74
Angus, Pastrami & Swiss	880	36	78
Angus, Roast, Beef & Cheese	770	32	73
BLT	550	22	71
Chicken & Pesto	550	13	71
Chicken Breast	490	5	75
Chipotle Chicken	530	11	71
Chipotle Grilled Chicken	540	12	74
Dijon Chicken	570	10	79
Dijon Grilled Chicken	580	10	82
Fresh Veggie	460	10	76
Grilled Chicken & Pesto	560	13	74
Grilled Chicken Breast	500	6	77
Homestyle Tuna	590	19	73
Mediterranean Tuna	520	10	75
Santa Fe Chicken	590	14	74
Santa Fe Grilled Chicken	600	14	77
Smoked Turkey Breast	490	7	75
Smoked Turkey Reuben	700	36	44
Texas Schlotzsky's	720	29	73
Turkey & Guacamole	540	11	78
Turkey Bacon Club	760	29	77
Original Style: The Original	750	33	74
Cheese	770	37	74
Deluxe	950	46	78
Ham & Cheese	690	25	75
Turkey	800	32	77
Panini: Classic Swiss & Tomato	610	26	63
Grilled Chicken Romano	540	16	64
Italiano	710	31	66
Mozzarella & Portobello	500	16	66
Smoked Ham Crostini	610	23	66
Smoked Turkey & Guacamole	590	22	70
Wraps: Asian Chicken	370	4	70
Feta & Portobello	490	32	45
Grilled Chicken & Guacamole	520	28	50
Homestyle Tuna	360	13	45
Mediterranean Tuna	310	7	47
Parmesan Chicken Caesar	490	26	47
Bread/Buns: Dark Rye, medium	330	2	68
Jalapeno Cheese, medium	340	4	63
Sourdough, medium	330	2	67
Wheat, medium	340	3	67

Continued Next Page ...

Fast - Foods & *Restaurants*

Schlotzsky's® cont...

8" Pizzas: Per Pizza	C	F	Cb
BBQ Chicken & Jalapeno	660	15	98
Baby Spinach Salad	460	8	82
Bacon, Tomato & Mushroom	620	25	75
Combination Special	640	26	75
Double Cheese	600	23	74
Fresh Tomato & Pesto	560	20	72
Grilled Chicken & Pesto	640	22	74
Mediterranean	550	20	72
Pepperoni & Double Cheese	690	31	74
Smoked Turkey & Jalapeno	640	20	77
Thai Chicken	680	23	84
Vegetarian Special	540	18	73

Salads: without Dressing/Croutons Unless Indicated			
Baby Spinach & Feta	210	16	9
Caesar Salad	100	5	10
Chicken Salad	270	14	13
Fruit Salad	100	0	25
Garden Salad	50	1.5	12
Greek Salad	130	8	13
Grilled Chicken Caesar w. Croutons	200	8	13
Ham & Turkey Chef Salad	240	12	15
Pasta Salad	60	3	10
Potato Salad	290	15	35
Side Salad	25	0.5	7
Turkey Chef Salad	300	17	15

Soups: Per Cup			
Boston Clam Chowder	200	12	21
Broccoli Cheese	180	13	13
Chicken Tortilla	150	6	13
Hearty Vegetable Beef	110	5	12
Old Fashioned Chicken Noodle	90	1.5	11
Potato w. Bacon	170	9	24
Timberline Chili	230	8	26
Vegetarian Vegetable	80	0.5	14
Wisconsin Cheese	280	22	23

Kid's Meals: without Cookie or Drink			
Cheese Pizza	480	13	72
Cheese Sandwich	390	14	48
Ham & Cheese Sandwich	420	15	49
Pepperoni Pizza	520	17	72

Desserts			
Brownie	410	24	47
Carrot Cake	485	28	52
Cheesecake	310	18	31
Cookies: Chocolate Chip	160	7	23
Fudge Chocolate Chip	160	6	22
Oatmeal Raisin	150	5	24
Sugar	150	7	22
White Choc Macadamia	170	6	22

Second Cup® ~ see CalorieKing.com

Shakey's®

Pizzas (12"): Per Slice (1/10 Pizza)	C	F	Cb
Cheese only:			
Thin Crust	135	5	13
Thick Crust	170	5	22
Homestyle Pan	305	14	31
Onion/Olives/Mushrooms:			
Thin Crust	125	5	14
Thick Crust	160	4	22
Homestyle Pan	320	15	32
Sausage Pepperoni:			
Thin Crust	165	8	13
Thick Crust	205	8	22
Homestyle Pan	375	20	31
Sausage Mushroom			
Thin Crust	140	6	13
Thick Crust	180	6	22
Homestyle Pan	340	17	31
Pepperoni:			
Thin Crust	150	7	13
Thick Crust	185	6	22
Homestyle Pan	345	15	31
Shakey's Special:			
Thin Crust	170	9	13
Thick Crust	210	8	22
Homestyle Pan	385	21	32

Other Items			
3-Piece Chicken & Potato	945	56	51
5-Piece Fried Chicken & Potato	1700	90	130
Hot Ham & Cheese Sandwich	550	21	56
Potato Wedges, 15 pieces	950	36	120
Shakey's Super Hot Hero	810	44	67
Spagh. w. Meat Sce/Garlic Bread	940	33	134

Sheetz®

Coffeez™: Per 16 fl.oz	C	F	Cb
Hot Chocolate, medium	190	3	39
Cupo'ccino®: Per Medium (16 fl.oz)			
Almond Amaretto; French Vanilla	220	8	34
Fat Free French Vanilla	225	0	47

M.T.O® Cold Subs:			
Per 6" Sub (No Cheese Unless Indicated)			
Cheese Sub w. American Cheese	320	12	41
Chicken Salad	405	12	51
Club Combo Sub	335	6	42
Cold Cut Sub	400	17	43
Cooked Ham Sub; Roast Beef, avg.	300	5	42
Egg Sub	270	7	42
Italian Sub	345	10	43
Tuna Salad	420	13	50
Turkey Sub	275	4	42
Veggie Sub	210	3	41

Sheetz® cont...

M.T.O® *Hot Subs:* Per 6" Sub	C	F	Cb
Buffalo/Rstd Chicken, no Cheese	355	6	42
Meatball, no Cheese	410	18	46
Pepperoni Sub	490	29	41
Steak, no Cheese, 10 oz	380	10	43

M.T.O® *Bagelz:* No Cheese Unless Indicated			
Cheese Bagel w. American Cheese	410	11	61
Chicken Salad	495	11	71
Club Combo	425	5	62
Cold Cut	490	17	63
Egg	360	6	62
Ham; Roast Beef, avg.	380	5	62
Italian	435	9	63
Tuna Salad	510	12	70
Turkey	565	3	62
Veggie	300	2	61

M.T.O® *Hot Dogs:* No Cheese			
¼ lb All Beef Big Dogz	550	34	43
Hot Dogz	270	15	23

M.T.O® *Nachos:* Per Serving			
Nachos Grande w. Cheese	520	32	42
Nachos Bueno, w. Cheese	520	32	42

M.T.O® *Salads:* No Cheese			
Caesar Salad	15	0	3
Chef Salad	100	3	5
Chicken Caesar; Roasted Chicken	205	4	3
Chicken Salad	215	9	14
Garden Salad	20	0	4
Oriental Chicken	430	12	37
Steak Salad	190	7	6
Taco Salad	210	9	27
Tuna Salad	230	10	13

M.T.O® *Breakfast* (Includes Cheese)			
Shmagels: Bacon & Egg Breakfast	410	10	62
Egg	470	15	62
Ham & Egg	560	18	64
Shmiscuits: Bacon	370	19	26
Egg	320	15	26
Ham & Egg	410	18	28
Sausage & Egg	460	28	26
Shmuffins: Egg	320	15	28
Bacon & Egg	370	19	28
Ham & Egg	410	18	30
Italian Meats & Egg	365	17	29

Shoney's®

Breakfast	C	F	Cb
All Star Breakfast, no extras	190	15	1.5
Deluxe Pancake Platter	1610	32	299
Half Stack Pancake Platter	930	14	187
Big Eater Steak Brkfast, no extras	630	41	1.5
Country Fried Steak Breakfast	990	66	49
Sunrise Breakfast	975	60	88
Sausage Biscuit (1)	540	34	42

Burgers			
All-American: Burger	690	32	44
Bacon Cheeseburger	890	49	44
Mushroom Swiss Burger	970	57	49
Famous Patty Melt	945	60	40
Half-O-Pound Burger	1350	53	130

Sandwiches			
Blackened Chicken	885	21	122
Charbroiled Chicken	895	22	122
Chicken Parmesan Sandwich	750	30	80
Corned Beef Reuben	795	53	37
Fish Sandwich	830	16	126
Fried Chicken Sandwich	560	14	77
Original Slim Jim Sandwich	1005	33	123
Raymond's French Dip	500	14	53
Turkey Club/Whole Wheat	945	52	47
Ultimate Grilled Cheese S'wich	895	46	77

Steaks			
BBQ Ribs	1520	78	124
Choice Sirloin, 6 oz	1225	51	127
Half-O-Pound w. Grilled Onions	1335	52	133
Half-O-Pound w. Grilled Mushr.	1320	52	127
Ribeye, 8 oz	1480	75	127
Southwest Half-O-Pound	1305	70	83
T-Bone, 12 oz	1810	100	127

Surf & Turf:			
Ribeye & 5 Fried Shrimp	1640	82	138
Ribeye & 6 Grilled Shrimp	1590	81	128
Sirloin & 5 Fried Shrimp	1380	58	138
Sirloin & 6 Grilled Shrimp	1330	57	128
T-Bone & 5 Fried Shrimp	1970	107	138
T-Bone & 6 Grilled Shrimp	1920	105	128

Rib Combos, w. Fries:			
¼ Rack & BBQ Chicken	1230	54	103
¼ Rack & Tenderloins	1370	70	120
¼ Rack & Fried Shrimp	1145	50	113
¼ Rack & Grilled Shrimp	1125	52	103

Continued Next Page ...

Fast - Foods & *Restaurants*

Shoney's® cont...

Blue Plate Specials	C	F	Cb
Cajun Whitefish	480	10	56
Baked Whitefish	510	8.5	58
Grandma's Meatloaf w. Glaze	1090	46	93
Grandma's Meatloaf w. Gravy	1090	48	87
Original Country Fried Steak	1150	62	103
Grilled Liver & Onions	710	22	79
Ham Steak Dinner (no veges)	665	25	60
Roast Beef Platter (no veges)	880	30	96
Pasta: Per Serving			
Chicken Alfredo	1705	78	170
Italian Feast	1435	45	204
Pasta Ya-Ya	1850	81	176
Shrimp Alfredo	1780	85	171
Seafood: Fish 'n' Shrimp	1100	39	129
Fried Fish Platter	1050	38	123
Grilled Cod/Salmon Lite, avg.	200	4	0
Grilled Salmon	750	19	95
Grilled Shrimp	720	20	96
Grilled Shrimp Lite	320	8	30
Shrimper's Feast	1030	39	128
Shrimp Stir Fry	875	19	131
Chicken: Chicken Stir Fry	1200	35	172
Charbroiled Blackened Chicken	830	26	100
Charbroiled Chicken Breast	800	23	99
Fried Chicken Tenderloins	1160	60	121
Monterey Chicken	910	40	83
Smothered Chicken	890	34	90
Junior Meals: Fish 'N Chips	310	11	29
Chicken Dinner	190	10	12
Sides: Baked Potato, Plain	350	6	67
French Fries, 4 oz	215	10	25
Onion Rings, 1 order (7 rings)	500	15	83
Desserts, Ice Cream, Sundaes			
Apple Pie: a la Mode	1205	53	174
w. NutraSweet	455	18	64
Cheesecake, 1 slice, 4 oz	365	25	23
Hot Fudge Sundae	600	30	75
Original Strawberry Pie, 1 slice	330	17	45
Ultimate Hot Fudge Cake	875	37	126
Cherry/Peach Pie w. Nutrasweet	480	20	68
Caramel Sundae	620	27	83
Chocolate Milk Shake	1080	51	141
Strawberry Sundae	610	27	85
Walnut Brownie a la Mode	575	34	60

Sizzler®

Hot Entrees: (No Sides)	C	F	Cb
Hamburger	625	33	36
Dakota Ranch Steak: 6 oz	315	20	0
8 oz	420	27	0
9½ oz	500	32	0
Hibachi Chicken Breast,	195	3	13
w. Pineapple			
Lemon-Herb Chicken Breast	140	3	0
Malibu Chicken Patty, each	310	19	11
Salmon	250	12	0
Santa Fe Chicken Breast	150	3	0
Shrimp: Broiled	150	6	0
Fried, 4 only	225	2	35
Mini	150	1	24
Shrimp Scampi	145	3	0
Swordfish	315	14	0
Low Carb Grill Menu			
Grilled Salmon w. Broccoli	405	19	14
Hibachi Chicken w. Broccoli	295	6	15
Petite Sizzler Steak w. Broccoli	520	26	11
Hot Bar			
Broccoli Chse Soup, 4 oz	140	9	10
Chicken Noodle Soup, 4 oz	30	1	4
Chicken Wings, 1 oz	75	4	4
Clam Chowder, 4 oz	120	6	11
Focaccia Bread, 2 pces	110	7	9
Meatballs, 4 balls	155	11	5
Minestrone Soup, 4 oz	35	0	7
Pasta: Fettucine, 2 oz	80	1	15
Spaghetti, 2 oz	80	0	16
Potato Skins, 2 oz	160	8	22
Refried Beans, ¼ cup	60	1	11
Saltine Crackers, 2 crackers	25	1	4
Taco Filling, 2 oz	105	9	3
Taco Shells, each	50	2	7
Dessert Bar: Chocolate Syrup, 1 oz	90	0	21
Choc/Vanilla Soft Serve, 4 oz	135	4	24
Strawberry Topping, 1 oz	70	0	18
Whipped Topping, 1 Tbsp	10	1	1
Salads & Toppings			
Prepared Salads: Per 2 oz			
Carrot & Raisin	130	10	10
Chinese Chicken; Teriyaki Beef	55	2	6
Mediterranean Minted Fruit	30	0	7
Mexican Fiesta	55	1	10
Old Fashioned Potato	85	5	10
Red Herb Potato	120	9	9
Seafood	55	3	4
Seafood Louis Pasta	65	2	9
Spicy Jicama	15	0	4
Tuna Pasta	135	10	6

Restaurants & Fast - Foods

Sizzler® cont...

Sides	C	F	Cb
Baked Potato, plain	220	0	50
Cottage Cheese, 2 oz	50	1	2
Eggs, 1 oz	45	3	0
Garbanzo Beans, ¼ cup	65	1	11
Kidney Beans, ¼ cup	50	0	10
Olives, 1 oz	60	6	1
Peaches, ¼ cup	35	0	9
Peas, ¼ cup	30	0	6
Real Bacon Bits, 1 Tbsp	30	2	2
Turkey Ham, 1 oz	60	5	0

Dressings: Per 2 Tbsp (1 oz)	C	F	Cb
Blue Cheese	110	12	1
Honey Mustard	160	16	4
Italian, Lite	15	0	2
Japanese Rice Vinegar, Fat Free	10	0	2
Parmesan Italian	100	10	2
Ranch	120	12	2
Ranch, Reduced-Calorie	90	8	4
Thousand Island	145	15	3

Skyline Chili®

Burritos	C	F	Cb
All Chili, burrito	560	30	37
All Chili Deluxe, burrito	650	35	45

Salads: Without Dressing	C	F	Cb
Buffalo Chicken Salad	150	7	7
Classic Chicken Salad	150	7	8
Garden Salad	80	5	6
Greek Chicken Salad	170	8	9
Greek Salad	60	3.5	5
Southwestern Chkn w. Tortilla Chips	760	44	66

Meals: Per Regular Serving	C	F	Cb
Coney w. Cheese	340	22	17
Coney, no Cheese	220	12	17
Black Bean & Rice, 3-Way	800	40	74
Black Bean & Rice, 4-Way	810	40	77
Black Bean & Rice, 5-Way	880	40	89
Black Bean & Rice, Spaghetti	490	12	79

Bowls: Chili	C	F	Cb
Chili Bean	270	12	17
Chili Cheese	440	30	6
Coney	870	69	9
Loaded Chili	580	40	18
Vegetarian Black Beans & Rice	320	9	46

Skyline Chili® cont...

Meals (Cont): Per Regular Serving	C	F	Cb
Chili Spaghetti: Regular	450	18	43
w. Bean & Onion	530	17	64
w. Bean	520	17	61
w. Onion	470	17	51
Steamed Potatoes: Plain	310	0	72
Cheddar	740	41	72
Chili	440	8	74
Sour Cream	570	27	72

Sandwiches & Burgers	C	F	Cb
Chili Cheese Sandwich	290	17	17
Wraps: Buffalo Chicken, no dressing	520	21	55
Classic/Greek Chicken, no Dressing	510	21	55
Southwestern Chicken, no Dr.	670	30	65

Fries: French Fries	C	F	Cb
Cheese Fries	630	33	79
Chili Fries	870	49	75
Chili Cheese Fries	780	38	78
	1010	57	78

Smoothie King®

Berry Smoothies: Per 21.6 oz	C	F	Cb
Blueberry Blast	410	3	98
Cranberry Crush	420	3.5	106
Raspberry Dream	520	2	123
Strawberry Patch	420	1	104
Very Berry	420	1.5	96

Classic Smoothies: Per 21.6 oz	C	F	Cb
Factory Original	300	0	73
The Mango Smoothie	450	5	92
The Original Factory, Original	330	0.5	81
Yogurt Yahoo	390	7	67

Protein Smoothies: Per 21.6 oz	C	F	Cb
After-Workout Formula	420	1	92
Factory Latte	520	4	93
Hercules	490	7	105
Just Peachy	280	0.5	62
Peanut Butter Powerhouse	590	9	95
Engineered Foods, packet only, (fruit not incl. in nutritional analysis)	280	2	24

Continued Next Page ...

Smoothie King® cont...

Specialty Smoothies: Per 21.6 oz

	C	F	Cb
Bulk Upper	1320	21	184
Energizer	340	5	75
Immune Booster	350	5	84
Light Delight	360	2	82
One's A Meal	510	6	77

Tropical Smoothies: Per 21.6 oz

Island Delight	410	5	103
Key Lime Splash	390	5	98
Pina Colada	560	90	117
Pineapple Passion	270	0	71
Tropical Squeeze	360	5	92

Kids Kups

Original	170	0	43
Strawberry Jr.	140	0	38

Snappy Tomato®

Large Pizzas: Per Slice (⅛ Pizza)

	C	F	Cb
Buffalo Grilled Chicken	250	8	32
Cheese Pizza	220	7	30
Hawaiian Pizza	370	18	33
Meat Topper Pizza	430	23	31
Pepperoni Pizza	340	17	31
Ranch Pizza	370	21	31
Snapperoni Pizza	390	22	31
Supreme Pizza	340	17	32
Veggie Pizza	240	8	33

Sides

Chicken Snappers, 2 pieces, 82g	150	5	12
Grilled Chicken Breast Hoagie, 87g	110	4.5	3
Hoagie Bun, 140.6g	380	6	68
Hoagie Patty (1),113g	290	22	5
Snappy Wings, 3 pieces, 74g	160	11	0

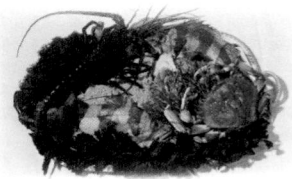

Sonic Drive-In®

Burgers

	C	F	Cb
Sonic Burger w. Mayonnaise	630	37	53
Sonic Burger w. Mustard	540	25	52
Cheeseburger w. Mayonnaise	700	42	55
Cheeseburger w. Mustard	600	31	54
Bacon Burger	770	47	55
SuperSonic Cheeseburger: w. Mayo	970	63	56
w. Mustard	870	52	55
Jr. Burger	320	16	29
Jr. Cheeseburger	380	21	30

Sandwiches/Coneys/Wraps

Coney: Extra-Long Cheese (1)	600	33	54
Corn Dog (1)	250	15	23
Sandwiches: Breaded Chicken	670	33	66
Grilled Chicken	330	11	32
Toaster Sandwiches: Chicken Club	690	35	64
Bacon Cheeseburger	690	37	58
Wraps: Chicken Strip	480	20	56
Fritos Chili Cheese	670	38	66
Grilled Chicken	380	11	44

Chicken

Chicken Strip Dinner	920	43	97
Jumbo Popcorn Chicken:			
Snack, no Sauce, 4 oz	370	21	27
Large, no Sauce, 6 oz	560	32	41
Popcorn Chicken Sauces: BBQ	45	0	11
Honey Mustard	90	7	7
Ranch	150	16	1

Fresh Tastes Salads: No Dressing

Grilled Chicken	310	14	19
Jumbo Popcorn Chicken	490	28	39
Santa Fe Grilled Chicken	370	15	29

Salad Dressings: Per Serving (2 oz)

Golden Italian Fat-Free	50	0	13
Honey Mustard	240	21	14
Original Ranch	260	28	0
Original Ranch Light	120	7	14

Sides

French Fries: Plain, regular, 2.6 oz	210	10	28
w. Cheese, regular, 3.3 oz	280	15	29
w. Chili & Cheese, regular, 4.3 oz	300	18	31
Mozzarella Sticks (5), no Sauce	410	21	35
Onion Rings, regular, 5 ½ oz	500	28	55
Tater Tots: Plain, regular, 3 oz	220	14	23
w. Cheese, regular, 3.6 oz	290	19	25
w. Chili & Cheese, regular, 4.6 oz	310	21	26

Sonic Drive-In®cont...

Breakfast	C	F	Cb
Burritos: Bacon Egg & Cheese	450	27	38
Ham Egg & Cheese	440	23	37
Sausage Egg & Cheese	570	39	39
SuperSonic	650	43	48
French Toast Sticks: w. Syrup (4)	580	26	80
no Syrup (4)	500	26	59
Breakfast Sandwiches			
Bistro: Bacon Egg & Cheese	470	27	35
Ham Egg & Cheese	430	21	35
Sausage Egg & Cheese	560	37	35
Toaster: Bacon Egg & Cheese	540	30	46
Ham Egg & Cheese	500	23	46
Sausage Egg & Cheese	630	39	46
Desserts (Frozen Favorites): *Per Regular*			
Banana Split	450	12	82
Vanilla Cone	180	6	30
Vanilla Dish	240	9	36
Cream Pie Shakes: Banana	690	23	113
Chocolate	750	23	127
Coconut	680	24	108
Strawberry	720	23	120
CreamSlush: Lemon-Berry; Strawb., avg.	460	12	85
Other varieties, average	440	13	77
Floats: Diet Coke; Diet Dr Pepper	220	8	33
Other varieties, avg.	300	8	56
Malts/Shakes, avg.: Banana	560	20	89
Chocolate	630	20	102
Pineapple; Strawberry	590	20	95
Vanilla	550	21	84
Sonic Blast: Butterfinger	670	31	89
M&M's; Oreo	660	28	95
Reese's Peanut Butter Cups	620	22	96
Sundaes: Chocolate	410	13	67
Hot Fudge	440	18	63
Pineapple; Strawberry	380	13	60
Drinks: Barq's Root Beer, large	305	0	82
Sunrise Breakfast: Regular	180	0	46
Large	230	0	60
Fruit Smoothie: Strawberry, 14 oz	460	0	113
Strawberry-Banana, reg., 14 oz	440	0	108
Tropical, reg., 14 oz	500	0	124

For Complete Nutritional Data ~ see CalorieKing.com

Souper Salad®

Soups: Per Serving (5 oz)	C	F	Cb
Adobe Rice & Chicken	100	5	10
Black Bean	90	2	20
Cherokee Joe's Cornbread	60	1.5	11
Chicken Noodle	90	3.5	9
Chicken Tortilla	70	2.5	7
Holiday Harvest	90	6	5
Mama Mia Chicken; Zucchini Chkn	80	3.5	8
Minestrone	80	1.5	13
Mr. B's Hot & Sour Chicken	60	1.5	8
Red French Onion, no Crouton	45	1.5	6
Seafood Bisque	120	8	8
Pasta Tortellini; Seafood Gumbo, avg.	110	4.5	14
Spicy Meatballs w. Rice	100	4.5	10
Vegetable Lentil	70	0	16
Vegetarian Vegetable	50	0.5	11
Other varieties, average	80	2.5	10
Bread			
Blueberry Bread, piece	320	2.5	29
Cornbread Muffin, muffin	150	4	26
Garlic Breadstick, piece	130	4.5	18
Gingerbread, piece	180	6	30
Tortilla Chips, serving, 5 pieces	70	3.5	9

For Complete Nutritional Data ~ see CalorieKing.com

Souplantation®

Soups: Per Cup	C	F	Cb
Low Fat: Chicken Tortilla	100	3	5
Classical Minestrone	120	2	20
Vegetable Medley	90	1	14
Regular Soup: *Per Cup*			
Chesapeake Corn Chowder	280	16	30
Cream of Mushroom	290	21	15
Irish Potato Leek	260	16	23
Manhattan Clam Chowder	130	4	16
Minestrone w. Italian Sausage	210	11	14
Navy Bean w. Ham	340	10	30
Vegetarian Harvest	190	8	23
Chili: Low-Fat Kettle House, 1 cup	230	3	26
Breads: Sourdough	150	0.5	27
Buttermilk Cornbread, 1 pce	140	2	27
Focaccia: Garlic Asiago	140	5	19
Tomatillo	140	6	16
Fresh Tossed Salads: *Per Cup*			
Antipasto Salad; BBQ, average	140	10	6
Caesar Salad Asiago	190	14	10
Won Ton Chicken Happiness	150	8	12

Continued Next Page ...

For Extra Menu Items + Full Nutritional Data ~ See Author's Website www.CalorieKing.com

Fast - Foods & *Restaurants*

Souplantation® cont...

Prepared Salads: Per ½ Cup	C	F	Cb
Aunt Doris' Red Pepper Slaw	70	0	18
Baja Bean & Cilantro	180	3	29
BBQ Potato	160	8	20
Carrot Raisin	90	3	17
Dijon Potato w. Garlic Dill Vinegar	150	12	9
Greek Couscous w. Feta Cheese	170	9	19
Oriental Ginger Slaw w. Krab	70	3	8
Southern Dill Potato	120	3	20
Thai Noodle w. Peanut Sauce	170	8	17
Zesty Tortellini	190	15	18
Dressing & Croutons: Per 2 Tbsp			
Balsamic Vinaigrette	180	19	1
Blue Cheese Dressing	140	14	3
Italian Dressing, creamy	120	13	1
Fat Free	20	0	5
Honey Mustard Dressing	150	13	8
Fat Free	45	0	10
Ranch Dressing	130	13	1
Fat Free	50	0	2
Thousand Island Dressing	110	11	3
Croutons, Garlic Parmesan, 5 pcs	40	3	2
Hot Tossed Pastas: Per Cup			
Bruschetta	260	4	41
Creamy Bruschetta	360	16	43
Garden Vegetable: w. Meatballs	270	7	42
w. Italian Sausage	300	10	42
Italian Vegetable Beef	270	6	43
Vegetarian Marinara w. Basil	260	4	44
Muffins: Chocolate Brownie	170	8	22
Georgia Peach Poppyseed	150	6	20
Tangy Lemon	140	4	24
Wildly Blue Blueberry, small	140	5	22
Fruit Medley Bran	80	0.5	17
Desserts			
Apple Cobbler, ½ Cup	350	10	64
Apple Medley (fat-free), ½ cup	70	0	18
Banana Royale (fat-free), ½ cup	80	0	20
Chocolate Chip Cookie, small	70	3	10
Chocolate Lava Cake, ½ cup	295	8	55
Jello, flavored, ½ cup	85	0	20
Rice Pudding, ½ cup	110	2	20
Vanilla Pudding, ½ cup	140	4	24
Chocolate Syrup, 2 Tbsp	70	0	18
Granola Topping, 2 Tbsp	110	4	19
Soft Serve: Chocolate, ½ cup	95	0	21
Vanilla Soft Serve (reduced fat)	140	4	22

For Complete Nutritional Data ~ see CalorieKing.com

Southern Tsunami®

Sushi: Per Pack	C	F	Cb
California Roll, 12 pieces	360	6	66
California Roll & Inari, 9 pieces	505	11	87
California Roll Plus	495	10	87
Cream Cheese Roll w. Salmon (12)	515	20	59
Crunchy Shrimp Roll, 12 pieces	510	21	64
Dragon Roll, 12 pieces	645	18	66
Eel Roll (Freshwater Eel), 12 pieces	495	16	65
Eel Roll (Sea Eel), 12 pieces	435	12	66
Futomaki	505	6	96
Inari, 4 pieces	420	9	73
Inari & Maki	560	9	102
M&M Roll: Shrimp & Avocado (16)	330	5	59
Tuna & Cucumber, 16 pieces	305	1	57
Nigiri: Cuttlefish, 1 piece	40	0	8.5
Egg Cake, 1 piece	75	1	13
Fish Roe, 1 piece	60	0.5	9
Fresh Salmon, 1 piece	70	1	9
Fresh Water Eel, 1 piece	110	5	11
Octopus, 1 piece	55	1	9
Sea Eel, 1 piece	90	3	11
Shrimp, 1 piece	45	0	8
Smoked Salmon, 1 piece	70	1	9
Tilapia, 1 piece	50	0.5	8
Tuna, 1 piece	60	0	8
Yellowtail, 1 piece	55	0.5	8
Ocean Crab Roll, 12 pieces	390	7	60
Orange Roll, 12 pieces	395	8	65
Rainbow Roll, 12 pieces	490	9	66
Snack Pack: Cucumber, 16 pieces	265	0	57
Imitation Crab & Cucumber (16)	290	1	61
Spicy Roll: Salmon, 12 pieces	485	16	59
Shrimp, 12 pieces	395	11	57
Tuna, 12 pieces	450	11	57
Tempura Roll, 12 pieces	530	11	82
Tofu Roll, 12 pieces	320	3	62
Tsunami Roll, 12 pieces	470	13	71
Vegetable Combo: 12 pieces	350	7	65
24 pieces	445	4	92
Combinations: Fullmoon, 12 pcs	425	13	64
Marina Plate, 6 pcs	380	8	52
Meteor Special, 14 pieces	385	3	69
Seaside, Tuna & Salmon, 16 pcs	360	3	58
Seaside, Tuna, Salmon, Shrimp, Eel	355	4	59
Shoreline, 12 pieces	480	8	78
Stardust, 16 pieces	540	12	94

Spaghetti Warehouse®

Lunch

	C	**F**	**Cb**
Minestrone Soup	80	1.5	12
Grilled Chicken Marinara	530	8	65
Seafood Marinara	385	5	65
Spaghetti: w. Tomato Sauce	425	5	82
w. Marinara Sauce #12	440	5	84
Spicy Marinara Sce Spaghetti	280	4	52
Vegetable Primavera	340	4	65

Dinner

	C	**F**	**Cb**
Minestrone, 1 bowl	110	2	18
Grilled Chicken Marinara	640	10	85
Grilled Halibut Dinner	880	14	106
Grilled Marinated Chicken Breast	910	17	116
Marinara Sauce #12	520	6	99
Seafood Marinara	520	8	86
Spaghetti w. Tomato Sauce	525	6	101
Spicy Marinara Sce Spaghetti	330	6	60
Vegetable Primavera	610	8	116

Starbuck's®

Figures Based on Grande (16 fl.oz)
Without Whip Unless Indicated

Drinks: Per 16 fl.oz

	C	**F**	**Cb**
Apple Juice	200	0	49
Caramel Apple Cider	305	0	73
Chocolate Milk, Whole Milk	295	13	36
Hot Chocolate, Whole Milk	360	14	50
Steamed Apple Cider	240	0	59
Vanilla Creme	335	14	39
White Hot Chocolate, Whole Milk	495	19	65
Steamed Milk, Whole	270	15	21
w. Nonfat Milk	160	0	23
w. Soy Milk	210	6	28
Caffe Misto/Au Lait, Whole Milk	145	7	11
Caffe Americano	20	0	3
Caffe Latte, Whole Milk	270	14	21
w. Nonfat Milk	170	0	24
w. Soy Milk	215	6.5	29
Breve	570	50	20
Caffe Mocha, Whole Milk	310	13	42
w. Nonfat Milk	230	2	43
w. Soy Milk	265	6.5	47
Breve	535	39	40

Hot Drinks: Per Grande (16 fl.oz)

	C	**F**	**Cb**
Cappuccino: w. Whole Milk	170	9	13
w Nonfat Milk	105	0	15
w. Soy Milk	130	3.5	17
Breve	345	30	13
Caramel Macchiato: w. Whole Milk	305	12	37
w. Nonfat Milk	225	1	40
w. Soy Milk	265	5.5	44
Breve	550	41	36
White Choc. Mocha: w. Whole Milk	425	15	57
w. Nonfat Milk	345	5	58
w. Soy Milk	375	10	62
Breve	640	41	55

Espresso (Hot): Per Serving

	C	**F**	**Cb**
Espresso: Doppio	10	0	2
Solo	5	0	1
Espresso con Panna: Doppio	110	9	4
Solo	110	9	3
Espresso Macchiato: Doppio	15	0	2
Solo	10	0	1

Continued Next Page ...

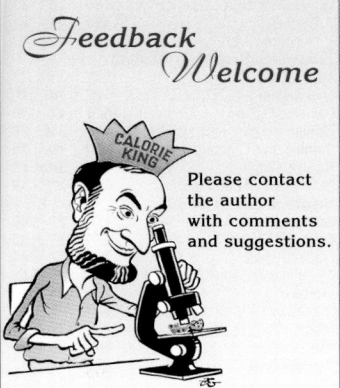

Feedback Welcome

Please contact the author with comments and suggestions.

Write to: Allan Borushek
1001 West 17th St, Costa Mesa CA 92627
Email: feedback@calorieking.com

Fast - Foods & *Restaurants*

Starbuck's® cont...

Figures Based on Grande (16 fl.oz)
Without Whip Unless Indicated

Iced Drinks: Per 16 fl.oz	C	F	Cb
Caffe Americano	20	0	3
Caffe Latte: w. Whole Milk	140	7	11
w. Nonfat Milk	90	0	13
w. Soy Milk	110	3	15
Caffe Mocha: w. Whole Milk	210	8	34
w. Nonfat Milk	175	2.5	35
w. Soy Milk	200	4.5	36
Caramel Macchiato, Whole Milk	235	9	30
Syrup Flavored Latte; Vanilla Latte	210	7	31
White Choc. Mocha, Whole Milk	350	11	55
Frappuccino® Blended Tea: *Per 16 fl.oz*			
Tazo® Chai Creme	340	2	71
Frappuccino® Blended Coffee: *Per 16 fl.oz*			
Caffe Vanilla	300	3	63
Caramel	260	3	53
Coffee	235	3	46
Espresso	210	3	41
Mocha varieties, average	270	4	54
Frappuccino® Light Blended Coffees: *Per 16 fl.oz*			
Caffe Vanilla	200	1	43
Caramel; Mocha	170	1.5	34
Coffee	135	1	26
Espresso	120	1	24
Java Chip	240	7	43
White Chocolate Mocha	210	2.5	40
Frappuccino® Blended Cremes: *Per 16 fl.oz*			
Double Chocolate Chip	395	8	73
Green Tea w. syrup	375	2.5	77
Strawberries & Creme	415	2	89
Vanilla Bean	315	2	64
Frappuccino® Juice Blends: *Per 16 fl.oz*			
Pomegranate	310	0.5	75
Tangerine	210	0	50
Tazo® Tea: *Per 16 fl.oz*			
Iced Tazo® Chai, Whole Milk	255	6	45
Tazo® Chai, Latte, Whole Milk	290	7	49
Drink Extras: *Per Serving*			
Flav. Sugar Free Syrup, 1 pump	0	0	0
Flavored Syrup, 1 pump	20	0	5
Mocha Syrup, 1 pump	25	0.5	6
Toppings: Chocolate, 4g	5	0	1
Caramel, 15g	15	0.5	2
Sprinkles	0	0	0
Whipped Cream Topping:			
Tall, 25g	90	9	2
Grande/Venti, 35g	130	12	2
Hot Beverage, 27g	100	9	2

Starbuck's® cont...

Note: Baked items below are approximate only, and vary between regions

Muffins	C	F	Cb
Banana Bran	390	13	66
Blueberry	500	20	71
Carrot Cake	680	40	75
Maple Streusel	370	19	53
Pumpkin	480	23	60
Zucchini Walnut	640	38	65
Scones: Blueberry	490	19	71
Cafe: Chocolate Chip; Vanilla	120	5	17
Cranberry Orange	460	20	67
Maple Oat Nut	520	25	68
Pumpkin	510	22	71
Loaf Cakes & Coffee Cakes			
Banana Walnut	390	16	58
Holiday Gingerbread	500	16	84
Lemon	420	17	66
Lemon Zucchini	380	16	49
Pineapple Passion	350	18	43
Pumpkin	360	11	59
Mini: Mixed Berry Cream Cheese	420	22	50
Whole Wheat Carrot	310	19	42
Whole Wheat Pumpkin	250	12	50
Reduced-Fat Coffee Cake: Banana	460	15	75
Blueberry	350	11	61
Cinnamon Swirl	330	10	62
Doughnuts, Sweet Rolls & Danish			
Apple Fritter	520	22	73
Cheese Danish	320	19	30
Cinnamon Crisp	620	42	56
Cinnamon Roll	480	15	79
Doughnut w. Chocolate Icing	370	16	50
Maple Doughnut	430	18	61
Old-Fashioned Doughnut	450	21	49
Brownies, Cookies & Bars			
Caramel Nut	450	29	40
Chocolate Chunk	430	19	61
Cranberry Bliss	330	17	43
Crispy Marshmallow Square	320	8	63
Espresso	370	21	43
Fruit Slice	370	19	47
Fudge	290	17	35
Mint	480	28	52
Oatmeal Raisin	410	15	65
Organic Blueberry	350	14	51
Pumpkin	390	19	51
Snowman	420	21	52
Toffee Almond,	430	21	56
White Chocolate Cranberry	380	18	53

Ice Cream & Ice Cream Bars ~ See Page 35, 38
For Bottled Drinks ~ See Page 164

Steak Escape®

Small Sandwiches (7"): No Cheese or Condiments	C	F	Cb
Grand Gobbler	380	2	67
Grand Escape	435	6	64
Grandest Chicken	425	5	64
Great Escape	430	6	63
Hambrosia	380	2	69
Ragin' Cajun Chicken	410	5	58
Turkey Club	380	2	62
Portabello Vegetarian	310	1	65
Wild West BBQ	455	6	60
Large Sandwiches (12"): *No Cheese or Condiments*			
Grand Gobbler	680	4	116
Grandest Chicken	770	10	110
Great Escape; Grand Escape	775	12	108
Hambrosia	685	4	119
Ragin' Cajun Chicken	630	10	80
Turkey Club	580	3	88
Portabello Vegetarian	440	2	93
Wild West BBQ	840	12	126
Fresh Salads: *No Cheese or Condiments*			
Side Salad	40	0.5	8
Grilled Salad: w. Chicken	175	5	11
w. Ham	130	2	8
w. Steak	185	6	11
w. Turkey	130	2	8
Smashed Potatoes: Plain, 14 oz	245	0	53
w. Chicken	385	4	56
w. Ham	340	2	59
w. Steak	395	5	56
w. Turkey	340	2	59
Loaded: Bacon & Cheddar	635	26	91
Ranch & Bacon	690	34	87
Fresh Cut Fries: *Per Serving*			
Small, 6 oz	500	26	67
Medium, 7.8 oz	650	34	87
Large, 11.3 oz	920	48	123
Loaded: Bacon & Cheddar	905	44	88
Ranch & Bacon	1045	71	84
Condiments			
Mayonnaise, 1 oz	100	11	0
BBQ Sauce, 1 oz	40	0	9
Cheddar Cheese, 1 oz	115	9	1

For Complete Nutritional Data ~ see CalorieKing.com

Steak 'n Shake®

Meals	C	F	Cb
All-American Melt Sandwich	1230	97	54
Chicken Fingers, no fries	615	46	22
Chili 3-Way	660	36	63
Chili 5-Way	1035	67	66
Chili Deluxe, 6 oz cup	480	36	17
Fish Fillet Sandwich w. Cheese	825	58	54
Frisco Melt Sandwich	1175	93	44
Grilled Cheese & Bacon Sandwich	790	61	41
Grilled Chicken Breast Sandwich	470	26	33
Original Dbl Steakburger w. Cheese	580	38	29
Original Single w. Cheese	400	23	29
Philadelphia Sandwich	850	52	63
Triple Steakburger	690	47	29
Turkey Melt Sandwich	950	70	47
Fries: French, reg, 5 oz	470	23	62
French, large, 7.25 oz	685	34	90
Cheddar Cheese, reg., 5 oz	580	31	67
Salads: Beef Taco Salad w. dress.	940	59	76
Chicken Chef Salad no dressing	470	32	10
Fried Chicken Salad w. dress.	1050	81	47
Soups: Chicken Gumbo, 6 fl.oz cup	85	2	10
Chicken Noodle, 6 fl.oz cup	70	1	8.5
Cream of Broccoli, 6 fl.oz cup	135	8	11
Vegetable Beef, 6 fl.oz cup	120	6.5	10
Breakfast: Bacon 'n Egg (1) Works	625	47	36
Biscuits, Gravy 'n Hash Browns	1585	99	154
Buttermilk Pancakes (2)	160	2.5	31
Country Scrambler (1)	660	53	16
Cinnamon Swirl French Tst, 3 sl.	265	7	44
One Egg, cooked w. Margarine	140	13	1
Silver Dollar Hash Browns	370	25	35
Steak 'n Eggs Breakfast	1015	80	30
Sandwich on Bagel: Egg & Chse	565	19	76
Egg, Cheese & Bacon	675	29	77
Desserts: Apple Cobbler	505	22	76
Hot Fudge Brownie	490	23	69
Hot Fudge Sundae	510	26	64
Outrageous Parfait, no cream	770	40	95
Pumpkin Pie, (⅛) w. topping	395	14	61
Beverages: Root Beer Float	555	22	87
Hot Chocolate, 7 fl.oz, no topping	140	3.5	27
Orange Freeze, regular	615	19	101
Shake: Chocolate, no Cream reg.	685	22	110
Banana; Vanilla, regular	670	21	106

Subway®

6" Sandwiches (6g Fat or Less)   C   F   Cb

Figures based on wheat bread and toppings: lettuce, tomato, onion, green peppers, olives and pickles. Cheese, oil or mayo not included.

	C	F	Cb
Ham; Roast Beef, average	290	5	46
Oven Roasted Chicken Breast	310	4	48
Subway Club	310	6	48
Sweet Onion Chicken Teriyaki	370	5	59
Turkey Breast	280	4.5	46
Turkey Breast & Ham	290	5	47
Veggie Delite	230	3	44

Other 6" Sandwiches

Figures based on wheat bread plus lettuce, tomato, onion, green peppers, olives, pickles and cheese.

	C	F	Cb
Chicken & Bacon Ranch	580	30	47
Cold Cut Combo	410	17	47
Italian BMT	450	21	47
Meatball Marinara	560	24	63
Spicy Italian	480	25	45
Steak & Cheese	530	31	44
Subway Melt	380	12	48
Tuna	530	31	44
Mini Subs (4"): Ham	180	3	30
Roast Beef	190	3.5	30
Tuna, with cheese	320	18	30
Turkey Breast	190	3	30
Deli Style Sandwich: Ham	210	4	36
Roast Beef	220	4.5	35
Tuna	350	18	35
Turkey Breast	210	3.5	36
Double Meat Subs (6"): Ham	350	7	50
Chipotle Southwest Steak & Chse	540	28	47
Cold Cut Combo	550	28	49
Italian BMT	630	35	49
Meatball Marinara	860	42	82
Oven Roasted Chicken	400	8	51
Roast Beef	360	7	46
Steak & Cheese	540	18	52
Subway Club	420	8	50
Sweet Onion Chicken Teriyaki	480	7	65
Turkey Breast & Ham	360	7	50
Turkey Breast	330	5	48

Pizza (8")

	C	F	Cb
Cheese	295	22	96
Cheese & Veggies	380	25	100
Pepperoni	790	32	96
Sausage	770	30	97

Breakfast Sandwiches   C   F   Cb

	C	F	Cb
6" Sub: Cheese	400	17	43
Chipotle Steak & Cheese	580	31	48
Double Bacon & Cheese	500	25	44
Honey Mustard Ham & Egg	460	19	51
Western with Cheese	440	18	45
Breakfast Wraps: Cheese	390	19	37
Chipotle Steak & Cheese	570	33	41
Double Bacon & Cheese	480	27	38
Honey Mustard Ham & Egg	450	21	45
Western w. Cheese	420	20	39

Salads (6g Fat or Less)

Includes lettuce, tomato, onions, green peppers, olives, carrot, cucumber. Dressing and croutons are not included in data.

	C	F	Cb
Ham	120	3	14
Oven Roasted Chicken Breast	140	2.5	11
Roast Beef	120	3	12
Subway Club	150	4	14
Sweet Onion Chicken Teriyaki	210	3	26
Turkey Breast	110	2.5	13
Turkey Breast & Ham	120	3	14
Veggie Delight	60	1	11

Salad Dressings: Per Package (2 oz)

	C	F	Cb
Fat-Free Italian	35	0	7
Ranch	320	35	3

Soups: Per Cup (10 oz)

	C	F	Cb
Chicken & Dumpling	170	5	23
Chili Con Carne	290	8	35
Cream of Broccoli	160	7	18
Cream of Potato w. Bacon	240	13	26
Golden Broccoli & Cheese	200	12	17
Minestrone	80	1	15
New England Style Clam Chowder	150	5	20
Roasted Chicken Noodle	80	2	11
Spanish Style Chicken w. Rice	110	2	17
Wild Rice w. Chicken	220	11	21

Breads: Wrap

	C	F	Cb
Wrap	190	4.5	33
6" Hearty Italian; Parmesan Oregano	220	3	41
6" Honey Oat	250	3.5	48
6" Italian Herbs & Chse; Monterey	250	5	40
6" Italian White	200	2	38
6" Wheat	200	2.5	40

Cookies & Desserts

	C	F	Cb
Cookies: Oatmeal Raisin (1)	200	8	30
Peanut Butter (1)	230	12	26
Sugar (1)	220	12	28
Chocolate varieties, avg. (1)	220	10	30
White Chip Macadamia Nut	220	11	29
Apple Pie, 2½ oz	245	10	37
Apple Slices, 1 package, 2.5 oz	35	0	9
Raisins, 1 package, 1½ oz	140	0	33

Subway® cont...

Sandwich Fillings (on 6" Sub or Salad) **C** **F** **Cb**

	C	F	Cb
Cheese Slices, ½ oz	45	3.5	1
Cucumber, Lettuce, Pickles, Peppers	0	0	0
Tomato (3 slices), Onion, Olives	5	0	2
Meats: Bacon, 2 strips	45	3.5	0
Ham, 2 oz	60	2	3
Italian BMT Meats, 2¼ oz	180	14	2
Meatballs, 7 oz	300	18	19
Roast Beef, 2 oz	70	2	1
Subway Club Meats, 3 oz	100	3	3
Tuna, 2½ oz	260	24	0
Turkey Breast, 2 oz	50	1	2
Sauces & Dressings:			
Chipotle Southwest, 1¼ Tbsp	95	10	1
Honey Mustard, fat-free, 1¼ Tbsp	30	0	7
Mayonnaise: Reg., 1 Tbsp, ½ oz	110	12	0
Light, 1 Tbsp, ½ oz	50	5	1
Mustard, Yellow or Brown, 2 tsp	5	0	1
Olive Oil Blend, 1 teaspoon	45	5	0
Ranch Dressing, 1¼ Tbsp	120	13	1
Red Wine Vinaigrette, 1¼ Tbsp	30	0	6
Sweet Onion Sauce, 1¼ tbsp	40	0	9
Vinegar, 1 teaspoon	0	0	0
Fruizle Express: Per Small Cup			
Berry Lishus	110	0	28
Berry Lishus w. Banana	140	0	35
Peach Pizzazz	100	0	26
Pineapple Delight	130	0	33
Pineapple Delight w. Banana	160	0	40
Sunrise Refresher	120	0	29

For Complete Nutritional Data ~ see CalorieKing.com

Jared Fogle lost over ²⁰⁰ lbs with low fat Subway® Sandwiches and lots of walking·

Sub Station®

Sandwiches **C** **F** **Cb**
Per ½ Sub (Incl. Oil, Vinegar, Salad)

	C	F	Cb
Ham & Cheese	580	36	48
Ham, Turkey & Cheese	605	37	49
Turkey & Cheese	600	37	48
Roast Beef & Cheese	630	40	44
Ham, Salami, Pepperoni, Cappicola, Bologna, Turkey & Cheese	825	57	43

Sweet Tomatoes®
~ Same Menu & Data as Souplantation (See Page 253) ~

Swiss Chalet®

Burgers: Includes Garnishes **C** **F** **Cb**

	C	F	Cb
Bacon Cheese Burger	870	46	45
Hamburger	730	49	44
Veggie Burger	430	13	51
Rotisserie Chicken: Meat Only			
Double Leg w. Skin	630	38	4
Half Chicken, no Skin	455	18	0
w. Skin	610	31	5
Quarter Chicken: Leg, no Skin	230	11	1
Leg meat w. Skin	310	19	2
Breast meat, no Skin	210	7	0
Breast meat w. Skin	300	11	3
Appetizers			
Baked Garlic Cheese Loaf, 9 oz	730	31	83
Chalet Chicken Wings, 8 wings	1030	59	38
Chicken Fingers, 4 strips	420	21	32
Perogies w. Cajun Sauce, 6.5 oz	420	10	69
Soup: Chalet Chicken, 1 cup	160	4	17
Side Salads: Garden	30	0	6
Caesar Salad	360	32	15
Meals: Chicken Pot Pie, 1 pie	640	33	52
From The Grill: *No Flatbread*			
BBQ Ribs: Regular Cut	630	38	4
Large Cut BBQ Ribs	1270	77	9
Feature Cut BBQ Ribs	420	26	3
Entree Salad: w. Chicken	410	25	13
Vegetable	270	21	14
Grilled Chicken Breast	130	1.5	41
Lighter Favorites: *Includes Salad & Vegetables*			
Quarter Chicken Breast Dinner	360	11	15
Quarter Chicken Leg Dinner	410	18	12
Santa Fe Grilled Chicken Salad	370	10	19
Vegetables Stir-Fry, no rice	270	2.5	54
w. Grilled Chkn Breast, no rice	400	4	55

Swiss Chalet®cont...

Sides	C	F	Cb
Baked Potato	220	0	48
Flatbread, 1.6 oz	120	1.5	23
Butter, ½ oz	100	11	0
Coleslaw Ramekin	70	4	6
Corn, 6 oz	140	2	24
French Fries, 6 oz	470	25	56
Gravy, 4 oz	40	1	7
Mashed Potatoes	160	5	21
Rice Pilaf	280	3.5	57
Sour Cream & Chives, 1½ oz	70	5	3
Vegetables, 6 oz	80	0	15
Sandwiches: No Sides			
Chicken Club Wrap	570	20	51
Chicken on Kaiser, white meat	440	8	31
Grilled Santa Fe Chicken	380	4	49
Messy Chicken, white meat	490	12	40
Salad Dressings: Light Italian, 15ml	35	2	3
1000 Isle Dressing, 15ml	55	6	2
Famous Chalet Sauce, 125ml	30	1	5
French Dressing, 15ml	65	6	2
Light Mayonnaise, 15ml	45	5	1
Raspberry Vinaigrette, 15ml	15	0	3
Dipping Sauce: BBQ, 33ml	55	0	13
Honey Mustard, 33ml	75	1	19
Plum, 28ml	50	0	13
Salsa, 50ml	20	0	13
Desserts: Apple Blossom	490	25	62
Apple Pie	330	14	49
Carrot Cake	700	45	70
Chocolate Eruption Cheesecake	820	55	72
Coconut Cream Pie	310	16	39
Colossal Caramel Fudge Chsecake	700	39	78
Cranberry, Raspberry Yogurt	120	2	23
Lemon Meringue Pie	280	9	47
Pecan Pie	530	28	63
Swiss Alps Choc Layer Cake	590	39	55
Ice Cream: Butter Pecan	150	7	21
Chocolate	115	5	17
Vanilla	125	6	16
Sauce: Butterscotch	100	0	26
Chocolate	80	0	20
Strawberry	40	0	9

For Complete Nutritional Data ~ see CalorieKing.com

Taco Bell®

Burritos	C	F	Cb
7-Layer Burrito	530	21	68
Bean Burrito	370	10	55
Burrito Supreme Beef, avg	440	18	52
Chili Cheese Burrito	390	18	40
Fiesta Burrito Beef	390	14	51
Fiesta Burrito Chicken; Steak, avg.	370	12	49
Grilled Stuft Beef	720	32	80
Grilled Stuft Chicken; Steak, avg.	680	27	77
Tacos: Taco, regular/Crunchy	170	10	13
Taco Supreme	220	14	14
Double Decker Taco Supreme	380	18	40
Soft Taco Beef	210	10	21
Soft Taco Ranchero Chicken	270	14	21
Soft Taco Supreme Beef	260	14	23
Crunch Wrap Supreme	550	23	69
Big Bell Value Menu: Per Serving			
Burrito, ½ lb Bean, Chsy Bean & Rice	490	21	61
Burrito, ½ lb Beef & Potato	540	25	66
Burrito, ½ lb Beef Combo	470	19	52
Burrito, Spicy Chicken	420	19	51
Caramel Apple Empanada	290	15	37
Cheesy Fiesta Potato	290	18	28
Double Decker Taco	340	14	39
Taco, Grande Soft	450	21	44
Taco, Spicy Chicken Soft	180	7	21
Gorditas: Gordita Baja Beef	350	19	31
Gordita Baja Chicken; Steak	320	16	29
Gordita Supreme Beef	310	16	30
Gordita Supreme Chicken; Steak	290	12	28
Gordita Nacho Cheese Beef	300	13	32
Gordita Nacho Cheese Chkn; Steak	270	10	30
Chalupas: Chalupa Baja Beef	430	28	32
Chalupa Baja Chicken; Steak	410	25	30
Chalupa Supreme Beef	400	24	31
Chalupa Supreme Chicken	370	21	29
Chalupa Supreme Steak	370	22	29
Chalupa Nacho Cheese Beef	380	22	33
Chalupa Nacho Cheese Chkn; Steak	360	20	31
Fresco Style (Less Than 10g Fat)			
Burritos: Bean	350	8	56
Fiesta Chicken	340	8	50
Supreme Chicken/Steak	350	9	50
Enchiritos: Beef	270	9	35
Chicken	250	5	34
Steak	250	7	34
Gordita Baja: Beef	250	9	31
Chicken; Steak, average	230	7	29
Tacos: Regular/Crunchy, average	150	7	14
Soft Taco Beef	190	8	22
Soft Beef Chicken/Steak	170	5	21
Tostada	200	6	30

Taco Bell® cont...

	C	F	Cb
Nachos and Sides: Nachos, 3.5 oz	320	20	32
Nachos Supreme	460	26	42
Nachos BellGrande	790	44	79
Pintos 'n Cheese, 4.5 oz	180	7	20
Mexican Rice, 4.6 oz	200	9	26
Cinnamon Twists, 1.25 oz	160	5	27
Specialities			
Border Bowl: Zesty Chicken	730	40	69
w/out Dressing	490	16	64
Southwest Steak	690	28	79
Crunshwrap Supreme	560	24	70
Enchirito: Beef	380	18	35
Chicken; Steak, avg.	350	16	33
Express Taco Salad with Chips	630	34	58
Fiesta Taco Salad with Shell	860	46	82
without Shell	490	25	43
MexiMelt	290	16	23
Mexican Pizza, 7½ oz	540	31	47
Quesadilla: Chicken	540	30	40
Steak	490	28	39
Tostada	250	10	29

For Complete Nutritional Data ~ see CalorieKing.com

Taco Cabana®

Grilled Chicken: Per Serving			
¼ Chicken White, 5 oz	295	14	1
No Skin, 4 oz	170	3	0
¼ Chicken Dark, 4.5 oz	300	18	0.5
No Skin, 3.5 oz	170	7	1
Fajitas: Beef, 4 oz	245	12	4
Chicken White, 4 oz	190	6	3
Chicken Dark, 4 oz	235	11	2
Sides: Black Beans, 4 oz	110	0.5	21
Borracho Beans, 4 oz	110	2.5	17
Chips, 2 oz	290	14	36
Guacamole, 1 oz; Sour Cream, 1 oz	50	4	2
Queso, 3 oz	170	12	7
Refried Beans, 4 oz	170	6	21
Salsa, all types, 1 oz	10	0	2
Spanish Rice, 4 oz	180	5	30
Tortillas: 6" Flour	130	3.5	22
6" Table Corn	60	1	11
Tortilla Soup: Small, 8.5 oz	250	8.5	26
Large, 19 oz	375	13	32
Tacos: Bean & Cheese	290	12	35
Black Bean	215	5	31
Carne Guisada	200	8	20
Crispy Beef	150	7	13
Soft Chicken	220	9	21

Taco Cabana® cont...

	C	F	Cb
Burritos			
Bean & Cheese	545	27	85
Beef/Chicken, average	485	24	76
Black Bean	465	11	95
Breakfast Tacos: Barbacoa	310	15	2
Chorizo & Egg	250	12	22

Taco John's®

Burritos: Bean Burrito	380	12	53
Bean Burrito, no Cheese	320	7	53
Beefy Burrito	430	20	41
Chicken & Potato Burrito	460	19	54
Combination Burrito	400	16	47
Crunchy Chicken & Potato Burrito	590	29	62
Meat & Potato	490	23	55
Super Burrito	450	20	49
Grilled Burrito: Steak	600	34	46
Beef; Chicken, avg.	590	32	49
Tacos: Bravo	340	14	39
Crispy Taco	180	10	13
Softshell Taco	220	10	21
Softshell Taco, Beef	190	8	19
Softshell Taco, Chicken	190	6	19
Taco Burger w. Cheese	280	12	28
Regional Menu Items			
Burrito: Ranch Beef	420	22	41
Ranch Chicken	390	18	40
Smothered	500	21	55
Chili Enchilada	310	16	24
Mexi Rolls w. Nacho Cheese	480	30	33
Potato Oles, Chili Cheese	610	36	59
Specialties: Cheese Quesadilla	480	28	39
Chicken Taco Salad, no Dressing	540	27	44
Chicken Festiva Salad, no Dressing	400	23	24
Fajitas: Grilled Chicken	850	31	99
Grilled Steak	850	32	100
Potato Oles Bravo	530	33	50
Potato Oles Super	1060	67	91
Super Nachos	830	51	73
Super Nachos Chicken	780	45	62
Taco Salad, no Dressing	580	32	46
Sides: Mexican Rice	240	8	36
Nachos	380	23	38
Potato Oles, medium	620	36	67
Refried Beans	400	14	50
Desserts: Apple Grande	240	9	36
Choco Taco	300	15	38
Churro	230	11	31

For Complete Nutritional Data ~ see CalorieKing.com

Fast - Foods & *Restaurants*

Taco Mayo®

Beans	C	F	Cb
Refried w. Cheese	300	9	43
No cheese	285	6.5	42
Burritos: Bean w. Cheese	470	13	72
No cheese	445	11	70
Chicken Supreme Burrito	410	16	39
No cheese & sour cream	345	12	38
Fajita Steak Grilled Burrito	520	24	42
No cheese	435	19	41
Taco: Crispy, with cheese	160	9.5	10
No cheese	135	7	10
Beef Soft Taco: with cheese	230	11	17
No cheese	200	9	16
Chicken Soft Taco: with cheese	185	6	16
No cheese	160	4	16
Extreme Fajita Chicken Soft Taco	260	10	19
No cheese & sour cream	195	6	18
Rice: Mexicali	160	1	35
Salads			
Fiesta Acapulco	725	53	33
No cheese, guacamole & corn stix	410	32	7.5
Fiesta Monterey	510	31	32
No corn stix	295	19	9
Fiesta Santa Fe	590	36	38
No cheese & corn stix	320	19	14

Target Food Court

	C	F	Cb
Breakfast: Pancakes (3) + Syrup	490	4	104
Breakfast Sandwich w. Bacon	380	20	29
Cinnamon Swirl French Toast, 2 slices	230	5	36
Pretzels (Cinnabon): Cinnamon, 5¾ oz	550	9	105
Mega Cinnamon, 6½ oz	650	15	115
Salted Pretzel, 5½ oz	435	3.5	89
Meals: Bowl of Chili, 9 oz cup	300	10	32
Chicken Breast Sandwich, 4 oz	280	9	31
Chicken Tenders, 5 strips, 3 oz	280	19	14
Hot Dog Meal: w. Chips & Soda	570	22	84
w. Apple Sauce & Soda	520	12	93
Hot Dog: Plain, 3½oz	260	12	28
All Beef Meat, 5 oz	350	20	30
Cheddar, 4 oz	310	16	38
Macaroni & Cheese: 8 oz	340	13	41
w. Apple Sauce & Soda Meal	600	13	106
w. Chips & Soda, Meal	650	23	97
Mini Pizza (6"), 5½ oz	360	14	42
Nachos w. Cheese, 40 chips, 4 oz	1100	59	132
Spaghetti O's Meal: w. Chips & Soda	490	11	93
w. Apple Sauce & Soda	440	1	102

For Complete Nutritional Data ~ see CalorieKing.com

Taco Time®

Burritos	C	F	Cb
Beef, Bean & Cheese	615	23	66
Big Juan Beef Burrito	640	25	71
Big Juan Chicken Burrito	620	24	69
Casita Burrito, Beef	645	31	54
Chicken & Black Bean	400	18	45
Chicken BLT	580	39	38
Crisp Burrito: Bean	425	18	53
Meat	550	30	39
Chicken	420	25	32
Soft Bean Burrito	380	10	58
Soft Meat Burrito	490	21	48
Veggie Burrito	490	16	70
Tacos			
Crisp Taco	295	17	16
½ lb Chicken Soft Taco	385	16	41
½ lb Soft Taco	510	23	46
Soft Taco	315	15	23
Super Soft Taco	510	23	50
Specialties			
Cheddar Fries, Medium, 7 oz	505	35	40
Cheddar Melt	205	11	17
Mexi Fries®, Medium, 6 oz	390	25	40
Mexi-Rice, 4 oz	160	2	30
Nachos: Regular, 10.5 oz	680	38	61
Deluxe, 15.25 oz	1050	57	91
Stuffed Fries, Medium, 6.2 oz	640	44	50
Refritos, 7 oz	325	10	44
Taco Cheeseburger	635	36	48
Salads: Per Serving			
Chicken Fiesta, 12 oz	390	19	35
Chicken Taco	370	21	27
Taco Salad, regular	480	28	30
Tostada Salad	630	33	48
Sauces & Dressings: Per 1 oz			
Green Sauce	10	0	2
Original Hot Sauce	10	0	2
Salsa Fresca	65	0	16
1000 Island Dressing	120	12	3
Desserts: Cinnamon Crustos	375	15	47
Fruit Filled Empanadas	250	9	37

For Complete Nutritional Data ~ see CalorieKing.com

Tacone®

Gourmet Wrapped Sandwiches	C	F	Cb
Campfire, ½ wrap	340	12	41
Malibu Melt, ½ wrap	360	17	25
Pilgrim, ½ wrap	260	14	21
Thai Cone, ½ wrap	300	9	35

For Complete Nutritional Data ~ see CalorieKing.com

TCBY®

	C	**F**	**Cb**
Soft Serve Frozen Yogurt: Average all Flavors			
96% Fat-Free: Kids Cup	110	2	18
Junior Cup	200	4	33
Small Cup	290	6	47
Regular Cup	370	8	60
Large Cup	450	10	74
Non-Fat: Junior Cup	160	0	33
Small Cup	220	0	46
Regular Cup	290	0	60
Large Cup	350	0	73
No Sugar Added/Non-Fat: Small	190	0	41
Regular Cup	240	0	53
Large Cup	290	0	65
Low-Carb Lovers: Small	170	10	25
Regular	300	18	45
Large Cup	360	22	56
Waffle Cones: Kids	70	1	15
Regular	110	2	22
Hand Scooped Frozen Yogurt: Average all Flavors			
Kids Cup	90	3	14
Junior Cup	140	5	22
Small Cup	180	6	28
Regular Cup	280	10	44
Large Cup	370	13	58
No Added Sugar, Vanilla:			
Small Cup	100	1	24
Regular Cup	160	1	38
Large Cup	210	1.5	50
Fruithead Smoothies: Per 20 fl.oz Cup			
A Lotta Colada: no Yogurt	380	12	69
w. Yogurt	550	17	99
Berry Slim: no Yogurt	300	0	75
w. Yogurt	410	3	95
Healthy Balance: no Yogurt	300	0	75
w. Yogurt	410	3	95
Holy-Cal: no Yogurt	360	0	94
w. Yogurt	470	3	114
Peachy Lean: no Yogurt	360	0	96
w. Yogurt	470	3	116
Raspberry DeLITE: no Yogurt	240	0	59
w. Yogurt	360	3	85
Raspberry Revitalizer: no Yogurt	300	0	79
w. Yogurt	370	3	84
Tropical Replenisher: no Yogurt	240	0	61
w. Yogurt	370	3	87
Workout Whey: no Yogurt	340	0	92
w. Yogurt	460	3	112

TCBY® cont...

	C	**F**	**Cb**
Sorbet: Average all Flavors			
Kids Cup	80	0	19
Junior Cup	150	0	35
Small Cup	200	0	49
Regular Cup	260	0	63
Large Cup	320	0	17
Frappe Chillers: Per 16 fl.oz Cup			
Caramel de Leche	240	9	32
Coffee	190	7	25
French Vanilla	200	9	23
Frozen Hot chocolate	230	9	32
Mocha	240	9	31

Teriyaki Stix®

	C	**F**	**Cb**
Bowls: Beef Bowl	620	7	102
Chicken Bowl; Hot & Spicy	730	15	101
Chicken Curry	680	17	92
Teriyaki Chicken Salad	360	13	26
Teriyaki Special	740	13	111
Veggie Bowl	440	1	99
Yakisoba	360	4.5	56

The Taco Maker®

	C	**F**	**Cb**
Burritos			
Bean	295	9	44
Beef	445	16	43
Chicken	375	12	44
Crisp Bean; Crisp Beef, avg.	420	27	30
Enchiladas: Beef	375	20	23
Cheese	585	38	25
Chicken	315	13	21
Nachos: Cheese	605	35	49
Chips 'n Beans	290	16	32
Macho Nacho w. Beef	815	50	57
Macho Nacho w. Guacamole	845	55	62
Salad: Chicken Fiesta	625	35	38
Taco	685	42	39
Tacos: Crisp	185	9	16
Crisp Super	310	15	24
Soft	180	6.5	20
Soft Super	390	15	43
Tater Gem Fries, Regular	485	30	48

Fast - Foods & *Restaurants*

Tim Hortons®

Sandwiches

	C	F	Cb
Tim's Own: Chicken Salad	380	9	55
Garden Vegetable w. Dressing	400	14	57
Ham & Swiss w. Tim's Own Dress.	440	12	56
Turkey Bacon Club w. Mustard	440	8	63
Turkey Breast w. Tim's Own Dress.	390	5	59

Soup: Per Bowl (10 oz)

Beef Stew	235	8	25
Chili	300	16	18
Cream of Broccoli	190	5	31
Creamy Mushroom	170	7	25
Hearty Vegetable	70	0	14
Tomato Florentine	95	2	18
Minestrone	120	3	24
Tim's Own, Chicken Noodle	120	2	18
Turkey Rice	120	1.5	21

Cookies

Chocolate Chip	150	7	21
M&M w. Chocolate Chips	160	7	22
Oatmeal Raisin	150	6	22
Peanut Butter	160	9	18
Peanut Butter Chocolate Chunk	170	10	19

Donuts: Per Donut

Cake: Chocolate Glazed	260	10	39
Old Fashion Plain	260	19	20
Sour Cream Plain	270	17	27
Filled: Blueberry	230	8	36
Boston Cream	250	9	38
Canadian Maple	260	9	41
Strawberry	230	8	36
Honey Cruller	320	19	37
Yeast: Apple Fritter	300	11	49
Other varieties, avg.	210	8	30

Baked Goods: Per Serving

Croissant: Butter	340	18	38
Cheese	370	20	37
Southern Country Biscuits, avg. (1)	470	19	68
Tea Biscuit: Plain, 3 oz	250	9	35
Raisin, 3 oz	290	10	45
Cinnamon Roll: Frosted	470	25	57
Glazed	420	23	50
Danish: Cherry Cheese	330	13	46
Chocolate	430	24	51
Maple Pecan	380	20	46

Bagels: Average all types

	305	3	59
Cream Cheese: Plain, 1½ oz	130	12	2
Plain Light, 1½ oz	85	6	3
Garden Vegetable; Strawb., 1½ oz	120	11	3

Tim Hortons® Cont...

Muffins: Per Muffin

	C	F	Cb
Blueberry Bran	340	10	56
Wheat Carrot	400	19	55
Cranberry Fruit	360	11	60
Chocolate Chip Plain	430	14	71
Fruit Explosion	350	10	61
Raisin Bran	380	9	67
Strawberry Sensation	370	11	62
Low-Fat varieties	290	2.5	62

Timbits, Low-Fat

Cake: Chocolate Glazed	70	2.5	10
Old Fashion Plain	70	2	5
Filled, all varieties	60	2	10
Yeast: Apple Fritter	50	1.5	9
Honey Dip	60	2	9

Desserts

Yogurt: Strawberry w. Berries	150	2.5	28
Creamy Vanilla w. Berries	160	2.5	32

Beverages: Per Serving

Cafe Mocha, 10 fl.oz	170	7	27
Cappuccino: Eng. Toffee, 10 fl.oz	220	6	40
French Vanilla, 10 fl.oz	240	7	39
Iced w. 2% Milk, 12 fl.oz	300	15	41
Coffee w. sugar/cream, 10 fl.oz	75	3.5	9
Hot Chocolate, 10 fl.oz	240	6	45
Iced Tea, 12 fl.oz	50	1	10

T.J. Cinnamons®

Bakery

Chocolate Twist, 2½ oz	250	12	34
Cinnachips			
50/50 blend of Pecan Chips, 10 oz	1130	50	157
Cinnamon Twist, 1 roll, 2½ oz	260	14	33
T.J. Icing, 1 oz	120	5	18
Original Roll: no icing, 5.3 oz	510	10	73
w. Cream Cheese Icing	650	17	95
Pecan Sticky Bun, 1 bun, 6½ oz	690	22	91

Beverages: Per Serving (12 fl.oz)

Coffee	0	0	0
Mocha Chill: no Whipped Cream	260	4	46
w. Whipped Cream	310	7	49

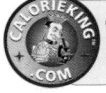

Restaurants & Fast - Foods

Togo's Eatery®

Sandwiches: Regular 6" Roll	C	F	Cb
Albacore Tuna	450	10	69
Avocado & Cucumber	590	26	79
Avocado & Turkey	670	27	78
Black Forest Ham & Cheese	630	24	67
Cheese Sandwich	660	30	70
Chunky Chicken & Almond Salad	750	43	64
Cold Roast Beef	680	22	68
Egg Salad & Cheese	650	28	69
Hummus	790	31	104
Salami & Cheese	760	37	70
The Italian	740	37	65
Turkey & Bacon Club	600	21	65
Turkey & Cheese	600	18	71
Turkey Ham & Cheese	600	19	70
Turkey Roast Beef & Cheese	670	23	70
BBQ Beef	530	13	64
California Roasted Chicken	620	15	68
French Onion Dip	640	16	66
Hot Pastrami	810	42	72
Meatballs in Zesty Tomato Sauce	690	23	80
Pastrami Reubin	650	25	68
Roast Beef	680	22	68
Savory BBQ Chicken	520	6	79
Sicilian Chicken	670	22	73

Large Size: Add 50% to Regular Size

Topz®

Burger: Ahi Fillet Burger	360	8	42
Cheeseburger	490	23	38
Chicken Breast	320	5	37
Double Cheeseburger	720	36	45
Garden Cheeseburger	490	17	62
Grilled Cheese Sandwich	440	20	50
Spicy Chicken Breast Burger	350	6	43
Topz Burger	420	15	44
Topz Jr Burger	230	9	21
Turkey Burger	390	11	38
Chili: Half Order, 4 oz	110	5	4
Fries: Aero, 5.6 oz	380	14	58
Chili Cheese, 9 oz	660	35	68
French Fries, 6 oz	500	22	68

Tropical Smoothie Cafe®

Sandwiches	C	F	Cb
American Albacore	725	30	86
Cheese BLT	715	37	72
Chicken Caesar	625	25	66
Chipotle Chicken	660	27	71
Club Sandwich	705	26	77
Ham & Cheese	605	19	78
Roast Beef	680	30	63
The Italian	750	39	71
Turkey Bacon Ranch	670	23	69
Tuscan Turkey	440	13	67
Wraps: Breakfast Wrap (Bacon)	535	23	55
Breakfast Wraps (Ham)	525	18	57
Buffalo Chicken	565	21	61
Cool Tuna Wrap	645	27	71
King Caesar	555	27	55
Sesame Chicken	755	24	103
Totally Turkey	655	27	58
Veggie Veggie	615	26	72
Western Wrap	535	18	59
Salads: No Cheese or Dressing			
Chef Salad	170	2	12
Garden Classic Salad	60	0.5	10
Sesame Chicken Salad	415	10	54
Thai Chicken Salad	355	4	54
Low Fat Smoothies (with Turbinado)			
Blimey Limey; Cool Breeze, avg.	410	0	102
Blue Lagoon	330	1	80
Hawaiian Breeze	360	0	88
Island Fever; Orange Passion, avg.	455	0.5	111
Rockin Raspberry	515	0.5	125
Strawberry Beach	450	0	109
Sunrise Sunset	390	0.5	96
Fat Buster	375	0.5	91
Health Nut	620	10	104
Lean Machine; Paradise Point, avg.	475	0.5	115
Muscle Blaster	595	3	119
Peanut Paradise	810	22	119
Dessert Smoothies (with Turbinado)			
Beach Bum, avg. all flavors	570	5.5	126
Chocolate Chiller	555	7	118
Coconut Royale	730	11	155
Mocha Madness	645	12	127
Peanut Butter Cup	840	24	142

With Splenda, deduct 200 calories & 50g carbs

Tubby's®

Subs: Per Regular Sandwich	C	F	Cb
Burger Subs: Big Tub	670	56	55
Burger Special	900	59	59
Cheeseburger	910	60	59
Pizza Burger	930	60	62
Taco Burger	825	47	67
Deli Style Subs: Ham & Cheese	570	30	54
Club Sub	700	41	53
Tubby's Famous	665	39	55
Turkey & Cheese	600	32	51
Turkey Club Sub	680	38	52
Specialty Subs: BLT	635	42	50
Cold Veggie	460	14	66
Italian Sausage	730	45	56
Tuna Salad	415	18	47
Veggie Stir Fry	650	27	90
Chicken Subs: Per Regular Sandwich			
Chicken & Broccoli	550	23	56
Chicken & Cheddar	545	23	54
Chicken Club Sub	705	41	53
Chicken Fajita Sub	445	12	57
Grilled Chicken	345	5	52
Steak Subs: Per Regular Sandwich			
Mushroom Steak	835	26	52
Pepper Steak	710	46	52
Pizza Steak	985	57	85
Steak & Cheese	825	56	51
Steak Special	745	46	58

Una Mas®

Burritos: No Sides/Chips	C	F	Cb
Bean & Cheese	755	39	56
Fresca	415	6.5	70
Gallito Griller	855	51	33
Grilled Fajita Burrito: Chicken	665	28	70
Steak	750	33	71
Pineapple Thai	560	16	70
San Lucas Fish, Baja Style	590	30	49
San Lucas Fish, Cabo Style	480	23	58
Tacos: Chicken Taco	230	6	30
Crispy Chicken Taco Plate	365	22	27
Steak Taco	255	7.5	30
Veggie Taco	210	5	34
Nachos, 1 serving, 24 oz	1890	110	180
Quesadillas			
Monterey Chicken	790	51	32
Monterey Steak	875	56	32

Uno Chicago Grill®

Entrees	C	F	Cb
Veggie Burger, no sides	500	11	71
Chicken Parmesan, no sides	940	21	140
Pasta Spinoccoli	1590	83	117
Flatbread Pizza: Individual			
Four Cheese	1570	56	93
Spinach, Mushroom & Gorgonzola	930	40	93
Soup: French Onion, 13 oz	230	12	19
Veggie, 12 oz	110	1.5	25
Salads: House, no dressing	120	1	25
Caesar w. dressing	430	35	21
Greek Salad, w. dressing	430	40	17
Honey Crisp Chicken w. dressing	760	38	65

For Complete Nutritional Data ~ see CalorieKing.com

Wahoo's Fish Taco®

Bowls	C	F	Cb
Carne Asada, Steak	760	22	90
Chicken, Skinless Breast	750	18	90
Fish of the Day	705	16	90
Classic Burrito (A la Carte)			
Fish, average	455	14	51
Chicken, average	545	17	50
Carne Asada	515	20	49
Carnitas	595	26	49
Shrimp	470	14	51
Veggie	600	14	98
Mushroom	415	17	57
Tacos: Carne Asada, Steak	195	7	18
Carnitas, Pork	230	10	18
Chicken, Skinless Breast	210	6	18
Fish of the Day	175	4	19
Veggie	200	4	33
Sides: Beans	445	2	80
Rice	475	6	94
Salads: Chips Not Included			
Carne Asada, Steak	555	33	13
Chicken, average	560	28	15
Fish, average	420	23	15

For Complete Nutritional Data ~ see CalorieKing.com

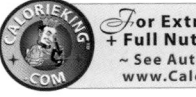

For Extra Menu Items + Full Nutritional Data
~ See Author's Website
www.CalorieKing.com

Restaurants & Fast - Foods

WAWA®

Breakfast & Baked Goods | **C** | **F** | **Cb**

	C	F	Cb
Bagel: Plain	285	1	61
w. Butter	495	23	64
w. Cream Cheese	425	13	67
Avg. other varieties	320	2	66
Bagel Melts: Ham & Cheese	485	13	67
Pepperoni & Cheese	740	38	67
Turkey Club w. Mayo	720	32	70
Breakfast Bowls: *Per Bowl*			
Creamed Chipped Beef on a Bisc.	475	25	54
Sausage Gravy on a Biscuit	515	29	53
Croissant, Regular, 2 oz	190	9	24
Hash Brown (1), 1.7 oz	90	5	10
Muffins: Banana Walnut, 6 oz	605	36	71
Blueberry, 6.2 oz	620	34	76
Chocolate Chip, 4 oz	450	24	55
Corn, 6 oz	650	31	83
Sizzli Bagels: Bacon Egg & Chse	460	19	53
Sausage Egg & Cheese	505	24	53
Sizzli Biscuits: Bacon Egg & Chse	540	34	45
Sausage Egg & Cheese	580	40	46
Sizzli Muffins: Bacon Egg & Chse	360	20	29
Sausage, Egg & Cheese	400	24	29
Hot Sandwiches: *No Cheese Unless Indicated*			
Chicken Breaded Club w. Cheese	710	36	56
Roasted Pork Kaiser	395	15	38
Classics: BBQ Pork w. Cheese	1090	48	112
Chicken Steak, no Dressing	515	10	61
Meatball w. Cheese	700	31	73
Roast Beef Homestyle w. Cheese	645	21	67
Cold Sandwiches: *No Cheese Unless Indicated*			
Italian w. Pesto & Rstd Peppers	725	32	67
Roast Beef Classic	595	10	62
Healthy Choice: Chicken	465	6	64
Ham on White	265	5	31
Smoked Turkey on White	265	4	31
Roast Beef on White	265	4	31
Turkey Carolina on White	290	2	28
Turkey on White	420	6	67
Roast Beef	375	7	37
Seafood Salad	455	22	53
Tuna Salad	575	36	45
Veggie	330	3	62
Veggie Supreme	515	16	71

WAWA® cont...

	C	F	Cb
Cold Shortis: American	435	18	40
BLT; Cheese, average	495	28	37
Chicken Salad	505	28	42
Egg Salad w. Cheese	630	40	43
Healthy Choice: Ham; Roast Beef	320	6	40
Honey Smoked Turkey	325	5	42
Hot Shortis: Chicken Steak	315	7	36
Meatball w. Cheese	440	21	45
Roast Beef Homestyle w. Cheese	400	14	40
Wraps: Buffalo Blue Chicken	365	16	33
Roast Beef & Pepper Jack	440	17	42
Roasted Chicken Caesar	415	20	33
Smoked Turkey Supreme	350	10	45
Turkey Bacon & Colby Jack	450	22	36
Hot Dogs: ¼ lb Beef Frank	390	28	23
All Beef Hot Dog	250	15	22
Big Bacon Cheese Dog	710	50	39
Hot Sausage	310	20	21
Kielbasa	290	16	21
Bowls: *Per 12 oz Bowl*			
Beef Stew	440	27	42
Chili	535	13	86
Chipotle Chicken Chili	530	11	88
Roasted Pork	545	35	38
Sides: *Per Medium*			
Beef Stew, 11 oz	265	12	22
Chili, 11 oz	220	8	28
Homestyle Chkn & Noodles, 11 oz	325	16	25
Macaroni & Cheese, 11 oz	460	22	50
Mashed Potatoes, 11 oz	470	31	47
Meatballs in a Cup, 4 oz	165	11	9
Shepherd's Pie, 11 oz	390	24	37
Soups: *Per Medium (11 oz)*			
Boston Clam Chowder	360	24	29
Chicken Corn Chowder	360	24	29
Potato w. Bacon	255	16	25
Vegetable Beef & Barley	150	5	19
Drinks: Cappuccino, 12 fl.oz	175	7	27
French Vanilla Cappuccino, 12 fl.oz	220	7	30
Fat Free Cappuccino, 12 fl.oz	160	0	37
Frozen Cappuccino, 12 fl.oz	250	7	47

Wendy's®

Sandwiches	C	F	Cb
Big Bacon Classic w. Mayo	590	30	46
Classic Single w. Mayo	420	20	37
Classic Double w. Cheese, Mayo	700	39	38
Classic Triple w. Cheese, Mayo	970	59	38
¼ lb Double Stack	420	20	34
¼ lb Deluxe Double Stack	470	24	36
Chicken Temptations: Ultimate	370	8	44
Spicy Fillet w. mayo	480	17	53
Homestyle Fillet	470	16	55
French Fries: Small, 5 oz	440	18	58
Medium, 5.6 oz	495	20	64
Large, 6.7 oz	590	24	77
Kids, 3.2 oz	285	12	37
Chicken: Crispy Nuggets, 5 pce	230	15	12
Homestyle Strips (3), no sauce	410	21	33
Sauce: Heartland Ranch, 1 pkt	200	22	1
Other varieties, avg., 1 pkt	175	17	5
Garden Sensations Salads			
Caesar Side Salad, no toppings	80	4.5	6
Caesar Chicken: no toppings	190	5	9
w. Dressing/Croutons	540	31	36
Chicken BLT Salad: no toppings	340	18	17
w. Croutons/Dressing	680	46	38
Mandarin Chicken: no toppings	170	2	18
w. Dressing/Nuts/Noodles	550	26	53
Side Salad, no Dressing	35	0	8
Southwest Taco: no toppings	440	22	32
w. Chips/Sour Cream/Dressing	710	41	51
Spinach Chicken: no toppings	260	12	9
w. Dressing/Croutons	450	16	42
Kids Meal: Hamburger only	270	9	33
Cheeseburger only	320	13	34
Chicken Nuggets, 4 pces, no sauce	190	12	10
Frosty, 4 oz	160	4	26
Baked Potatoes: Plain, 10 oz	270	0	61
Bacon & Cheese	460	13	78
Broccoli & Cheese	340	3.5	69
Sour Cream & Chives	320	4	63
Buttery Spread, 1 pkg	50	6	0
Sides: Chili, small, 8 oz	220	6	23
Chili, large, 12 oz	330	9	35
Cheddar Cheese, shredded, 2 Tbsp	70	6	1
Hot Chili Seasoning, 1 pkg	5	0	2
Mandarin Oranges, 5 oz	80	0	20
Saltine Crackers (2)	25	0.5	4
Yogurt w. Granola Cup	250	6	42
Chocolate Chip Cookie, 2 oz	270	12	37
Frosty: Large, 14 oz	520	13	86

For Complete Nutritional Data ~ see CalorieKing.com

WesterN SizzliN®

Steaks (Meat Only, Raw Wts)	C	F	Cb
New York Strip, 14 oz	900	60	0
Ribeye, 10 oz	520	28	0
Sirloin: 8 oz Steak	540	33	0
16 oz Steak	1080	66	0
T-Bone, 20 oz	1230	99	0
Baked Potato, plain, 8 oz	245	0	58

Wienerschnitzel®

Breakfast	C	F	Cb
Biscuit: w. Egg	280	18	20
Egg & Bacon	360	25	20
Egg, Bacon & Cheese	410	29	20
Egg, Sausage & Cheese	510	38	24
Burrito: Egg, Bacon & Cheese	530	28	39
Chili Cheese	510	24	44
Country Breakfast, 10.1 oz	630	45	31
French Toast Sticks	500	30	50
Hash Browns, 2.8 oz	290	25	14
Platter w. Bacon	640	43	40
Burgers: Chili Cheeseburger	350	13	32
Deluxe Cheeseburger	450	23	33
Deluxe Hamburger	400	19	33
Double Chili Cheeseburger	560	24	35
Fries: Regular, 4.6 oz	340	25	28
Large, 6.4 oz	470	34	39
Chili Cheese, 8.1 oz	540	38	39
Hot Dogs: Chili Dog	290	13	31
Chili Cheese Dog	340	17	31
Deluxe; Kraut; Mustard; Relish, avg.	270	12	30
All Beef: Chili Dog	380	21	33
Chili Cheese Dog	430	25	33
Other varieties, avg.	365	20	31
Turkey: Chili Dog	270	11	31
Chili Cheese Dog	320	15	31
Other varieties, average	250	10	28
For Pretzel Bun add extra	145	3	26
Sandwiches: Bacon Ranch Chkn	420	20	39
Italian Sausage	350	17	31
Pastrami	580	35	38
Polish Sausage	490	29	39
Sides: Onion Straws, 3.4 oz	430	35	25
Ranch Dressing, 1.2 oz	120	12	2
Desserts: Freezee, average	565	22	87
Banana Split	780	23	141
Chocolate Dipped Cone	420	26	45
Plain Cone	230	8	36

Whataburger®

Burgers/Sandwiches	C	F	Cb
Whataburger	615	31	61
No Bun	270	18	4
Double Meat Whataburger	845	48	61
Whataburger w. Bacon/Cheese	775	43	62
Triple Meat Whataburger	1065	66	61
Justaburger	310	16	30
Whatacatch	490	30	42
Whatachick'n	510	19	59
Whataburger Jr.	320	16	32
Grilled Chicken S'wich: w. Dressing	460	19	45
No Bun	190	7	10
Grilled Chicken Fajita Taco	365	13	36
Whatameals: Includes Drink & Fries (medium)			
Whataburger Meal	1320	51	191
Whataburger w. Bacon & Chse	1480	63	192
Chicken Strips (3)	1280	57	164
Double Meat Whataburger	1550	68	191
Grilled Chicken S'wich Meal	1160	39	175
WhataChick'N S'wich Meal	1200	39	190
French Fries: Small, 3 oz	260	13	31
Medium, 4½ oz	400	20	47
Large, 6 oz	530	27	63
Onion Rings: Medium, 4.3 oz	420	27	37
Large, 6.4 oz	630	40	55
Chicken & Salads			
Chicken Strips (2)	390	25	23
Chicken Strips Salad	580	39	35
w. Cheddar Cheese, no Bacon	600	39	32
Garden Salad	60	0	12
w. Cheddar Cheese, no Bacon	220	15	11
Grilled Chicken Salad	230	7	19
w. Cheddar Cheese, no Bacon	400	22	19
Dressings: Ranch, 2 oz	310	33	3
Reduced-Fat Ranch, 2 oz	230	22	6
Low-Fat Vinaigrette, 2 oz	40	1.5	6
Thousand Island, 2 oz	150	13	11
Shakes			
Chocolate; Strawberry:			
Small, 20 fl oz	615	16	100
Medium, 32 fl oz	905	25	146
Vanilla: Small, 20 fl oz	535	17	81
Medium, 32 fl oz	800	26	122
Breakfast			
Bacon, 1 slice	75	5.5	0
Cinnamon Roll	400	7	80
Hashbrown Sticks (4)	200	12	20
Texas Toast, 1 slice	180	8	25

Whataburger® cont...

Breakfast (Cont)	C	F	Cb
Biscuit: Buttermilk	300	17	32
w. Bacon	350	21	32
w. Bacon, Egg, Cheese	505	33	33
w. Egg & Cheese	445	27	35
w. Sausage	540	38	32
w. Sausage Gravy	510	35	49
w. Sausage, Egg, Cheese	695	50	33
Breakfast-On-A-Bun: w. Bacon	400	23	29
w. Sausage	585	40	29
Breakfast Platters (Biscuit/Eggs/Hash Brown):			
w. Bacon, 2 slices	740	46	53
w. Sausage, 1 patty	930	63	53
Pancakes: Plain (3)	580	8	112
w. Bacon, 2 slices	630	12	112
w. Sausage, 1 patty	820	29	112
Taquito: Bacon & Egg	380	12	27
Potato & Egg	560	37	37
Sausage & Egg	410	24	27
Desserts: Hot Apple Pie	225	11	29
Chocolate Chunk Cookie, 2 oz	230	11	33
White Choc Macadamia Cookie	250	14	30

Winchell's®

Baked Products	C	F	Cb
Croissant	260	17	28
Cake Donuts: Chocolate Iced	230	15	28
Traditional Cake	215	14	26
Yeast Raised Donuts: Per Donut			
Chocolate Bar	240	16	29
Chocolate Round/Twist	240	16	29
Glazed Round/Twist	230	15	27

White Castle®

Beverages: Per Medium (20 oz) Unless Indicated	C	F	Cb
Barq's Red Cream Soda	250	0	70
Coca-Cola, Classic/Cherry, avg.	230	0	61
Hot Chocolate, medium, 12 fl.oz	140	4	26
Iced Tea	170	0	46
Icee, all varieties	145	0	42
Orange Juice, 6 fl.oz	80	0	20
Choc./Strawberry Shake, avg.	400	4	82

White Castle® Cont...

Sandwiches & Burgers	C	F	Cb
Bacon Cheeseburger	200	12	13
Cheeseburger	160	9	13
Chicken Supreme	230	10	22
Double Bacon Cheeseburger	360	23	20
Double Cheeseburger	290	18	19
Double Jalapeno Cheeseburger	320	20	20
Double White Castle	250	14	19
Fish w. Cheese Sandwich	180	8	18
Jalapeno Cheeseburger	170	10	13
Chicken Breast w. Cheese Sandwich	210	8	21
Chicken Ring Sandwich w. Cheese	190	10	17
Surf & Turf Sandwich	390	22	27
White Castle Burger	140	7	13
Sides: Chicken Rings, 6 rings	340	23	15
Clam Strips, 4 oz	250	22	5
Fish Nibblers, 14 pieces	280	16	24
French Fries, 3.8 oz	310	15	39
Mozzarella Cheese Sticks, 3 sticks	250	14	22
Onion Rings, 13 rings	750	39	91
Sauces: Cheese Sauce, 1½ oz	130	10	6
Honey Mustard Fat-Free, 1 oz	50	0	13
Horseradish Mustard, 5.5g pkg	5	0	0
Marinara Sauce, 1 oz	15	0	3
Nacho Cheese Sauce, 1.6 oz	50	4	3
White Castle Zesty Zing, 1 oz	120	11	4

Yoshinoya®

Bowls	C	F	Cb
Beef Bowl: Regular	840	30	109
Large	1160	41	153
Chicken Bowl: Regular	760	15	125
Large	1110	22	180
Combo Bowl: Regular	750	19	117
Large	1220	36	171
Shrimp & Beef Bowl, Regular	1280	34	184
Kids Meal Bowl	340	11	48
Vegetable Beef Bowl: Regular	770	23	114
Large	1090	32	163
Vegetable Bowl: Regular	530	3.5	116
Large	780	5	169
Side Orders: Beef	370	28	6
Chicken & Vegetables	300	12	21
Rice	460	2.5	104
Vegetables	60	0.5	12
Desserts: Cheesecake	280	15	31
Chocolate Cake	330	17	44
Flan	230	7	35
Strawberry Shortcake	290	15	37

Note: Yoshinoya Beef Bowl Restaurants are based in California.

Zoup!®

Soups: Per Cup (8 fl.oz)	C	F	Cb
Chicken Potpie	200	8	21
Cream of Broccoli	160	11	12
Fire Roasted Tomato Bisque	290	22	22
Ginger Butternut Squash	240	15	28
Jamaican Gumbo; Chkn w. Garlic, avg.	130	2.5	19
New England Clam Chowder	200	5	22
Seafood Bisque	150	6	12
Tomato Spinach/Rice; Tom. Chili, avg.	100	3	19
Vegetable Bounty	90	1.5	33
Vegetarian Split Pea	140	1.5	25
White Chkn Chili; Chkn Chowder, avg.	160	3	23
Other varieties, average	140	7	17
Paninis: Turkey Club, ½ sandwich	470	28	22
Italian Chicken, ½ sandwich	370	21	23
Smoked Ham and Swiss, ½ s'wich	190	8	18
Bread: Per Piece (2 oz)			
Extra Low-Carb French, 2 oz	105	2	7
Extra Multigrain, 2 oz	190	4	30
Extra Sourdough, 2 oz	170	1.5	31

Zero's Subs®

Oven Baked Subs (6")	C	F	Cb
(Includes cheese, lettuce, tomato, onions, oil & vinegar)			
BLT	410	19	48
BLT, no Mayo	330	12	43
Cosmo Vegetarian	470	23	46
Cosmo Deluxe	490	25	48
Grinder	560	31	48
Grinder, Multigrain	560	32	50
Ham & Cheese	440	19	44
Meatball & Cheese	565	30	50
without Cheese	465	22	50
Pepperoni & Cheese	545	31	42
without Cheese	345	15	41
Roast Beef & Cheese	460	19	45
The Club	515	23	44
Tuna & Cheese	520	26	47
Turkey & Cheese	455	17	44
12" Size Subs: Double the figures for 6" size			
6" Subs From The Grill			
Grilled Veggie	395	14	52
Hot Italian Sausage & Cheese	665	37	45
Philly Chicken & Cheese	400	10	48
w. Mushrooms/Green Peppers	500	21	50
without Cheese	330	4	47

Notes on Cholesterol

- **Cholesterol** is a white waxy substance produced mainly by our liver. It is also found in animal food products. Plant foods have no cholesterol.

- **Cholesterol is essential to life.** It is a structural part of every body cell wall and is the building block for vitamin D, sex hormones, and bile acids which help in the digestion of dietary fats.

- **The body makes sufficient cholesterol** for its needs and does not rely on cholesterol in the diet. Dietary fats have a major influence on blood cholesterol levels - more so than dietary cholesterol.

- **A high blood cholesterol increases** the risk of atherosclerosis - the thickening of arteries that can reduce or block blood flow to the heart muscle, brain, eyes, kidneys, sex organs and other body parts.

  This in turn increases the risk of heart attack, stroke, blindness, kidney failure, impotence and other blood circulatory problems.

  Other risk factors which increase the risk of atherosclerosis include high blood pressure, tobacco smoking, obesity and diabetes (uncontrolled).

BLOOD CHOLESTEROL

Check Your Risk!

Cholesterol Level (mg/dL)	Risk of Heart Attack
240 and above ~	High Risk
200 - 239 ~	Borderline/High
Below 200 ~	Desirable

♥ Know your cholesterol level, particularly if there is a family history of heart disease or stroke. If high, see your doctor.

♥ All adults should have their cholesterol, HDL and triglycerides tested at least every 5 years.

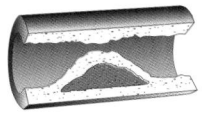

▲ Atherosclerosis can clog arteries and impede blood flow to the heart muscle or other body organs.

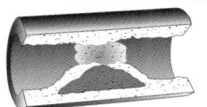

▼ A thrombus (blood clot) can form on unstable, festering atherosclerotic plaque and rapidly block blood flow. A heart attack or stroke can result.

HEART ATTACK WARNING SIGNALS

Many victims die before reaching hospital by ignoring warning signals and delaying medical help.

Symptoms vary and commonly include:

- **Chest pain**, vice-like squeezing or burning sensation in centre of chest or between shoulder blades, or feeling of severe indigestion.

- **Pain** may spread to shoulders, neck, jaw or arms.

- **Sweating**, nausea, dizziness, shortness of breath, irregular pulse.

If you experience any of the above symptoms seek IMMEDIATE medical attention!

Every minute counts.

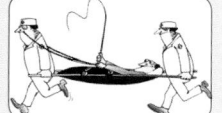

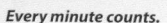

Fats & Cholesterol Guide

The amount and type of dietary fat has the greatest influence on blood cholesterol levels.

Fats in food are a mixture of 3 basic types: saturated, monounsaturated, and polyunsaturated. Animal fats are mainly saturated while plant oils and fish oils are mainly mono- and polyunsaturated.

Saturated fats have subgroups known as long chain, medium chain, and short chain fats. Most of the long chain fats raise blood cholesterol; and increase the risk of blood clots and thrombosis leading to artery blockage.

Long chain saturated fats are found mainly in full cream milk, cheese, butter, cream, fatty meats and sausages, and processed foods.

Monounsaturated fats tend to more selectively lower 'bad' LDL-cholesterol and maintain the protective 'good' HDL-cholesterol in the bloodstream - but only if they replace saturated fats in the diet.

Foods rich in monounsaturates include canola and olive oils, canola margarine, peanuts, and avocados.

Polyunsaturated fats consist of two main classes. **Omega-6** polyunsaturates tend to lower blood cholesterol. Rich sources include safflower, sunflower and corn oils.

Omega-3 polyunsaturated fats can lower blood cholesterol, and also confer extra benefits by lowering blood triglycerides, and reducing the risk of thrombosis, heart arrhythmias, and artery spasm.

Best practical omega-3 sources include canola oil and margarine, soybean oil and fish. (See adjoining chart)

A balanced intake of the two omega classes is important for optimal health. Increasing slightly omega-3 intake by Americans would help to attain a more ideal balance. Adequate vitamin E intake is also important.

> **All fats are high in calories and need to be limited for weight control.**

DIETARY FATS COMPARISON

■ Saturated Fat ■ Monounsaturated Fat
Polyunsaturated Fats:
☐ Linoleic (Omega-6) ☐ Alpha-Linolenic (Omega-3)

OILS — PERCENTAGE CONTENT

Oil	Saturated Fat	Monounsaturated Fat	Linoleic (Omega-6)	Alpha-Linolenic (Omega-3)
CANOLA OIL	7	63	20	10
LINSEED/FLAX OIL	9	19	17	55
SAFFLOWER OIL	9	14	77	
GRAPESEED OIL	10	22	68	
SUNFLOWER OIL	11	23	66	
CORN OIL	14	32	52	2
OLIVE OIL	14	76	10	
SOYBEAN OIL	15	23	54	8
PEANUT OIL	19	45	34	2
COTTONSEED OIL	26	16	58	
PALM OIL	51	39	10	

SPREADS & FATS

Saturated Fat includes 'Trans Fats'   ☐ WATER CONTENT

Spread/Fat	Saturated Fat	Monounsaturated	Linoleic	Alpha-Linolenic	Water Content
LIGHT MARGARINE	14	14	21		51
CANOLA MARGARINE	18	45	12	6	19
POLYUNSATURATED MARG	24	20	36		20
BUTTER	57	18	2		24
LARD	41	47	12		
BEEF FAT	44	37	4		15

Good Sources Of Omega-3 Fats

Plant Sources	Omega-3 Fats (Grams)
Canola Oil, 1 Tbsp, ½ fl.oz	1.5g
Flaxseed Oil, 1 Tbsp	8g
Soybean Oil, 1 Tbsp	1.2g
Canola Margarine, 1 Tbsp, ½ oz	1g
Soybeans, cooked, ½ cup, 4 oz	0.5g
Walnuts, ½ oz	0.5g

FISH - Per 4 oz Serving

High Content: Salmon (Chinook), Tuna, Trout (Lake), Sardines, Herring, Mackerel — 3g

Medium Content:
Salmon, (Pink/Red/Coho), 4 oz — 2g

Fair Content: Per 4 oz Serving
Bass, Catfish, Cod, Grouper, Hake, Halibut, Kingfish, Perch, Pollock, Shark, Trout (Rainbow), Tuna (Skipjack), Crab, Oysters, Blue Mussel, Shrimp, Squid } 0.5-1g

How Much Is Needed?

As little as 1-2 grams daily of omega-3 fats may promote general health. High doses of fish oil supplements should only be taken as directed by your doctor.

Cholesterol in Food

Dietary Cholesterol

Cholesterol in food varies in its effect on blood cholesterol level (BCL) from person to person. Much depends on the amount and type of fat, and fiber eaten at the same meal.

Any elevating effect of dietary cholesterol on BCL is more likely to occur when the diet is high in saturated fat. Little elevation, if any, generally occurs when dietary fats are balanced in favor of mono- and polyunsaturated fats (including omega-3 fats).

For example, while fish does contain cholesterol, the omega-3 fats can prevent any increase in BCL. Conversely, a meal containing no cholesterol but rich in saturated fat, may result in a significant increase in BCL.

Consequently, the need to be overly concerned about dietary cholesterol is being de-emphasized in favor of a stricter approach to limiting total fats, as well as saturated fat and trans fats in particular.

The liver usually cuts back its own cholesterol production in response to cholesterol in the diet. Many people can consume normal amounts of high cholesterol foods without concern.

However, it is difficult to identify just who is at risk - the so-called 'hyper-responders' - and because over 50% of Americans have a BCL above ideal levels, the **American Heart Association** advises all Americans to be prudent and limit their cholesterol intake to less than 300mg daily – as well as adopting a heart-healthy diet.

This limitation still allows the inclusion of most foods regularly eaten - even the overly maligned egg.

> Note: Eggs contain a modest 5 grams of fat per large egg of which barely 2 grams are saturated, the rest being mono- and polyunsaturated.
>
> By comparison, a cup of whole milk has almost 10g fat of which 6g are saturated.

CHOLESTEROL COUNTER

Cholesterol is found only in foods of animal origin. Plant foods contain no cholesterol.
AHA recommends limiting dietary cholesterol to less than 300mg/day.

	Chol mg
Meat - Average all types:	
Lean Meat, cooked, 4 oz	70
Fatty Meat, cooked, 4 oz	105
Fat, thick strip, 2 oz	35

(Note: While lean meat and fat have similar amounts of cholesterol, choose lean meat to limit fat intake.)

	Chol mg
Chicken/Turkey: average, 4 oz	90
Organ Meats: Liver, fried, 4 oz	500
Brains, beef, pan fried, 3 oz	1700
Sausages: Frankfurter, 1.5 oz	25
Salami, 2 slices, 2 oz	40
Bacon: 3 slices, cooked, 1 oz	20
Fish: Fish fillets, average, ckd, 4 oz	70
Tuna/Salmon, canned, 3 oz	30
Scallops, 9 medium, 3 oz	30
Shrimp, 12 large, raw, 3 oz	130
Oysters, raw, 6 medium, 3 oz	45
Lobster, Crab, raw, 3 oz	80
Eggs (Chicken), 1 large	210
1 medium	180
Egg White, *Egg Beaters*	0
Milk/Yogurt: Whole, 1 cup, 8 fl.oz	35
1% Milk, 1 cup	10
Skim/Non-fat, 1 cup	5
Soy Milk, Tofu, Tempeh	0
Cheese: Natural/Hard/Cream, 1 oz	30
Cottage, lowfat, 4 oz	5
Ricotta, part skim, 4 oz	25
Fats: Butter, 2 Tbsp, 1 oz	60
Margarine, Oils (vegetable)	0
Mayonnaise, 1 Tbsp	10
Cream: Heavy, whipping, 2 T, 1 oz	40
Half & Half/Sour, 2 Tbsp, 1 oz	10
Icecream: Regular, ½ cup, 4 fl.oz	30
Fruit, Vegetables, Avocados	0
Nuts, Seeds, Grains	0
Coffee, Tea, Soda, Beer, Wine	0

For Comprehensive Food Listings ~ see CalorieKing.com

Blood Cholesterol ~ Diet Hints

DIETARY HINTS TO LOWER BLOOD CHOLESTEROL

1. **Maintain a healthy weight.**
   If overweight, lose weight with lowfat eating and daily exercise.

2. **Reduce saturated fat intake by:**
   (a) eating less dairy fat. Choose lowfat or fat-reduced varieties of milk, yogurt, soy drinks, cheese, and icecream.

   (b) replacing saturated fats with fats and oils rich in mono- and polyunsaturated fats. Choose vegetable oils such as canola, olive, sunflower and soybean. Avoid solid frying fats.

   Take Control and *Benecol* (spreads) contain plant stanol esters which can lower total and LDL cholesterol.

   (c) eating less fat from meat and poultry. Choose lean cuts of meat and skinless chicken. Go easy on luncheon meats, salamis and fatty sausages. Enjoy fish.

   (d) eating less saturated and trans fats from baked and fried fast-foods. Avoid deep-fried foods. Avoid donuts, cakes, pastries and cookies unless made with healthier fats and oils.

3. **Increase your 'soluble' fiber intake.**
   Foods rich in 'soluble' fiber include dried beans, baked beans, lentils, chick peas, hummus, nuts, seeds, psyllium seed husks and psyllium fiber supplements. Oat bran, rice bran and barley are also useful, as are fruit, veggies and avocados.

4. **Eat more soya bean products** such as: soy drinks, tofu, tempeh (cultured soya beans), soy flour and soy vegetarian foods. Soy protein in place of animal protein can significantly decrease high blood cholesterol levels - as well as 'bad' LDL-cholesterol and blood triglycerides. Good HDL-cholesterol is maintained. For best results, eat at least 25g of soy protein per day (from 3-4 servings).

5. **Eat more fruit and vegetables and wholegrains** in place of high-fat foods. Aim for 2 fruits and 5 servings of vegetables per day. They also contain valuable antioxidants. The fat of avocados (and most nuts) is mainly unsaturated and can lower blood cholesterol levels.

6. **Limit cholesterol to 300mg per day.**
   (Extra Notes ~ See Previous Page)

7. **Avoid brewed unfiltered coffee** (espresso; plunger-style). Several cups per day may raise blood cholesterol. American-style filtered coffee is fine.

8. **Spread your food intake over the day.**
   Have 5-6 small meals per day rather than just 2-3 large meals. Nibbling, versus gorging, favors lower blood cholesterol.

ALCOHOL - WINE

Alcohol is a mixed bag. Moderate amounts of 1-2 drinks daily appear to reduce the risk of heart attack and ischaemic stroke in older persons.

However, larger amounts increase the risk of high blood pressure, obesity, heart failure and hemorrhagic stroke; and can aggravate hypertriglyceridemia - as well as many other health hazards. *(See Alcohol Guide – Page 166)*

The speculative benefits of moderate alcohol intake have been overstated in the media. The over-riding harmful effects of excess alcohol do not allow its recommendation for any aspects of health promotion.

Fruit, Vegetables & Tea Also Protect:
Red wine and red grapes (more so than white) contains antioxidants which may help protect cholesterol in the blood from becoming oxidized.

Many fruits, vegetables, grains, nuts and tea also contain protective antioxidants.

How Fats Affect Blood Flow

Fats in the diet not only affect blood cholesterol levels. They can also strongly influence blood clot formation and thrombosis, as well as blood flow and ultimate oxygen delivery to body parts and organs.

While advanced atherosclerosis can impede blood flow to the heart and other organs, it is thrombosis (complete blockage by blood clots) or arterial spasm which commonly result in a heart attack or stroke.

Plant and fish oils rich in omega-3 fats lessen the risk of blood clots, thrombus formation and artery spasm by reducing platelet stickiness and adhesion to artery walls. This reduces the risk of atherosclerotic plaque becoming unstable and reactive.

Omega-3 fats also improve blood flow by reducing blood viscosity; and increasing the flexibility of red blood cells (RBC) that need to flex and twist on themselves in order to squeeze through tiny narrow capillaries often half their diameter.

A diet high in saturated fats has the opposite effect by stiffening RBC membranes and increasing blood viscosity thereby hindering blood flow. The stiffening of the RBC membrane also reduces its ability to release vital oxygen to body cells and take up carbon dioxide.

Stiff red blood cells may also form aggregates like coin stacks. In narrow blood vessels, this further impedes blood flow and impairs oxygen release through the much lessened surface area of red blood cell membranes exposed to blood. (Smoking, lack of exercise, and stress can have similar adverse effects on thrombosis, red blood cell flexibility and blood flow.)

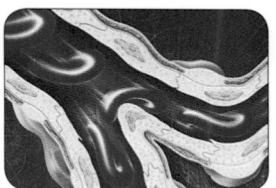

▲ **Picture of Healthy Blood Flow**

Flexible red blood cells twist and slide through tiny capillaries - often half the diameter of red blood cells.

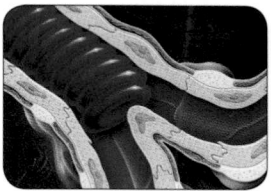

▲ **A Not-So-Healthy Picture!**

Red blood cells have lost their flexibility and ability to twist and slip through capillaries. They are stacked up thereby impeding blood flow.

A diet high in saturated fats can contribute to this picture - as can smoking, lack of exercise and stress.

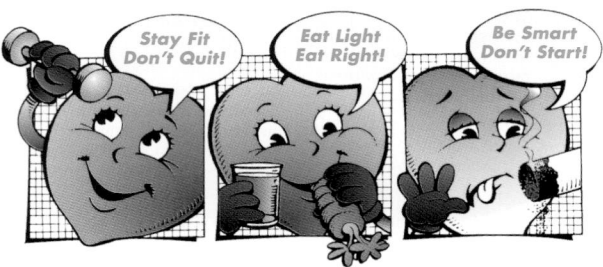

Stay Fit Don't Quit!

Eat Light Eat Right!

Be Smart Don't Start!

Fiber Guide

Introduction

Fiber is the general term for those parts of **plant** food that we cannot digest (although bacteria in the large bowel partly digests fiber through fermentation). It is not found in foods of animal origin (meats, dairy products).

Fiber promotes intestinal health, bowel regularity, can benefit diabetes and blood cholesterol levels, and may help prevent colon cancer. High fiber foods also assist weight control.

Most Americans don't eat enough fiber - less than 20 grams/day - instead of a healthier **25 to 35 grams/day.**

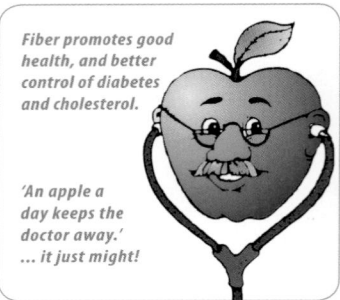

Fiber promotes good health, and better control of diabetes and cholesterol.

'An apple a day keeps the doctor away.' ... it just might!

Types of Fiber

Plant foods contain a mixture of different fibers in varying proportions. Insoluble and soluble fiber categories are based on their solubility in water. All types of fiber are beneficial to the body.

◆ **Insoluble fibers** (cellulose, hemi-celluloses, lignin) make up the structural parts of plant cell walls.

  Best food sources are wheat bran, corn bran, rice bran, wholegrain cereals and breads, dried beans and peas, nuts, seeds and the skins of fruits and vegetables.

These fibers absorb many times their own weight in water. They create a soft bulk and hasten the passage of waste products through the intestines.

They promote bowel regularity, and aid in the prevention and treatment of uncomplicated forms of **constipation, diverticulosis and haemorrhoids.**

The risk of colon cancer may also be reduced by fiber's diluting effect of potentially harmful substances.

◆ **Soluble fibers** (pectin, gums, mucilages) are found mainly within plant cells, soy milk (whole bean) and products.

Types of Fiber (Cont)

Best Sources of Soluble Fiber:
Fruits and vegetables, oat bran, barley, dried beans and peas, psyllium and flax seed.

These fibers form a gel which slows both stomach emptying and the absorption of sugars from the intestines. This helps to control **blood sugar** levels.

Weight control is also aided by the slower emptying of the stomach and the feeling of **fullness provided by soluble fiber.**

Some soluble fibers can lower **blood cholesterol** by binding bile acids and excreting them. More body cholesterol must then be broken down to supply bile acids for emulsification of dietary fats. **Rice bran, while not high in soluble fiber can also lower blood cholesterol.**

◆ **Resistant starch** is that part of starchy foods (approx. 10%) which is tightly bound by fiber and resists normal digestion. Friendly bacteria in the large bowel ferment and change the resistant starch into short-chain fatty acids which are important to bowel health and may protect against colon cancer.

Starchy foods include bread, cereals, rice, pasta, potatoes and legumes.

Fiber & Weight Control

Fiber can assist weight control in several ways. Fiber-rich foods such as fresh fruit and vegetables, potatoes and whole-grain bread contain few calories for their large volume (due to their lowfat, high water content).

Their bulk fills the stomach and satisfies appetite much earlier than fiber-depleted foods. The extra chewing time also contributes to satiety, and gives the stomach time to register a feeling of fullness. Excessive calories are less likely to be consumed.

Fiber-depleted foods and drinks are more concentrated in calories; e.g. fats, sugar, candy, soft drinks, fruit juices, alcohol. They require little or no chewing. Large amounts with excessive calories can be consumed before appetite is satisfied.

Example: Whereas one fresh apple might satisfy our appetite, an apple juice drink with the equivalent sugars and calories of 2-3 apples does little to satisfy appetite. (See illustration below.)

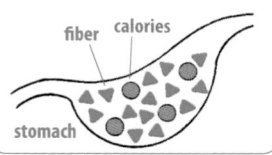

High Fiber Foods fill the stomach. Fewer calories are consumed.

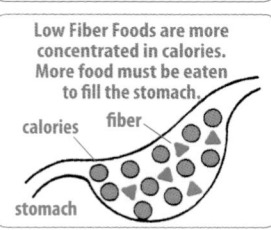

Low Fiber Foods are more concentrated in calories. More food must be eaten to fill the stomach.

EFFECTS OF REMOVING FIBER FROM FOOD

2-3 pieces of fresh fruit produces 1 glass of fruit juice. The removal of fiber concentrates the sugar and calories.

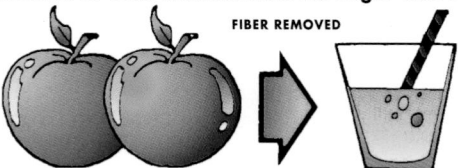

FIBER REMOVED

Fresh Fruit		Fruit Juice
High Fiber	←	Negligible Fiber
Low Calorie Density	←	High Calorie Density
Long Eating Time	←	No Eating Time (Drink)
Satisfies Hunger	←	Does Not Satisfy Hunger
Sugar Slowly Absorbed	←	Sugar More Quickly Absorbed
Less Insulin Required	←	More Insulin Required

Fiber Guide - Constipation

Constipation

Constipation can reasonably be defined as a failure to have a bowel movement at least every second day – and just as importantly, without straining or pain.

Typically, stools are too hard, too narrow and too small.

The **main cause** is simply a lack of dietary fiber. Other contributing factors include insufficient fluids, too little exercise, emotional stress, gastro-intestinal disease, lack of proper dentition to chew high-fiber foods, and some medications (e.g. some antacids, antidepressants, tranquilizers).

Note: Check with your doctor to rule out any underlying medical problem – especially if you have a change in bowel habits in middle-age or later years.

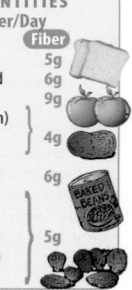

DESIRABLE FIBER INTAKE
Adults: 25-35gm per day
Children (under 18): Age + 5gm
Example: 6-year old (6 + 5)= 11gm

SAMPLE FOOD QUANTITIES
For 35 Grams of Fiber/Day

	Fiber
Breakfast Cereal (higher-fiber)	5g
plus 4 slices wholegrain Bread	6g
plus 3 servings fresh Fruit	9g
plus 1 medium Potato (w. skin)	
or 1 cup Brown Rice	4g
or ½ cup wholegrain Pasta	
plus 3-4 servings Veges/Salad	6g
plus 1 cup Bean Soup	
or ¼ cup Baked/Soy Beans	
or ½ cup Corn/Peas/Lentils	5g
or 1¼ oz Almonds (natural)	
or 3 medium Figs	

HINTS TO INCREASE FIBER AND AVOID CONSTIPATION

1. **Breakfast is an important** contributor to daily fiber intake. Eat high-fiber breakfast cereals (bran-based cereals, oatmeal etc.). Add 1-2 tablespoons of unprocessed bran (wheat/ barley/ rice) and wheat germ if required.

   Dried fruits, chopped nuts, soy grits, and seeds are also excellent additions to cereals.

   Note: A gradual increase in fiber will prevent bloating, gas or pain. People intolerant to bran may benefit from psyllium-based fiber supplements and cereals.

2. **Drink 6-8 glasses of water daily.** Fiber works by absorbing many times its own weight of water.

3. **Eat whole-grain breads,** or fiber-enriched breads. One slice of wholegrain bread has over double the fiber of regular white bread.

4. **Enjoy fruit as fresh fruit** with skins rather than as fruit juice. Enjoy wholegrain pasta, barley, brown rice, nuts and seeds.

5. **Eat more vegetables,** salads and legumes – especially dried beans, baked beans, lentils, potatoes with skins, avocado, broccoli, brussel sprouts, cabbage, carrots, celery and peas.

6. **Add bran** (barley/rice/wheat) or soy grits to soups, casseroles, yogurt, desserts, cookies, cakes. Also use wholemeal flour or soy flour in place of white flour. Use nuts and seeds.

7. **Snack** on fresh or dried fruits, carrot or celery sticks, popcorn, nuts or seeds, wholegrain crackers, high-fiber bars (low-fat). Limit amounts if overweight.

8. **Exercise regularly** to strengthen abdominal muscles and stimulate the gut. Keep up fluids, especially in warm weather.

9. **Avoid** indiscriminate and regular use of harsh laxatives. They can overstimulate the intestinal muscles and may make normal bowel activity impossible. It may take several weeks to restore normal bowel function.

FOODS WITH ZERO FIBER

- **Dairy Products (Milk, Cheese, etc)**
- **Meats, Poultry, Fish, Eggs**
- **Fats/Oils, Sugar/Syrups**

(Only foods of plant origin contain fiber.)

Breakfast Cereals

	Fiber
General Mills:	
Basic 4, 1 cup, 2 oz	3
Cheerios (Honey Nut; Multigrain), 1 c., 1 oz	3
Multi-Bran Chex, 1 cup, 2 oz	7
Oatmeal Crisp Almond, 1 cup, 2 oz	4
Raisin Nut Bran, 1¼ cup, 2 oz	5
Total, average all types, ¾ cup, 1 oz	3
Wheat Chex, 1 cup, 2 oz	5
Wheaties Energy Crunch, 2 oz	3
Health Valley:	
Amaranth Flakes, ¾ cup, 1 oz	4
Crunches & Flakes, ¾ cup, 2 oz	4
Fiber 7 Flakes, ¾ cup, 1 oz	4
Golden Flax, ¾ cup, 1.8 oz	6
Granola (Low-Fat), ⅔ cup, 2 oz	6
Healthy Fiber Flakes, ¾ cup, 1 oz	4
Oat Bran Flakes, all types, ¾ cup, 1 oz	4
Oat Bran O's, ¾ cup, 1 oz	3
Real Oat Bran, ½ cup, 1.7 oz	5
Kellogg's: All-Bran, ½ cup, 1 oz	10
All-Bran w. Extra Fiber, ½ cup, 1 oz	13
All-Bran Bran Buds, ⅓ cup, 1 oz	13
Corn Flakes, Fruit Loops, Smacks, ¾ cup, 1 oz	1
Cocoa/Rice Krispies Treats, ¾ cup, 1 oz	0
Complete: Wheatbran Flakes, ¾ c., 1 oz	5
Oatbran Flakes, ¾ cup, 1.1 oz	4
Corn Pops, 1 cup, 1 oz	0.5
Cracklin' Oat Bran, ¾ cup, 1.7oz	6
Crunchy Blends: Granola w. Raisins, ⅔ cup	3
Muesli, ⅔ cup, 2 oz	4
Frosted Mini Wheats, 24 bisc., 2 oz	5
Nutri-Grain Cereal Bars, 1 bar, 1.3 oz	1
Raisin Bran, 1 cup, 2 oz	7
Smart Start: Healthy Heart, 1¼ cups, 2 oz	5
Soy Protein, 1 cup, 2 oz	4
Product 19, 1 cup, 1.1 oz	1
Special K, 1 cup, 1.1 oz	0.5

Fiber ~ Fiber (grams)

Breakfast Cereals (Cont)

	Fiber
Kashi: GoLEAN Cereal, 1 cup, 1.8 oz	10
GoLEAN Crunch!, 1 cup, 1.9 oz	8
GoLEAN Bars, avg. (1)	4
Good Friends: 1 cup, 1.9 oz	12
Cinna-Raisin Crunch, 1 cup, 1.8 oz	8
Heart to Heart, ¾ cup, 1.2 oz	5
7 Whole Grain Pilaf, ½ cup, cooked, 5 oz	6
7 Whole Grain Puffs, 1 cup, 0.7 oz	1
Quaker: Captain Crunch, ¾ cup, 1 oz	1
100% Natural Granola, average, ⅔ cup, 1.9 oz	3
Crunchy Corn Bran, ¾ cup, 1 oz	5
Fruitangy Oh's, 1 cup, 1 oz	1
Honey Nut Oats, ¾ cup, 1 oz	1
Life Cereal, ¾ cup, 1.1 oz	2
Oat Bran, ½ cup, 1.4 oz	6
Oatmeal, average, 1 packet	3
Puffed Rice, 1 cup, ½ oz	0
Puffed Wheat, 1 cup, ½ oz	1
Shredded Wheat, 3 biscuits, 2.2 oz	7
Post: 100% Bran, ⅓ cup, 1 oz	9
Alpha Bits, 1 cup, 1 oz	3
Blueberry Morning, 1 cup, 2 oz	3
Cocoa/Fruity Pebbles, 1 cup, 1 oz	3
Cranberry Almond Crunch, 1 cup, 2 oz	3
Fruit & Bran, 1 cup, 2 oz	6
Grape-Nuts, ½ cup, 2 oz	6
Great Grains, ⅔ cup, 1.9 oz	4
Honey Bunches of Oats, ¾ cup, 1 oz	2
Shredded Wheat 'n Bran, ½ cup, 2 oz	8

Brans & Supplements

Oat Bran: 1 Tbsp (level)	1
⅓ cup, (5⅓ Tbsp), 1 oz	4.4
Rice Bran, raw. ¼ cup, 1 oz	6
Wheat Bran (unprocessed): Raw, 1 Tbsp	1.5
2 Tbsp (level), ¼ oz	3
¼ cup, (4 Tbsp), ½ oz	6.5
½ cup, 1 oz	13
Corn Germ: Raw, ¼ cup, 1 oz	5
Wheat Germ: Raw, ¼ cup, 1 oz	4
Psyllium Seed Husks, 2 Tbsp	8
Metamucil, 1 dose	3.4

Hot Cereals, Oatmeal

Bulgur (cracked Wheat), ckd, 1 cup	8
Corn/Hominy Grits, dry, 3 Tbsp, 1 oz	0.5
Cream of Wheat, cooked, ¾ cup	1
Oatmeal (uncooked ⅓ cup), ckd, ⅔ cup	2.5

Fiber Guide

Breads & Crackers | Fiber

Bread: White, 1 slice, 1 oz	0.6
Whole-wheat, 1 slice, 1 oz	1.5
Whole-grain, 1 slice, 1 oz	2
Rye, Pumpernickel, 1 oz	1.5
Bagel/Roll/Bun, 1 medium, 2 oz	1.5
Pita, whole wheat, 6½" pocket	4.5
Crackers: Graham, average, 2	0.4
Saltine, 4 crackers	0.4
Crispbreads (Rye), average, 2	4
Matzo 1 board, 1 oz	1
Rice Cakes, average, 1 cake	0.3
Tortilla: Regular, 6"	0.5
Whole-wheat, 6"	1.3

Barley, Pasta, Rice & Flours

Barley, pearled, raw, ¼ cup, 1.7 oz	8
Rice: White, cooked, 1 cup	0.6
Brown, cooked, 1 cup	3.5
Rice-A-Roni, average, 1 cup, prepared	1.5
Spaghetti/Noodles: Cooked, 1 cup	2
Whole-Wheat, cooked, 1 cup	4
Flour: Wheat, All-purpose, 1 cup, 4½ oz	3.5
Whole-Wheat, 1 cup, 4½ oz	15
Cornmeal, stone ground, 1 cup, 4½ oz	13
Carob Flour, 1 cup, 3½ oz	41
Rye Flour, 1 cup, 3½ oz	15
Soy Flour: Defatted, 1 cup, 3½ oz	17
Full-fat, raw, 1 cup, 3 oz	8
Soy Meal, defatted, 1 cup, 4½ oz	14

Frozen Entrees & Dinners

Average All Brands: *Per Serving*	
Beans/Chili base, average	6-10
Potato/Pasta base, average	4-6
Vegetable base, average	3
Meat/Chicken base, average	2-3
Pizzas, ¼ large, average	3
Vegetarian Soy Burgers, 1 pattie	4

Soups

Chicken Noodle, 1 cup	0.5
Tomato Soup, average, 1 cup	0.5
Vegetable Soup, average, 1 cup	3
Health Valley: *Per 1 Cup Serving*	
Black Bean; Minestrone	8
Tomato	1
5-Bean Vegetable; Lentil & Carrots	10
Mushroom Barley; Vegetable	4
Split Pea	8

Fast Foods & Restaurants | Fiber

Hamburgers: Small, average	1.5
Large/Whopper, average	2.5
Hot Dog, Regular	1.5
French Fries: Small serving, 2½ oz	2.5
Regular/Medium, 3½ oz	3.5
Chicken Nuggets, 6 pack	0.5
Chicken Sandwich, average	2
Taco, average	4
Sundaes, Shakes, Soft Drinks	0
Arby's: Baked Potato w. Broc. & Cheese	8
Roast Beef Sandwich, regular	2
Denny's: Grilled Chicken Salad, no bread	4
Classic Burger, no fries	4
Club Sandwich, no fries	4
Grilled Chicken Sandwich, no fries	4
Domino's (Classic): Vegi Feast, 1 sl. (12")	2
Hawaiian Feast, 1 slice, (12")	2
Pepperoni Feast, 1 slice (12")	2
McDonald's: Big Mac	3
Hamburger; Cheeseburger; Quarter Pounder	1
Egg McMuffin	2
Grilled Chicken Caesar Salad	3
McVeggie Burger on Wheat Bun	8
Pizza Hut: *Per 1 Slice, Medium*	
Pan Pizza: Cheese, Pepperoni	1
Supreme	2
Thin'n Crispy, Supreme	2
Hand-Tossed, average all varieties	2
Subway: Sandwich, white roll, avg.	4
w. Honey Wheat Roll, average	3.2
Footlong w. Wheat Roll, average	8
Salads, average	4

Cakes, Cookies, Snack Bars

Apple/Fruit Pie, 1 serving, 4 oz	2
Cake: w. plain flour, 1 serving, 3.4 oz	1.5
w. whole-wheat flour, 1 serving	3
Carrot Cake, 1 serving, 1.2 oz	2
Cookies, oatmeal, (3 small/1 large)	1
Donuts, Medium, 1.7 oz	0.7
Fruit Cake, 1 serving, 1½ oz	2
Fig Bars, 1 cookie, ½ oz	0.7
Muffins, Oat Bran (2 small, 1 large), 4 oz	5
Granola Bars, average, 1 bar	2
Atkins Advantage Bars, average	7
Clif Bars, 2.5 oz	5
Fi-Bar Chewy & Nutty 1 bar	5
Health Valley: Fruit/Granola Bars	1
Cereal Bars	1
Luna Bars, avg., 1.7 oz	3

Chocolate, Chips, Popcorn | Fiber
Cheese Balls/Curls/Twists	1
Chocolate, Hard Candy, 1 oz	0
Chocolate with nuts/fruit, 2 oz bar	1.5
Mars Bar, 1.8 oz	1
Potato Chips, corn chips, 1 oz	1
Popcorn, 3 cups	3
Pretzels, Twists (6)	1

Nuts, Seeds
Almonds: Natural, 25 kernels, 1 oz	3.5
Blanched (skins removed), 1 oz	3
Cashews, Filberts, Pecans, 1 oz	1.7
Peanuts, Mixed Nuts, Coconut, 1 oz	2.5
Peanut Butter, 2 Tbsp, 1 oz	2
Pistachio Nuts, dried, shelled, 1 oz	3
Walnuts, Black/English, dried, 1 oz	2
Seeds: Amaranth, 2½ Tbsp, 1 oz	3.5
Flax Seeds, 3 Tbsp, 1 oz	7
Psyllium Seed Husks, 5 Tbsp, 1 oz	20
Quinoa Seeds, 3 Tbsp, 1 oz	1.7
Sesame Seeds, whole, 1 oz	3.4
Sesame Butter/Tahini, 2 Tbsp, 1.1 oz	1.4
Sunflower kernels, ¼ cup, 1 oz	3.8
Teff Seeds, 1 oz	3.8

Fruit – Fresh
Apples: 1 medium, 5½ oz (whole)	
with skin + core	3.7
with skin, no core	3.2
without skin, no core	1.7
Apricots, 2 medium, 4 oz	1.5
Avocado, average, ½ medium	6.7
Banana, 1 medium, 6 oz (w. skin)	3
Blueberries, raw, ½ cup, 2½ oz	1.7
Cherries, sweet, raw, 8 fruits, 1.6 oz	1
Grapefruit, average, ½ fruit, 10 oz	1.4
Grapes, 1 medium bunch, seedless, 7 oz	2
Kiwifruit, 1 medium, 2.7 oz	2.3
Mango, 1 medium, 11 oz (whole)	1.6
Melons: Cantaloupe, 4 oz (edible)	1
Nectarine, 1 medium, 4 oz	1.9
Olives, average all types, 7 jumbo, 2 oz	1.5
Oranges, 1 medium (7-8 oz w. skin)	
5½ oz (peeled)	3.8
Passionfruit, 2 medium, 2½ oz	5
Peaches, 1 large, 6 oz	2
Pears, raw, 1 medium, 6 oz	4.5
Pineapple, 1 slice, 3 oz	1.2
Plums, 2 medium, 6 oz	1.8
Strawberries, 6 medium/3 large, 2 oz	1
Watermelon, 4 oz (edible)	0.5

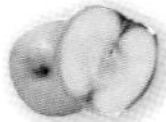

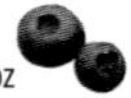

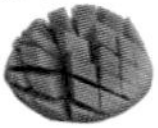

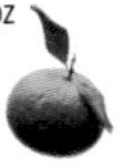

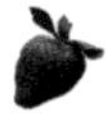

Fruit – Dried, Juice | Fiber
Dried Fruit: Apricots, 8 halves, 1 oz	2.2
Dates (3 med); Raisins (2 Tbsp), 1 oz	1.5
Figs, 3 medium, 1½ oz	5
Prunes, 4 medium, 1 oz	2
Fruit Juice: Orange/Apple etc, 1 glass	<0.5
Prune Juice, 5 oz	1.4
Carrot Juice, 8 oz	1.8

Vegetables
Asparagus, 4 medium spears	1.3
Bean Sprouts, ½ cup, 2 oz	1
Beans: Snap/Green, ½ cup, 2 oz	2
Baked Beans in Tom Sce, ½ c, 4½ oz	5
Dried Beans, ckd, average, ½ cup	7
Beets, ckd, slices, ½ cup, 3 oz	1.7
Broccoli, cooked, ½ cup, 3 oz	2.4
Brussels Sprouts, ckd, ½ cup, 3 oz	3.5
Cabbage: White, ckd, ½ cup, 2½ oz	1
Red, ckd, ½ cup, 2½ oz	2
Carrots, 1 medium (7½"), ½ cup, 3 oz	2.5
Cauliflower, cooked, 3 flowerets, 2 oz	1.5
Celery, raw, diced, 1 cup, 3½ oz	1.6
Chick Peas (Garbanzos), ckd, ½ c., 3 oz	6.5
Corn, kernels, ckd, ½ cup, 2½ oz	2.5
Cream-style, ½ cup, 2½ oz	1.5
Cucumber/Lettuce/Mushrooms, 2 oz	0.5
Eggplant, raw, sliced, ½ cup , 1½ oz	2
Lentils, cooked, ½ cup, 3½ oz	8
Mixed Vegetables, frozen, cooked, ½ cup	3
Onions: Raw, 1 medium, 4 oz	1.5
Spring Onions, chop., ¼ cup, 1 oz	0.7
Peas: Green, Raw, 2½ oz	3.7
Cowpeas (Black-eyed), ckd, ½ cup	10
Split Peas, ckd, ½ cup, 3½ oz	8
Peppers, sweet, raw, 1 large, 6 oz	3
Potatoes, 1 medium, with skin, 5 oz	4
without skin	2.5
½ cup mashed, 3½ oz	1.5
French Fries, small, 2.6 oz	3
Spinach, cooked, ½ cup, 3 oz	2.2
Squash: Summer, cooked, ½ cup, 3 oz	2.5
Winter, cooked, ½ cup, 3½ oz	2.4
Tomatoes: 1 medium, 4½ oz	1.5
Tomato Sauce, 1 cup	0.3
Soybean Products: Miso, ½ c., 5 oz	7.4
Tempeh, cooked, 1 piece, 3 oz	4
Tofu, ½ cup, 4.4 oz	0.4

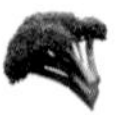

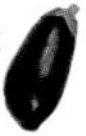

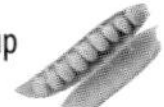

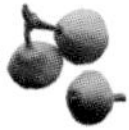

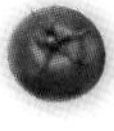

Salads: Side Salad, average
Bean Salad, ½ cup	5
Coleslaw, ½ cup	1
Potato Salad, ½ cup	2

Protein Guide

General Notes

- **Protein has many important body functions.** It builds and repairs muscle, and is the basis of our body's organs, hormones, enzymes, and antibodies to fight infection.

- **Protein is also an emergency fuel** in the absence of sufficient carbohydrate and fats. For this reason, weight loss should be gradual so as to preserve protein levels in muscle, the heart and other body organs.

- **It is easy to obtain sufficient protein**, even if vegetarian. **Plant proteins are not inferior to animal proteins.** In fact, eating more soy and other plant proteins, and less animal protein, may help to build stronger bones and prevent osteoporosis; and may help to control blood cholesterol levels.

- **When changing to a vegetarian diet**, include soybeans, and other dried beans, soy milk drinks (calcium-enriched), lentils, tofu, tempeh, nuts, and wholegrain breads and cereals. Milk, yogurt, cheese and eggs can enhance nutrient intake.

Protein & Muscle

- Although muscles are built of protein, protein is not a special fuel for working muscle cells - carbohydrates and fats are.

- In fact, a diet high in protein (and fat) and low in carbohydrate, can significantly reduce the performance of endurance sports athletes. **Carbohydrate** is the best fuel for muscles exercised for long periods.

- Any **extra protein** required by athletes and body-builders, can easily be obtained from the extra food eaten to satisfy hunger and energy needs.

- Remember, **excessive protein** intake will not build bigger muscles. Any excess is converted and stored as fat. Excess protein can also strain the kidneys which excrete the waste products of protein metabolism.

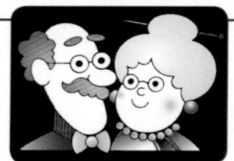

Elderly people (and dieters) must eat sufficient food to ensure adequate protein intake.

Inadequate protein leads to a drop in immune response with greater susceptibility to illness and infections. Muscle strength and muscle mass also drop.

Protein needs are easily met with sensible eating. Athletes who eat enough food for their energy needs, can obtain sufficient protein.

PROTEIN

RECOMMENDED DAILY PROTEIN INTAKE ~ HEALTHY RANGE ~
(Lower figure is RDA)

		PRO
Children:	1-3 yrs	13g-26g
	4-8 yrs	19g-38g
	9-13 yrs	34g-64g
Males:	14-18 yrs	52g-120g
	19+	56g-120g
Females:	14+	46g-110g
Pregnancy:		71g-120g
Breastfeeding:		71g-120g

Note: On lower calorie diets, aim for higher amounts of protein within the Healthy Range.

Iron & Anemia Guide

- **Iron deficiency** is one of the most common nutritional deficiencies in women. The risk is increased in dieters who do not eat well-balanced meals. Chronic shortage of iron leads to anemia.

- **Women** between 11 and 50 years of age are at greater risk because of the monthly loss of menstrual blood. Pregnancy, growth, and endurance sports also demand extra iron.

- In **red blood cells**, iron combines with protein to form **hemoglobin** - the red pigment which carries oxygen in the blood. A lack of iron limits the production of hemoglobin and hence the amount of vital oxygen delivered to body cells.

Note: A blood test will tell you if your Hb and Iron stores (ferritin) are adequate. (Iron stores can be low even when Hb is normal.)

- **Vitamin C** (in fruits/veges/salads) enhances absorption of 'non-heme' iron in bread, cereals, milk, vegetables, nuts, eggs and iron supplements. Small amounts of meat, fish or poultry also help. (They contain 'heme' iron).

- **Iron absorption is lessened** by up to 60% when high calcium foods are consumed with iron-rich main meals. Tea, coffee, phytates (in bran) and oxalates lessen absorption of non-heme iron.

- **For infants to 1 year**, use iron-fortified milk/soy formula if not breast-feeding. Introduce iron-fortified baby cereals at 4-6 mths.

Note: Iron deficiency in children (even without anemia), can result in lethargy, irritability, repeated infections, and developmental problems.

Iron Supplements

- **Most people** can obtain adequate iron from their diet. A **wide variety** of animal and plant foods contain iron. (See Iron Counter)

- **Iron supplements** are only recommended for women with heavy menstrual blood losses, during pregnancy (if tests show a low-iron status), endurance athletes with low blood ferritin (iron stores) and for persons with diagnosed anemia. Check with your doctor.

- While the 5 mg of iron in multi-vitamin/mineral supplements is safe for most people, large amounts can be toxic, (especially in persons with hemochromatosis iron-overload condition).

ANEMIA SYMPTOMS

Anemia reduces the amount of oxygen carried in the blood. The body tissues become starved of oxygen. Symptoms include:

- **Pale skin; brittle finger nails (may turn up into spoon shape)**
- **Excessive tiredness or fatigue**
- **Breathlessness**
- **Feeling of malaise and irritability**
- **Always feel cold**
- **Decrease in attention span**

Note: Other medical conditions may also cause similar symptoms. Check with your doctor.

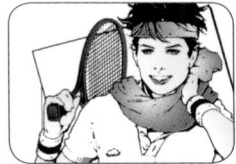

A nutritious diet with adequate iron is important - particularly for women and athletes.

RECOMMENDED DAILY IRON INTAKE (mg)		Iron
Infants (0-6 mths):		
	Breastfed ~	0.5mg
	Bottlefed ~	3mg
	6-12 mths ~	11mg
Children:	1-11 yrs ~	7-10mg
Males:	12-18 yrs ~	11mg
	19+ yrs ~	8mg
Females:	12-18yrs ~	15mg
	19-50yrs ~	18mg
	51+ yrs ~	8mg
	Pregnancy ~	27mg
	Breastfeeding ~	12-16mg

Protein & Iron Counter

Pro ~ Protein (grams)

Meat

	Pro	Iron
Steak: Average all cuts, lean (no fat)		
Small (4 oz raw/3 oz ckd)	23	2.3
Medium (6 oz raw/4¼ oz ckd)	34	3.4
Large (10 oz raw/7¼ oz ckd)	57	5.7
Roast Beef, lean, 2 slices, 3 oz	24	2.5
Ground Beef patty, lean, ckd, 3 oz	21	2
Lamb chop, broiled, 3 oz	22	1.5
Liver, cooked, 3 oz	23	5.5
Veal cutlet, 1 medium	23	1
Pork, cooked, lean, 3 oz	24	1
Bacon, 3 medium slices	6	0.3
Ham, roasted, 2 pieces, 3 oz	18	1
Ham, luncheon, 2 slices, 1½ oz	7	0.3
Pastrami (Oscar Mayer), 3 sl., 1¾ oz	10	1.3
Sausages: Bologna, 2 sl., 2 oz	7	1
Braunschweiger, 2 sl., 2 oz	8	5.3
Pork link, thick, 2 oz	6	0.4
Frankfurter, 1⅓ oz	5	0.5
Salami, hard, 3 slices, 1 oz	7	0.5
Vegetarian (Boca Burger), 1 pattie	13	2

Chicken/Turkey (Without Skin)

	Pro	Iron
Chicken, ckd; Breast, Roasted, 4 oz	36	1.5
Leg/Thigh,Roasted, 2 oz	14	0.5
½ Whole Chicken	60	2.5
Drumstick, Roasted, 1 medium, 3 oz	13	0.6
Turkey, cooked: Light meat, 3 oz	28	2
Dark meat, lean, 3 oz	24	2

Fish

	Pro	Iron
Fresh Fish: Per 4 oz, cooked		
Cod, Flounder/Sole, Pollock	28	0.5
Catfish, Haddock, Halibut, M/Mahi	28	1.3
Ocean Perch, Swordf., Orange Roughy	28	1.3
Canned Fish: Tuna, Light, 3 oz	25	1.5
White, 3 oz	23	0.5
Salmon, pink, 3 oz	17	0.7
Salmon, red, 3 oz	17	1
Sardines, 3 whole (3"), 1¼ oz	9	1
Anchovies, 1 can, 1½ oz	13	2
Shellfish: Crabmeat, 3 oz	17.5	0.7
Clams, raw, 4 large/9 sml, 3 oz	11	12
Crayfish, cooked, 3 oz	20	2.7
Lobster, cooked, 3 oz	17	0.5
Oysters, raw, 6 medium, 3 oz	7	5
Scallops, 2 lge/5 small, 1 oz	5	0.1
Shrimp, raw, 6 large, 1½ oz	8.5	1
Fish Products: Fish Sticks, 4 sticks	10	0.5
Fish Portions, in batter, 4 oz	13	0.6
Gefilte Fish, 1 medium ball, 2 oz	8	1

Iron ~ Iron (mg)

Eggs

	Pro	Iron
1 Large Egg, whole	6	0.7
Egg Yolk	3	0.7
Egg White	3	0
Omelet: Plain, 2 eggs	13	1.7
Ham & cheese	17	3
Egg Substitutes (liquid):		
Eggbeaters, 1 egg equiv.	4.5	1
Better 'n Eggs/Scramblers, ¼ cup, 2 oz	6	0.7

Milk, Yogurt, Icecream

	Pro	Iron
Milk: Whole/Lowfat/Skim, 8 fl.oz cup	8	0.1
Protein Enriched, 1 cup	10	0.1
Carb Countdown (2% or Fat Free), 1 c.	8	0
Chocolate Milk, 1 cup	8	0.6
Thick Shake, Chocolate, 10 oz	9	1
Vanilla, 10 oz	11	0.3
Soymilk (fortified), average, 1 cup	7	1
Yogurt: Plain, 6 oz	10	0.1
Fruit flavors: 6 oz	8	0.3
8 oz	11	0.5
Ice-Cream: Rich, ½ cup	2	0
Regular, Vanilla, ½ cup	2.5	0
Sherbet, ½ cup	1	0
Custard, baked, ½ cup	7	0.5

Cheese

	Pro	Iron
Hard Cheeses, average, 1 oz	7	0.2
4 oz piece	28	0.8
Cottage Cheese, ½ cup	13	0.3
Ricotta, part skim, ½ cup	14	1

Bread, Bagels, Biscuits

	Pro	Iron
Bread (w. enriched flour): 1 slice, 1 oz	2	1
4 slices, 4 oz	8	4
4 thick slices, 6 oz	1.2	6
Bagel, plain 2 oz	6	1.5
Biscuits, 1 oz	2	0.7
Pita Bread, 1 pita, 1½ oz	4	1
Pumpernickel, 1 slice, 1 oz	3	1

Infant/Baby Foods

Infant Formula Milk:	Pro	Iron
Enfamil/Gerber/Similac, 5 fl.oz		
Regular/Low Iron	2.2	0.2
With Iron	2.2	1.8
Isomil/Nursoy/ProSobee	3	1.8
Baby Cereals: Average All Brands		
Dry, 4 Tbsp, ½ oz	1	7
Jars (w. fruit), 4½ oz	1	7

Breakfast Cereals

	Pro	Iron
Hot Type, cooked:		
Bulgur, cooked, 1 cup, 5 oz	9	2
Oatmeal: Reg., non-fortified, 1 cup	6	1.5
Instant, fortified, average, 1 pkt	4	8
Quaker, all flavors, ½ cup	5	18
McCann's, Steelcut, ¼ cup dry	4	18
Corn/Hominy Grits: Reg., 1 cup	3	1.5
Quaker: Reg., 3 Tbsp, 1 oz	2	0.8
Instant White, 1 packet	2	8
Cream of Wheat, 1 cup	4	10
Ready-To-Eat: *Per 1 oz Serving Unless Shown*		
Arrowhead: Average, all varieties	3	1
General Mills: Basic 4, 1 cup, 2 oz	4	4.5
Cheerios, regular, 1 cup, 1 oz	3	8
Cocoa Puffs, 1 cup, 1 oz	1	4.5
Kix, 1⅓ cups, 1 oz	1	8
Multi-Bran Chex, 1 cup, 2 oz	4	16
Country Corn Flakes, 1 cup, 1.2 oz	2	8
Total Raisin Bran, 1 cup, 2 oz	3	18
Wheaties ¾ cup, 1 oz	3	8
Health Valley: Oat Bran O's, ¾ cup	3	0.7
Amaranth Flakes, ¾ cup, 1 oz	3	0.7
Bran Flakes w. Raisins, ¾ cup	3	0.7
Low-Fat Granola, ⅔ cup, 2 oz	5	1.4
Real Oat Bran; Alm. Crunch, ½ cup, 1.7 oz	6	0.7
Golden Flax, ¾ cup, 1.8 oz	6	1
Kashi GoLean: 1 cup, 1.8 oz	13	1.8
GoLean Crunch!, 1 cup, 1.9 oz	9	1.8
7 Whole Grain Flakes, 1 cup, 1.7 oz	6	1.4
Kellogg's: All-Bran, ½ cup, 1 oz	4	4.5
Complete Oatbran Flakes, ¾ cup, 1 oz	3	18
Cocoa Krispies, ¾ cup, 1 oz	1	4.5
Corn Flakes, 1 cup	2	8
Just Right, ¾ cup, 1.8 oz	4	9
Product 19, 1 cup, 1 oz	2	18
Raisin Bran, 1 cup, 2 oz	5	4.5
Rice Krispies, 1¼ cup, 1.1 oz	2	9
Special K: Regular, 1 cup, 1.1 oz	7	8
Low Carb, ¾ cup, 1 oz	10	8
Post: Raisin Bran, ⅔ cup, 2 oz	4	11
Grape Nuts, ½ cup, 2 oz	7	16
Quaker: Crunchy Corn Bran, 1 cup, 1 oz	1	8
100% Natural Granola, ⅔ cup, 2 oz	5	1.4
Life, ¾ cup, 1.1 oz	3	8
Cap'n Crunch, ¾ cup, 1 oz	1	4.5
Oat Bran, ½ cup, 1.4 oz	7	2.7

Brans & Wheatgerm

	Pro	Iron
Oat Bran, raw, 1 Tbsp	2	0.5
Rice Bran, raw, 2 Tbsp	1	1
Wheat Bran, unprocessed, 2 Tbsp	1	1
Wheat Germ, 2 Tbsp, ½ oz	4	1.3

Grains & Flours

	Pro	Iron
Amaranth, 1 cup, ½ oz	10	3
Barley, ½ cup, 3½ oz	8	2
Buckwheat Flour: Dark, 1 cup	11.5	2.7
Light, 1 cup	6	1
Carob Flour, 1 cup	5	3
Corn Flour, 1 cup, 4 oz	9	2
Corn Meal, enriched, 1 cup	11	3.5
Flour: White, enriched, 1 cup, 4½ oz	13	6
Wholegrain, 1 cup, 4¼ oz	16	5
Millet, wholegrain, 1 cup, 3½ oz	10	7
Rye Flour: Dark, 1 cup, 4½ oz	21	6
Light, 1 cup, 3½ oz	10	1
Soy Flour, full fat, 1 cup, 3 oz	32	5.5
Yeast: Brewer's, dry, 1 Tbsp	3	1.5

Rice, Spaghetti

	Pro	Iron
Rice: Brown/White, average		
1 cup cooked, 6½ oz	5	1
Spaghetti/Macaroni/Noodles (enriched):		
Cooked, 1 cup, 4½ oz	7	2
Canned: in Tomato Sauce, ½ cup	2	0.5
w. Meatballs, 1 cup, 8 oz	9	2

Soups

	Pro	Iron
With Noodles/Vegetables, 1 cup	3	0.5
With Meat/Beans/Peas, 1 cup	8	1.5

Fruit

	Pro	Iron
Fresh/Canned: Average, all types, 1 serving		
1 medium/2 small fruit	1	0.5
Avocado, ½ medium	2	1
Dried Fruit: Apricots, 8 halves, 1 oz	1	1.3
Dates, 6 dates, 2 oz	1.5	0.7
Figs, 4 medium figs, 2 oz	2	1.7
Prunes, 5 medium, 1½ oz	1	1
Raisins, 1 oz	1	0.7
Fruit Juice: Average, 1 cup	0.5	0.5
Prune Juice, 6 fl.oz	1	2.5
Tomato Juice, 6 fl.oz	0.5	1

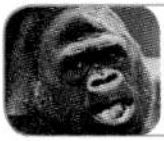

King Kong was a vegetarian!

Protein & Iron Counter

Vegetables	Pro	Iron
Beans: Snap/green, ½ cup, 2 oz	1	0.8
Dried: Average all types, cooked, ½ cup	7	2.5
Baked Beans, ½ cup 4½ oz	5	2
Bean Sprouts, mung, 1 cup, 4 oz	3	1
Broccoli, 3raw, ½ cup, 1½ oz	1.5	0.7
Cabbage; Cauliflower, raw, 1 c. 3 oz	1.5	0.6
Corn, raw, ½ cup kernels, 3 oz	2.5	0.3
1 ear trimmed to 3½"	2	0.4
Lentils, cooked, ½ cup, 3½ oz	9	3.3
Mushrooms, raw, ½ cup, sliced	1	0.3
Peas: Green, raw, ½ cup, 2½ oz	4	1.2
Split Peas, cooked, 1 cup, 7 oz	16	2.5
Potatoes, cooked:		
1 medium, with skin, 5 oz	3.3	2
without skin, 4 oz	2.3	1
French Fries, small, 2.6 oz	2	1
Potato Salad, ½ cup, 4 oz	3.5	2.5
Pumpkin, ½ cup mashed, 4.3 oz	1	1
Seaweed, kelp, 1 oz	<1	2.5
Spinach, cooked, ½ cup, 3 oz	2.7	3.5
Squash, ckd, all types, ½ cup	1	0.3
Tomatoes, 1 medium, 4½ oz	1	0.6
Vegetables, mixed, ckd, 1 cup	2.5	0.7
Soybeans, cooked, ½ cup, 3 oz	14	4.4
Tofu, Tempeh, Miso		
Tofu, raw, firm, ½ cup, 4½ oz	10	1.5
Tempeh, ½ cup, 3 oz	16	2
Miso, ½ cup, 5 oz	16	4
Miso Soup, 1 cup	3	0.4
Soybean Protein (TVP), 1 oz	18	3
Cakes, Pastries, Pies		
(Made with enriched flour)		
Carrot w. cream cheese frosting, 4 oz	4	1.3
Cheesecake, 1 piece, 4 oz	6	0.5
Chocolate, 1 piece, 2 oz	2	2
Fruitcake, 1 piece, 3 oz	4	2
Plain, 1 piece, 3 oz	4	1.2
Croissant, plain, 2 oz	5	2
Danish Pastry, 1 pastry, 2¼ oz	4	1.3
Donuts, average, 2 oz	4	1.2
Muffins, average, 1 medium, 1½ oz	3	1
Pancakes, 4" diam., two, 2 oz	4	1
Pies: Fruit, 1 piece, 5½ oz	4	1.5
Pecan, 1 piece, 5 oz	7	4.5
Puddings, average, ½ cup, 4½ oz	4	0.3
Waffles, 1 large, 2½ oz	7	1.5

Peanut Butter	Pro	Iron
Regular: 2 Tbsp, 1.1 oz	8	0.5
Peter Pan Plus, 2 Tbsp, 1.1 oz	8	4.5
Sugar, Honey, Jam		
Sugar: White	0	0
Brown, 1 Tbsp	0	0.3
Molasses: Light/Medium, 1 Tbsp	0	1
Blackstrap, 1 Tbsp, ¾ oz	0	3
Corn Syrup, 1 Tbsp, ¾ oz	0	1
Honey, Jams, Jelly	0	0.2
Candy, Chocolate, Carob		
Candy, sugar-based	0	0
Chocolate: Plain, 2 oz bar	4	0.8
with nuts, 2 oz bar	6	0.8
Carob, plain, 2 oz	6	0.7
Cookies, Crackers, Chips		
Cookies, average, 4 cookies	2	1
Crackers, Graham, 2½" sq., (2)	1	0
Rice Cakes, average, one	1	0
Corn/Potato Chips, 1 oz	2	0.3
Nuts: Almonds, shelled, 20-25 nuts	6	1
Brazil Nuts, 7-8 medium nuts, 1 oz	4	1
Cashews, 12-16 nuts, 1 oz	5	1.5
Macadamias, 1 oz	2	0.5
Peanuts, dry roasted, 40 nuts, 1 oz	6	0.6
Pecans, 24 halves, 1 oz	2	0.5
Walnuts, 15 halves, 1 oz	4	0.7
Seeds: Sesame Seeds, dry, 1 Tbsp	2	0.6
Pumpkin Kernels, dry, hulled, 1 oz	7	4.2
Sunflower Seeds, dried, hulled, 1 oz	6	2
Tahini, 1 Tbsp, ½ oz	2.5	1.4
Granola & Food/Protein Bars		
Granola Bars, average, 1 bar, 2 oz	2	0.5
Atkins Advantage Bar, avg., 2.1 oz	20	1.8
Balance Bars, Original, 1.76 oz	14	4.5
Bariatrix Proti-Bars (1), 1.4 oz	15	0.7
Dr Soy Protein Bars, 1.76 oz	11	18
Ensure Nutrition Energy Bar, 2.1 oz	9	3.6
GeniSoy Bar, 1.5 oz	14	4.5
Jenny Craig Bars, 1.97 oz	10	3.6
Met-Rx "Big 100", 3.5 oz	27	7.2
Myoplex Carb Sense Bar, 2.5 oz	26	2
Planters Carb Well Bar, 1.4 oz	6	1
PowerBar: Performance Bar, 2.3 oz	10	6.3
ProteinPlus, 1 bar, avg., 2.75 oz	24	8
Slim-Fast Optima Diet Bar, 2 oz	8	2.7

Nutritional & High Protein Drinks

	Pro	Iron
Atkins Shakes, 11 fl.oz can	20	2.7
Bariatrix Shakes, dry, 1 oz	15	3.6
Very High Protein, 1 pkt	35	6.3
Boost Ready To Drink, 8 oz can	10	3.5
Carnation Instant Breakfast, 10 oz	13	4.5
Curves Protein Drink, 2 scoops, dry	15	18
Ensure Plus, 8 oz can	13	2.3
GeniSoy Shake, 1 scoop, 1 oz	25	3.6
Kashi GoLean Shake (RTD), 11 oz can	15	2.7
Kindercal, 8 fl.oz	7	2.5
Met-Rx Protein Shake, 11 oz	35	4.5
Myoplex (EAS), Nutrition Shake, 1 pkt	42	5.4
Nature's Best, Protein Shake, 1 scoop	22	3.6
Optifast 800, made-up, 8 oz	14	3.6
Resource (Novartis) Standard, 8 fl.oz	9	4.5
Revival Soy, Plain, 58g pkt	20	3
Slim-Fast Shakes, 325 ml can	10	3.6
Ultra Slim-Fast, 1 can	7	6.3
Usana Soya Max, 2 scoops, 1 oz	24	6
Walgreens Slim For Less, 11 oz can	10	2.7
Weider Lean Pro, 2 scoops	20	6

Coffee, Tea, Soda

Coffee, Coffee Substitutes, 1 cup	0	0.1
Tea (all types); Soft Drinks/Soda	0	0
Hot Chocolate, 6 fl.oz	2	2.2

Beer, Wine, Spirits

Beer, 12 fl.oz	1	0
Wines, red/white, 1 glass	0	0.4
Spirits/Liquor	0	0

Fast-Foods/Burgers

For extra listings ~ see CalorieKing.com

Pancakes: Average all outlets, 3	8	2
Shakes, Chocolate	12	0.4
Sundaes: Average all outlets	7	0.3
Arby's: Roast Beef Sandwich, reg.	21	3.6
Roast Beef Sandwich, Super	21	3.8
Roast Chicken Club Salad	33	3.8
Burger King: Whopper S/wich	28	5.4
Hamburger	15	2.7
Bacon Double Cheeseburger	33	4.5
BK Big Fish Sandwich	24	4.5
Carl's Jr: Famous Star Hamburger	24	2
Ranch Crispy Chicken	24	2
Super Star Hamburger	41	3
Charbroiled Chicken Club Sandwich	42	3

Fast Foods/Burgers (Cont)

	Pro	Iron
Domino's Pizza: Deep Dish (12"), 1 sl.		
Cheese, 2 slices	13	2
Pepperoni, Sausage, Ham	14	2
Extravaganza	14	2.4
KFC: Original, Breast	40	1
3-Pce. Dinner, Original	72	0.6
Crispy Strips, 3 strips	29	1.8
Snacker, Regular	14	2.7
McDonald's: Big Mac	25	4
Cheeseburger	15	3
Chicken McNuggets (6)	15	1
Crispy Chicken Classic Burger	27	3
Filet-O-Fish	14	2
Grilled Chicken Caesar Salad	30	2
Hamburger	13	3
Quarter Pounder w. Cheese	29	5
French Fries: Small, 2.6 oz	2	0.4
Large, 6 oz	4.5	1
Breakfast: Egg McMuffin	17	3
Bacon, Egg & Cheese McGriddles	20	2
Ham, Egg & Cheese Bagel	28	4
Sausage McMuffin w. Egg	20	3
Pizza Hut: Per Medium, 1 slice		
Carb Tracker (6") average	41	4
Fit n' Delicious, Ham/Pineapple	8	1
Hand Tossed, Pepperoni	12	1.5
Pan Pizzas, average	14	2
Thin 'n Crispy, Supreme	11	1
Subway (6" Subs): Average	20	2
Cheese Steak	24	8
Meatball Marinara	24	7
Roast Chicken Breast	24	3.5
Subway Club	24	7
Taco Bell: Bean Burrito	14	2.7
Chicken Quesadilla	28	1.8
Chicken/Steak Enchirito	14	1.8
Gordita Baja Beef	13	2.7
Steak Burrito Supreme	17	2.7
Taco Supreme	9	1
Tostado	11	1.5
Wendy's: Single Sandwich w. Everything	25	4.5
Big Bacon Classic Sandwich	35	5.4
Club Frescata Sandwich	23	3.6
Hamburger (Kid's Meal)	15	3.6

High Blood Pressure

High Blood Pressure

Many American adults have hypertension (high blood pressure), and are unaware of it. It is generally symptomless, so **have your blood pressure checked annually** - particularly if it runs in the family.

Untreated hypertension overworks the heart, damages arteries and promotes atherosclerosis. This in turn greatly increases the risk of heart disease, stroke, blindness, kidney disease and impotence. The earlier hypertension is detected, the sooner it can be brought under control.

BLOOD PRESSURE CLASSIFICATIONS

National High Blood Pressure Educ. Prog. (2003)

	DIASTOLIC		SYSTOLIC
Normal ➤	Below 80	and	Below 120
Prehypertension			
➤	80-89	or	120-139
Stage 1 ➤	90-99	or	140-159
Stage 2 ➤	100 or more	or	160 or more

Treating Hypertension

Prehypertension (in the chart above) means you don't have high blood pressure now but are likely to develop it in the future.

You can take steps to prevent it with healthy lifestyle habits: reducing sodium intake, eating adequate fruit and vegetables, losing weight if overweight, limiting alcohol to 2 drinks or less daily, quitting smoking, exercising regularly, and managing stress.

Stage 1 hypertension can often be treated with the above lifestyle changes.

Stage 2 hypertension usually requires drug therapy. However, salt restriction, abstaining from alcohol and the above lifestyle changes will improve the success of drug therapy, and enable smaller drug doses to be prescribed.

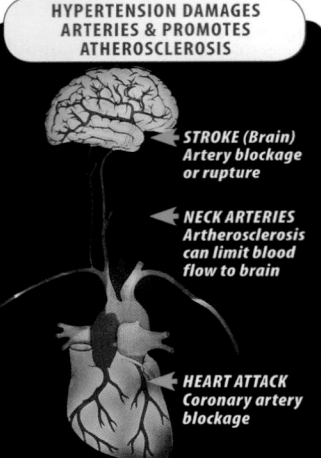

HYPERTENSION DAMAGES ARTERIES & PROMOTES ATHEROSCLEROSIS

STROKE (Brain) Artery blockage or rupture

NECK ARTERIES Artherosclerosis can limit blood flow to brain

HEART ATTACK Coronary artery blockage

STROKE
KNOW THE WARNING SIGNS!

If you notice one or more of these signs, **call your doctor immediately**. They may be signalling a possible stroke or transient ischemic attack:

- **Sudden weakness** or numbness in your face, arm or leg on one side of your body.

- **Sudden dimness**, blurring or loss of vision, particularly in one eye.

- **Loss of speech**, or trouble talking or understanding speech.

- **Sudden severe headache** - 'a bolt out of the blue' - with no apparent cause.

- **Unexplained dizziness**, unsteadiness or a sudden fall, especially if accompanied by any of the other symptoms.

Salt Sodium Guide

Salt & Sodium

- **Sodium is a mineral element** most commonly found in salt (sodium chloride). It also occurs naturally in much smaller amounts in animal and plant foods, and water - normally sufficient for our needs without having to add salt.

- **Sodium is required** for nerve and muscle function as well as to balance the amount of fluid in our tissues and blood.

  Sodium acts like a sponge to attract and hold fluids in body tissues.

- **Excess sodium** can cause water retention, and increase the risk of developing hypertension. Very high salt intake may also increase the risk of stomach cancer.

- **Too little sodium** may cause low blood pressure (hypotension), and decrease blood flow to the heart, brain and kidneys - especially during exercise. (A certain blood volume is required to sustain the blood pressure needed for adequate blood flow in the capillaries).

Salt-Sensitive Persons

- **Normally, our kidneys** excrete excess dietary sodium. The thirst we feel after a salty meal is the body calling for water to dilute the sodium, and enable the kidneys to flush out excess sodium.

- **However, 'salt - sensitive'** persons (up to 50% of adults) tend to retain excess sodium (above approximately 3000mg daily) instead of excreting it. Such persons are more likely to develop hypertension and would most benefit from sodium restriction. Assume you are susceptible if there is a family history of hypertension.

- **Although not everyone will benefit, all Americans are being asked to moderate their salt and sodium intake** as a public health measure - particularly that so many do not know whether or not they have hypertension; and also because we do not know just who is salt-sensitive.

SAFE SODIUM LEVELS

The American Heart Association recommends a **maximum sodium intake of 2300mg per day** for adults with normal blood pressure. However, people who consume less than 1500mg sodium have the lowest blood pressure levels.

Persons with hypertension and kidney ailments are usually restricted to as little as **1000mg sodium per day.** Your doctor will discuss the correct sodium level for you.

Persons with Menière's Disease (chronic attacks of vertigo, dizziness, hearing loss, imbalance), often benefit from lower sodium intake of less than 2000mg/day; as well as even distribution of food and fluids over the day (to prevent fluctuations in body fluids and pressure in the inner ear). Also avoid caffeine and MSG. Limit sugar and alcohol.

further info: www.calorieKing.com

FINDING HIDDEN SODIUM

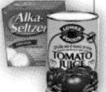

On average, **less than one third of our sodium intake comes from the salt shaker.** The rest is hidden in processed foods that have salt added during manufacture.

Sodium compounds added to food or medicinals can also contribute significant sodium.

Sodium bicarbonate in particular is widely used in antacid tablets (such as Alka Seltzer) and powders. Sodium bicarbonate contains 27% sodium by weight. Each gram contributes 270mg sodium. Large amounts of sodium can be unwittingly consumed - up to 600mg per tablet. (See Antacids ~ Page 293)

Example: 2 Alka-Seltzer Tablets = 1000mg sodium

Other sodium compounds include monosodium glutamate (MSG), sodium ascorbate, sodium nitrite, and sodium citrate.

ALCOHOL DANGER

Excessive alcohol intake contributes to hypertension. Susceptible persons should limit alcohol intake to 1-2 drinks per day.

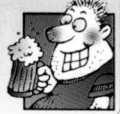

Salt Sodium Guide

Sodium accounts for only 40% of the weight of salt (sodium chloride). Examples:
1 gram (1000mg) Salt has 400mg Sodium
1 teaspoon (5g) Salt has 2000mg Sodium

Hints to Reduce Sodium

- **Watch the salt shaker.** Start with an easy 50% cut in sodium by using Lite Salt (*Morton*) or *Cardia* Salt. Then gradually cut back until you can leave the salt shaker off the table.

- **Taste your food before salting.** Use the pepper shaker (small holes) for more controlled sprinkling of salt.

- **Choose low sodium,** sodium free, and reduced sodium products in place of regular salted products.

- **Check food labels for sodium levels.** FDA Guidelines for sodium descriptors are:
  - **Reduced Sodium:** At least 25% less sodium than the original product
  - **Low Sodium:** 140 mg or less/serving
  - **Very Low Sodium:** 35mg or less/serving
  - **Sodium Free:** Less than 5mg/serving
  - **No Salt Added:** Made without the salt normally added, but still contains the sodium that is a natural part of the food

- **Use reduced-sodium breads,** butter and margarine. Regular varieties contain up to 2% salt. This is considered high in view of their significant contribution to our diet.

- **Go easy on condiments and sauces** such as tomato ketchup, mustard, soy sauce and spaghetti sauces, plus salad dressings. Use low sodium varieties.

- **Limit pizzas and salty fast-foods.** Check *CalorieKing.com* food database.

- **Avoid salty snack foods** such as potato chips, corn chips, salted nuts, pretzels and cheesy-flavored snacks. **Choose unsalted** popcorn, nuts or seeds. Eat more fruit.

- **Don't salt children's food** to your taste.

- **Limit or avoid antacids and saline powders with** sodium bicarbonate (such as *Alka-Seltzer*). They are high in sodium.

FOODS HIGH IN SODIUM

- Cheese, Butter, Margarine
- Pickles, Sauerkraut, Olives
- Condiments, Sauces
- Salad Dressings
- Canned vegetables/salads/beans
- Deli Salads (with dressing)
- Frozen/Packaged Meals/Entrees
- Soups: Canned/dry; bouillon cubes
- Meats: Ham, bacon, sausage, luncheon meats, smoked meats
- Canned Fish (in brine/salt)
- Sea Salt, Garlic/Celery Salt
- Snack Foods (potato chips, pretzels)
- Tomato Juice (Canned), V8 Vegetable Juice
- Fast Foods: Pizza, Burgers, Chicken
- *Alka-Seltzer* Antacid

MODERATE SODIUM

- Bread (Reduced Salt)
- Meat, Fish, Poultry - Unprocessed
- Milk, Yogurt, Soy Drinks, Eggs
- Peanut Butter
- Breakfast Cereals (less than 200mg/serving)
- Chocolate Candy, Fruit/Nut Bars
- *Reduced Sodium & Low Sodium Products*

FOODS LOW IN SODIUM

- Products labelled *Very Low Sodium*, or *Sodium Free*
- Fresh fruits and vegetables
- Canned and Dried Fruits
- Potatoes, Rice, Pasta
- Dried Beans & Lentils, Tofu
- Nuts & Seeds (unsalted)
- Corn & Popcorn (unsalted)
- Pepper, Spices, Herbs
- Jam, Honey, Syrup
- Candy, Gum
- Hard & Jelly Candy
- Coffee, Tea, Alcohol
- Fresh Fruit Juices, Water

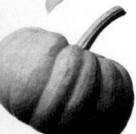

The American Heart Association recommends a sodium intake of **less than 2300mg/day**

Sodium ~ Sodium (mg)

Milk & Dairy Products

	Sodium
Milk: Whole/lowfat/skim, average	
1 cup, 8 fl.oz	120
Whole, low sodium, 1 cup	5
Choc Milk *(Hershey's)*, 1 cup	130
Soy Milk, 8 fl.oz	30
Buttermilk, cultured, 8 fl.oz	250
Dry/Powder, skim, ¼ cup, 1 oz	110
Yogurt, with fruit average, 8 oz	130
Cheese: Blue, 1 oz	330
Parmesan, 1 oz	450
Kraft Cheddar, 2% milk, 1 oz	230
Philadelphia Cream Cheese, 1 oz	90
Process Cheese., average,1 oz	430
Swiss, 1 oz	40
Cottage Cheese, ½ cup, 4 oz	450
Ricotta Cheese, ½ cup, 4 oz	150

Icecream, Frozen Yogurt

Icecream, average,½ cup	50
Frozen Yogurt, ½ cup	50

Fats/Oils

Butter/Margarine:	
Regular, 2 Tbsp, 1 oz	230
Unsalted, reg., 2 Tbsp, 1 oz	5
Mayonnaise, aver., 2 Tbsp, 1 oz	160
Oils/Lard/Dripping	0
Cream, average, 1 Tbsp	6
Coffee-Mate: Powdered, 1 tsp	2
Liquid, 1 Tbsp	5

Eggs

Whole, 1 large	70
Omelet, 2 egg, plain	220
w. cheese	400
Egg Beaters (Fleischmann's), ¼ cup	115

Meats

Meat, average all types, cooked	
(Beef/Lamb/Veal/Pork), 4 oz	80
Corned Beef, cooked, 3 oz	800
Bacon, cooked, 2 slices, ½ oz	270
Ham, 3 oz	1100

Chicken & Turkey

Chicken/Turkey, cooked, unsalted, 4 oz	80
Stuffing Mixes, average., ½ cup	500

Sausages & Meats

	Sodium
Bologna, 1 oz	280
Frankfurter, 2 oz	640
Ham, chopped, ¾ oz slice	290
Liverwurst (Braunschweiger), 1 oz	320
Pepperoni, 5 slices, 1 oz	570
Salami, cooked, 1 oz	350
dry/hard, 1 oz	600
Sausage, 1 oz link	220
Pork, 2 oz patty	260
Turkey Roll, 1 oz	160

Fish: Fresh Fish, average, plain	
Cooked, 4 oz (no bone)	60
Broiled w. butter, 4 oz	150
Breaded & fried, 4 oz	320
Fish fillets, batter-dipped 3 oz	350
Fish sticks, 1 oz stick	160
Gefilte Fish (w. broth), 1 pce, 1½ oz	220
Herring, pickled, 2 pces, 1 oz	260
Lobster, meat only, 4 oz	180
Oysters, fresh, 6 med., 3 oz	95
Salmon: Canned, 3 oz	460
No Salt Added, 3 oz	65
Smoked fish, average, 3 oz	650
Tuna: Canned, 3 oz	330
No Added Salt, 3 oz	40

Entrees & Meals

Frozen Meals, average	600-900
Lean Cuisine, average	700
Stouffer's, average	580
Dinners, average	900-1200
Side Dishes, average	400-600
Pizza, frozen, ¼ large, 6 oz	800-1200
Microwave Cup Meals	900-1200
Cup O'Noodles, average	1500

Fast-Foods & Restaurants

Cheeseburger	750
Chicken Dinner (3 piece)	2200
Chicken Nuggets w. Sauce	800
Fish/Chicken Sandwich	1000
French Fries, small, 2½ oz	150
Hamburger: Regular	500
Large with cheese	1100
Hot Dog (Frankfurter)	800
Pizza, 2 medium slices	1200
Shake, chocolate	250
Taco	400

Extra Listings ~ see CalorieKing.com

Sodium Counter

Sodium ~ Sodium (mg)	Sodium
Soups: Condensed, 1 c., 8 oz	800-1000
Low Sodium	70
Chicken Noodle, 1 cup	900
Bouillon Cube, average	950
Cup-A-Soup: Average	850
Lite, average	450
Soup Mixes, average, 1 cup	900
Condiments, Sauces, Dressings	
A-1 Sauce, 1 Tbsp	280
Barbecue Sauce, 1 Tbsp	130
Bragg Liquid Aminos, 1 tsp	220
Chili Sauce, 1 Tbsp	230
Ketchup: Tomato, 1 Tbsp	180
Low Sodium, 1 Tbsp	20
Mayonnaise, 1 Tbsp	80
Mustard, 1 tsp	70
Pizza Sauce, ½ cup	700
Salad Dressings, 2 Tbsp, 1 oz	160-400
Spaghetti Sauce, ½ cup	500
Soy Sauce: 1 Tbsp	900
Lite *(Kikkoman),* 1 Tbsp	600
Sweet & Sour, ½ cup	250
Tabasco, 1 tsp	25
Vinegar, Lemon Juice	0
Worcestershire, 1 Tbsp	200
Tomato: Sauce, 1 cup	1200
Paste/Puree (salted), ½ cup	1000
No Salt Added, ½ cup	25
Salt & Salt Substitutes	
Table Salt: 1 teaspoon, 6g	2400
Single Serve package, 1 g	400
Cardia Salt, 1 teaspoon	1080
Lite Salt *(Morton),* 1 teaspoon, 6g	1200
Morton **Salt Substitute**	5
No Salt Salt Substitute, 1 teaspoon	5
Garlic/Seasoned Salt 1 teaspoon, 4g	1300
Sea Salt, 1 teaspoon, 5g	2250
Seasonings, Herbs & Spices	
Baking Powder, 1 tsp, 3g	340
Baking Soda (Sodium bicarb), 1 tsp, 3g	810
Accent (Flavor Enhancer), 1 tsp	600
Chili Powder, 1 tsp, 3g	25
Curry Powder	0
Lemon Pepper *(Lawry's),* 1 tsp	340
Meat Tenderizer, 1 tsp, 5g	1750
MSG (Monosodium glutamate), 5g	500
Mrs Dash (Herb/Spice Blend), 1 tsp	0
Pepper, Mustard (dry), 1 tsp	1
Yeast, Nutritional, 1 Tbsp	10

Breakfast Cereals	Sodium
Kellogg's:	
All-Bran, ½ cup, 1 oz	80
Oatbran Flakes, ¾ cup, 1 oz	210
Corn Flakes, 1 cup, 1 oz	200
Just Right, ¾ cup, 2 oz	240
Mini Wheats Frosted, 24 bisc., 1.8 oz	5
Health Valley Cereals, 1 serving	5
Quaker: Cap'n Crunch, ¾ cup, 1 oz	200
Crunchy Corn Bran, ¾ cup, 1 oz	230
100% Natural Granola, ½ cup, 1 oz	15
Puffed Rice/Wheat, 2 cups, 1 oz	1
General Mills: Total, ¾ cup, 1 oz	190
Oatmeal: Regular, ¾ cup	1
Instant *(Quaker),* ⅔ cup (1 pkt)	270
Breads, Bagels, Crackers	
Bread: Average all types, 1 oz	140
Low Sodium, 1 oz	10
Bagels: Plain, 2 oz	200
Sara Lee, 3 oz	500
Biscuits, average, 1 oz	180
Bun/Roll, 1 medium, 1½ oz	200
Crackers: Saltine, 2 crackers	70
Low Salt *(Premium),* 2	25
Graham, 2 regular	50
Croissant, average, 2 oz	280
Rice Cakes, average	25
Ry-Krisp Crispbread, Sesame, 2	100
Cookies, Cakes, Desserts	
Cookies: Average, 2-3 cookies, 1 oz	100
Mrs Fields', average, 2½ oz	180
Baked Custard, ½ cup	100
Brownie, ¼ oz piece	75
Cake, average, 3 oz piece	250
Cinnamon Sweet Roll, 2 oz	250
Danish, Apple	250
Donut, average	150
Muffins: 1 medium, 2 oz	150
Pancakes, 3 x 4"	360
Pie, average 1/6 of 9" pie	300
Pudding: Average, ½ cup	160
Jell-O (Mix), Instant, ½ cup	400
Waffles:	
Home-made, 7", 2½ oz	350
Frozen: Average, 1¼ oz	260
Aunt Jemima, avg, 2½ oz	565

Fruit & Juices

	Sodium
Fresh Fruit, average all types, 1 serving	1
Dried/Canned Fruit, ½ cup	1
Fruit Juice: Fresh, sqz'd, 6 fl.oz	1
Commercial, aver., 6 fl.oz	20
Carrot Juice (Ferraro's), 8 fl.oz	230
Tomato Juice (Campbell's), 6 fl.oz	570
Low Sodium (No Salt Added)	20
V8 Vegetable (Campbell's), 6 fl.oz	600
(No Salt Added), 6 fl.oz	45

Vegetables

Fresh/Frozen (No Salt Added): Per ½ Cup

Asparagus, Bean Sprouts, Corn	3
Beets, Carrots, Celery, ½ cup	40
Broccoli, Cabbage, Cauliflower	10
Cucumber, Green Beans, Mushroom, Okra	3
Onions, Peas, Potato, Pumpkin, Squash	3
Peppers, Hot Chili, raw, each	3
Spinach, Turnips, ½ cup, ckd	40
Tomato, 1 medium, 5 oz	10
Canned: Asparagus, 4 spears	300
Beans, baked in tomato sauce	450
Beets, ½ cup, 3 oz	240
Corn Kernels, ½ cup, 3 oz	190
Creamed, ½ cup, 4½ oz	330
Mushrooms w. butter sce, 2oz	550
Peas, ½ cup, 3 oz	250
Sauerkraut, ½ cup, 4 oz	750

Pickles, Olives

Olives, pickled: Green, 1 large	90
Ripe/black, 1 large	40
Pickles: Bread & Butter, 4 sl., 1 oz	200
Dill, 1 pickle, 2½ oz	900
Sweet, 1 gherkin, ½ oz	130

Soybean Products

Miso (Soy Paste), ¼ c., 2½ oz	2500
Soybean Protein Isolate, 1 oz	280
Tempeh, ½ cup, 3 oz	5
Tofu, average, ½ cup, 4 oz	5

Jam, Honey, Syrups

Jam/Jelly, 1 Tbsp	2
Honey/Maple Syrup, 1 Tbsp	1
Log Cabin Syrup, 1 fl.oz	35
Lite, 1 fl.oz	90

Peanut Butter

Peanut Butter, regular, 1 Tbsp	70
Unsalted, 1 Tbsp	1

Snacks, Nuts

	Sodium
Cheese Balls/Curls, 1 oz	280
Corn/Tortilla Chips, average, 1 oz	220
Granola bars, average, 1 bar	80
Nuts: Plain, unsalted, 1 oz	1
Lightly salted, 1 oz	80
Salted or Honey Roasted, 1 oz	160
Popcorn: Plain (unsalted), 1 cup	1
Flavored, average, 1 cup	60
Salt added, 1 cup	180
Potato Chips: Plain, 1 oz	160
Flavored, 1 oz	250
Pretzels, regular, 3, 1 oz	450

Candy, Chocolate

Chocolate, milk, 1 oz	30
Carob Milk Bar, 1 oz	55
Fudge, chocolate, 1 oz	55
Candy Bars, average, 1½ oz	60
Hard Candy, Jelly Beans, 1 oz	10
Licorice, 1 oz	30

Beverages, Alcohol

Coffee (& Substitutes), Tea, 1 cup	1
Cocoa, dry, plain, 1 Tbsp	0
Mix, average, 1 envelope	120
Quik (Nestle), 2 tsp	35
Soft Drinks, average, 8 fl.oz	20
Mineral Water, Perrier, 8 fl.oz	5
Gatorade Thirst Quencher, 8 fl.oz	110
Water: Average, 1 cup, 8 fl.oz	5
Drier regions, 1 cup	20+
Alcohol: Beer, 12 fl.oz	15
Wines, average, 4 fl.oz	10
Spirits (distilled), 1½ fl.oz	1

Antacids – Alka-Seltzer

	Sodium
Alka-Seltzer (Per Tablet):	
Alka-Seltzer P.M., 1 tablet	500
Original (Light Blue Box)	570
Extra Strength (Dark Blue Box)	590
Flavored Lemon/Lime & Cherry	500
Antacid (yellow Box)	310
Gelatine Capsule, 1	0
Alka-Mints, chewable	0
Bromo Seltzer, ¾ capful	760
Rolaids, All types	0
Tums, Regular/Extra Strength	0
Sodium Bicarbonate (27% sodium), 1g	270

Index A - B

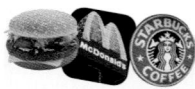

FAST-FOOD RESTAURANTS INDEX
~ SEE PAGE 183 ~

Index C - E

Index P - S

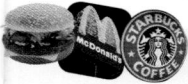

FAST-FOOD RESTAURANTS INDEX
~ SEE PAGE 183 ~

Index U - Z

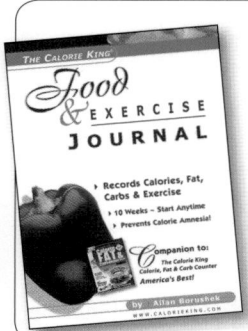